Core Curriculum for the Dialysis Technician

A Comprehensive Review of Hemodialysis

SIXTH EDITION

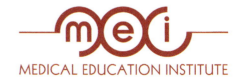

Core Curriculum for the Dialysis Technician

SIXTH EDITION

Copyright © 2018 Medical Education Institute, Inc. All rights reserved. No part of this book may be reproduced in any form or by any electronic or mechanical means, including information storage and retrieval systems, without permission in writing from the Medical Education Institute, Inc.

Contact Information:
Medical Education Institute, Inc.
414 D'Onofrio Drive, Suite 200
Madison, WI 53719
Phone: 608-833-8033
Email: info@meiresearch.org
Website: www.meiresearch.org.

Printed in the U.S.

Library of Congress Control Number: 2017955619

ISBN 978-1-937886-05-9

Legal Disclaimer

This sixth edition of the **Core Curriculum for the Dialysis Technician** is offered as a general educational guide for dialysis technicians and other medical professionals. When using this or any other educational guide, the reader must be aware that:

- This **Core Curriculum** is not to be used as a substitute for professional training, clinical practice guidelines, or policies and procedures of the hospital or clinic providing dialysis. Hospital or clinical policies may differ from those discussed in this **Core Curriculum**, and local, state, and federal regulations imposed on dialysis technicians, hospitals, or clinics may require different practices from those outlined in this **Core Curriculum**. (For example, the curriculum may represent a higher standard of care than set by basic regulations.) Consult the product label for any pharmaceutical or medical device referenced in this **Core Curriculum**.

- Educational curricula such as this **Core Curriculum** can only draw from the information available as of the date of publication. Although the authors and reviewers of these materials used considerable effort to assure that the information contained herein is accurate and complete as of the date of publication, no guarantees of accuracy or completeness can be provided. In addition, the sponsors of the **Core Curriculum** have no role in creation or review of curriculum content whatsoever. The authors, editors, publisher and sponsors are not responsible for errors or omissions or for any consequences from application of the information in this book and make no warranty, expressed or implied, with respect to the currency, completeness, or accuracy of the contents of the publication. Application of this information in a particular situation remains the professional responsibility of the practitioner.

- Neither the Medical Education Institute, Inc., the authors, the reviewers, nor the sponsors are under any obligation to update the information contained herein. Future medical advances; product information; or revisions to legislative, administrative, or court law may affect or change the information provided in this **Core Curriculum**. Technicians and other medical professionals using this **Core Curriculum** are responsible to monitor for ongoing medical advances relating to dialysis and adapt their practices as needed. This **Core Curriculum** is provided with the understanding that neither it nor its authors, reviewers, nor sponsors are engaged in rendering medical or other professional advice. If medical advice or other expert assistance is required, the reader is herein advised to seek the advice of a competent professional.

- The reader must recognize that dialysis involves certain risks, including the risk of death, which cannot be completely eliminated, even when the dialysis procedure is undertaken under expert supervision. Use of these materials indicates acknowledgment that neither the Medical Education Institute, Inc., the authors, the reviewers, nor the sponsors will be responsible for any loss or injury, including death, sustained in connection with, or as a result of, the use of this **Core Curriculum**.

SUPPORTERS

The Medical Education Institute would like to thank the following companies for their unrestricted educational grant support of the Core Curriculum for the Dialysis Technician.

GOLD

Serving our Students with Excellence and Passion
WWW.AHIMIAMI.COM

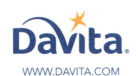
WWW.DAVITA.COM

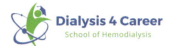
Leading Careers In Patient Care
WWW.DIALYSIS4CAREER.COM

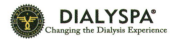
Changing the Dialysis Experience
WWW.DIALYSPA.COM

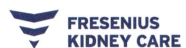
FRESENIUSKIDNEYCARE.COM

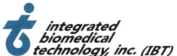
Manufacturer of innovative test strips
WWW.IBTBIOMED.COM

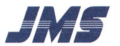
SysLocMINI, WingEater, & Harmony AVF Needle Sets
WWW.JMSNA.NET

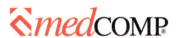
Medcomp. Access. Excellence.
WWW.MEDCOMPNET.COM

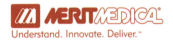
Understand. Innovate. Deliver.™
WWW.MERIT.COM

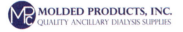
Access, Recirculation, Clamps & Protection
WWW.MOLDEDPRODUCTS.COM

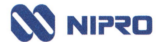
The Link Between Patient and Care
WWW.NIPRO.COM

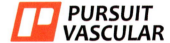
Prevent Catheter-Related Bloodstream Infections
WWW.PURSUITVASCULAR.COM

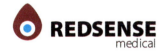
Saving lives by detecting blood loss using light
WWW.REDSENSEMEDICAL.COM

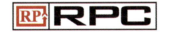
A leading innovator of technical dialysis products
WWW.RPC-RABRENCO.COM

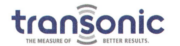
Helping Providers Save Patient Lives and Accesses
WWW.TRANSONIC.COM

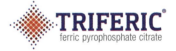
Triferic: A new way to treat your Anemia
WWW.TRIFERIC.COM

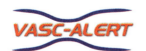
Prevent clots and conversions by timely referrals
WWW.VASC-ALERT.COM

Endotoxin Specific LAL Reagents and Accessories
WWW.WAKOPYROSTAR.COM

SILVER

B. Braun Medical Inc.
Sharing Expertise - Hemodialysis System Supplier
WWW.BBRAUNUSA.COM/DIALYSIS

CVInsight® Patient Monitoring by InteloMed
Meaningful Monitoring of Dialysis Tolerance
WWW.INTELOMED.COM

Dialysis Clinic, Inc. (DCI)
A non-profit corporation
WWW.DCIINC.ORG

Independent Dialysis Foundation
Proudly supporting this valuable education tool
WWW.IDFDN.ORG

TNT Moborg International LTD
Immobile: Providing a Sense of Security Since 1995
WWW.TNTMOBORG.COM

Utopia Health Career Center, LLC
Building a New Breed of Healthcare Professionals
WWW.UTOPIAHCC.COM

Acknowledgment

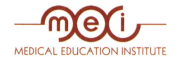

Welcome to the sixth edition of the **Core Curriculum for the Dialysis Technician**! Having spent half my life in nephrology, it has been quite a journey to *see* our community seek and find new ways to improve dialysis. This book is a way to share the best approaches to care for our patients—to help them live better, fuller, longer lives. The non-profit Medical Education Institute spends a full year out of every five to update this book to help YOU become the most caring, informed, professional dialysis technician you can be.

In this edition, we added content to help you see how vital it is for dialysis to be done *gently*, to avoid harm to patients' hearts. The book is full-color to aid learning and in print and e-book formats. We added an *Emergency Planning* module and set up a website for posttest questions—see the box below. Patient artists did the cover art for each module, and patient quotes give you a sense of what it is like to be in your patients' shoes.

We thank the American Nephrology Nurses Association (ANNA) and the National Association of Nephrology Technicians/Technologists (NANT) for their long tradition of working with us on this book. Their members' tireless efforts as authors and reviewers ensure that what you learn is accurate, complete, up-to-the-minute, and will help you in a real dialysis clinic. We profoundly appreciate their help.

Updating this book is an *enormous* task, and I would like to acknowledge the huge contributions made by:

- **John Sadler**, **MD**, esteemed nephrologist and Chair of the MEI Board of Directors, who has run dialysis clinics for decades, and was kind enough to do a thorough medical review on a tight deadline.
- **Darlene Rodgers, BSN, RN, CNN, CPHQ**, who worked tirelessly to coordinate author input, answer questions, find citations, and review modules—all with a smile.
- **Nancy Gallagher, CNN, RN**, who reviewed each module with an eye to technician certification.
- **Vern Taafe, President/CEO of RPC**, who graciously provided his decades of expertise to review the technical content of the modules and answer our numerous questions.
- **Priti Patel, MD; Nicole Rae Gualandi, MS, MPH, RN**, and **Christi Lines, MPH** at the Centers for Disease Control & Prevention (CDC) who reviewed the infection control and vascular access content.
- **Jeff Boyd, CHT** and **Rosa Watson Albert, CHT, CCHT**, who thoroughly read each module to write and double-check posttest questions and answers for each one.
- **Kellen Johnston**, who created and edited the graphics througout the book.
- **The MEI team: Kristi Klicko, Director of Operations**, who managed the project from start to finish, **Rob Poehnelt, Marketing Communications Manager**, who made the final layout and text changes, and **Karen Honer, Project Manager**, who proofread each reference and every module.

I could not be prouder of this sixth edition and the team of experts who came together to make it possible, and hope that learning to become a dialysis technician will be the start of a fulfilling career for you.

Dori Schatell

Executive Director, Medical Education Institute

Prepare for your certification exam!
Practice test questions: www.MEIresearch.org/cc6

Foreword

The fundamental goal for all nephrology caregivers is to achieve excellence in care for patients living with kidney disease. Passion combined with expertise has shown to be a successful pathway in achieving this goal.

All kidney patients deserve excellent care, from the newly diagnosed with renal disease to the patient living with the diagnosis for decades. From the young adult to the frail elderly patient, the care we provide must be at an optimal level.

Providing outstanding care requires teamwork, knowledge, passion and a commitment for excellence from the entire interdisciplinary team; nurses, physicians, social workers, dietitians. The dialysis technician directly interacts with the patient and provides their valuable insight to the interdisciplinary team, which is necessary for creating a plan of care that is individualized, patient-based, and produces the intended outcomes.

For dialysis technicians to be optimally effective in their work, there exists an essential need for comprehensive training. Current, evidence-based practice information is crucial and will provide the avenue for dialysis technicians to be successful in their work and career. The sixth edition of the *Core Curriculum for the Dialysis Technician* will assist in providing this knowledge.

Similar to previous editions, the *Core Curriculum* will serve as a comprehensive source of information on multiple aspects of dialysis, including scientific principles, devices, water treatment, and more.

Producing this edition was a collaborative effort. Many dialysis nurses and other professionals spent countless hours updating the contents, illustrations, and references to reflect the most state-of-the-art dialysis practices.

On behalf of the ANNA members involved in this publication, I can assure you that we take pride in our contributions. Our work on the *Core Curriculum* is a reflection of our longstanding commitment to improve educational opportunities for dialysis technicians.

Nephrology nurses and certified dialysis technicians share a common goal: To provide safe, effective dialysis that enables our patients to enjoy their lives to the fullest extent.

Alice Hellebrand MSN, RN, CNN
American Nephrology Nurses Association
President 2017-2018

Though dialysis basics were said to have been found thousands of years ago, the treatment as we know it now did not start until the 1960s. Since then, both the equipment and our knowledge have improved exponentially. Today, more than 650,000 patients in the United States and more than two million in the world have kidney failure. Each patient is unique and has a specific set of goals and needs. But, there is one thing they can *all* appreciate: dialysis gives them a chance to live more normal and productive lives! The goal of this *Core Curriculum* is to improve the preparation, professionalism, education, and proficiency of patient care staff. Our aim is to make dialysis safer and more comfortable for each patient.

As technology and medicine evolve, the *Core Curriculum* needs updates. Like the first five versions, this one has the most up-to-date concepts and practices about all aspects of dialysis. In it, you will find the facts about kidneys and kidney disease, nursing care, and all of the aspects of treatment. Many nephrology professionals devoted long hours to make sure this book was as helpful to you as it could be.

It is an honor and privilege to take part in updating this *Core Curriculum*. Writing this Foreword has given me time to reflect on the mentors who have been instrumental to me. Two who come to mind are Cheryl Winterich and the late and much-missed Dr. Peter DeOreo. Cheryl believed in me enough to give me the chance to begin my journey in the dialysis field, which is turning out to be an amazing career. Dr. Peter DeOreo was a great mentor who helped me take my knowledge to a higher level by helping with nephrology research. His contributions to the field and unique ability to share clinical medicine in an understandable and inspiring way were truly admired by his colleagues, staff, and patients.

This 6th edition is useful for *all* nephrology nurses and technicians. Both beginners and seasoned professionals can learn from it. As the President of BONENT *and* as a Fluid Manager, I refer staff to the book to brush up on their knowledge and prepare to take certification exams.

BONENT's main focus is to promote excellence in the kidney patient care in the U.S. and around the world. Like BONENT, the *Core Curriculum* strives to teach all members of the dialysis community—which, in turn, will produce better nurses and technicians who can deliver safer and more effective patient care.

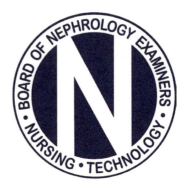

RJ Picciano, BA, CHT, OCDT, CHBT
BONENT President and Centers for Dialysis Care Fluid Manager

Back in the mid-seventies when I started my dialysis career there was little to no formal training for a Dialysis Technician. All the knowledge was passed from the physician to the nurse, then to the technician. I started as an equipment tech, but learned the dialysis procedures from the dedicated nurses I worked with. I learned the "How to", but, in most cases not the "Why". I was fortunate to work at a university based teaching hospital dialysis unit and eventually, I accumulated the background information I needed from reading, seminars, lectures from the doctors, and on-the-job experiences to become certified and a more educated caregiver.

As I advanced in my career I realized that other Dialysis Technicians were only taught what the clinics required them to know to do their jobs and little else. Then in the early nineties, Amgen published the first *Core Curriculum for the Dialysis Technician*. Authored by leaders in their respective fields, we now had the first standardized learning tool for dialysis. It is used extensively for training nurses and technicians alike and is a great reference for the other members of the multi-disciplinary team.

Of course, with all of the changes in treatment modalities, techniques, regulations, technology, standards of care, and the focus on outcomes over the years, the *Core Curriculum* had to be updated to remain the premier learning tool that it started out to be. The mandatory certification of Dialysis Technicians by CMS made it even more important that the information in the *Core Curriculum* be up to date and relevant.

My "hat is off" and I express my thanks to the authors of the first edition and to the many authors through the years who gave of their time and expertise to contribute to follow-up editions. The same goes to the authors and contributors of this sixth edition of the *Core Curriculum*. This well-researched information is up to date with the technology, current practices, techniques, and regulations we need to know and even looks a bit into the future of new and exciting things to come.

Even though things have changed over the years and will always continue to change and improve, our number one commitment as a dialysis caregiver will always be to the safety and the quality of care for our patients. This Sixth Edition will keep us moving forward to that end.

Charles H. Johnson, CHT
President, National Association of Nephrology Technicians/Technologists (NANT)

Table of Contents

1 TODAY'S DIALYSIS ENVIRONMENT

- Objectives 2
- Introduction 3
- Overview of Kidney Failure and Dialysis 3
  - Dialysis is Partial Kidney Replacement 4
- Payment for Dialysis and Transplant 6
- Quality in Dialysis 9
  - ESRD Networks 9
  - Guidelines for Dialysis Care 9
  - ESRD Quality Improvement Initiative 10
  - Quality Standards for Dialysis 10
  - Continuous Quality Improvement in Dialysis 11
- Dialysis Technician Professionalism 12
  - Professional Boundaries 13
  - Groups You Can Join 14
- Technician Certification 14
  - Certified Clinical Hemodialysis Technician Exam 14
  - Certified Clinical Hemodialysis Technician - Advanced Exam 15
  - Certified Hemodialysis Technician Exam 15
  - Certified in Clinical Nephrology Technology and Certified in Biomedical Nephrology Technology Exams 15
  - Certified Dialysis Water Specialists Exam 16
- Conclusion 16
- References 16

2 THE PERSON WITH KIDNEY FAILURE

- Objectives 20
- Introduction 21
- Kidney Structure 22
  - Nephrons 22
  - Glomeruli 23
  - Tubular System 23
- Kidney Functions 23
  - Excretory Functions 23
  - Endocrine Functions 24
  - Electrolyte Balance 24
  - Blood Pressure Control 24
  - Acid-base Balance 24
- Types of Kidney Failure 24
  - Acute Kidney Failure 25
  - Chronic Kidney Disease 25
- Causes of Kidney Failure 25
  - Diabetes 26
  - High Blood Pressure 26
  - Glomerular Diseases 27
  - Polycystic Kidney Disease 27
  - Other Causes of CKD 27
- Problems Caused by Kidney Failure 27
  - Electrolyte Imbalances 27
  - Uremia 29
  - Anemia 30
  - Left Ventricular Hypertrophy 31
  - Pericarditis 33
  - Mineral Bone Disorder 33
  - Dialysis-Related Amyloidosis 34
  - Neuropathy 35
  - Pruritus 35
  - Sleep Problems 36
  - Bleeding Problems 36
- Common Dialysis Blood Tests 37
- Treatment Options 37
  - Transplant 37
  - Dialysis 41
  - Peritoneal Dialysis 42
  - Hemodialysis 45
  - Medical Management Without Dialysis 48
- HD Care Team 49
  - Patient 49
  - Family Members 49
  - Nephrologist 50
  - Nurses 50
  - Social Workers 50
  - Dialysis Technicians 50
  - Renal Dietitians/Nutritionists 50
  - Starting Standard In-Center HD: The Risky First 90 Days 51
  - Safe Vascular Access 51
  - Avoiding Malnutrition 51
  - Tailoring the First Dialysis Treatments 51
- Nutrition for People on Standard In-Center HD 52
  - Calories and Malnutrition 52
  - Obesity 53
  - Fluid Intake and Water Weight 53
  - Sodium 56
  - Potassium 57
  - Calcium 57
  - Phosphorus 58
  - Vitamins 59
- Helping Patients Cope 59
  - Life Changes and Empathy 60

Money Concerns 61	Fluid Dynamics in Hemodialysis 94
Travel 61	Hemodiafiltration 95
Body Image 62	Applying Scientific Principles
Sexuality and Fertility. 62	to Peritoneal Dialysis 96
Pain 63	Diffusion in Peritoneal Dialysis 97
Mood 63	Osmosis in Peritoneal Dialysis. 97
The Health Insurance Portability and Accountability	Convection in Peritoneal Dialysis 98
Act and Patient Confidentiality 64	Adsorption in Peritoneal Dialysis 98
Active Listening 64	Conclusion. 98

Rehabilitation 65
    Self-Management—Not Compliance. 65
Patient Education: Creating Expert Patients 66
    Attitude 66
    Answers. 66
    Action 68
Special Challenges. 70
    Challenges and What You Can Do 70
    Coping with Patient Deaths. 71
Patient Resources. 72
    Website Resources 72
    Patient Organizations. 73
    Government Resources 74
Conclusion 74
References. 75

3 PRINCIPLES OF DIALYSIS

Objectives 82
Introduction 83
Basic Concepts and Principles. 83
    Solutions 83
    Solubility 83
    Diffusion 84
    Convection 85
    Osmosis. 85
    Adsorption 86
    Hydraulic Pressure 86
    Fluid Dynamics 86
    Filtration and Ultrafiltration 87
    Fluid Compartments
        in the Human Body 87
Applying Scientific Principles to Hemodialysis 87
    Solutions in Hemodialysis: Blood and Dialysate 88
    Dialyzers and Diffusion in Hemodialysis 89
    Osmosis, Ultrafiltration, and Organ Stunning in
        Hemodialysis 90
    Convection in Hemodialysis 94
    Adsorption in Hemodialysis 94

Appendix A:
    Metric System and Temperature Conversions. . . 99
References. 99

4 HEMODIALYSIS DEVICES 101

Objectives 102
Introduction. 103
Dialyzers and How They Work 103
    Membrane Materials 104
    Patient Reactions to Dialyzers During HD 105
    Membrane Surface Area 106
    Membrane Pores 107
    Clearance 107
    Mass Transfer Coefficient 109
    Ultrafiltration Coefficients. 110
    Testing Dialyzer Clearance 110
Dialysate. 111
    Dialysate Conductivity 111
    Mixing Dialysate Concentrates 112
Hemodialysis Machines 112
    Dialysate Circuit 113
    Dialysate Mixing. 113
    Dialysate Delivery 113
    Monitors and Alarms 114
    Ultrafiltration Control. 117
    Advanced Options. 121
Extracorporeal Circuit 122
    Blood Tubing 122
    Transducer Protectors 123
    Blood Pump 124
    Heparin Pump 125
    Venous Line Clamp 126
    Safety Monitors 126
Waste Disposal and "Green" Dialysis 130
    Medical Waste 130
    Dialysis Water. 130
Conclusion. 130
References. 131

5 DIALYZER REPROCESSING 133
Objectives 134
Introduction. 135
History of Dialyzer Reprocessing. 135
    Hollow Fiber Dialyzers and Reuse. 135
    Dialyzer Reuse Numbers 136
Why Dialyzers are Reused. 136
    Saving Dollars and Reducing Medical Waste 136
Safety of Reuse 136
    Reuse and Exposure to Pathogens 137
    Reuse and Exposure to Germicides 137
    Reuse and Dialyzer Efficiency. 138
Rules for Dialyzer Reprocessing 138
    Dialyzer Labeling for Reuse 138
    Automated Versus Manual Reprocessing 139
Preparing a Dialyzer for First Use 139
    Preprocessing. 140
After Dialysis 140
    Pre-clean the Dialyzer 140
    Clean and Disinfect the Header. 141
    Test Dialyzer Performance. 141
    Rejecting a Dialyzer 142
    Disinfect the Dialyzer 142
Handling Hazardous Materials. 142
    Safety Training 143
    Peracetic Acid Safety 143
    Formaldehyde Safety 143
    Glutaraldehyde Safety 143
Storage of Reprocessed Dialyzers. 144
Prepare for the Next Use. .144
    Inspect the Dialyzer 144
    Remove the Germicide. 144
Check the Dialyzer Prior to Treatment 145
Documentation 145
Quality Assurance and Quality Control 145
Conclusion 147
References 147

6 VASCULAR ACCESS 149
Objectives 150
Introduction. 151
Types of Access 151
    Fistula Basics 151
    Graft Basics. 152
    Catheter Basics 153
Access Planning 154
Fistulas in Detail. 155
    How Fistulas are Made. 155
    Body Image and Patient Resistance to Fistulas 156
    Vessel Mapping and Fistula Surgery. 156
    Assessing Fistula Maturity. 157
Starting HD with a Mature Fistula. 158
    Wash Your Hands. 159
    Examine the Fistula 159
    Prepare the Access Skin. 160
    Apply a Tourniquet 161
    Place the Needles 161
    Rope Ladder Technique. 162
    Avoid Needle Stick Injuries 165
    Buttonhole Technique 165
    Tape the Needles After Insertion. 167
    Monitor Arterial Pressure 168
Help Patients with Needle Fear 169
    Reduce Pain from Needle Insertion 169
Fistula Care After a Treatment. 171
Grafts in Detail 172
    How Grafts are Placed 172
Starting HD with a Graft 173
    Prepare the Access Skin. 174
    Wash Your Hands. 174
    Examine the Graft 174
    Find the Direction of Blood Flow. 174
    Inserting Sharp Needles in a Graft 174
    Graft Care After an HD Treatment 175
Complications of Fistulas and Grafts During Use . . 175
    Infiltration. 175
    Bleeding During HD 176
    Bleeding After HD 177
    Recirculation 178
    Steal Syndrome 178
Longer Term Complications of Fistulas and Grafts .178
    Aneurysms 179
    Pseudoaneurysms. 179
    Stenosis. 180
    Thrombosis 181
    Access Monitoring and Surveillance 182
    Infection 185
HD Catheters in Detail. 187
    Catheter Placement 187
    How HD Catheters Work 187
    Veins Used for Catheters 188
    Care of Hemodialysis Catheters. 189
    Starting HD with a Catheter 189
Complications of HD Catheters 191
    Infection 191

Catheter Disconnection 192
Catheter Loss 192
Central Venous Stenosis 192
Slow Blood Flow Rate 192
Improving Vascular Access Outcomes 192
Continuous Quality Improvement 192
Clinical Practice Guidelines 193
Conclusion 195
References 196
Appendix A: Teaching Buttonhole 198

7 HEMODIALYSIS PROCEDURES AND COMPLICATIONS 207

Objectives 208
Introduction 209
Infection Control 209
How Infections Spread 209
Hemodialysis Infection Control Precautions 210
Hand Hygiene 210
When and How to Use Aseptic Technique 211
Personal Protective Equipment 213
Safe Handling of Equipment and Supplies After Treatment 213
Bloodborne Diseases 214
Hemodialysis Procedures and Complications 215
Antibiotic-resistant Bacteria 216
Other Infection Concerns 217
Giving Medications and Solutions 218
Needles 218
Syringes 218
Safe Use of Syringes and Needles 218
Drawing Up Medicine 219
Using IV Solutions 220
Body Mechanics 220
Lifting and Carrying 220
Patient Transfers 221
Patients with Walkers 221
Chair-to-Chair Transfers 222
Stand and Pivot Technique 222
Using a Slide Board 222
Portable Lift Devices 223
Stretcher-to-Chair Transfers 223
Stretcher-to-Bed Transfers 223
Documentation 223
Electronic Charting 224
Paper Charting: Writing an Entry in the Medical Record 224

Predialysis Treatment Procedures 224
The Treatment Plan 224
Conduct an Alarm Safety Check 227
Evaluate the Patient 227
Weigh the Patient 228
Check for Edema 230
Take the Patient's Pulse 230
Take the Patient's Blood Pressure 230
Count the Respiration Rate 232
Take the Patient's Temperature 232
Check the Vascular Access 233
Ask About General Physical and Emotional Health 233
Starting a Dialysis Treatment .234
Calculate How Much Water to Remove 234
Cannulate or Connect the Patient's Access 239
Draw Blood for Laboratory Testing 239
Start the Dialysis Machine 241
Monitoring During Dialysis 242
Vascular Access 243
General Patient Condition 243
Giving Medicines 243
Patient Comfort and Safety 244
Anticoagulation 245
Machine Monitoring 246
Hemodialysis Complications 247
Clinical Complications 247
Technical Complications 261
Post-dialysis Procedures 263
End the Dialysis Treatment 263
Take the Patient's Vital Signs and Weight 263
Document the Treatment 264
Clean Up the Equipment 264
Measuring Dialysis Adequacy .264
Urea Kinetic Modeling 265
Drawing Pre- and Post-dialysis BUN 265
Minimum Delivered and Prescribed Dose of Dialysis . .266
Factors that Affect the Dialysis Treatment 266
Dialysis Dose and Patient Well-Being 267
Conclusion 267
References 268

8 WATER TREATMENT 271

Objectives 272
Introduction 273
Water Supply 273
Drinking Water Contaminants .273
Drinking Water Standards 273

Tap Water Treatment 274
Dialysis Water 275
    AAMI Standards for Dialysis Water 275
Design of a Dialysis Water Treatment System 277
    Pretreatment Components........................278
    Purification Components.........................278
    Distribution System 278
Parts of a Water Treatment System................280
    Reverse Osmosis (RO) 280
    Pretreatment Components 281
    Purification Components.........................284
    Distribution System 284
Monitoring a Water Treatment System............287
    How to Monitor and Maintain Water Treatment
        System Components 287
Analyze Water Quality 293
    RO Water Quality...............................293
    DI Water Quality................................293
    Monitor Water for Bacteria and Endotoxins..........295
    Monitor Water for Chemicals 296
Patient Monitoring 299
Conclusion 299
Appendix A: EPA Tap Water Standards 300
References 302

9 EMERGENCY PLANNING AND RESPONSE 305

Objectives 306
Introduction....................................307
Regulations and Oversight
    of Dialysis Emergencies......................308
    Conditions for Coverage 308
    The Joint Commission 308
    Local and State Rules............................308
    Kidney Community Emergency Response Program ...308
Types of Emergencies 310
Prepare for Emergencies........................310
    Anticipate, Plan, Train............................310
    Know Your Part in the Communication Plan..........310
    Plan for Clinic-level Events 311
    Plan for Area or Regional Events...................313
Patient Education for Emergencies................314
Responding to Emergencies.....................315
    Set Up a Command Center 315
    Triage 315
    Assess Damage to the Building and Equipment 315
    Maintain Staffing................................316
Recovering from an Emergency..................316
    Plan for Patient Care.............................316
    Physical Plant Safety 317
    Emotional Recovery After a Disaster 318
Quality Improvement............................319
Conclusion 320
Appendix A: Resources 321
Appendix B: 3-Day Emergency Diet Plan
    for Dialysis Patients 322
References.....................................324

GLOSSARY AND INDEX............325
Acronyms 326
Glossary 333

1 Today's Dialysis Environment

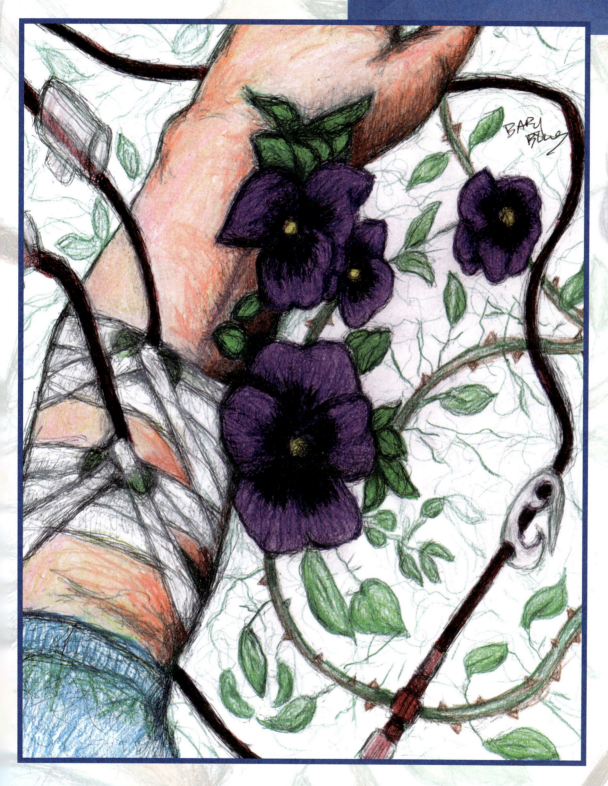

Anyone who has lived through CKD, transplants, dialysis, etc., knows it is not easy. It is a never ending road of complications and trials, and takes courage to overcome, be positive, and live life to the fullest!

Artist, Rebecca Schirmer

"I feel very lucky. I've been doing 7-hour nighttime treatments for almost 2 years and I love my nurse and techs. We have had a couple come and go but mostly we have had the same three the whole time I have been there. I can't say enough about these guys; I owe them my life."

Objectives

MODULE AUTHORS
Tony Messana, BS
Darlene Rodgers, BSN, RN, CNN, CPHQ
Dori Schatell, MS

MODULE REVIEWERS
Nancy M. Gallagher, BS, RN, CNN
Glenda M. Payne, MS RN, CNN
Darlene Rodgers, BSN, RN, CNN, CPHQ
John H. Sadler, MD
Dori Schatell, MS
Vern Taaffe, BS, CBNT, CDWS

1. State the main job of healthy kidneys.
2. Explain how dialysis is paid for in the United States.
3. List two quality standards for dialysis.
4. Describe the four main steps of continuous quality improvement (CQI).
5. Define what it means to be a professional and give three examples of professional behavior.
6. Discuss why and how a dialysis technician becomes certified.

An acronym list can be found in the Glossary.

Practice Test Questions at:
www.meiresearch.org/cc6

Introduction

As a dialysis technician, your job will be to help give safe and effective dialysis treatments to people whose kidneys have failed. To do this well, you will have a lot to learn, starting with the topics in this module:

- What dialysis is and a brief history
- How dialysis is paid for
- How to ensure high quality care for patients
- How to behave in a professional way
- Why and how dialysis technicians get certified

Dialysis is complex. An entire team is needed to help meet patients' needs for treatment, nutrition, medications, and social support. Team members include technicians, nurses, dietitians, social workers, and doctors. Others, such as physical therapists, pharmacists, exercise physiologists, and clergy, may be called on as well.

Patients do best on dialysis if they take an active role in their own care. No one can eat, drink, or take medicines for someone else—each patient needs to do this for him or herself. It is part of the care team's job to *engage* patients in their own care: to help them learn how to take an active role in their treatment. Care teams can engage patients by treating them with respect, *encouraging* their questions, and helping them to learn about their dialysis and all of the treatment options. In fact, engagement in healthcare is a life and death matter: those who don't understand kidney disease and dialysis are much more likely to die sooner.[1]

"Dialysis is a part-time job. So is a family, so is a puppy, so is raking up your leaves every fall... I owned my own business as a contractor, marketed myself, worked long hours in construction doing everything from roofing to windows, trained a puppy, made my own meals, never let my labs slip, and never missed a treatment."

We do dialysis to *help people live as fully as they can.* Helping your patients reach this goal can be one of the *best* parts of your job. This is something you can feel proud of, and it makes being a technician much more than just getting a paycheck. Many patients who get good dialysis *do* lead full and active lives. For others, having a good quality of life is harder. How someone feels on dialysis depends on many things, including:

- Age
- How active s/he was before kidney failure
- Other illnesses (such as diabetes, high blood pressure, lung disease)
- How well dialysis treatments are managed (for example, how gently water is removed during dialysis)
- Attitude toward dialysis
- Support from loved ones

As a technician, you have a chance each day to help patients feel their best—and this can lead to a rewarding career.

Overview of Kidney Failure and Dialysis

"As a 9 year old with kidney failure, I was surrounded by the most caring nurses and technicians I will ever know. I didn't ask to be treated differently nor did I let anyone do that. But many of us have lost something that has been a part of us our entire lives. We feel fear, sadness, and anger from what we lost, whether it be freedom or time or money. It takes its toll. As a technician you have to put yourself in that chair and imagine what was lost."

The main job of healthy kidneys is to help keep the body in homeostasis: a constant, minute-to-minute balance of water, minerals, electrolytes, and other substances. To do this, they:

- **Remove water and wastes.** Kidneys test and filter each drop of blood, and send wastes and extra water to the bladder as urine.
- **Keep salt and other electrolytes in balance.** Electrolytes carry signals between nerves and muscles.
- **Control blood pressure.** Kidneys keep water/salts in balance and make an enzyme called renin that can raise blood pressure if it drops too low.
- **Keep bones strong.** Kidneys help convert vitamin D into an active form (calcitriol) so calcium can be absorbed.
- **Maintain acid-base balance.** Kidneys help keep our blood and bodies at the pH level that lets our organs work as well as possible.
- **Help ensure the right level of red blood cells.** Kidneys sense if there are enough red blood cells in the blood. Not enough? They send a hormone (erythropoietin) to the bone marrow to make more.

Module 1

"[When my kidneys failed] I lost my appetite, lost a lot of weight, strength, stamina. I had that metallic taste in my mouth and couldn't stand the smell or taste of food. After a while [on dialysis], I could eat and sleep again and soon went back to work, in another profession."

When kidneys fail, the balance fails, too. As a result, people may retain water in their lungs and feel short of breath. (Some think they have asthma or pneumonia and are shocked to learn they have kidney failure.) They may have swelling in their hands or feet or under their eyes. Their blood pressure may soar. They may feel exhausted and cold all the time from *anemia*, a shortage of red blood cells.

There is no cure for kidney failure that is caused by a *chronic* (long-term) disease. People whose kidneys do not work will die—unless they get treatment to replace at least some kidney function. These are the treatment options:

- A **transplant** gives someone a new kidney from a living or deceased donor. Transplant does the best job of replacing all of the functions of healthy kidneys. Sometimes people whose kidneys are failing will get a *"preemptive"* kidney transplant before they need to start dialysis. But, most people will have to start dialysis and wait for a kidney.
- **Dialysis** removes some water and wastes from the body. There are two main types: **hemodialysis** (HD) and **peritoneal dialysis** (PD). HD (in all its forms) is the most common (89.9% of U.S. dialysis patients).[2] Technicians may help with both HD and PD treatments.
- **Conservative management** does not prolong life, it treats only the symptoms of kidney failure without dialysis or a kidney transplant.

Dialysis is Partial Kidney Replacement

Dialysis—no matter what kind—can only do *part* of the work of healthy kidneys. The treatments remove some of the excess water and wastes. But, as soon as a treatment is over, wastes and water start to build up until the next time. Patients may need to strictly limit their fluids and diet so less water and fewer wastes build up. *The more urine someone still makes and the more dialysis s/he gets, the more freedom s/he will have in fluid intake and diet.* Dialysis cannot make hormones or enzymes, so these are given as medicines.

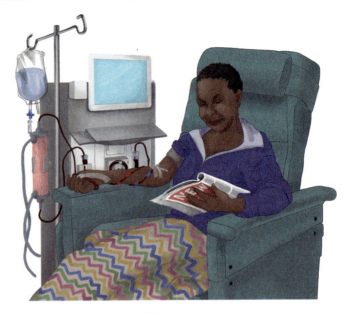

Figure 1: Person Receiving HD Treatment

HEMODIALYSIS (HD)

HD treatments pass a patient's blood through a filter on a dialysis machine (an artificial kidney, or *dialyzer*) that is designed to remove water and wastes. To reach the blood, a pathway called a *vascular access* is created by a surgeon. Tubing is connected to the access to carry the blood to the filter and then back to the patient in a closed loop, called an *extracorporeal* (outside the body) *circuit*. With each pass through the filter, the blood gets a bit cleaner (see Figure 1). There are three main types of HD access. You will learn about each type in Module 6: *Vascular Access*.

During an HD treatment, a blood pump pulls blood out of the patient through one needle and pushes it to a dialyzer. Or, blood will be pulled through one side, or *lumen*, of a catheter. Inside the dialyzer, blood is filtered and cleaned: wastes and water pass out of the blood through hollow hair-like fibers in the dialyzer and into a cleansing fluid called *dialysate*. Then, the blood goes back to the patient through another needle (or other catheter lumen). Used dialysate is sent to a drain. (Dialysate has most of the same chemicals as blood plasma. We use it to balance the content of the plasma and remove wastes.) The dialysis machine sets the rate of blood flow, and mixes purified water concentrates to make and deliver dialysate. There are many safety checks and alarms on the machine to make sure that the treatment is being done right.

How many dialysis treatments does a patient need? And, how long should the treatments be? There are several different HD schedules (see Table 1).

Table 1: HD Schedules

Type & Location	# Days or Nights/Week	# Hours/Treatment	# Hours/Week
Standard *in-center*	3	3–4	9–12
Nocturnal *in-center*	3	8	24
Self-care *in-center*	3	3–4	9–12
Standard *home*	3 or every other day	4–6	12–21
Short daily *home**	4–6	2.5–4	10–24
Nocturnal *home*	3–6	7–8	21–48

*Very rarely, this option is offered in-center as well.

In the U.S., about 88% of dialysis patients follow a standard in-center treatment schedule with technicians like you providing their treatments.[2] Patients who dialyze in-center may also choose to do some or even all of their own care, an option called *in-center self-care*. Their dialysis clinics provide the training and the clinic staff provides support, as needed. It can be rewarding for you to see your patients becoming more self-sufficient and taking pride in what they learn. You may choose to work in one clinic. Or, as you learn more, you may choose to travel and take temporary assignments with an agency.

Some HD patients choose to dialyze at home, or for more hours than the "standard" in-center treatment. Why? Healthy kidneys work 24 hours a day, 7 days a week—168 hours a week. Longer or more frequent HD can feel more like having healthy kidneys did, because it is gentler and causes fewer symptoms—and it can help patients live longer.[3] A treatment that can be done at night does not take time out of the day, so it may feel like less of a burden (for patients who are able to sleep through it). And, home treatments give patients back a sense of control that kidney failure can take away from them, which some people prefer. When patients do HD at home, a nurse trains them, and the clinic provides the machine and supplies. Patients do not have to buy them. There are roles for technicians with home dialysis as well.

PERITONEAL DIALYSIS (PD)

PD is a home treatment that removes water and wastes *inside* the body. (Rarely, PD is started or done in-center.) The abdominal cavity is filled with dialysate fluid. The tiny *capillary* blood vessels in the *peritoneum* that line the inside of the abdomen act as filters. Wastes and excess water flow out of the blood in the capillaries and into the dialysate.

Your Job with In-center HD

When patients receive HD treatments, technicians may work under the supervision of a nurse to:

- Set up a clean, safe dialysis station and machine for patients
- Talk to patients about how they are feeling, take their vital signs, and draw blood for tests
- Explain to patients what you are doing, answer questions or find someone who can
- Put in dialysis needles safely, enter the machine settings correctly, and closely monitor the treatment
- Teach patients to place their own needles and learn how to set up and run the machine
- Help patients with problems or symptoms during treatment, trips to the bathroom, etc.
- Alert other staff to patients' needs, as appropriate
- Remove needles carefully, ensure that bleeding has stopped and it is safe to let the patient leave the clinic
- Open and close the center and order supplies

Your Job with Home HD

- Help set up patients' homes for home dialysis treatments and troubleshoot any challenges
- Provide respite treatments to those doing home HD
- Prepare the equipment, supplies, and dialysate for home HD training
- Help home HD patients arrange supplies and put in needles

After a "dwell" time of a few hours, used dialysate fluid is drained out and fresh dialysate is added (see Figure 2). This sterile process of removing spent fluid and replacing it with fresh fluid is called an *exchange*. To get dialysate into the abdomen, the "access" is a *catheter* (tube) placed through the wall of the belly or chest wall (*presternal*). A nurse teaches the patient how to safely use the catheter to fill the belly with dialysate. In the U.S., about 9.7% of dialysis patients do PD.[2]

Module 1

Whenever there is dialysate in the abdomen, PD is working to remove water and wastes. For most patients, this means that PD goes on 7 days a week. PD is very gentle—but it is also much less efficient than HD. About 80% of patients who do PD use a cycler machine at home to do exchanges at night while they sleep. The rest do PD by hand, most often four times a day.[2] Manual PD can be done at home, at work, or while traveling, and each exchange takes about 30 minutes.

Your Job with PD

When patients receive PD treatments, technicians may work under the supervision of a nurse to:

- Check patients into an exam room for clinic visits (check vital signs, draw blood, etc.)
- Observe or reinforce PD tasks after the nurse has done training
- Manage phone lines, schedule patients
- File paperwork, track Plan of Care documents, and help set up referrals and hospital stays
- Enter data into electronic medical records and government report databases
- Manage supply inventory, including emergency evacuation supplies
- Irrigate new PD catheters and assist with PD exchanges for patients who are new/training
- Open and close the clinic (pull charts for the next day, etc.)

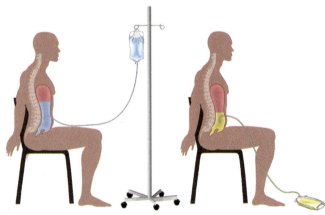

The peritoneal cavity is filled with dialysate, using gravity

At the end of the exchange, the dialysate is drained into the bag, again using gravity

Figure 2: Peritoneal Dialysis

Payment for Dialysis and Transplant

"My husband was just approved for Medicare Part B. Why would he have a monthly payment of $120? Am I misunderstanding this? I thought it paid for 80% of his health care. And then my insurance will pick up the other 20%. I'm confused..."

What if we had the knowledge and technology to save the lives of people with kidney failure—but not enough machines or money to pay for them? Who would decide which patients would get dialysis and live and which would die? Before 1973, this difficult scenario happened all across the U.S.

Early U.S. dialysis programs were in Veteran's Administration and other hospitals. Some had "Life and Death" committees with psychologists, social workers, physicians, and clergy to choose who would get the scarce, costly treatment.[4] These committees chose patients based on age, maturity, education, whether they had children, could pay for their care, and how much they might give back to the world if they lived. For those who were chosen, the costs of treatment were high. Insurance companies said dialysis was "experimental," and would not pay for it.

People with kidney disease fought to get the U.S. government to pay for dialysis. One patient, Shep Glazer, even did a few minutes of HD on the floor of Congress.[4] In 1972, Congress was convinced that it made sense to help pay for treatments that would allow patients to remain working, tax-paying citizens. Public Law 92-603, the **Medicare End-Stage Renal Disease (ESRD) Program**, took effect in 1973. This program gives coverage to patients who have worked enough to qualify for Social Security, or to their dependents.[5] Today, Medicare (a program run by the **Centers for Medicare & Medicaid Services, or CMS**) pays 80% of the cost of dialysis and kidney transplants. Medicare has several parts. Part A covers hospitalization, and is free for those who qualify. Part B covers outpatient care, such as dialysis. Patients must pay a premium for Part B. There is also a Part D, which helps pay for medicines. Patients need to have a second health plan along with Medicare, such as Medicaid or Medigap, to pay the balance that Medicare does not cover. See how Medicare changed dialysis in Table 2.

Today's Dialysis Environment

Table 2: Dialysis Before and After the Medicare ESRD Program

Before the Medicare ESRD Program	After the Medicare ESRD Program
About 40% of patients did their treatments at home.[4]	More clinics began to open and most people got their treatments in a clinic.
There were only a few dialysis clinics.	Today, there are about 6,500 clinics.[8] Most (about 70%) are owned by for-profit dialysis companies.[9] DaVita and Fresenius, two for-profit large dialysis organizations (LDOs) dominate the U.S. dialysis market.[10]
People chosen for dialysis were young—under 45—and healthy, apart from kidney failure. Most were married, white men.[5]	Older and sicker people get dialysis, too. About half of patients are under age 60 and half are over.[11]

Kidney failure is one of just two diseases with its own Medicare program.* CMS makes rules that all dialysis clinics must follow if they want to be paid. These rules are called the **Conditions for Coverage for End-Stage Renal Disease (ESRD) Facilities**.[6] The *Conditions* were updated in 2008 for the first time in 32 years. Dialysis is still very costly, and some people still start treatment with no health plan.

*U.S. citizens with amyotrophic lateral sclerosis (ALS, or Lou Gehrig's disease) can also get Medicare when their disability payments start.[7]

Some patients have employer group health plans (EGHP) through their own job or a spouse's job. EGHPs are *primary*: they pay first for the first 30 months after a patient can get Medicare. Medicare is *secondary* during those 30 months, and may pay some or all of what the EGHP does not cover. After the 30 months are up, insurance coverage switches: Medicare becomes primary and an EGHP is secondary. EGHPs tend to pay much more than Medicare. This means that dialysis clinics can bring in more revenue when patients keep their jobs and EGHP health plans. Clinics that offer PD and home HD treatment options can help patients keep their jobs.[12]

Choosing how to pay for dialysis—and which type of insurance plan will be best for a particular patient—can be complicated. Patients may want to seek advice from an independent expert to help them understand all the options and make an informed decision.[13] Dialysis clinics may have financial counselors to help patients. The social worker may also be a resource for financial questions.

When Medicare Starts to Pay

Patients who don't have Medicare when they start dialysis must wait 3 full months for it to start to pay—IF they do in-center HD. But, if they train for PD, home HD, or in-center self-care, Medicare starts to pay on the first day of their first month of dialysis.[14] Medicare will also pay for a kidney transplant. Choosing a home treatment or in-center self-care before the first day of the *fourth month can save patients tens of thousands of dollars*. Patients often don't know this, so if they are worried about money, you can tell them to ask their social worker or use the Medicare Start Date Calculator on the Home Dialysis Central website, at: www.homedialysis.org/home-dialysis-basics/calculator.

For decades, Medicare paid for dialysis with a **composite rate** for each treatment. Set in 1983 at $130 per treatment, the composite rate paid for overhead, staff, machines, patient rehabilitation efforts, and some drugs.[6] Other drugs and lab tests were billed separately.

In January 2011, Medicare changed over to a *new* way to pay for dialysis: the **ESRD Prospective Payment System (PPS)**, also called the "bundle." The PPS "bundles" what was in the composite rate *plus* lab tests, some drugs, and a home training add-on (when used) into one payment.[15] The rate now differs for each patient based on age, weight, height, and some other illnesses, and it differs across the U.S. based on local wages. It may help your patients to know that Medicare pays for kidney transplant surgery and 3 years of post-transplant care as well. Three years after a successful transplant, Medicare will stop, and the patient will need other health insurance.

The PPS has had a big effect on the budgets of most dialysis clinics. Before the PPS, clinics owned by large companies used to make extra money by giving medications and doing lab tests. Now, these *cost* the clinic money instead. Gentler or more intensive treatment options like PD, home HD, and nocturnal in-center HD often let patients use fewer medications. That's good news for the patients who can use these options *and* for the clinics that offer them.

In January 2012, CMS made a second change to dialysis payment. A **Quality Incentive Program (QIP)** started that will reduce a clinic's Medicare payments by up to 2% if it does not meet certain measures.[16] The goal of QIP is to improve care by paying less when outcomes are poor. The whole care team needs to help the clinic meet these measures (see Table 3).

Table 3: 2017 and 2018 Quality Incentive Program Measures

2017 QIP Measures[17]	
Topic	**Measure**
Adequate Dialysis Dose	■ % of HD patient months with a Kt/V ≥ 1.2 ■ % of PD patient months with a Kt/V ≥ 1.7
HD Fistulas	■ % of patient months when the last HD treatment used a fistula
HD Catheters	■ % of patient months when the last HD treatment used a catheter that had been in place for 90 days or more
Blood Calcium Levels	■ % of patient months with a 3-month uncorrected average serum calcium > 10.2 mg/dL
Bloodstream Infections	■ # of HD outpatients with positive blood cultures per 100 HD patient months
Hospital Readmissions	■ Ratio of the # of actual, unplanned to expected, unplanned readmissions
Bone Mineral Blood Tests	■ # of months a clinic reports serum phosphorus values for each Medicare patient
Anemia	■ # of months a clinic reports ESA medicine dose and hemoglobin or hematocrit blood levels for each Medicare patient at least once a month
Patient Experience of Care	■ Patients are given the ICH CAHPS survey twice a year and the results are sent to CMS
2018 QIP Measures Include the 2017 Measures, Plus:[18]	
Topic	**Measure**
Blood Transfusions	■ Ratio of actual to expected blood transfusions in a clinic
Pain Management	■ Clinics report whether pain is assessed, is documented, and a follow-up plan is made
Depression Screening	■ Clinics report whether depression is assessed, is documented, and a follow-up plan is made
Staff Flu Vaccines	■ Clinics report whether staff have been vaccinated for the flu
Patient Experience of Care	■ % of completed ICH CAHPS surveys (minimum 30) and reporting of composite test scores

Quality in Dialysis

"I had a chance to speak with a state dialysis inspector. I told her that many members of a group I am in were told that their machines could not be turned towards them. And, they could not be taught how to self-cannulate or it was against state law for them to learn to run their machines. We had this talk while I was setting up and putting myself on the machine in my center. She made it very clear to me that the government and the state encourage patients to participate in their care."

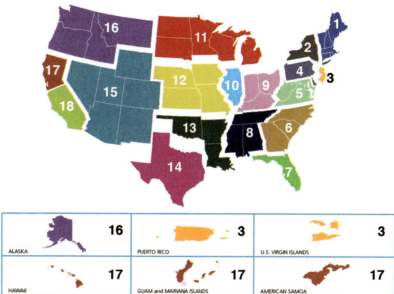

Figure 3: ESRD Network Map

Used with permission from ESRD National Coordinating Center (NCC) at esrdncc.org

The quality of dialysis has been a focus of the Medicare ESRD Program since it was created by Congress in 1972. The goals of dialysis were to help patients *stay active, work, and pay taxes—not* just keep them alive. Once there were enough resources to treat all of the people with kidney failure, we were able to focus on this goal. Congress wants to know that the Medicare ESRD Program is successful and worth its high cost. We do this, in part, by showing that centers give high quality care.

ESRD Networks

In 1978, Congress set up ESRD Networks to oversee the quality of dialysis care in the U.S. There are 18 ESRD Networks covering all U.S. states and territories. The Centers for Medicare & Medicaid Services (CMS) contracts with organizations to do the Network tasks the government requires (see Figure 3). Networks:

- Encourage patient and family engagement at the dialysis clinic
- Collect and report data about dialysis outcomes
- Do quality improvement projects and foster safe practices
- Evaluate and help resolve patient grievances
- Help clinics deal with conflict
- Provide resources to staff and patients

Dialysis clinics are required by Medicare statute to work with the Networks.

Guidelines for Dialysis Care

To measure the quality of care in a center, we look at *outcomes* or results of care. Outcomes like *morbidity* (sickness) and *mortality* (death) vary from clinic to clinic. This can be due to differences in patients, in care, or both. How can we improve outcomes for all patients? One way is to find the best ways to do dialysis and require clinics to use them. Clinical practice guidelines are efforts to do just that.

RENAL PHYSICIANS ASSOCIATION (RPA)

In 1993, the first clinical practice guideline for kidney failure came from *nephrologists* (kidney doctors) in the RPA. It suggested a minimum dose of HD. Other RPA guidelines include care of people with kidney disease who are not on dialysis, when to start and end dialysis, and many more. RPA guidelines can be found at www.renalmd.org/End-Stage-Renal-Disease/.

NATIONAL KIDNEY FOUNDATION (NKF)

The **Dialysis Outcomes Quality Initiative (DOQI)** was formed in 1995.[19] Teams of experts wrote sets of guidelines for:[20]

- Anemia
- HD adequacy
- PD adequacy
- Vascular access

Since 1997, the scope of the DOQI has grown to cover all stages of kidney disease. Now it is called the **NKF Kidney Disease Outcomes Quality Initiative (KDOQI™)**. The goal of the KDOQI Guidelines is to improve the care and outcomes of all people with kidney disease in the U.S. In 2003, a new NKF program called **Kidney Disease: Improving Global Outcomes (KDIGO)** began work to improve the care of kidney patients around the world.

Updates and new guidelines are always in development. You will need to stay aware of these changes and how they may affect your center. To work, guidelines must be used each day. As a dialysis technician, you are a key member of a team that puts the guidelines into practice and helps patients understand them. The *Core Curriculum for the Dialysis Technician*, sixth edition, will help you learn more about how to do this.

DIALYSIS OUTCOMES AND PRACTICE PATTERNS STUDY (DOPPS)

The **DOPPS** is a series of long-term studies of patients with chronic kidney disease. Started in 1996, the DOPPS now tracks more than 70,000 patients in more than 20 countries. The goal of DOPPS is to improve patients' lives by looking at practice patterns that can be linked to better outcomes.[21]

ESRD Quality Improvement Initiative

In 2004, the **ESRD Quality Improvement Initiative** was launched by CMS to improve the quality of dialysis care. Parts of the program are:

- **Dialysis Facility Compare** – a website with quality data on dialysis clinics to help patients choose between them.[22]
- **Star Ratings** – a 0–5 star scale in Dialysis Facility Compare that sums up clinic data for patients and families.[23] As of this writing, the star system may be revised.
- **Fistula First Catheter Last** – a program to increase the use of better types of HD vascular access and reduce the use of risky types. Their website has sections for patients and professionals.[24]
- **ESRD Conditions for Coverage** – rules dialysis clinics must follow to obtain payment from Medicare.[7]
- **In-Center Hemodialysis CAHPS Survey** – a survey that measures how satisfied dialysis patients are with their care (an experience-of-care survey).[25]
- **Consolidated Renal Operations in a Web-enabled Network (CROWNWeb)** – a database of information about patients reported by dialysis clinics.[26]
- **Quality Incentive Program** – bases clinic payments on standard measures of quality care.[27]

Quality Standards for Dialysis

State Surveyors inspect clinics for Medicare to be sure they follow the rules in the *ESRD Conditions for Coverage*. The surveyors observe care, review patient charts, talk to patients and staff, and use a checklist of the rules called the **Measures Assessment Tool (MAT)**. Clinics that do not follow all of the rules must make a Plan of Correction. A new survey may be done to make sure the clinic has fixed any problems. In severe cases, clinics can lose their Medicare funding, or even be closed.

The same surveyors who inspect dialysis clinics may also review nursing homes and mental health centers. Each of these must be inspected once a year, but there is no such rule for dialysis. This means that years may go by between surveys. However, each clinic should *always* be ready for a surprise survey and work each day as if it will be inspected.

Many other dialysis standards exist as well:

- Each ESRD Network has a **Medical Review Board (MRB)** to collect patient and clinic data, and measure outcomes. CMS may also require specific quality improvement efforts by clinics.
- **The Joint Commission** has standards for hospital-based dialysis programs.
- The **Association for the Advancement of Medical Instrumentation (AAMI)** has standards for dialysis water treatment, dialysate fluid, dialyzer reuse, and medical equipment. Since the AAMI standards are approved by the American National Standards Institute, ANSI, you will often see AAMI/ANSI. CMS includes some of the AAMI/ANSI standards in the *Conditions for Coverage*.
- The **Centers for Disease Control and Prevention (CDC)** standards cover infection control in dialysis clinics.
- **Food and Drug Administration (FDA)** oversees all medical devices. In 1991, the FDA put out *Quality Assurance Guidelines for Hemodialysis Devices*.[28] These guidelines cover dialyzers, blood tubing, alarms, dialysis machines, dialyzer reprocessing equipment, water treatment, and all other devices. Updates to these guidelines can be found on this site: www.fda.gov/RegulatoryInformation/Guidances/default.htm.[29] The FDA requires clinics to fill out reports to tell manufacturers and the FDA about problems with devices and equipment, as well as adverse events.[28]

Today's Dialysis Environment

- **United States Renal Data System (USRDS)** puts out a report each year that compiles data from all U.S. dialysis clinics. Data include the number of patients, death rates, cost of care, and much more. The results help us to see if outcomes for all patients are getting better or worse. Clinics can compare the U.S. data with their own outcomes.

Continuous Quality Improvement (CQI) in Dialysis

CQI is a way to look at what is going on in a system (like a dialysis clinic), find problems, and fix them. CQI can be both "top-down" and "bottom-up." Top-down means *management* commits to a CQI culture and uses resources to help CQI succeed. Bottom-up means *workers* find ways to make changes to improve care. CQI projects can be:

- **Clinical** – e.g., anemia, dialysis dose, access problems
- **Technical** – e.g., water treatment, dialyzer reuse
- **Organizational** – e.g., policies and procedures, patient safety
- **Process** – e.g., scheduling, location of hand sanitizer

CQI PROCESS

Dialysis rules require the doctor, nurse, dietitian and social worker on the team to do CQI. As a technician, you will be included as needed. Different CQI models exist, but their goals are the same. All dialysis organizations have quality programs that are used in their clinics. Figure 4 is an example of a four-step CQI process.[30] Steps I–III are where other CQI models may differ.

I. Identify Improvement Needs

The goal of this step is to find something that needs to be improved. There are four sub-steps:

1. Collect data
2. Analyze the data
3. Identify the problem/need for improvement
4. Prioritize next steps

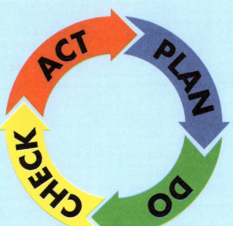

Figure 4: Plan, Do, Check, Act Cycle

II. Analyze the Process

1. **Choose a team** – include members of the care team based on the problem: doctors, nurses, dietitians, technicians, social workers, and patients.
2. **Review the data** – look at the data from the first step.
3. **Study the process/problem** – try to identify all the factors/steps in the process/problem. Review the literature on the problem to see if there are standards or guidelines that apply.
4. **Look for patterns and trends** – think about reasons for the problem, using the data.

III. Identify Root Causes

From research, discussion, and data, decide the causes of the problem.

IV. Implement the "Plan, Do, Check, Act" (PDCA) Cycle

The last step is to use the PDCA cycle. The four steps in the PDCA cycle are:
1. **Plan** – make a plan to address the problem. Include outcomes, ways to solve the problem, a task list for each team member, and a time frame.
2. **Do** – try the action plan.
3. **Check** – monitor the results of the plan, assess results after the plan is done, and evaluate the plan for any needed changes.
4. **Act** – adopt the plan in the clinic on a formal basis and continue to check progress.

The PDCA cycle is an ongoing process. Once a solution to the problem is started in the clinic, you can't assume that the problem is solved. The new process needs to be verified to be sure it is being used in day-to-day care and is working to create the change the team wanted. When one part of a process changes, other parts may be affected (sometimes in ways you did not expect). So, the whole process must be watched carefully.

CQI is part of a larger quality effort that goes on in dialysis clinics. The Conditions for Coverage require formal quality improvement efforts. Each dialysis clinic must have a **Quality Assessment and Performance Improvement (QAPI)** program.[7] All services (e.g., HD, PD, water treatment) given by a dialysis clinic must be included. A QAPI program needs to use a PDCA approach and:
- Use clinical practice guidelines to track health outcomes
- Find, prevent, and reduce medical errors
- Take action to improve outcomes that do not meet the target levels
- Measure patient satisfaction

Dialysis Technician Professionalism

"The technician who trained me to self-cannulate is like a mother to me. Her daughter went to my college. I watched her grow from technician to clinical manager. I guarantee she would agree that professionalism is important!"

As a dialysis technician, you are a member of a *team* that cares for patients at your clinic. You will have more direct contact with patients than any other staff member, and you represent the clinic to your patients and their families. So, you need to know what it means to do your job in a professional way.

A professional should:
- Know the field *and* the job: become an expert
- Provide safe and effective treatments to achieve the best outcomes for patients
- Do high-quality work
- Follow a high standard of ethics
- Have good work morale and motivation
- Respect patients and colleagues

How can *you* behave in a professional way?
- **Keep learning**. Ask questions, read, take classes.
- **Take pride in your work**. Arrive on time, dressed for work, and well groomed.
- **Learn and follow your clinic's policies and procedures**.
- **Be prepared**. Have all equipment ready and working when the patient arrives.
- **Be organized**. Keep the patient care area clean, set up so you can find what you need, and free of blood.
- **Wash your hands and put on clean gloves before you touch a patient**! Infection control is one of *the most* important ways to be a professional. We will talk more about this in other modules.
- **Talk to your patients**. When you enter a patient's treatment space, tell him or her what you are doing

and why. Help patients learn and treat them like people, not work to be done.

- **Use patients' titles** (i.e., Mrs. Smith). Use first names or nicknames only if the patient asks you to.
- **Maintain your patients' dignity**. Always introduce yourself and other members of the team to new patients so they feel more comfortable in the clinic. Use the privacy curtains when needed. Never uncover patients' private areas in front of other patients or staff.
- **Protect everyone's privacy and confidential information**. Speak quietly and do not yell across the patient care floor. Do not talk about one patient in front of another.
- **Speak the clinic's language on the patient floor**. Speak to your coworkers in the language used for business in the clinic. When you use a language patients don't understand, they may think you are talking about them or being rude.
- **Remember your manners**. Say "please" and "thank you" when you talk to patients, families, and other staff members, and "excuse me" if you interrupt someone.
- **Don't stand around with other staff members**. Patients will assume that you are not being attentive to their care and safety.
- **Avoid distractions**. Cell phones, TV and other things can take your attention away from your patients. Your patients' safety is your top priority.

Professional Boundaries

Psychological boundaries are the rules people use to form the right kinds of relationships with each other. In a dialysis clinic, you may spend 40 hours a week with patients, and may see the same patients for years. Staff become very close to patients and to each other. We do need to care about our patients—but there is a danger if staff become too attached to patients, and vice versa.

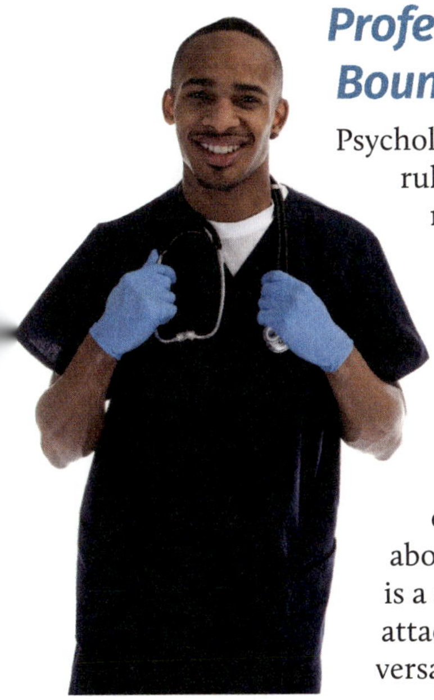

Figure 5: Dialysis Technician

As a technician, you need to always be sure you are keeping your relationship with your patients *professional*.

Patients are not your friends and family, though they may seem close enough to be. You may need to remind yourself each day to keep a professional (not personal) relationship with your patients. Your supervisor can help you with this. Ask patients about their lives, their families, and what they like to do, so you know what motivates them. But, focus all talk on the patient—*not on your own life*. You cannot solve everyone's problems. Most of the time you can only be there to offer support. Patients may express their feelings to you, and you will need to stay calm no matter what they say. To stay on the right track, **DO NOT**:

- Give patients your phone number
- Share personal details about your life outside of work
- Tell them about your problems
- Date patients or touch them in a sexual way
- Go to patients' homes, invite them over, or see them outside of the clinic
- Give patients a ride or run errands for them
- Send texts, emails, or tweets, or follow or "friend" them on social media sites
- Give patients advice that has nothing to do with dialysis (e.g., refer them to a lawyer, real estate agent, etc.)
- Loan, borrow, or accept money from patients (your clinic has a policy about gifts)
- Send personal greeting cards, give gifts, or buy anything for patients
- Sell patients anything (e.g., Avon, Tupperware, school fund drives, etc.)

Acting unprofessionally can harm your patient. For example, if a patient gets mad at you due to something you said, he might skip a treatment. You could also get into legal trouble with your clinic or the state if you don't act professionally with patients.

Your nurse manager and social worker can help if there is a conflict with a patient, or if two patients are having an issue with each other. It is important for you to stay calm in these situations, be professional toward patients, and seek support from your nurse and social worker if you need it.

Another key issue is confidentiality—maintaining patient privacy. Your clinic will train you about privacy and the rules of the **Health Insurance Portability and Accountability Act (HIPAA)** law. HIPAA gives federal protection for personal health information (PHI), which can be used only for patient care and billing. HIPAA allows the federal government to fine dialysis clinics that do not follow the law.

Groups You Can Join

Joining a group of dialysis technicians can help you learn and advance in your profession. You can share knowledge and ideas on how to do things better or more efficiently. You can also build a network of colleagues. It takes time and discipline to learn all you will need to know, but you will reap the rewards in many ways. The following two groups can help you learn more about dialysis.

NATIONAL ASSOCIATION OF NEPHROLOGY TECHNICIANS/TECHNOLOGISTS (NANT)

NANT is a national, non-profit, professional organization founded in 1983. NANT's goals are to ensure that technicians are included in decision making for dialysis care, maintain safety and quality, help the renal community improve technology, and provide education. NANT is the only U.S. group just for dialysis technicians. It has an elected Board of Directors and 1,500 members. To learn more about NANT, call (877) 607-NANT, or visit www.dialysistech.net.

COUNCIL OF NEPHROLOGY NURSES AND TECHNICIANS (CNNT)

CNNT is a professional council of the National Kidney Foundation (NKF). Its focus is on advising the NKF about health policies that affect nurses and technicians, promoting education, helping to develop clinical or research training, and conducting public service projects to prevent and detect kidney disease and support national organ donation programs. CNNT advocates and contributes to the professional development of its members. To learn more about CNNT, call (800) 622-9010, or visit www.kidney.org/professionals/CNNT/aboutcnnt.

ONLINE TECHNICIAN DISCUSSIONS

RenalWEB has an online discussion forum for dialysis technicians at www.renalweb.com. Many professional organizations are turning to social media to reach and have conversations with dialysis professionals. Look for conversations taking place on Facebook and Linkedin.

Technician Certification

CMS requires that all dialysis technicians be certified. This means you will need to pass a test given by an approved state or national program.[31] Your clinic will help you find out which programs are approved in your state. The **national** certification programs are:

Certified Clinical Hemodialysis Technician (CCHT) Exam

The Nephrology Nursing Certification Commission (NNCC) offers this 150-question exam. The CCHT content comes from four HD practice areas: clinical (50%), technical (23%), environmental (15%), and role (12%).[32]

The content of the CCHT exam is based on a national job role analysis survey done by the Center for Nursing Education and Testing (C-NET). The NNCC's Clinical and Technical Board reviews survey data and suggests changes to the test and who can take it. To take the CCHT exam, you will need to pay a fee and:

- Have at least a high school diploma or a GED
- Pass a training program that has classroom learning *and* supervised work in a clinic
- Have a preceptor or supervisor sign a form to verify your training and clinic time
- Follow all of the federal and state laws that apply in your area
- Meet the training and experience rules in the *Conditions for Coverage* and for your state

The CCHT exam is nationally accredited by two organizations:
- The National Commission for Certifying Agencies (NCCA)
- The Accreditation Board for Specialty Nursing Certification (ABSNC)

NNCC suggests (but does not require) that you work for 6 months full time (about 1,000 hours), including training, before you take the exam. The certification lasts 3 years, and then you must renew it. To learn more about the exam and how to prepare for it, see the exam website at www.nncc-exam.org.

Certified Clinical Hemodialysis Technician – Advanced (CCHT-A) Exam

The Nephrology Nursing Certification Commission (NNCC) offers this 150-question exam for technicians with 5 years of continuous employment and at least 5,000 hours as a clinical dialysis technician. To learn about the CCHT-A exam, see the exam website at www.nncc-exam.org.

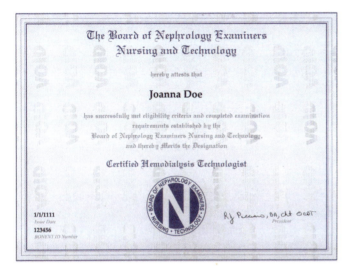

Figure 6: Sample BONENT Certification Certificate
Image courtesy of the Board of Nephrology Examiners Nursing and Technology (BONENT)

Certified Hemodialysis Technician (CHT) Exam

The Board of Nephrology Examiners Nursing and Technology (BONENT) (www.bonent.org) offers a 150-question exam to become certified. You can put CHT after your name when you pass. The exam tests your knowledge of five major areas: patient care (45%), machine technology (12%), water treatment (15%), infection control (18%), and education/personal development (10%).

To take the CHT exam, you must pay a fee and:
- Have at least a high school diploma or a GED. You will need a copy of your diploma or transcript with a school seal or principal's signature. If you don't have proof of a diploma or GED, 4 years of work as a dialysis technician can be used instead.
- Have one year of dialysis patient care *or* complete a BONENT-approved dialysis technician training program within the past 2 years.
- Have two signed letters of reference, with one being from your supervisor. The other letter can be from a peer or a mentor in dialysis.

You can take the exam on paper in English or Spanish, or on a computer in English only. You have three chances to pass the BONENT exam in 12 months. If you do not pass, you will need 8 more hours of continuing education in dialysis or a passing grade in a nephrology-related educational program. The CHT certification is good for 4 years, and then you must renew it. To learn more or take an online practice exam, visit the BONENT website at www.bonent.org.

Certified in Clinical Nephrology Technology (CCNT) and Certified in Biomedical Nephrology Technology (CBNT) Exams

The National Nephrology Certification Organization, Inc. (NNCO) offers these exams:

1. **Clinical Nephrology Technology** – you can put CCNT after your name if you pass. The CCNT exam tests your knowledge of seven areas: principles of dialysis (10%), patient care (18%), dialysis procedures and documentation (17%), complications during dialysis (15%), water treatment and dialysate preparation (15%), infection control and safety (20%), and dialyzer reprocessing (5%).
2. **Biomedical Nephrology Technology** – you can put CBNT after your name if you pass. The CBNT exam measures knowledge in seven main areas: principles of dialysis (25%), scientific concepts (10%), electronic applications (10%), water treatment (20%), equipment functions (13%), environmental/regulatory issues (12%), and dialyzer reuse/reprocessing (10%).

To take the CCNT or CBNT exams, you must pay a fee and:
- Have at least a high school diploma, GED, or 4 years of work as a dialysis technician.
- Complete a total of one year in a training program, work as a technician, or a combination of both. (In Ohio, you must have completed 12 months of patient care to take these exams.)

Certified Dialysis Water Specialists (CDWS) Exam

The NNCO also offers this exam. You can put CDWS after your name if you pass. The CDWS exam measures knowledge in seven main areas: water quality standards (15%), water treatment terminology and acronyms (5%), basic water and water quality (15%), risks and hazards of poorly treated water (15%), water treatment equipment (20%), water system performance and monitoring (15%), and disinfection strategies and prevention practices (15%).

To take the CDWS exam, you must pay a fee and meet ONE of the following eligibility options:

- Have a high school diploma or GED certificate and 3 years of dialysis water experience
- Have an Associate's Degree or some college and 2 years of dialysis water experience
- Have a college degree or higher or a healthcare credential (e.g., nursing, physician assistant, pharmacist) and 1 year of dialysis water experience
- Have current CCNT or CBNT certification and 1 year of dialysis water experience

To learn more about the exams, visit the NNCO website at www.ptcny.com/clients/nnco/#ccnt-pt.

Conclusion

The history of dialysis and how it is paid for are important context for your job. Knowing the system of care and how you fit into it can help you to do a better job of what *really* matters: helping your patients live as fully as they can.

"Today is a bittersweet day. It was the last day of my favorite technician, who was the best technician in the clinic. She has played a huge role in making my last 3 years of dialysis bearable. She has exhibited the utmost professionalism, care, and compassion since I've known her. I'm happy she's moving on to a better job in another clinic, but will miss her tremendously."

When you act in a professional way, you help your patients feel safe and can give them better care, and your coworkers will know that they can rely on you.

And, finally, the more you learn—through training, networking, and certification—the more you can grow professionally. As you have seen, technicians can work in one dialysis clinic, or travel to many. You can work with in-center patients or with PD or home HD patients. You may even be able to work in hospital dialysis. Some people make a lifelong career out of being a dialysis technician. Others use the job as a jumping-off point for nursing school, social work, administration, or other work in or outside of healthcare.

References

1. Cavanaugh KL, Wingard RL, Hakim RM, et al. Low health literacy associates with increased mortality in ESRD. *J Am Soc Nephrol.* 2010;21:1979-85
2. United States Renal Data System. *2015 USRDS Annual Data Report: Epidemiology of kidney disease in the United States.* National Institutes of Health, National Institute of Diabetes and Digestive and Kidney Diseases. Bethesda, MD, 2015 (Reference Tables, Volume 2, Table D.1). Available at www.usrds.org/reference.aspx. Accessed August 2016
3. Kliger AS. More intensive hemodialysis. *Clin J Am Soc Nephrol.* 2009;4:S121-4
4. Blagg CR. The early history of dialysis for chronic renal failure in the United States: A view from Seattle. *Am J Kidney Dis.* 2007;49(3):482-96
5. Lockridge RS. The direction of end-stage renal disease reimbursement in the United States. *Semin Dial.* 2004;17(2):125-30
6. Centers for Medicare and Medicaid Services. *Conditions for Coverage for End-Stage Renal Disease Facilities: Final Rule,* 73 *Federal Register* 73 (15 April 2008), p. 20484. Available at www.cms.gov/Regulations-and-Guidance/Legislation/CFCsAndCoPs/downloads/esrdfinalrule0415.pdf. Accessed September 2016
7. Centers for Medicare and Medicaid Services. *Medicare Basics.* CMS Pub 11034. Available at www.medicare.gov/Pubs/pdf/11034.pdf. Accessed June 2016
8. United States Renal Data System. *2015 USRDS Annual Data Report: Epidemiology of kidney disease in the United States.* National Institutes of Health, National Institute of Diabetes and Digestive and Kidney Diseases. Bethesda, MD, 2015 (Reference Tables, Volume 2, Table J.1). Available at www.usrds.org/reference.aspx. Accessed August 2016

9. United States Renal Data System. *USRDS 2015 Annual Data Report: Epidemiology of kidney disease in the United States.* National Institutes of Health, National Institute of Diabetes and Digestive and Kidney Diseases. Bethesda, MD, 2015 (Volume 2, Table J.5). Available at www.usrds.org/reference.aspx. Accessed September 2016
10. Neumann ME. Annual renal provider survey. *Nephrol News Issues.* 2016;30(8):26-29
11. United States Renal Data System. *2015 USRDS Annual Data Report: Epidemiology of kidney disease in the United States.* National Institutes of Health, National Institute of Diabetes and Digestive and Kidney Diseases. Bethesda, MD, 2015 (Reference Tables, Volume 2, Table A.1). Available at www.usrds.org/reference.aspx. Accessed August 2016
12. Dunn D, Evans D, Mutell R, et al. Employment status among end-stage renal disease patients by treatment modality. Abstract and poster presented at the National Kidney Foundation Spring Clinical Meetings, April 27-May 1, 2016, Boston, MA
13. Neumann ME. Steering dialysis patients away from Medicare will hurt ESRD program in the long run. *Nephrol News Issues.* Sept 7, 2016. Available at: www.nephrologynews.com/steering-dialysis-patients-away-medicare-will-hurt-esrd-program-long-run/
14. Centers for Medicare and Medicaid Services. *Medicare Coverage of Kidney Dialysis & Kidney Transplant Services.* CMS Product No. 10128. Available at www.medicare.gov/Pubs/pdf/10128-Medicare-Coverage-ESRD.pdf. Accessed September 2016
15. Centers for Medicare and Medicaid Services. *ESRD Prospective Payment System (PPS) Overview.* Available at https://www.cms.gov/Medicare/Medicare-Fee-for-Service-Payment/ESRDpayment/index.html. Accessed September 2016
16. Centers for Medicare and Medicaid Services. *ESRD QIP Payment Year 2017 Program Details.* Available at https://www.cms.gov/Medicare/Quality-Initiatives-Patient-Assessment-Instruments/ESRDQIP/Downloads/PY-2017-Program-Details.pdf. Accessed September 2016
17. Centers for Medicare and Medicaid Services. *Quality Incentive Program Payment Year 2017 Measure Technical Specifications.* Available at https://www.cms.gov/Medicare/Quality-Initiatives-Patient-Assessment-Instruments/ESRDQIP/Downloads/PY-2017-Technical-Measure-Specifications.pdf. Accessed September 2016
18. Centers for Medicare and Medicaid Services. *Quality Incentive Program Payment Year 2018 Measure Technical Specifications.* Available at https://www.cms.gov/Medicare/Quality-Initiatives-Patient-Assessment-Instruments/ESRDQIP/Downloads/PY-2018-Technical-Measure-Specifications.pdf. Accessed September 2016
19. National Kidney Foundation. *KDOQI History.* Available at https://www.kidney.org/professionals/KDOQI/abouthistory. Accessed September 2016
20. National Kidney Foundation. *Guidelines and commentaries.* Available at https://www.kidney.org/professionals/guidelines/guidelines_commentaries. Accessed September 2016
21. Dialysis Outcomes and Practice Patterns Study Program. *About the program.* Available at https://www.dopps.org/OurStudies/HemodialysisDOPPS.aspx. Accessed September 2016
22. Medicare Dialysis Facility Compare. Available at https://www.medicare.gov/dialysisfacilitycompare/. Accessed September 2016
23. Medicare Dialysis Facility Compare. *Star ratings.* Available at https://www.medicare.gov/dialysisfacilitycompare/#data/star-ratings-system. Accessed September 2016
24. ESRD National Coordinating Center. *Fistula First Catheter Last.* Available at http://www.esrdncc.org/en/professionals/. Accessed September 2016
25. In-Center Hemodialysis CAHPS Survey. Available at https://ichcahps.org/. Accessed September 2016
26. CrownWeb. Available at mycrownweb.org/. Accessed September 2016
27. Centers for Medicare and Medicaid Services. *ESRD Quality Incentive Program.* Available at https://www.cms.gov/Medicare/Quality-Initiatives-Patient-Assessment-Instruments/ESRDQIP/. Accessed September 2016
28. Vlchek DS, Burrows-Hudson S, Pressly NA. *Quality assurance guidelines for hemodialysis devices.* HHS Publication FDA 91-4161. Washington, DC, Health and Human Services, 1991, pp. 1-3 and 13-4 –13-6
29. U.S. Food and Drug Administration. Available at www.fda.gov/RegulatoryInformation/Guidances/default.htm. Accessed September 2016.
30. Wick G. Continuous quality improvement: a problem solving approach (Part 1). *Nephrol Nurs Today.* 1993;3(1):1-8
31. Neumann ME. Time running out for technicians. *Nephrol News Issues.* 2010;24(3):8-9
32. Nephrology Nursing Certification Commission. Certified clinical hemodialysis technician examination. Available at https://www.nncc-exam.org/sites/default/files/specifications/cchtSpecifications.pdf. Accessed September 2016

2 The Person with Kidney Failure

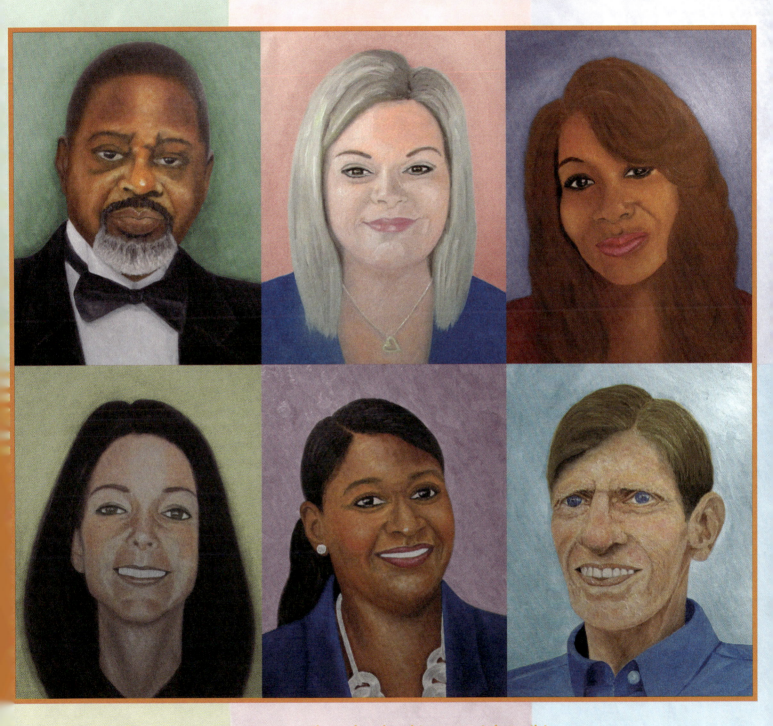

Katrina Parker Williams, a graduate of East Carolina University with a Master's in English Education in 1998, taught English at a community college for more than 20 years until kidney disease forced her to leave teaching in 2013. Today, she is a writer and self-taught artist. These images are of strong people with kidney disease who live productive lives and the staff who care for them. Visit www.katrinaparkerwilliams.weebly.com to view more artwork or commission a painting.

"I've been on dialysis more than half my lifetime. I raised my boys, put them through college, worked two jobs, remarried, and now have grandkids, all in 32 years with ESRD. I am surviving, being an advocate, and hopefully an inspiration to others who [wrongly] believe that this is a death sentence."

Objectives

MODULE AUTHORS
Teri Browne, PhD, MSW, NSW-C
Lesley McPhatter, MS, RDN, CSR
Vickie Peters, MSN, MAEd, RN, CPHQ
Dori Schatell, MS
Lyle Smith, RN, BSN, CNN, CDPN
Beth Witten, MSW, ACSW, LSCSW

MODULE REVIEWERS
Nancy M. Gallagher, BS, RN, CNN
Darlene Rodgers, BSN, RN, CNN, CPHQ
John H. Sadler, MD
Vern Taaffe, BS, CBNT, CDWS
Tamyra Warmack, RN
Beth Witten, MSW, ACSW, LSCSW

After you complete this module, you will be able to:

1. Label the structures and list the functions of a normal kidney.
2. Define uremia and list at least five symptoms of it.
3. List at least four health problems that often occur due to kidney failure.
4. Describe each of the treatment options for kidney failure.
5. Discuss the value of empathy and explain three techniques to help provide empathetic care.
6. Describe the three key aspects of rehabilitation for people with kidney failure.

An acronym list can be found in the Glossary.

Practice Test Questions at:
www.meiresearch.org/cc6

Introduction

People whose kidneys fail need dialysis or a kidney transplant to live. There are several types of treatment, and the choice of a treatment will have a major impact on patients' day-to-day lives, including:

- What they can eat and drink
- How well they sleep
- Their activity and employment
- How many medications they need to take
- How they spend their time
- Their ability to have children

The person on dialysis is the focus of care. S/he is the one whose life can be made better by good dialysis—or harmed by errors or poor treatment. Some patients will take an active role in their care and learn all they can. Respect this interest and encourage it! Others may not be as active, but they need your support and help, too.

Some people give up on life when they need dialysis, and others view their treatment as just one part of their lives. They may be teachers, bus drivers, lawyers, homemakers, real estate agents, tool and die makers, students, parents, retirees, artists, and much more. Either way, those on dialysis are more than just "patients." **They are *people* first—*just like you***. They never wanted kidney failure, they never asked for it, they may not have done anything to cause it, and they *all* have lives they would much rather be out living.

"I graduated college, got a full-time job that I love, married my best friend, bought a house, raised three dogs and chickens, and became a part of the patient family advisory council at our hospital to share my experiences to help improve patient care!"

The goal of caring for people with kidney failure is to help each one reach his or her highest level of function and health. Your patients have just one thing in common—kidneys that do not work. When you check vitals, perform a step in the treatment, or do machine checks, talk with your patients and learn about them. Ask about their families, jobs, and things they enjoy doing. Ask what they know about the cause of their kidney disease and about dialysis. Learn what they want to be able to do in the future. You may find that the person who looks depressed and dejected was very independent not so long ago.

Dialysis is like a tidal wave in patients' lives—it can wash away everything they are used to. They may wonder how long and how well they can live—and if they can handle all the changes dialysis brings. They may *assume* that they can no longer do things they used to love, and never ask to see if this is really true. Tell them that it is possible to live a long time without working kidneys. There are people who have lived 50 or more years after their kidneys failed, with dialysis and transplants. Unless patients have *hope* and believe they have a future, they will not be able to learn. Help your new patients understand that taking an active role in their care can help them feel better and live longer. Messages like these can give patients hope and help them improve their own outcomes.

You will learn about how patients cope later in this module. People with kidney failure may tell you they feel anxious, depressed, or angry. Or, they may not be able to express their feelings at all. They may *seem* to be coping well—until something triggers an outburst. Tell the social worker when you hear or see something that concerns you. Ask him or her to teach you ways to support your patients. How you and the rest of the staff treat patients affects how they experience their care at your clinic. Treat each patient with respect. Think about how you or your loved ones would want to be treated. Keep this in mind each day so you can give the best care to all of your patients.

"I danced ballroom four nights a week and competed the entire time I was on dialysis."

As a dialysis technician, *you* are the eyes and ears of the care team, and you have the closest contact with each patient. Try to learn about your patients and share insights with the rest of the team to improve care. Patients will ask questions and expect you to know the answers—or refer them to someone who can help. This means you need to know about kidney disease, what causes it, how it affects the body, treatment options, who does what on the care team, and more. It is okay not to have all of the answers, but patients still need help with their questions. If you do not know something, find someone who does.

This module covers:

- Normal kidney function
- Acute and chronic kidney disease
- Problems caused by kidney failure
- Treatment options for kidney failure

Module 2

- The role of the care team
- *Renal* (related to the kidneys) nutrition
- How to help patients cope with kidney disease
- Communication skills
- Rehabilitation
- Coping with patient deaths

What you learn will help you understand your patients so you can give them the best care.

Kidney Structure

Most people have two kidneys (see Figure 1). Each is about the size of a fist and weighs about five ounces. Kidneys are in the back of the body, just above the waist. Pads of fat and the bones of the rib cage protect them.

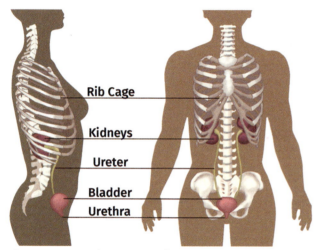

Figure 1: Location of the Kidneys

A tough, fibrous outer capsule surrounds each kidney (see Figure 2). Just inside the capsule is a layer of cells called the *cortex*. If you cut a kidney in half, you would see that under the cortex, the kidney has sections:

- The inner part of the kidney, or *medulla*, is made up of pie-shaped wedges called *pyramids*. Each pyramid and the cortex above it is called a *lobe*.
- Each point of the "pie" is called a *papilla* (plural: *papillae*).
- Each papilla points into a cup-shaped opening called a *calyx* (plural: *calyces*).
- Each calyx sends drops of urine into the *renal pelvis*.
- The renal pelvis of each kidney links to a *ureter* (a tube that sends the urine to the *bladder*).
- Both ureters empty into the *bladder*.
- The bladder stores urine until it leaves the body through a tube called the *urethra*.

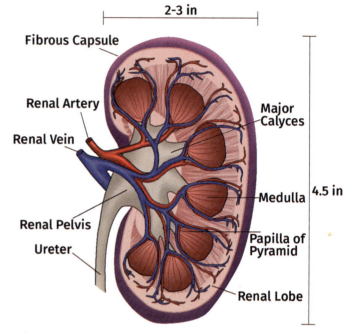

Figure 2: Cross Section of the Kidney

Nephrons

Each beat of the heart pumps blood through the aorta—the largest artery—and right to the *renal* (kidney) arteries. Smaller blood vessels then keep a constant renal blood flow. *Capillaries*—some so small that just one red blood cell can pass through at a time—bring blood to the *nephrons* inside each kidney (see Figure 3). A million or so nephrons in each kidney filter out excess water and wastes, and keep what the body needs. Nephrons start in the renal cortex and extend into the medulla. Each is made up of a *glomerulus* and a set of *tubules*.

Tubular System

Each glomerulus sends filtrate into a series of *tubules*:

- The *proximal* (near) convoluted tubule
- The loop of Henle
- The *distal* (far) convoluted tubule
- The collecting tubule

Inside the tubules, chemicals and water that the body still needs pass back into the blood. Wastes and extra water empty into the calyces. From there, they flow into the renal pelvis and then the ureter to become urine.[1]

A normal adult makes about 125 mL of glomerular filtrate each minute, which is about 180 liters per day.[1] Nearly all of the filtrate is *reabsorbed* in the tubules. Blood goes back to the bloodstream through the *efferent* (away from the organ) arteriole. Only 1% or so of the water in the glomerular filtrate—about 1–2 liters—becomes urine.[1]

Kidney Functions

The main job of kidneys is to keep a constant internal balance in the body at all times: *homeostasis*. By choosing what to reabsorb and what to release into urine, kidneys help keep a tight balance of water and minerals in the blood. To maintain homeostasis, the kidneys:

- Remove water and wastes
- Keep salt and other electrolytes in balance
- Control blood pressure
- Make hormones
- Maintain acid-base balance

Excretory Functions

Kidneys *excrete* (get rid of) wastes and excess water as urine. If you work outside on a hot day and sweat a lot without drinking, your kidneys will make less urine. If you drink a quart of lemonade, your kidneys will make more. Urine is excess body water, with a high level of wastes that come from:

- Foods or drugs that are *metabolized* (broken apart into pieces the body can use)
- Breakdown of tissue due to normal muscle use
- Toxins and acids

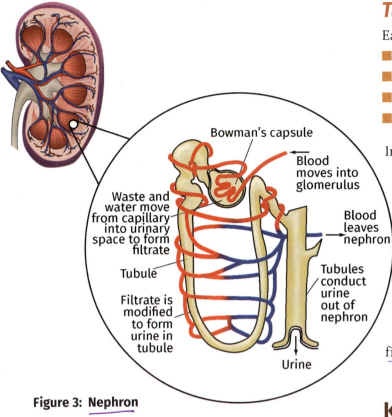

Figure 3: Nephron

Glomeruli

A *glomerulus* is a ball of capillaries in a sac called *Bowman's capsule*. (The plural of glomerulus is *glomeruli*.) Capillary walls are *semipermeable membranes*. Pores in the walls let small substances pass through, but hold larger ones in.

Kidneys work a little like a coffee maker. A filter keeps large coffee grounds in, but lets liquid coffee pass through. If the filter is torn, grounds will leak into your coffee.

Like a coffee filter, pores in healthy glomerulus walls keep in large cells, like blood cells and proteins, and let water and smaller substances pass through. Blood enters each glomerulus from an *afferent* (toward the organ) *arteriole* (small artery). The blood pressure created by each heartbeat forces water out of the blood—through tiny slits—into "Bowman's space." Small wastes and more water pass through the pores as *glomerular filtrate*. If there is nephron damage, large cells can leak through, too.

Endocrine Functions

A *hormone* is a chemical made in one part of the body that acts on other cells or organs.[2] Hormones act as messages to turn functions on and off in another part of the body. The kidneys have an *endocrine* function—they act as glands and secrete two hormones and an enzyme into the blood (see Figure 4):

- **Erythropoietin** tells the bone marrow to make red blood cells.
- **Calcitriol** (active vitamin D) lets the gut absorb calcium from food.
- **Renin**, an *enzyme* (protein that causes an effect), helps control blood pressure.

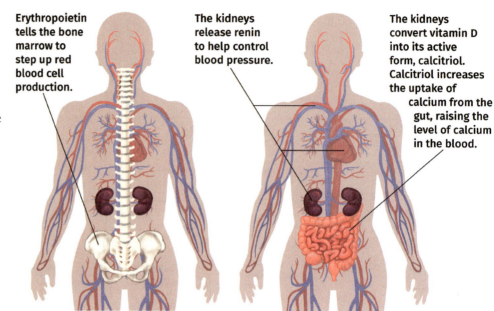

Figure 4: Hormones Made by the Kidneys

Electrolyte Balance

Electrolytes form *ions* (charged particles) when they dissolve in water. Ions conduct electricity. Blood has seven major electrolytes: sodium, chloride, calcium, bicarbonate, magnesium, phosphate, and potassium. The kidneys absorb or release these to keep the right level of each one in the blood at all times.

Blood Pressure Control

Healthy kidneys help control blood pressure in two main ways:[3]

1. Kidneys retain or release water on a moment-to-moment basis. Having a correct, constant volume of water in the blood helps keep blood pressure stable. When blood water volume *rises*—so does blood pressure. When blood water volume *drops*—so does blood pressure. Having constant water levels also helps keep levels of blood electrolytes in the safe range.

2. Kidneys need a strong, constant blood supply to function. Special cells on the renal arteries track the pressure of blood as it enters the kidneys. Each time blood pressure drops, kidneys secrete the enzyme renin. The body uses renin to help form angiotensin, a powerful *vasoconstrictor* that raises blood pressure by making blood vessels more narrow. Angiotensin also tells the kidneys to hold onto salt and water.

Acid-base Balance

Pure water has a neutral pH (7): it is neither acidic (pH less than 7) nor basic (pH greater than 7; alkaline means "basic.") To sustain life, body fluids must remain in a pH range of 7.35 to 7.45, which is a bit alkaline. Healthy kidneys help maintain acid-base balance.[4] They take extra acid out of the blood and remove it in the urine, and help make bicarbonate, a buffer that helps keep acid-base levels in the right range. If body fluids become too acidic (a problem common in kidney patients called *metabolic acidosis*), proteins break down and enzymes stop working. Patients who have this condition may feel weak and tired, breathe rapidly, and have a racing heartbeat. They may also have headaches and confusion.

Types of Kidney Failure

Kidneys can fail quickly due to an *acute* (sudden) event, or they can fail slowly over a period of years, during which the patient may or may not know that something is wrong.

Table 1: Stages of CKD, *Albuminuria* (protein in the urine), and Risk of ESRD*

CKD Stage	eGFR (mL/min/1.73 m^2)		Level of Albuminuria		
			Normal to mild increase < 30 mg/g	Moderate increase 30–300 mg/g	Severe increase > 300 mg/g
1	90+	Normal or high			
2	60–89	Mild decrease			
3A	45–59	Mild to moderate decrease			
3B	30–44	Moderate to severe decrease			
4	15–29	Severe decrease			
5	< 15	Kidney failure			

*Reprinted from Kidney International Supplement. Vol 3. Kidney Disease: Improving Global Outcomes (KDIGO) CKD Work Group. KDIGO 2012 clinical practice guideline for the evaluation and management of chronic kidney disease. Pages 1-150, 2013 with permission from Elsevier.

Acute Kidney Failure

Acute kidney injury (AKI), a sudden, severe loss of kidney function, can cause acute kidney failure.[5] Causes of AKI may include dehydration or loss of fluid (such as severe blood loss), toxins (such as medicines), and *sepsis* (severe blood infection).[6] We need kidney function to live, and its loss—even for a short time—can be fatal. In a study of 156 patients with AKI, more than half of those who needed dialysis died in the hospital. Of those who made it home, just over 40% lived for 5 years.[6] Among AKI patients in an intensive care unit with other health problems, the rate of death was as high as 80%.[6] And, about 1 in 10 of those who lived went on to have chronic kidney failure in the future.[6]

Chronic Kidney Disease (CKD)

CKD is a long, slow process of nephron loss. Kidneys can have so many nephrons that people may feel healthy even when more than half of their nephrons are not working. People may not notice early symptoms of CKD, or may notice them, but not realize that they are due to a kidney problem. Or, they may have some or all of the signs of *uremia* (toxins in the blood) that we will talk about in a later section.

It can take months or years for CKD to cause kidney failure, if it ever does. Most people with CKD—as many as 95%—will die of other causes, like heart disease, before their kidneys ever fail.[7] Many people with CKD also have heart problems or other illnesses.

Routine medical exams that include a urine test and blood pressure check are good screening tools for CKD. A blood test for *creatinine* (a waste that healthy kidneys remove) may find CKD early, when treatment to slow nephron loss will work best.

People with CKD can help slow the loss of kidney function if they:[8]

- Keep their blood sugar in the target range
- Keep their blood pressure in the target range
- Avoid pain pills called NSAIDS (non-steroidal anti-inflammatory medicines, like naproxen and ibuprofen)
- Quit smoking, if they smoke
- Ask the doctor to take steps to protect their kidneys if they need imaging tests with contrast (dye), like X-rays or CT scans

The National Kidney Foundation (NKF) defines five stages of CKD based on *estimated glomerular filtration rate* (eGFR), a formula for how well the kidneys are filtering, that uses age, gender, race, and level of creatinine in the blood. Stage 5 CKD is the most severe. The risk that CKD will progress to kidney failure is greater when there is more *albumin* (a type of protein) in the urine. (See Table 1 for CKD Stages and Level of Albuminuria. Green is the lowest risk, dark red is the highest.) Dialysis or a kidney transplant is needed when the GFR drops below about 10—but should be based on patient symptoms, not just on blood test results.[9-12]

Causes of Kidney Failure

Kidney failure was caused by diabetes, high blood pressure, or glomerular diseases in 83.5% of people who started dialysis in the U.S. between 2010 and 2014.[13]

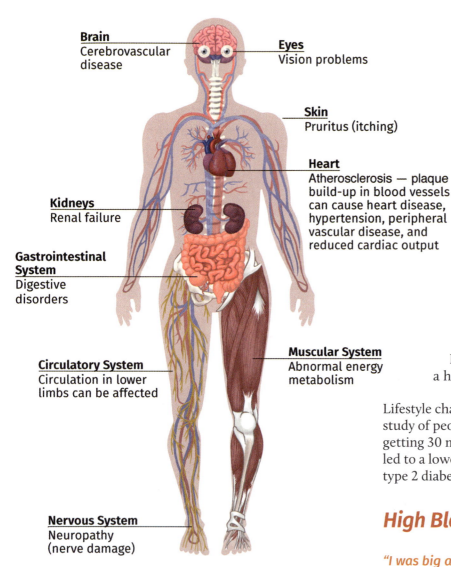

Figure 5: Possible Complications of Diabetes

- In **type 1**, the immune system kills the *beta cells* in the pancreas that make insulin.
- In **type 2**, the pancreas does not make enough insulin, or the body cannot use what it does make.

Type 2 diabetes is the number one cause of kidney failure in this country; more than 9 out of 10 adult Americans with diabetes have type 2. Between 2010 and 2014, 45.9% of all kidney failure in the U.S. was due to diabetes—42.1% of it from type 2.[13]

Diabetes harms the heart, blood vessels, and nerves, and is the leading cause of blindness, limb loss—and kidney failure (see Figure 5).[15] Some ethnic groups—African-Americans, Hispanics, and Native Americans—are at a higher risk for type 2 diabetes.[16]

Lifestyle changes can help prevent diabetes. In a large study of people at risk, losing 5% of body weight and getting 30 minutes of exercise 5 or more days a week led to a lower risk. These changes reduced the rate of type 2 diabetes by 34%, even 10 years later.[17]

Diabetes

"As someone with diabetes for over 20 years, and who didn't take care of it for the first 10, I can say that while I was informed of the consequences of uncontrolled diabetes, I really didn't believe any of those awful things would happen to me."

Diabetes, a disease that causes higher than normal blood sugar levels, affects as many as 29 million Americans and is the seventh leading cause of death in the U.S. Another 86 million Americans have pre-diabetes and are at risk for diabetes.[14]

There are two main types of diabetes, and *both* can harm the kidneys:

High Blood Pressure

"I was big and had high blood pressure and didn't know the signs. I would get a headache and just pop a pill. I passed out one day and ended up in the ER with my BP 200/167. They gave me meds to help protect my kidneys, but I knew that at some point I would need dialysis. I started dialysis a few months after I had my baby."

The second leading cause of kidney disease in the U.S. is *hypertension* (high blood pressure). From 2010 to 2014, 29.4% of those on dialysis had kidney failure due to high blood pressure.[13] High blood pressure can harm the blood vessels that lead to the kidneys and damage the tiny glomeruli. People with high blood pressure may not have symptoms, so they may not get treatment. Or, they may know, but not take blood pressure medicines due to cost or side effects.

There are two types of high blood pressure:

1. **Primary or essential** hypertension – unknown

cause of high blood pressure. Treatments may include diet (such as limits on salt and processed foods), exercise, and blood pressure medicines (*antihypertensives*). Essential hypertension often runs in families, so a family history of this problem can be important.

2. **Secondary hypertension** – the cause of high blood pressure is another health problem or a reaction to a drug. Surgery can fix some problems, like a birth defect in the aorta, or narrowing of the renal artery.[18]

Glomerular Diseases

"I felt sick and had swelling in my legs, so I went to go see my doctor. He tested my urine, and I expected him to tell me I might have a flu or something mild, but he had a really worried look on his face, and it freaked me out. This was my family doctor that took care of me ever since I was a child. He told me I had to see a kidney specialist—that's where I learned I had FSGS [a glomerular disease], and I was super shocked and stunned."

Diseases of the glomeruli include illnesses like:
- *Glomerulonephritis* (inflammation of the glomeruli)
- *Glomerulosclerosis* (hardening of the glomeruli)

These illnesses may have a slow or a fast onset. From 2010 to 2014, 8.2% of people with kidney failure had glomerular diseases.[13]

Polycystic Kidney Disease (PKD)

"I have PKD and my kidneys are enormous. In fact they are so large that they have to be removed before I can receive a transplant."

PKD is a genetic disease that causes fluid-filled cysts that can grow in the kidneys (and sometimes in the liver). Kidney cysts can crowd out healthy tissue, so the kidneys may fail. In most cases, patients with PKD are otherwise healthy and stable, and tend to do well. There are medicines that can help slow the progress of PKD to end-stage. From 2010 to 2014, 2.2% of those whose kidneys failed had some type of cystic disease.[13]

Other Causes of CKD

"I have Lupus and hypertension that was undetected for too long. The scarring shut my kidneys down and I ended up on dialysis!"

There are many other, less common causes of kidney failure, too:[13]
- Birth defects
- Frequent or large kidney stones
- Systemic lupus erythematosus (SLE)
- Drug abuse
- Kidney infections
- Cancer
- HIV/AIDS
- Sickle cell disease
- Unknown

No matter what made the kidneys fail, the treatment options are the same.

Problems Caused by Kidney Failure

Now you know that the kidneys have a number of complex jobs in the body, and as they start to fail, they stop doing these vital tasks (see Figure 6). For this reason, kidney failure affects most body systems.

Electrolyte Imbalances

"My husband's potassium levels were creeping up, even though he thought he was following his diet pretty closely. Then he had a seizure, was taken to [the] ER, was unconscious in the ICU and on life support for 5 days, and in the hospital for 12 days."

Electrolytes are minerals that break apart into ions when they dissolve. The body uses them to send signals from nerves to muscles. Healthy kidneys keep electrolytes in balance, but that function is disturbed by CKD. When the blood level of any electrolyte is too high or low, the effects can harm—or even kill—your patients. Dialysate is composed to mimic normal plasma water. This allows dialysis to balance normal products and remove wastes.

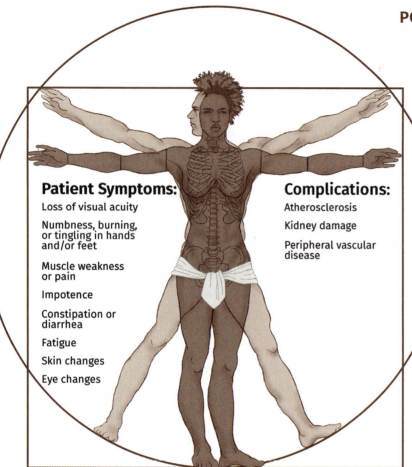

Figure 6: Complications of CKD

Patient Symptoms:
- Loss of visual acuity
- Numbness, burning, or tingling in hands and/or feet
- Muscle weakness or pain
- Impotence
- Constipation or diarrhea
- Fatigue
- Skin changes
- Eye changes

Complications:
- Atherosclerosis
- Kidney damage
- Peripheral vascular disease

SODIUM (Na⁺)

Sodium helps keep body water in balance and helps send nerve signals.

- **Hypernatremia** is *too much* sodium in the blood. This is not common in dialysis, but can occur if someone is dehydrated (loses too much water) or if both water *and* salt are lost (e.g., from a severe virus or a lot of bleeding). Symptoms can include intense thirst, confusion, seizures, and death.[19]

- **Hyponatremia** is *too little* sodium in the blood. In the general public, contests where people drink large volumes of water have led to this problem. Hyponatremia can occur if dialysate is incorrectly mixed and not tested. Symptoms can include muscle cramps, restlessness, confusion, headache, fatigue, and nausea. In severe cases, fatal brain swelling can occur.[20] In patients with heart failure, potassium levels may be too high at the same time that sodium levels are too low.[21]

POTASSIUM (K⁺)

"Before my doctor switched the potassium in my dialysate, I had to watch each crumb of veggie or fruit. I maybe had one serving a day and panicked about it. My potassium was at the high end all the time, especially in summer when I would have a fresh veggie from the garden or some nice fresh fruit. Since it was changed, I can enjoy a tomato and some cantaloupe or strawberries (which I LOVE) and not worry. I eat 1-3 servings of veggies or fruit a day."

Potassium helps control nerves and muscles, including the heart. It also helps the body keep water in balance and use glucose. Most potassium in the body is inside the cells—not in the blood. A small, constant level of potassium is needed in the blood, and this level is tightly controlled by healthy kidneys.

- **Hyperkalemia** is *too much* potassium in the blood. Those on dialysis may eat too many high-potassium foods. Other causes include severe blood loss, crush injuries, trauma, *hemolysis* (breakdown of red blood cells), and missed treatments. Hyperkalemia can change heart rhythm, which can be deadly. Symptoms may include changes in heart rhythm, weakness, and skipped heartbeats. Or, the heart may just stop.[1]

- **Hypokalemia** is *too little* potassium in the blood. This is less common on dialysis. It can occur if the patient has some kidney function, vomits, has diarrhea, does not eat enough foods with potassium, or dialysis removes too much. Hypokalemia can cause tingling or numbness, fatigue, weak muscles, muscle damage, fainting, and changes in heart rhythms.[22]

Dialysate ("bath") potassium levels are most often kept in the range of 2–3 mEq/L to help protect patients' hearts. This level has been shown to reduce potassium shifts that could raise the risk of sudden cardiac death—*in those whose predialysis levels are < 5 mEq/L*. But, patients who *do* eat a lot of fruits and vegetables *and* have levels > 5.5 mEq/L may be a rare exception.[23]

The nephrologist prescribes the potassium level in the dialysate. Patients can ask their doctors about the potassium level if they prefer to eat a lot of fruits and vegetables.

CALCIUM (Ca++)

Calcium, mainly found in the bones and teeth, is needed in the blood and body fluids at all times to control blood clotting, enzymes, hormones, nerves, and muscles.

- **Hypercalcemia** is *too much* calcium in the blood. This can have many causes, such as too much calcium (from phosphate binder medicines) or too much vitamin D. Symptoms may include fatigue, vomiting, weakness, muscle twitches, and confusion.[24]
- **Hypocalcemia** is *too little* calcium in the blood. This can occur when the gut cannot absorb calcium. Or, if phosphorus levels are too high, calcium levels drop. Some medicines can change blood calcium levels. Symptoms may include muscle cramps, irregular heartbeat, and tetany (tremors, facial twitches, muscle spasms, and muscle pain).[19]

PHOSPHORUS (P)

"My dietitian told me that longer treatments give my body the chance to pull the phosphorus stored in my cells out and into my bloodstream so it can be dialyzed off."

Like calcium, phosphorus is mainly found inside the cells of the bones and teeth. It plays a vital role in the body's use of energy.

- **Hyperphosphatemia** is *too much* phosphorus in the blood. Failed kidneys do not remove as much phosphorus as healthy ones. Standard in-center hemodialysis (HD) does not remove much phosphorus either, so it can build up in the blood. In the short term, the patient may have severe itching if blood levels of phosphorus are high.[25] In the long term, bone disease can develop. If both calcium and phosphorus blood levels are high at the same time, the two minerals can bond, and sharp calcium phosphate crystals may form in the skin, eyes, lungs, heart, and joints, and block blood vessels. Patients can lose fingers, limbs, or even their lives if this rare problem, called *calciphylaxis* or *calcific uremic arteriolopathy* (*CUA*), occurs.[26] Standard in-center HD patients must take phosphate binders with each meal and snack. These attach to phosphate in the gut, so less is absorbed in the bloodstream. Patients must also limit phosphorus in what they eat and drink.
- **Hypophosphatemia** is *not enough* phosphorus in the blood. This is not common on dialysis and can be due to having some remaining kidney function, a poor diet, or taking too many binders. Symptoms are often not seen until phosphorus is < 2 mg/dL and may include muscle weakness, coma, and/or problems with the function of red blood cells.[19]

> **Your Role in Electrolyte Management**
> - Report all symptoms to the nurse.
> - Verify that the right dialysate is given to each patient.
> - If you mix dialysate, double check with another staff person to be sure it is correct.
> - Urge patients to follow their prescribed meal plans and fluid limits.
> - Learn to do dialysate and water treatment system checks, and start treatment only after they are correct.

Uremia

"I gained 20 pounds almost overnight. I couldn't breathe and could barely walk a half a block, and my whole body itched. I knew something was terribly wrong. I was vomiting and was getting nosebleeds."

"I was being seen by my primary, but after months of swollen ankles and uncontrollable high BP, I went to the ER. They ran some simple tests and told me I was at a Stage 4. It was a shock!"

People whose kidneys fail have uremia (a build-up of wastes in the blood). The word uremia comes from *urea*, a waste that is used to measure the dose of dialysis. Urea is not the only waste that builds up and causes symptoms, or even the most toxic, but it is easy and inexpensive to measure. A health history and a physical exam (with some lab tests) can help diagnose kidney disease and uremia. Symptoms of uremia can come on so slowly that patients may not notice them. Or, patients may have symptoms but not know it, because they do not know what to look for (see Table 2).[27] Most people do not have pain around the kidneys as their kidneys fail, but people with polycystic kidney disease, infection, or kidney stones may have pain.

Table 2: Symptoms of Kidney Failure and Why They Happen

Kidney Failure and Uremic Symptoms[1]	Why They Happen
Edema (swelling) in the feet, hands, and/or face	Water build-up in the tissues
Trouble breathing	Water build-up in the lungs
Making more or less urine; getting up at night to urinate (*nocturia*)	Kidneys make more urine at night (or when someone is lying down)
Foamy or bubbly urine	Protein leaks out into the urine
Pruritus - itching that may be severe	Wastes build-up in the body, such as urea, phosphorus, and potassium
Ammonia breath, metal taste in the mouth, nausea, avoidance of protein foods	
Yellow skin tone	
Sleep or sexual problems	

Your Role in Uremia Management

Dialysis can help many of the symptoms of uremia. But, standard in-center HD three times a week replaces only a small fraction of the function of healthy kidneys. A normal eGFR in a healthy person is **90–120** mL/min/1.73 m².[28] When eGFR falls to the range of about **6–12**, dialysis may be started, depending on symptoms. How much eGFR does HD provide?[29]

- **Three** (standard) treatments per week: about **16.8** mL/min/1.73m²
- **Four** treatments per week: about **21.0** mL/min/1.73m²
- **Five** treatments per week: about **26.6** mL/min/1.73m²
- **Six** treatments per week: about **33.6** mL/min/1.73m²

Healthy kidneys make *erythropoietin* (EPO). EPO signals the bone marrow to make more red blood cells. As the kidneys fail, they make less EPO, which leads to *anemia*—a shortage of red blood cells (see Figure 7). To test for anemia, we measure the blood level of *hemoglobin* (Hgb), the oxygen-carrying protein that gives red blood cells their color.

With fewer red blood cells, the tissues are starved for oxygen when someone has anemia, which can lead to symptoms like:

- Fatigue
- Weakness and lack of energy
- Feeling cold all the time
- Mental confusion
- Pale skin, gums, and fingernail beds

So, patients may have uremic symptoms even on dialysis, if they do not get enough treatment.

You can help if you:

- Learn the symptoms of uremia
- Ask patients if they have these symptoms (they may not know what to look for)
- Report symptoms to the nurse so the patient's treatment can be assessed

Anemia

"It's kind of hard to have any enthusiasm if you're just stuck and you don't have enough energy. I mean, I might have an idea or want to do something, but I just can't do it. I don't have the energy and I get kind of depressed because the things I like to do, I just can't do."

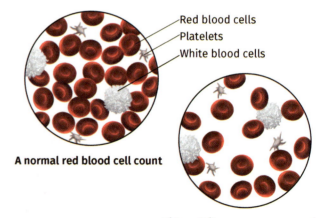

Figure 7: Normal Blood and Anemia

Doctors diagnose and monitor anemia by measuring Hgb levels. If a patient's Hgb level falls too low, there are treatments:

- **Iron**. The building block of red blood cells, iron is most often given to patients in oral or intravenous (IV) forms. However, oral iron can cause stomach upset and constipation.[30] IV iron may cause severe, even life-threatening allergies.[31] And, excess iron has been shown to build up in patients' livers[32], and toxic levels of iron may raise the risk of heart disease and death.[31] Now, there is a third option. Nephrologists may prescribe a form of iron that is added to the dialysate fluid. This drug, Triferic®, replaces just the amount of iron that is lost at each treatment (when blood is lost, iron is lost with it), brings iron to the bone marrow where it is needed, and does not cause excess iron to build up in the liver.[33] Since the drug is added to the dialysate, you may have a role in giving it to patients, depending on your state laws.

- **Erythrocyte stimulating agents (ESAs)**. These synthetic forms of EPO came on the market in the late 1980s to treat anemia *without* the need for blood transfusions. Since then, studies have linked high-dose ESAs to a higher risk of strokes and heart problems. In 2011, the U.S. Food and Drug Administration (FDA) put limits on ESAs for people on dialysis:[34]
  - Begin ESA treatment when the Hgb level is less than 10 g/dL.
  - Reduce or interrupt the dose of ESA if the Hgb level approaches or exceeds 11 g/dL.

The nephrologist must balance each patient's symptoms and need for ESAs with the need to avoid blood transfusions, especially in those who want a transplant. There are a number of ESAs. Most dialysis anemia protocols use iron to try to raise Hgb levels before giving ESAs.

- **Blood transfusions**. Giving patients donor blood may be done when Hgb levels drop quickly, since transfusions raise Hgb right away. But, blood is a living substance that contains antibodies from the donor. These antibodies, part of the immune system, can "sensitize" a patient's immune system so it would attack a new kidney—which can make it much harder to get a kidney transplant in the future. When possible, it is safest to treat anemia with iron and ESAs. Blood transfusion rates in the U.S. have gone up since Medicare went to "bundled" payment for dialysis and medicines.[35] The average use of ESAs has dropped, and clinicians are working to find out what the right dose of ESAs should be for patients.

Good anemia care takes a team effort. Your clinic may have an **Anemia Management Plan**. A nurse or dietitian may be the Anemia Manager. S/he follows the plan, looks at trends in Hgb levels, and works with each patient to assess symptoms and report them to his or her doctor. Ask who the Anemia Manager is in your clinic. You can work with him or her to help ensure that your patients get good anemia care.

> **Your Role in Anemia Management**
> - Rinse back as much of the patient's blood as you can at each treatment.
> - Tell the nurse about any unusual bleeding. Blood loss makes anemia worse.
> - Tell the nurse if the patient has an infection. Inflammation in the body can cause resistance to EPO, so the dose has to be much higher.
> - Use pediatric (child-sized) blood tubes for blood tests, if the lab will take them.
> - If your clinic reuses dialyzers, tell the nurse if a dialyzer does not pass the tests.
> - Urge your patients to come for each treatment and stay for the full time.
> - In some states, you may add Triferic® to the dialysate when a doctor prescribes it.

Left Ventricular Hypertrophy (LVH)

"Friday morning I had trouble breathing. I was gasping for air and afraid I was dying. I called 911. The ER gave me oxygen and some medicine to ease my panic. They took X-rays, etc. Too much fluid in my lungs, and there may be damage to a part of my heart. My blood pressure was up to 200 over 125."

The heart pumps oxygenated blood from the lungs to every cell in the body. LVH is a heart problem in which damaged muscle in the left ventricle—the heart's main pumping chamber—becomes flabby and overgrown, and fibrosis may occur. The weak, stiff heart muscle that is left is bigger, but cannot pump blood as strongly, *and* there is less room in the chamber to fit the volume of blood the body needs (see Figure 8).[36] When the heart is large and weak, blood can back up into the lungs (congestive heart failure), and the body is starved of oxygen.

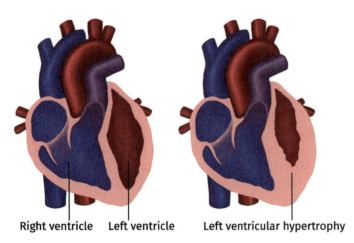

Figure 8: Heart with LVH

What harms the muscle fibers in the left ventricle? There are several factors, all of which can lead to less oxygen getting to the heart during dialysis, such as:

- **Anemia** – fewer red blood cells means less oxygen is in the blood.[37]
- **Aggressive water removal (*ultrafiltration*, or *UF*)** during hemodialysis that causes blood pressure to drop.[38] See Module 3: *Principles of Dialysis* to learn about ultrafiltration.
- **Blockage of the coronary arteries**.[39]

Kidney failure and heart disease tend to go hand-in-hand. In an almost 10-year study of 1,268 people with stage 3 or greater CKD, just 5% went on to have kidney failure, but 61% died—mostly from heart problems.[7] By the time people start dialysis, 80% have some degree of heart problems.[37]

ORGAN STUNNING DURING STANDARD IN-CENTER HEMODIALYSIS

Most body water is not in the blood—it is inside the cells and in the spaces between them. Pulling too much water out of the blood during HD, or pulling it out too quickly, can "stun" patients' organs. This is one reason why patient fluid overload can be so dangerous.

- Stunning damage occurs when blood pressure drops during HD, a problem called *intradialytic hypotension*, or *IDH*.
- This blood pressure drop causes *ischemia* (less blood flow starves tissues of oxygen).
- Patients' hearts, brains, and the kidney function they have left are harmed by stunning.

When the rate of water removal (UF) is higher than the patient can tolerate, s/he can have small heart *attacks during treatment*. We know this, because a substance (Troponin T) is found in the blood—which only occurs when the heart muscle is damaged.[40] The body makes repairs through *fibrosis*: it makes repair fibers that do not work like muscle does, but take up more space. This process, found in 2/3 of standard in-center HD patients in one study, leads to left ventricular hypertrophy (LVH). And, LVH causes heart failure and sudden death, a leading cause of death on dialysis.[38]

Other organs besides the heart can also be stunned by too-fast UF rates. The white matter of the brain can be damaged. It is known that many people who do standard in-center HD may not think as well as they used to and are likely to be depressed. Brain stunning could be one reason for this.[41] Those who do standard in-center HD also lose their remaining kidney function faster than those who do peritoneal dialysis or are left untreated. Kidney stunning could be the reason. Since these patients must constantly rebuild their tissues, they age faster than people of the same age who are not on HD. Stunning is not the only reason for these changes, but it is one that we can prevent.

Organ stunning does not occur when the UF rate is less than 10 mL/kg/hr.[42] It does not occur with peritoneal dialysis.[43] Short daily or nocturnal HD are far less likely to stun organs.[44] These approaches all remove water more gently.

In 2013, a CMS Technical Expert Panel said clinics should measure the UF rate (UFR). The group noted that in the United Kingdom, the UFR should not exceed 10 milliliters per kilogram of body weight per hour (mL/kg/hr).[45] If so much water must be removed that the UFR would be higher than 13 mL/kg/hr, tell the nurse. The patient may need longer treatments or an extra one to remove the water safely. In the U.S., CMS has set an upper limit on UFR of 13 mL/kg/hr, but perhaps this will change over time.

> **Your Role in LVH Management**
> - Report any complaints of shortness of breath or chest pain to the nurse.
> - Gentle water removal during dialysis can help avoid making LVH worse.
> - If the nephrologist prescribes it, using slightly cool dialysate (1/2° C below core body temperature) can help prevent "stunning" damage caused by rapid ultrafiltration.[41]

Pericarditis

"I had pericarditis about 20 years ago. So much chest pain, I thought I was going to die. It started as cold/flu-like symptoms, then settled in my chest, and then the chest pain became immense. It hurt to move. I was treated with IV antibiotics in the ER after they ruled out a heart attack."

Patients with kidney failure may develop *pericarditis* (swelling of the sac around the heart). In those with CKD, this problem is most often due to uremic toxins. It may occur before or after the start of dialysis.[46] Symptoms of pericarditis may include:

- Constant pain in the center of the chest that may spread out to other places. The pain may be sharp and stabbing. It is often worse when lying down and may be better when sitting up—or patients may not have symptoms at all. People on dialysis are less likely to have pain due to pericarditis than others.[46]
- Fever
- Dry cough
- Fatigue
- Low blood pressure
- Irregular heartbeat

A nurse or doctor can listen for a "pericardial friction rub" through a stethoscope to help find the problem. Treatment includes pain pills, anti-inflammatory drugs, antibiotics, and/or intensive dialysis (longer and/or more frequent treatments). In some cases, the sac can squeeze the heart so it cannot beat as well. Surgery may be needed to reduce pressure so the heart can function.

> **Your Role in Pericarditis Management**
> - Report any and all complaints of chest pain to the nurse right away.
> - If a patient has chest pain before dialysis, do not start the treatment until the nurse has seen the patient.
> - If a patient starts to have chest pain during a treatment, tell the nurse right away.
> - Be sure to give patients their full treatments—do not cut their time for bathroom trips, alarms, or other reasons.

Mineral Bone Disorder (MBD)

"My bone problems continue to get worse. I am in a great deal of pain all the time, with many fractures, especially of ribs and vertebrae. I have quite a curvature to my spine now. I am only 43 years old. The rib fractures make it hard for me to breathe."

In people with CKD, MBD occurs when bone minerals (calcium and phosphorus) and parathyroid hormone (PTH) are out of balance. This imbalance can cause one or more problems for patients, such as:[47]

- The body cannot use bone minerals, PTH, and active vitamin D correctly
- Bones are not formed well and are not as strong
- Blood vessels and soft tissues *calcify* (turn to bone)
- Severe itching can occur, when sharp crystals of calcium phosphate deposit in the tissues

MBD starts when calcium and phosphorus balance is lost (see Figure 9). *Why* are calcium and phosphorus levels out of balance?

1. Healthy kidneys convert vitamin D into its active form, a hormone called *calcitriol*.
2. Active vitamin D lets the gut absorb the mineral calcium from food.
3. Failing kidneys convert less active vitamin D.
4. Without enough active vitamin D, the gut absorbs less calcium.
5. With the gut absorbing less calcium, there is less calcium in the blood.
6. A drop in blood calcium tells the parathyroid glands to release parathyroid hormone (PTH).
7. PTH steals calcium out of the bones to keep blood calcium levels up.
8. Since there is *still* not enough active vitamin D, the glands *keep* sending out PTH.
9. In time, the glands grow so large they *cannot* shut off (*secondary hyperparathyroidism*). They may have to be surgically removed.

High PTH levels cause bone disease and other problems. Patients with MBD may not have symptoms. Or, they may have joint pain, bone pain, or muscle pain and weakness that can make it hard to walk. To remain strong, healthy bone must "remodel" all the

Module 2

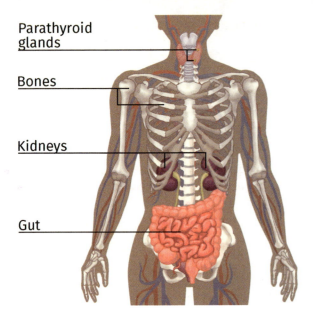

Figure 9: Body Parts Involved in Phosphorus-Calcium Imbalance in ESRD

the body continuously breaks down and removes old bone and builds new bone. There are three main types of MBD, each of which can be diagnosed with a bone biopsy (a sample of bone is analyzed under a microscope):

1. **Low turnover (*adynamic*) bone disease**. The bone is *underactive*. It is not built up as it should be, and can become thin, weak, and likely to fracture. This problem used to be seen much more often when aluminum-based phosphate binders were in use.

2. **High turnover bone disease**. The bone is *overactive* due to constant bombarding with PTH when a patient has secondary hyperparathyroidism. Too much tearing down and rebuilding occurs, so the new bone is not well made and can be prone to fracture.

3. **Mixed bone disease**. The bone can be both underactive *and* overactive at the same time.

Problems with MBD may be linked with calcium phosphate deposits on the heart and blood vessels as well.[48] These deposits raise the risk that a patient will have a heart attack or a stroke. Calcium phosphate deposits can also form in soft tissues, causing wounds that will not heal. This problem, called *calciphylaxis* or *calcific uremic arteriolopathy (CUA)*, can cause limb loss, or may be fatal. People on dialysis take medicines to treat MBD.

Your Role in MBD Management

- Listen to your patients and report all of their symptoms to the nurse.
- Reinforce what the doctor, nurses, and dietitians teach patients about bone minerals.
- Urge patients to take their medicines as prescribed and follow their meal plans.

Dialysis-Related Amyloidosis (DRA)

"My first symptoms were shoulder pain, carpal tunnel syndrome, and arthritis that made me feel achy all over, especially in the morning. As the years passed I began to have problems with pain in my hips, hands, and neck."

DRA occurs when a waxy protein builds up in patients' soft tissues, bones, and joints. The protein, beta-2-microglobulin (β_2M), belongs on cells and in body fluids, and healthy kidneys remove any excess. When the kidneys fail, β_2M levels start to rise. The protein then forms into long fibrils of amyloid and enters tissues where it does not belong.[49]

DRA can cause:
- *Carpal tunnel syndrome* (painful compression of a nerve in the wrist)
- Joint pain
- Tendinitis
- Bone cysts and fractures
- Bowel obstructions

No one knows exactly how often DRA occurs, but it may be common among those on dialysis who live long enough to develop it. In one study amyloid was found by X-ray in about:[50]
- 20% of patients after 10 years of hemodialysis
- 30–50% of patients after 15 years
- 80–100% of patients after 20 years or more

Some types of dialyzer membranes remove more β_2M than others, but since β_2M is being generated all the time, no dialyzer can clear it all.[51] Longer and/or more frequent hemodialysis (HD) treatments remove more β_2M.[52]

> **Your Role in DRA Management**
> - Report any and all complaints of pain, skin sores, or tissue lumps to the nurse.
> - Learn about all of the types of dialysis and their impact on DRA—more hours of HD can help prevent or even reverse this problem.
> - Be sure that patients receive their full treatments.

Neuropathy (Nerve Damage)

"My husband has neuropathy from dialysis. Once the damage is done there is nothing that can be done about it. Better dialysis will slow down the progression. He describes it as walking on wadded up socks. He also has had tremendous pain—even the weight of the blankets on the bed hurts his toes."

Patients may develop nerve damage in the hands and/or feet (*peripheral neuropathy*). It may begin before they start dialysis. Neuropathy is most common in those who have diabetes, though others can have it as well. Symptoms of neuropathy may include:

- Burning and pain in the hands and/or feet
- Numbness or a "pins and needles" feeling in the hands and/or feet
- Muscle weakness
- Erectile dysfunction in men
- Trouble walking

No one yet knows what causes nerve damage in people on dialysis. Wastes that are not removed well by dialysis may build up in the body and kill off nerve cells.[53] Nerve damage does occur most often when the GFR falls below 12 mL/min/1.73m².[54] And, in one case study, severe nerve damage improved when a patient switched to long HD treatments during sleep (nocturnal HD).[55] A lack of vitamins or other substances may be part of the problem as well. An older study found that taking vitamin B6 helped ease nerve pain in people on dialysis—and this may suggest a lack of the vitamin.[56,57] Or, both problems may occur at the same time.

Neuropathy with numbness in the feet is a risk factor for limb loss. When someone cannot feel his or her feet, an injury can occur and not be noticed or felt. In patients whose blood flow may be poor (such as with diabetes), wound healing is slow—or may not happen at all. People with stage 4 and 5 CKD and those on dialysis are at higher risk for foot ulcers and major amputation than those with stage 3 CKD.[58]

There are some treatments that can help ease nerve pain. In patients with diabetes, alpha-lipoic acid supplements have been shown to relieve pain[59] and even help slow progression of nerve damage.[60] Patients should *only* take vitamins or supplements that their doctors approve. Some prescription drugs can help treat nerve pain as well.

> **Your Role in Neuropathy Management**
> - Tell the nurse if patients complain of weakness, numbness, burning, or hand or foot pain.
> - Notice whether your patients are having trouble walking and ask them about it.
> - Suggest that patients ask their doctors about treatment for nerve damage and pain, including more dialysis.
> - Urge your patients with diabetes or nerve damage to wear shoes or slippers all the time and look at their feet each day for wounds they may not feel. Some clinics perform foot checks on patients who may not be able to see their own feet.

Pruritus (Itching)

"I had terrible itching the first 2 years. I tried everything, but the only thing that worked for me was to not scratch and apply high quality lotion after every single shower while my skin was still wet. It took a lot of practice to develop a resistance to the urge to scratch, but once I did – it stopped bothering me as much."

Severe and constant itching is common in people with kidney failure. In one large study, 42% of patients had itching.[61] Itching can make it hard to sleep, reduce patients' quality of life, and raise the risk of hospital stays and death.[61] Several treatments may help:

- Dry skin can cause itching, since patients may have poor nutrition and less sweating. If this is the case, lotions can help.
- Treating MBD may help if itching is due to hyperphosphatemia; a common cause.

- Itching may improve after surgery to remove the parathyroid glands or after a kidney transplant.

Itching with *hives* (raised welts) that only happens *during* dialysis may be due to an allergy. *Contact dermatitis* is an allergy to something that touches the skin. The culprit might be laundry soap or bleach used to clean the treatment chairs. Allergies to drugs (e.g., heparin) or chemicals used to make or sterilize a new dialyzer can also cause hives during a treatment.

> **Your Role in Pruritus Management**
> - Ask the nurse if oatmeal baths or Aveeno® soap might be options for the patient to try.
> - Ask the nurse and dietitian if you should talk with the patient about phosphate binders.
> - Urge patients to come for each treatment and stay the whole time.

Sleep Problems

"I cannot sleep for more than 4 hours at a time. The doctors gave me medicine but it does not help, I am still up every 4 hours and I get so sleepy in the day. I take a nap only for an hour or so. The rest of the time I walk around so tired I don't know what to do..."

Trouble falling or staying asleep is common in people with kidney failure—and other chronic diseases, such as depression. Sleep *apnea* (brief periods of not breathing) is also common. Patients whose partners report that the patient snores loudly or stops breathing should be tested for sleep apnea. The condition can cause or worsen some heart problems.[62]

Sleep problems often start during CKD, and the reasons for them are not clear. Sleep problems may be worse if patients sleep during a daytime treatment. A problem called restless legs syndrome (RLS) can make it hard to fall asleep or stay asleep. RLS may occur in as many as 1 in 4 people with kidney failure. Patients may have a "creepy-crawly" feeling in their legs, almost as if insects are crawling on them. They are compelled to move their legs—which can disturb both the patient and a partner. Dialysis patients with RLS have been found to be at a much higher risk of death.[63]

Some patients take prescription sleeping pills or supplements to improve their sleep, and these may help—at least in the short term.[64] Of course, all supplements must be cleared by the nephrologist.

Small studies have found that *nocturnal* HD (a longer treatment, done during sleep at home or in a clinic) may improve sleep quality by:

- Making the throat less narrow so breathing is easier[65]
- Bringing back the normal rhythm of melatonin, a sleep hormone[65]

> **Your Role in Sleeping Problems Management**
> - Ask your patients about how well they are sleeping.
> - Report sleep problems, including RLS, to the nurse.
> - Learn about all of the types of dialysis and their impact on sleep.

Bleeding Problems

"Today was the pits!!!! I left the center at noon after my treatment. On the way home my arm started bleeding pretty bad, all over the car and my clothes. When I got home I was able to stop it, and took it easy on my arm all afternoon. But, at about 4:00, it started bleeding again! This time it was even worse. Blood everywhere. I had to go to the ER."

Bleeding problems in those on dialysis can have a number of causes:

- Using too much heparin
- Use of Warfarin or other blood thinners along with heparin
- *Stenosis* (narrowing) in a fistula or graft can cause prolonged bleeding after the needles are removed, or bleeding after dialysis
- Changes in the blood itself. With kidney failure, *platelets* (blood clotting cells), do not "clump" as they should. Other aspects of blood clotting may not work as well, either. Signs of clotting problems may include easy bruising, gastrointestinal (GI) bleeding, blood in the stool, and nosebleeds.[67]

The Person with Kidney Failure

> **Your Role in Bleeding Problems Management**
> - Ask patients if they have any bleeding between treatments—if yes, tell the nurse.
> - If you are allowed to give heparin in your state, always be sure the dose is right.
> - If bleeding occurs, ask the nurse how the heparin dose should be changed.
> - Tell the nurse if there is a lot of clotting in a patient's dialyzer.

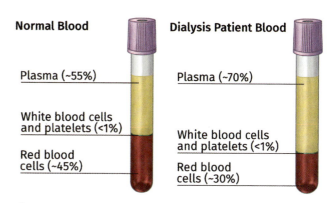

Figure 10: Blood Components

Common Dialysis Blood Tests

"Keep in mind that lab tests are a snapshot of what happened at THAT treatment. If my numbers don't look as good as they do normally, perhaps my time was shorter that day for some reason, or the needle placement made me get lower than normal blood flows, etc. I look at the trends."

Lab tests are a vital window into the patient's body to assess health, find problems, and check how much treatment they are getting. In fact, blood test results can even predict whether patients will survive on dialysis. Patients in one large study (13,792 people) were 89% more likely to live if they met the targets for all six of these blood tests *at the same time*:[68]

- **Single-pool Kt/V** – measures the dose of dialysis
- **Red blood cell count** (RBC) – number of red blood cells
- **Serum albumin** – protein in the blood
- **Calcium** – bone mineral balance
- **Phosphorus** – bone mineral balance
- **PTH** – parathyroid hormone level

Routine blood tests are done each week, month, and quarter, or as the doctor orders. Table 3 lists common blood tests. When you know why these are done and what "normal" is, you can support the care team's patient teaching and answer patients' questions. Blood tests may be run on whole blood, red blood cells only, or serum (part of plasma) (see Figure 10). Read Module 7: *Hemodialysis Procedures and Complications* to learn about how to draw and process blood tests.

Treatment Options

If the kidneys fail, a kidney transplant or dialysis treatments can sustain life—sometimes for decades. Treatment for kidney failure affects *all* aspects of life. For patients to feel their best and live as fully as they can, they need to choose a treatment that is a good fit for how they want to live. In this section, you will learn about transplants and all of the ways to do dialysis.

Transplant

"A transplant is the closest we will ever have to "normal." Most of us would trade in dialysis for a kidney and consider ourselves blessed—despite the higher chance that we will get cancer or other side effects. Kind of an eye opener isn't it? Let's face it...none of us will live a record-breaking long life, but it would be nice if we had quality of life and freedom while alive."

A kidney transplant gives a patient one healthy kidney from a donor (see Figure 11). Patients must pass health and psychological tests to be sure they are healthy and strong enough for a transplant. Each transplant program has its own rules for who can qualify. So, a patient who is turned down by one clinic due to age, weight, or some other cause can try a different program.

Table 3: Common Blood Tests Performed on People with ESRD

Blood Test	How Often	Target Value (NOTE: varies with lab)	What the Test Means
Albumin A type of protein	Monthly	General: 3.5–5.5 g/dL Dialysis: ≥ 4.0 g/dL[69]	**If low:** May mean malnutrition, inflammation or infection. Some health problems, like diabetes, can affect levels.[70] Patients tend to live longer with levels greater than 3.5g/dL.
Blood Cultures A test for bacteria in the blood	As needed	Negative, or no growth	**If positive:** Confirms infection. Testing also helps show which bacteria cause an infection so a doctor can prescribe the best antibiotic. (The doctor may still treat if negative, based on signs or symptoms.)
Blood Urea Nitrogen (BUN) An easy way to measure waste	Monthly[71] (pre- and post-dialysis)	General: 10–20 mg/dL[70] Dialysis: 60–80 mg/dL[70]	**If low:** May mean the patient is not eating enough protein. **If high:** May mean not enough dialysis. BUN is used to calculate Kt/V (the dose of dialysis).[70]
Calcium (Ca^{++}) An electrolyte	Monthly[69]	General: 9.0–10.5 mg/dL[70] Dialysis: Within normal range[72] Hypercalcemia (Levels > 10.2) must be addressed[73]	**If low:** May be caused by lack of vitamin D, malabsorption, or not enough PTH. **If high:** May be caused by too much Vitamin D, too much PTH, cancer, or some forms of MBD.[70]
Complete Blood Count (CBC) A basic screening of red, white, and other blood cells	Monthly	Depends on type of cell being monitored	Abnormal levels can mean immune cell problems, anemia, infection, and/or inflammation.
Creatinine A waste that forms when we move our muscles	Monthly[69]	General: 0.7–1.3 mg/dL[70] Dialysis: 2–15 mg/dL, based on muscle mass, GFR/dialysis[70]	A level that is higher or lower than usual: Can mean a change in the patient's muscle mass or dialysis dose.
Serum ferritin Stored iron	Monthly (at start of ESA therapy or if low), then quarterly[70]	General: 15–200 ng/mL[70] PD: ≥ 100 ng/mL[70] HD: 200-500 ng/ml[69]	**If low:** May mean iron deficiency. **If high:** May be due to high iron intake (from supplements), blood transfusions, or inflammation.[70]
Glucose Blood sugar	Monthly	General: 70–105 mg/dL (fasting)[70] Dialysis: ≤ 200 (non-fasting)[70]	**If low** (hypoglycemia): May be due to too much insulin in someone with diabetes. **If high** (hyperglycemia): May be due to poor diabetes control.[70]
Hemoglobin (HgB) Protein in red blood cells that carries oxygen	Monthly[69]	General male: 14–17 g/dL[70] General female: 12–16 g/dL[70] Dialysis: 10–11.0 g/dL (at least 9 g/dL)	**If low:** May mean anemia, chronic blood loss, or can occur in early CKD. **If high:** May mean dehydration, too much ESA therapy, newly diagnosed or poorly controlled diabetes.[70]
Hepatitis B[70] Anti-HBc (antibody to hepatitis B core antigen). A test for infection.	Prior to start of dialysis	General: Negative	**If positive:** Suggests a previous or ongoing hepatitis infection.

Table 3: CONTINUED

Blood Test	How Often	Target Value (NOTE: varies with lab)	What the Test Means
Anti-HBs[69] (antibody to hepatitis B surface antigen). A test for immunity.	Prior to start of dialysis. Further testing depends on immune status.	General: Negative Immunized: Positive	**If positive:** Patient is immune due to a vaccination. If both Anti-HBs and Anti-HBc are positive and HBsAg is negative, immunity is due to a previous infection.
HBsAg[69] (hepatitis B surface antigen). A test for infection.	Prior to start of dialysis and monthly for susceptible patients.	General: Negative	**If positive:** The patient is contagious and must be isolated. If HBsAg and both antibody tests are negative, the person is susceptible and may develop hepatitis B if exposed to the virus.
Hepatitis C[69] Anti-HCV – shows infection with the hepatitis C virus	Prior to start of dialysis. Further testing per clinic protocol.	General: Negative	**If positive:** Must report as required by state and local health authorities. Isolation of patients infected with HCV is not necessary.
Magnesium (Mg^{++}) An electrolyte	At start of dialysis and then as needed.	General: 1.5–2.4 mEq/L[70] Dialysis: normal limits[70]	**If low:** May mean malnutrition. **If high:** May mean excess magnesium intake from water, dialysate, antacids, or laxatives.[70]
Plasma intact parathyroid hormone (PTH) A hormone released when blood calcium levels drop	1–3 months	General: 10–65 pg/mL[70] Dialysis: 2–9 times the upper limit of normal[66] (approx. 130–600 pg/mL)	**If low:** May mean too much calcium, too much vitamin D, or not enough magnesium. **If high:** May mean hyperparathyroidism, not enough vitamin D, or low calcium.[70]
Phosphorus (P) An electrolyte	Monthly[75]	General: 3.0–4.5 mg/dL[70] Dialysis: Within normal range[66]	**If low** (rare): Suggests not enough vitamin D, low phosphorus intake, too many binders, or bone disease. **If high:** May mean too many high phosphate foods, not enough binders, too much vitamin D, or bone disease.[70]
Potassium (K^+) An electrolyte	Monthly	General: 3.5–5.0 mEq/L[70] Dialysis: within normal limits[70]	**If low:** May be due to diarrhea, vomiting, or antibiotics. **If high:** May be caused by not enough dialysis, wrong dialysate, or use of salt substitutes/low sodium spice mixes.[70]
Sodium (Na^+) An electrolyte	Monthly	General: 136–145 mEq/L[70] Dialysis: within normal limits[70]	**If low:** May be due to overhydration, inappropriate diuretic use, or diabetic acidosis. **If high:** May be due to dehydration, diabetes, or masked water retention.[70]
Transferrin saturation (TSAT) How much iron is in the body to form red blood cells[74]	1–3 months Monthly with anemia; every 3 months if no anemia (varies based on ESA or iron therapy)[75]	General: 20–50%[70] Dialysis: KDOQI target: > 20%[74]	**If low:** Suggests iron deficiency (perhaps due to blood loss) or malnutrition. **If high:** Suggests iron overload (perhaps due to IV iron), acute hepatitis,[70] or hemochromatosis, a genetic disorder.

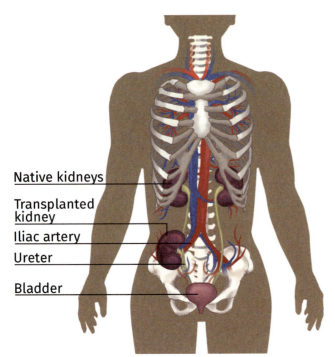

Figure 11: Location of Transplanted kidney

A transplant *does not cure kidney failure*; it is a treatment option, with pros and cons. Lifestyle with a transplant can be close to normal for as long as the new kidney lasts. A transplant may not work at all—or it may last 5, 10, 20, or even more years. About 92% of deceased donor kidneys work one year after transplant, about 71% work 5 years later, and about 45% still work 10 years later.[76] *Rejection* can occur at any time—the patient's immune system sees the new organ(s) as "foreign" and attacks.

Immunosuppressant drugs are used to try to keep the immune system from attacking the transplant and causing it to fail. People who get a transplant must take these drugs for as long as they have the new kidney. These costly drugs have side effects that may include:

- Weight gain
- Stomach irritation
- High cholesterol
- High blood pressure
- Cataracts
- Bone disease or joint problems
- Infection
- Diabetes
- Cancer

All of these side effects can be managed. Transplant patients may have a diet that limits calories, fat, and salt, but have many fewer diet limits than those on standard in-center HD. Each year in the U.S., more than 120,000 people reach kidney failure,[77] and more than 17,000 have transplants.[78] Patients go on dialysis while they wait, and, if a transplant fails, they can go back on dialysis again. They may be able to get another transplant.

Kidneys for transplant come from three sources:

1. **Someone who has died (deceased donor)**. Getting on the list for a deceased donor kidney is *not* automatic. A patient who wants a kidney must be evaluated by a transplant center to get on the list. The United Network for Organ Sharing (UNOS) keeps the national transplant list.
There are not enough deceased donor organs to meet the need, so those who want one may have to wait a few years—or seek a living donor.

2. **A blood relative** (living, related donor).

3. **A *non*-blood relative, spouse, or friend** (living, non-related donor).

People who are in good health can volunteer to donate a kidney. Donors must have blood tests to see if their blood and tissue type match the patient's. If they match, they will be tested to see if they are suited—physically and emotionally—to donate a kidney. Donors can live normal lives with one kidney. Unrelated kidney donors tend to live longer than the general public because they are often healthier to start. But, living kidney donors *who are related to their recipients* have a higher risk of death and kidney failure, though the risk is still quite small.[79] A long-term study began in 2016 to follow donors and compare them to healthy non-donors, so we should know more in the future.[80]

> ### *Kidney-Pancreas Transplant*
> Some patients with diabetes and kidney failure may be able to get *two* new organs. A kidney-pancreas (KP) transplant means no more dialysis—or insulin—while the organs work. And, without diabetes, a new kidney may last longer. About 75% of the time, the kidney and pancreas come from the same deceased donor at the same time. In most cases, transplant programs offer KP transplants to people under age 55 with type 1 diabetes. Diabetic damage to the eyes, nerves, and heart may improve after a KP transplant.[81] Many patients with diabetes are not aware of the KP transplant option, and you can tell them about it so they can ask their doctors.

Once a patient is on the transplant list, wait list time will start as of the first day of dialysis. A *preemptive* transplant is also possible once the GFR is 20 or less. This means someone gets a transplant before they start dialysis. Because of the timing, preemptive transplant is most likely with a living donor.

Updated transplant rules may help shorten the wait:

- **The United Network for Organ Sharing wrote new rules in 2014 for how to distribute kidneys**. Now, kidneys are matched so they have the best chance to last a long time: younger people get younger kidneys; older people get older ones. Each donated kidney is given a Kidney Donor Profile Index (KDPI) score that predicts how long it will last, based on the donor's age, height and weight, cause of death, and other factors. And, each patient who wants a kidney is given an Estimated Post-Transplant Survival (EPTS) score. This score predicts how long someone may live after they receive a kidney.[82] Early results suggest that the new approach is working.[83]
- **ABO (blood type) *incompatible* transplants let patients get a kidney from a donor with a blood type that does not match**. The patient's immune system is "desensitized" with drugs before and after the transplant to make this work.[84]
- **A *paired donor exchange* can help when two or more patients each have someone who is willing to donate a kidney—but who is not a match for them**. Each donor gives a kidney to a different patient who *is* a match.[85]
- **A *chain donation*** can start when an altruistic donor gives a kidney to someone. Then, the recipient's donor (who did not match) gives a kidney to someone else. These kidney "swaps" may include more than a dozen people.

As a technician, it is vital for you to know that the hope of one day getting a transplant is what keeps many dialysis patients going from day to day. Some who learn that they cannot have a transplant are so devastated that they may even want to stop treatment. Knowing that there are other forms of dialysis that can make them feel better may help you to help them. Ask the social worker to talk to patients who are upset after they learn that a transplant is not in their future. The social worker may have another patient who has been down the same road and has coped well. Talk to them.

Dialysis

"It may be an inconvenience at times, but I know many fellow dialysis patients who live busy, active lives despite dialysis. Sure we have our ups and downs, but the alternative without dialysis is death. Not an option for me!"

Dialysis removes some of the wastes and water that build up in the body when the kidneys fail. Blood is sent through a filter. Wastes and excess water pass through microscopic pores in a *membrane* (a thin film) and into a special dialysis fluid called *dialysate*.

Dialysis cannot *fully* remove wastes and excess water. The human body does adjust, to some degree, but the goal of dialysis is to help keep people feeling as well as they can. Table 4 compares normal kidney function to dialysis.

Table 4: Normal Kidney Function Compared to Dialysis

Normal Kidney Function	Dialysis
Removes all excess water each day	Removes *some* water on *treatment days*
Removes *all* waste products *each* day	Removes *some* wastes on *treatment days*
Controls electrolyte and acid-base balance	Helps restore electrolyte and acid-base balance
Fully controls blood pressure by keeping water and sodium in balance	Helps controls blood pressure by removing some water and helping balance sodium on *treatment days*
Makes erythropoietin, which tells the bone marrow to make red blood cells	Dialysis patients may not make erythropoietin, so an ESA can be given by injection.
Controls calcium/phosphorus balance *each* day	■ Can change serum calcium levels somewhat on *treatment days* by adjusting calcium in dialysate ■ Can remove some phosphorus, but not as well as healthy kidneys
Activates vitamin D	Cannot activate vitamin D, so active vitamin D is given by mouth or injection

A well-dialyzed patient who is otherwise healthy can have:
- Enough energy to work, pursue hobbies, and enjoy life
- A good appetite and good sleep
- A sex drive and intimacy with a partner
- Blood pressure that is near normal with few (or no) medicines
- Blood tests that are in the target range (for dialysis)
- A healthy heart, blood vessels, bones, and joints

Patients' treatments should be comfortable and leave them feeling well. *They should not have painful muscle cramps or low blood pressure.* While these events may be common, they are *not* normal—or acceptable. Patients should have few, if any, problems, and no treatment-related accidents.

Dialysis is an intensive treatment. It gives people the chance to live after their kidneys have failed—but it takes a lot of time. Keep in mind that patients had full lives just like you before they had kidney failure. Choosing a treatment option that will let them keep what matters most to them may help reduce depression. Here are some things to think about:
- Each year, half of all Americans who start dialysis are between 18 and 64 years old: working age.[77] Work pays much more than disability and helps people keep their self-esteem and social contacts, and feel useful in the world. An employer group health plan can help pay for dialysis, and tends to pay far more than Medicare. To keep their jobs, patients need to have their symptoms managed and get "*work-friendly*" treatments that give them enough energy to work and allow them to control their schedules. Work-friendly dialysis might be done at night, for example, so patients' days are free.
- Patients who care for children or elders may find that their lives work better if they do their treatments at home instead of in-center.
- Those who love to eat and drink may feel better with a treatment that gives them fewer limits on diet and fluids.
- If travel is what a patient lives for, a portable treatment can work best.
- When women want to have babies, a transplant or *much* more dialysis can help make that goal possible.

Patients may ask *you* about their options. When a patient wants to change treatments, suggest that he or she speak to the home training nurse or doctor.

In most of the modules of this *Core Curriculum*, we only cover in-center hemodialysis (HD), because you are most likely to work with these patients. In this module, we cover *all* of the options, so you can help answer patients' questions. **NOTE**: With more than 477,000 people on dialysis in the U.S.[86] and about 6,500 clinics[87] caring for them in-center and at home, you do not have to worry about your job if some patients choose to do home treatments. There are *lots* of patients! And, there can be roles for you with *any* type of dialysis, in-center or at home.

All told, there are seven ways to do dialysis, each of which we will explain below:
1. **Peritoneal dialysis (PD) by hand (at home or at work)**
2. **PD using a cycler machine at night during sleep (at home)**
3. **Standard HD in a clinic**
4. ***Nocturnal* (nighttime) HD in a clinic**
5. **Standard home HD**
6. **Daily home HD**
7. **Nocturnal home HD**

"If what your clinic offers is the best option for you, that's fine, but if there's another option, especially a better option out there, then they should at least give you the chance to make your own choice, even if they don't offer it themselves!"

Peritoneal Dialysis (PD)

"We were told about PD in our first nephrology visit, but in-center HD seemed to be their main push. I did a lot of research on PD, kept asking questions of whoever I could, and searched online. Since we had clinic visits for 3 years we had a lot of time to find out how to do the option I wanted."

PD is a daily self-care treatment patients can do alone, at home, or at work. Training by a nurse takes 1–2 weeks, and some companies have PD technicians to help patients. Patients may choose PD because it:
- Is work-friendly, flexible, and portable
- Allows a more normal diet with fewer fluid limits than in-center HD
- Is an option that does not require needles
- Lets people feel like they are not "sick"[88]

How You Can Help Your Patients Choose a Treatment Option

Most patients do not know how their treatment will affect their lives—or that they can change treatments if they are not happy with their first choice. Here are some tips to help them.

- **Find out more yourself.** Learn about all of the home options and in-center nocturnal HD at Home Dialysis Central: www.homedialysis.org.
- **Watch for "teachable moments."** A patient may complain about the meal plan, thirst, taking so many meds, or tell you they worry about losing their jobs, homes, or partners. Use these moments as a chance to point out options that would not limit them as much in these areas.
- **Help patients solve problems.** Patients who gain too much fluid, live far from the clinic, or have children or elders to care for may do better at home than in the clinic.
- **Teach patients to put in their own needles.** CMS gives patients the right to be as involved as they want to be in their dialysis—including putting in their own needles.[89]
- **Help patients feel confident.** Assure them that if they choose a home treatment, a nurse will train them and provide 24/7 support. Both the patient and the training nurse must be confident that the patient can succeed. (NOTE: It is best if a patient does as much as possible of a home treatment, rather than placing the whole burden on a care partner.)
- **Encourage patients to learn more.** Talking with others who have had transplants or do home treatments can help them get a better sense of what to expect.

- **Point patients to a free, online decision aid.** Built by the non-profit Medical Education Institute and endorsed by the American Association of Kidney Patients and Home Dialyzors United, this tool will help them match an option to their lives: www.mydialysischoice.org

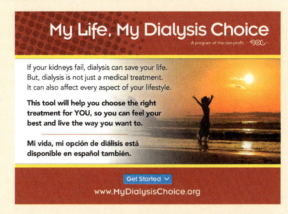

Do not:

- Scare patients away from home treatments. You would want to know all of the options in an unbiased way if you or a loved one had kidney disease. Your patients want to know, too.
- Give out wrong information. If you are not sure of an answer, say, "*Great question! Let me find out for you.*" Ask the nurse.
- Tell patients things like, "*You can't go home, you are my favorite patient! I would miss you!*" Or, "*Who will help you if you have a problem?*" Both the patient and the training nurse need to be confident of success before anyone goes home.

PD uses the patient's own *peritoneum*, which lines the inner abdomen, as a membrane to clean the blood. This lining is full of capillary blood vessels that act as filters. (See Module 3 to learn more about how PD works.) Those who choose PD have a *catheter* (tube) placed in the belly by a surgeon (see Figure 12). Less commonly, a chest wall (*presternal*) PD catheter may be used, which may reduce the chance of infection[90] (see Figure 13).

A nurse will teach the patient how to use the PD catheter to fill the belly with sterile fluid (*dialysate*). Wastes and water from the blood slowly shift into the dialysate. After the dialysate "dwells" in the belly for a few hours, the patient drains it out and fills up the belly again with fresh dialysate in a sterile process called an *exchange*.

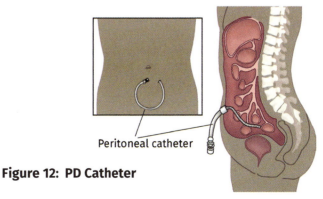

Figure 12: PD Catheter

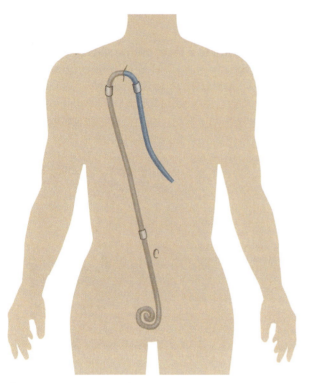

Figure 13: Presternal PD catheter

The most common problem for those on PD is a painful infection called *peritonitis*. Infection can scar the peritoneum, so PD may no longer be possible. Patients can prevent peritonitis if they wash their hands, wear a mask, and use aseptic technique to do the exchange steps just as they are taught. Infections of the PD catheter can also occur. Patients who want to do PD must have space in their homes to store enough fluid bags for a month.

Many people on PD have at least a little bit of *residual* (remaining) kidney function, which also helps remove water and wastes from the blood. Over time, residual function may slow down or end, and the peritoneum can become less efficient, so some patients may have to switch to HD. Patients who use PD must have regular adequacy tests done to ensure that they are getting enough treatment.[91] Just over half of the people who start PD (51.5%) will live for 5 years using this option.[92]

There are two ways to do PD: CAPD and CCPD/APD. As of 2017, 2,464 clinics offer CAPD and 2,461 offer CCPD/APD.[93]

CAPD

"I am blind, and am excited and nervous as I hold the connectors in my hands and join them, knowing if I do it wrong it could be extremely serious. I practice time after time with dummy lines. We devise ways I can do it all by touch or with the amazing technology at my disposal, and I feel more each day like I hold my life in my hands again. It is a wonderful, freeing, empowering feeling."

Continuous ambulatory (walking around) *PD* (CAPD) means the patient does PD exchanges (most often four a day) by hand (see Figure 14). The patient may do an exchange at breakfast time, lunch time, dinner time, and bed time, and can shift the timing a bit to fit his or her life—but must do all of them. Each exchange takes about 20–30 minutes. The patient must wash his or her hands, control airflow to the room, wear a mask, and carefully use aseptic technique to avoid infection. Pets must be kept out of the room during an exchange. When the patient's belly is always full of dialysate, treatment goes on all the time.

The United States Renal Data System (USRDS) reported that 1.9% of people with kidney failure in the U.S. were using CAPD in 2014.[94] Dialysis clinics train patients and monitor their care.

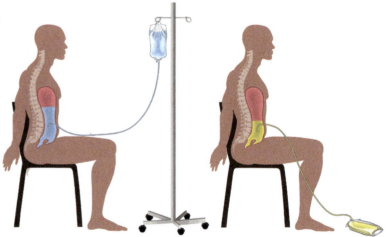

The peritoneal cavity is filled with dialysate, using gravity

At the end of the exchange, the dialysate is drained into the bag, again using gravity

Figure 14: Performing a CAPD Exchange

CCPD/APD

"I am on cycler PD and work full time. It's not bad except for the early bedtime so I can connect no later than 8:30 pm and be done in time for work. I start my job at 7:00 am, so some mornings it is tough, but it works for me."

Continuous cycling PD (CCPD) or *automated PD* (APD) uses a cycler machine at night (see Figure 15). Long tubing lines can allow patients to move around after connecting before it is time to go to sleep, or to use the bathroom during the night. This way, a patient can do PD exchanges for 8–10 hours each night while s/he sleeps, so days are free for work or other tasks. Some patients use a cycler and also do one or two day-time exchanges by hand to get more treatment. Per the USRDS, 7.8% of U.S. patients were using CCPD in 2014.[94]

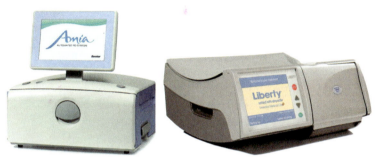

Figure 15: PD Cyclers
Amia Cycler – Image used with permission from Baxter Healthcare Corporation. Liberty Cycler – Image used with permission from Fresenius Medical Care North America.

Hemodialysis (HD)

HD is the most common treatment in the U.S. for kidney failure, and the one you are most likely to work with. It is done in homes, clinics, and hospitals all over the world. To do HD, blood is pumped out of the patient's body, through a filter called a *dialyzer* or *artificial kidney,* and then back into the patient (see Figure 16).

The dialyzer packs thousands of hollow fibers, each as thin as a hair, into a clear plastic cylinder (see Figure 17). During a treatment, the patient's blood flows through the inside of the fibers, while dialysate bathes the outside of the fibers. Water and some wastes pass through microscopic pores in the fibers, into the dialysate, and down the drain. Only about half a cup of blood is outside of the patient's body at any time.

How does blood get to the dialyzer? The patient needs a *vascular access*—a way to get blood out of the body. There are three types of access:

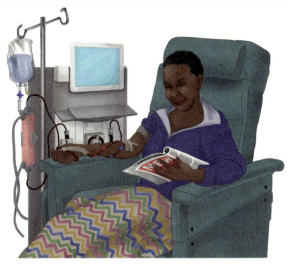

Figure 16: Hemodialysis

1. **If the patient's blood vessels will support it,** a surgeon will link a patient's own artery and vein together under the skin of an arm (or, rarely, a leg). This is an **arteriovenous fistula**. When it is possible for a patient to have one, a fistula is the best choice.

2. An **arteriovenous graft** links a patient's artery and vein together with a piece of man-made tubing. A graft may be the next best choice for someone who cannot have a fistula.

3. An **HD catheter** is a tube placed into a large, central vein in the neck, chest, or groin with the tip ending in the vena cava of the heart. If a patient needs dialysis right away, or has poor blood vessels, it may be the only choice. But, catheters often have problems, like infections and poor blood flow rates.

To do HD, two needles are placed into the fistula or graft and each is connected to a bloodline that takes the patient's blood to or from the dialyzer. Or, the bloodlines are connected to an HD catheter, with no needles used. For nocturnal HD only, a single needle is available. See Module 6: *Vascular Access*, to learn more.

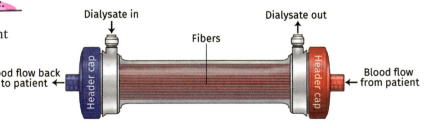

Figure 17: Dialyzer

45

STANDARD IN-CENTER HD

"I leave dialysis at the clinic! I don't see anything at home to remind me of dialysis, and it allows me to live a somewhat normal life. Going to dialysis is like a job, and my wife lets the clinic worry about me. I've been doing dialysis for 14 years."

Most HD in the U.S. today is done in a dialysis clinic ("in-center"). Treatments are done at the same time of day, three times a week, on a Monday, Wednesday, and Friday or a Tuesday, Thursday, and Saturday. While healthy kidneys work 24 hours a day, 7 days a week (168 hours), standard HD treatments provide only about 10.8 hours of treatment each week (3.6 hour/treatment x 3 = 10.8 hours).[95] A study of more than 22,000 HD patients from seven countries found that longer HD treatments saved lives: patients were 30% less likely to die when treatments were at least 4 hours long than if they were shorter. And, each extra 30 minutes of HD beyond 4 hours further reduced the risk of death by 7%.[96] This is helpful information to know when your patients say they want shorter treatments or if they do not come on time or ask to leave early.

There are some benefits to doing HD in a clinic. Some patients feel safer getting treatment in a clinic with nurses and technicians on hand to help if there is a problem. Older people who do not have family nearby to support them may be lonely and appreciate the chance to meet others who also need dialysis, and make friends at the clinic. Doing treatments in a clinic means the home is free of medical supplies, too. And, no partner is needed.

On the other hand, when a patient starts in-center HD, the clinic may not have a shift time that fits his or her life. A time slot that is a better fit may open up in a few weeks—or months—but this may be too late for someone to keep a job or stay in school. Patients who do not have their own vehicles may have a hard time finding a ride to and from the clinic three times a week. Those with young children may not be able to find or pay for childcare during school breaks.

Standard in-center HD places the most limits on what patients can eat and drink, requires the most medicines to take and pay for, and causes the most symptoms of any option. Since it is the smallest dose of dialysis, it also has the poorest 5-year survival rate: 40.2%.[97] (In comparison, the 5-year American survival rate for breast cancer is 91%, and for colon cancer is 65%.[98]) In the U.S. in 2014, 88% of those on dialysis used standard in-center HD,[94] and many said they were not told about other options.[99] In contrast, when nephrologists were asked which type of dialysis they would choose if their own kidneys failed, just 6% said they would do standard in-center HD.[100]

The "Killer Gap"

The "killer gap" (a term coined by Dr. Carl Kjellstrand), is the 2 days without treatment for patients who dialyze 3 days a week. After a weekend, a patient comes in with the most water weight and out-of-balance electrolytes. Going 2 days with no water or waste removal is linked with more hospital stays and death rates than dialyzing more often; in fact, research has found that the risk of death for in-center HD patients is 39% to 41% higher on a Monday or a Tuesday than on any other day of the week.[101] In a keynote address at the Annual Dialysis Conference in February of 2014, Dr. Kjellstrand estimated that more than 10,000 dialysis deaths occur each year in the U.S. just due to the "killer gap."

The care team may try on a Monday or a Tuesday to get a patient all the way back to his or her target weight. But instead, it may be wiser to use all three of the weekly treatments to catch up, so patients do not take off more than 10 mL of water per kilogram per hour. A doctor would need to order this, of course.

The best approach would be to do HD at least every other day so there is no 2-day gap. This is far more possible for patients on home HD, as few clinics are able to stay open seven days a week.

NOCTURNAL IN-CENTER HD

"I go three times a week for 8 hours at a time and find that since I started nocturnal, I feel better than I can remember in years. I have been on dialysis for 15 months, 6 of them on nocturnal."

As of 2017, 156 of the 6,500 or so clinics across the U.S. offer in-center HD at night.[93] Patients come to the clinic after the day shifts end, often around 8:00–9:00 pm, 3 nights a week. Staff like you do the treatments for 7–8 hours while the patients sleep. Some staff report they like working nights when the clinic is less fast-paced and quieter.

With in-center nocturnal HD:

- Patients get twice as much HD as with standard treatments. So, they have fewer limits on what they can eat and drink, and may not need to take as many medicines.
- Water removal is slow and gentle. Cramps are rare, and the treatments are easy on the heart. One study of 655 patients who used this option found they were less likely to be in the hospital than those who did standard HD.[102]
- Longer HD removes much more $\beta_2 M$, the protein that causes amyloidosis.[103]
- The treatments are work-friendly, since patients have their days free.
- Those who do not have a partner for home HD or who do not want an HD machine in their home may find this option a good fit.

Studies have found from 25%[104] to 72%[105] better survival with nighttime HD in-center than with standard HD in-center.

STANDARD HOME HD

"After a year or so of in-center treatment I went home, using a Fresenius 4008B machine, about the size of a small refrigerator. For me the greatest advantage of home dialysis is being able to juggle my treatment around my social life."

When dialysis first started in the U.S., 40% of patients were on home HD.[106] A small number still do home HD today on a standard (3 times a week) schedule, or some do treatments every other day. As of 2017, standard home HD was offered by 896 clinics across the country.[93] Patients and/or their partners are trained for a few weeks to learn how to:

- Put in needles
- Order supplies
- Run the machine
- Prevent infection
- Give prescribed medicines
- Take vital signs and blood samples
- Report problems
- Take care of emergencies
- Dispose of waste

In effect, they become their own technicians. Most home patients do well with this self-care treatment. They are in charge of their day-to-day care and can choose their own schedules. Their treatment fits into their lives. Home HD is work-friendly, so patients may be more likely to keep their jobs or stay in school.

Patients may do longer or every other day treatments to feel better and have fewer symptoms. Most clinics that offer home HD want patients to have a care partner who will train with them and be on hand for treatments. They also need space in their homes to store the machine and supplies. Some machines require plumbing or wiring changes to the home. Not every patient can meet these requirements.

DAILY HOME HD

"My husband was ALWAYS sick in-center. By the time he would start to feel okay it would be time to drive him back for another treatment. But, after 6 weeks at home, he had no more headaches, no more upset stomach all the time. His BP and pulse are normal for the first time in 7 years. The best part for me is that he is no longer in that 'fog.' He thinks clearer. We have normal conversations, when before he was too tired to talk for more than a half hour. I can't say enough good about home hemo. It's the best thing we ever did. I feel like I have him back again."

Healthy kidneys work 7 days a week, and this is what the body is used to. Daily home HD treatments last about 2.5 to 4 hours, and are done 5 or 6 days a week, most often at home, since it can be difficult to fit these treatments into a clinic day, and travel to and from a clinic every day would be burdensome. Daily home HD is the newest type of treatment in the U.S.— and the fastest growing. In 2017, nearly 1,000 clinics offered daily home HD, up from just 37 in 2004.[93] Machines built for patient use are smaller, fast and easy to set up and clean up, and make short treatments more practical. In 2017, the FDA approved solo patient use of the NxStage machine for daytime home HD, with no partner.

As with any type of home HD, patients and/or care partners are trained by a nurse to do the treatments. The shorter daily treatments can fit well into family and work life. They can be done in the morning before work or during a couple of TV shows at night. After a year of daily HD, patients slept better and had fewer episodes of restless legs syndrome.[107]

The Frequent Hemodialysis Network study compared 125 people who were randomly assigned to daily HD treatments (in-center) to 120 on standard HD.[108] The study found that those who did daily HD:

- Had healthier hearts
- Felt better physically
- Had lower blood pressure
- Had lower phosphorus levels

Another study of 1,873 people who used daily HD found that their survival was 13% better than that of 9,365 matched controls who did standard in-center HD.[109]

NOCTURNAL HOME HD

"I switched to nocturnal HD 5+ years ago. Better water removal lets me breathe deeper. Now, I can take longer strides, walk faster, and jump to my feet without joint or bone pain or balance issues. I can sweep, mop floors, wash dishes, etc., without shortness of breath or the need to rest. I need less sleep, have a better appetite, words come more quickly, I can joke around better, etc."

Patients and care partners can learn to do nighttime HD treatments at home, too. As of 2017, 290 clinics offered this option.[93] Most often, people dialyze 3–7 nights each week for 7–8 hours while they sleep. The dialysis needles and blood tubing are well taped, so they do not come out or pull apart. Alarms under the access arm and the dialyzer can detect even a drop of blood and wake the patient up. Clinics run by the U.S. Veterans Administration, use the Redsense™ alarm, which was made for this purpose. Others may use the Fresenius WetAlert™ or HemoDialert™ alarms. And, since blood flow rates for nocturnal HD are quite slow, there is time to safely deal with a blood leak, if there is one. In some programs, the dialysis machine is linked by a modem to the clinic, so a nurse or technician can follow each treatment.

Studies of nocturnal home HD in the U.S. and other countries have found improvements in important outcomes. Patients had higher blood albumin levels than those on standard HD, and they did not need phosphate binders to reduce the phosphorus levels in their blood.[110] Most had no fluid limits.[111] They felt more in control and reported better quality of life.[112] In addition, heart damage that occurred while on standard HD *improved* when people switched to nocturnal treatments[113]—which can help some patients to qualify for a kidney transplant. Those who do nocturnal home HD may live about as long as those who get deceased donor transplants: 5-year survival is 84.5%[114] Patients who live far from a clinic or who want to keep their days free for other things—like working or caring for small children—may want to think about doing nocturnal home HD.

Medical Management Without Dialysis

"I have always had a positive attitude to life on dialysis, and this acceptance of death is the most positive statement I have ever made. I'm making the right choice at the right time in the right place and for the right reasons."

Without treatment, kidney failure will ultimately lead to death. And, this may be a choice that makes sense, if someone's health is very poor. Patients who have other illnesses or are in a lot of pain may opt not to treat kidney failure. Or, they may start a "trial" of treatment and stop if they do not feel better or their quality of life is still poor. Most major religions think of this as letting natural death occur—not as suicide. People who are older than 80 and have other illnesses may not live any longer with dialysis than they would without it. So, it can be a kindness to forego dialysis, and people may still live for a year or two.[115]

"I have always regarded the ability to choose the time, the hour, the place and the manner of our death as the greatest privilege that dialysis gives us. And it is unique to us. So I'm grabbing the opportunity with both hands. I wish I had a third to embrace it even harder."

When a patient wants to stop treatment, the care team will make sure that s/he has thought through the choice and will offer support. If a patient is depressed, counseling, medicine, or a switch to another treatment option may help him or her see that there is still hope for a good life. Patients who do choose to end treatment will get active care to treat their symptoms. Hospice services can help the patient and family. Having someone stop treatment is difficult. But, as hard as it may be, helping someone to have a peaceful death can be rewarding.

The doctor, nurse, or social worker will talk with patients about what care they would or would not want for a health crisis. These wishes are called *advance directives*. Patients have the right to complete an advance directive and to know whether their clinic will honor it. It can be hard to talk about this, but most patients value the chance to have their say and know that their wishes will be respected.

HD Care Team

To obtain good healthcare and quality of life outcomes for patients, the whole team must work together (see Figure 18). Since 2008, CMS has required the care team to hold meetings and share information to make each patient's *Plan of Care* work as well as it can.[89] Below, you can learn about the responsibilities of each of the team members. When you know this information, you can guide your patients to the right person to help them if they have a question or problem.

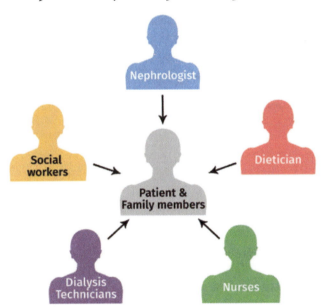

Figure 18: HD Care Team Members

Patient

As the person with a chronic disease, the patient has a *job*. He or she needs to:

- Learn about kidney failure and its treatment
- Have input into the care plan, then follow it (meal plan, fluid limits, drugs, dialysis)
- Tell the care team about any symptoms or problems
- Take as active a role in their day-to-day care as s/he prefers
- Know his or her rights and responsibilities

Patients spend far more of their time outside of the dialysis clinic than in it, and good treatment lets them spend that time doing things they value and enjoy. Patients have the best chance of a good life if they learn all they can and are active partners in their care. *CMS gives patients the right to be as involved as they want to be, up to and including putting in their own dialysis needles and running the machine.* You and the rest of the care team can help them get up to speed so they can take care of themselves. In some cases, family members will help with care or speak for patients who cannot speak for themselves.

Your patients will have dialysis in common, but sometimes not much else. They may be old or young: about half are age 60 or older, while half are younger. They are men, women—or may not identify as either. They may be straight or gay, black, white, Hispanic, or from any country on Earth. They may practice one of many religions, or none at all. They may or may not speak English. They may be friendly and funny and nice, or sullen, angry, and hostile. Patients may be able-bodied or not able to move at all by themselves. **Each patient must be treated with dignity—the way you or your loved one would want to be treated.** CMS requires that all patients be treated with respect, and your clinic can be cited by Medicare surveyors if patients say that this is not the case.

If you do not understand someone's culture, ask—the patient is likely to be happy to tell you about it. Some patients may be prejudiced against you because of your gender, color, or race, but you also deserve to be treated with respect. Talk to the social worker if you run into challenges with patients over any of these issues.

Family Members

Patients' families can be a source of support. It is the patient's right to choose how involved his or her loved ones can be and what they are told about the care plan. Involved families can help patients feel normal and adjust to their changed lives. And, the patient's health and treatment impact the family as well—emotionally, financially, socially, etc. Family may pick up the slack for tasks at home that a patient no longer feels well enough to do. And, patients who have other illnesses, such as diabetes with blindness, may need a lot of hands-on care each day from family members to even get to their treatments.

Unfortunately, some patients find that their family and friends fade away when they start dialysis.

Perhaps their loved ones do not know what to say, or are afraid of being asked for a kidney. Patients who do not feel support from others have a lower quality of life, do not follow their treatment plans as well, and are more likely to die.[116] We cannot fix our patients' families and make them supportive when they are not. But, we can encourage patients to reach out to their loved ones, to be specific about what they need, and to seek other sources of help, like in-person or online support groups. And, we can be our patients' cheerleaders if no one else will.

Nephrologist

A nephrologist is a doctor who is a specialist in kidney disease. S/he sets up the patient's plan of care with the other care team members. The doctor prescribes treatments and drugs and orders tests. Each clinic is required to have a Medical Director, who is a board-certified nephrologist. The Medical Director's job is ensure that staff are trained and competent, and that policies and procedures are followed to assure safe, high-quality care.

Nurses

The nurse coordinates each patient's care with the other members of the care team. S/he will put the plan of care into action, teach patients, give them medications, assess them before and after each treatment, do direct patient care, and train staff. CMS requires each clinic to have a full-time registered nurse (RN) manager with 12 months of clinical experience. At least one RN must be present on each dialysis shift as well. In some states, nurses must also connect patients with catheters to their dialysis machines. Nurses may have many different levels of credentials:

- Licensed Practical Nurse (LPN)
- Licensed Vocational Nurse (LVN)
- Registered Nurse (RN)
- Clinical Nurse Specialist (CNS)
- Bachelor of Science in Nursing (BSN)
- Master of Science in Nursing (MSN)
- Doctor of Nursing Practice (DNP)
- Nurse Practitioner (NP)
- Advanced Practice Registered Nurse (APRN)
- Certified Nephrology Nurse (CNN)

Social Workers

Social workers help patients cope with kidney disease and the life changes that treatment for kidney failure may require. The social worker counsels patients and their loved ones to help them sort out and handle their feelings. S/he can put patients in touch with local financial help, housing, rides to and from the clinic, drug assistance programs, job training, and more. S/he may be able to answer questions about health insurance or refer patients to someone who can. You can ask the social worker for help to deal with a patient whose behavior is challenging. Or, if a patient seems depressed, tell the social worker. Social workers can also work with technicians and the rest of the care team to help patients self-manage their care. CMS requires each dialysis clinic to have a social worker with a master's degree in social work.

Dialysis Technicians

In a dialysis clinic, you may be the one most likely to spend one-on-one time with the patient at each treatment. You have a chance to get to know patients and to observe whether they are doing better—or worse—so you can alert the rest of the care team. You can build trust with your patients by acting in a professional way, knowing your job, and treating them respectfully.

In some clinics, technicians take on multiple roles. In others, there may be as many as four different types of technician:

1. *Patient care technicians* take care of patients on dialysis, working under a registered nurse.
2. *Biomedical equipment technicians* maintain and fix the machines.
3. *Reuse technicians* label, clean, and reprocess dialyzers so they can be used again.
4. *Water treatment technicians* care for the water treatment system.

Renal Dietitians/Nutritionists (RD/RDN)

The renal dietitian works with patients, families, and the care team to develop a nutrition plan to meet each patient's dietary needs and limits. The plan is tailored to include foods the patient likes to eat in safe amounts. Part of the dietitian's role is to teach patients and their loved ones how to best meet the patients' nutritional needs. S/he will go over monthly lab test results with each patient and help explain how diet affects each result. CMS requires each dialysis clinic to have a renal dietitian with at least one year of experience on staff.

Starting Standard In-Center HD: The Risky First 90 Days

The first 90 days of dialysis are a period of high risk of death for patients. The patient and family are dealing with new challenges, like fears about what kidney failure will mean to them. They may not yet know much about the treatment or what they should or should not do. **In research, patients in their first 90 days of dialysis were twice as likely to die as those who had been doing treatment longer.** Those who were older and sicker were at a higher risk of death than younger, healthier patients.[117] A renal community program to improve the care patients receive at the start of dialysis cut this death rate by 34% at 4 months and 22% at a year.[118] Education before dialysis starts can also help patients live longer.[119]

Patience and repetition can help people through this stressful time. You may need to explain things more than once, such as why patients need to come to dialysis, why they need a permanent access, and what their treatment options are. Patients are afraid—*and people who are afraid cannot learn*.[120] And, patients may still be uremic, which can make it hard for them to remember. Some dialysis providers have first 90-day programs for their patients, such as IMPACT by DaVita, RightStart from Fresenius, and Optimal Start from Satellite.

Safe Vascular Access

Patients who start dialysis with a fistula or graft for vascular access are more likely to live than those who have an HD catheter.[121] So, it is best to help patients to get a fistula or graft as soon as possible. They will need a referral to have vessel mapping and to see a vascular surgeon. The care team needs to explain to the patient and family what to expect at these appointments. Then, they need to explain how to care for the new access once it is in place and when it is ready to use. You can learn more about vascular access for dialysis in Module 6: *Vascular Access*.

Avoiding Malnutrition

Many new patients who start dialysis are malnourished, because uremia can reduce appetite and cause a bad taste in the mouth and/or nausea and vomiting.[122] Along with high levels of inflammation, a first serum *albumin* (protein) level of less than 3.5 g/dL predicts death.[123] (The whole care team needs to address nutrition often in the first 90 days. Read the Nutrition section of this module to learn more.)

Tailoring the First Dialysis Treatments

In the first 90 days, *pulmonary edema* (a build-up of water in the lungs) or *hyperkalemia* (too much potassium in the blood) need urgent action. But, in most cases, the uremic toxins and excess water do not build up overnight. So, we should not try to remove them all with just one or two treatments. Trying to correct uremia too quickly can cause *dialysis disequilibrium syndrome* and brain swelling. (To learn more, see Module 7: *Hemodialysis Procedures and Complications*.) *Organ stunning* occurs when water is removed too quickly, and can cause loss of remaining kidney function and damage to the heart and brain.

The nephrologist can adapt a patient's first dialysis treatments to be more gentle by ordering:

- Minimal water removal until the patient is used to HD, never more than 13 mL/kg/hr, and ideally, not more than 10 mL/kg/hr.[45] Patients who still make urine may not need to have water removed. In any case, it is vital to avoid making the patient's blood pressure drop, since this can cause organ stunning.
- Less heparin, because CKD slows blood clotting, and bleeding could occur in other parts of the body.
- Dialysate potassium that is a bit higher than it is for longer-term patients; removing potassium too quickly can change heart rhythms.
- Dialysate sodium based on a patient's blood tests and set so the treatments will take off sodium—or at least not add any.
- Shorter treatment time to start, adding 15–30 minutes at each treatment.
- Treatments for a few days in a row (most often in the hospital) to fix problems without the need for big changes during any one treatment.
- An ESA for anemia, which may take 6–8 weeks to raise the red blood cell count. The patient may need a transfusion in the meantime.

Nutrition for People on Standard In-Center HD

"My greatest challenge has been diet. All the things I love are on the danger list. I was a very healthy eater until I got sick."

Healthy kidneys work 24 hours a day to remove the water and wastes from the body that build up mainly from the food we eat. They include urea, creatinine, potassium, sodium, phosphorus, and water. Dialysis, as you have just learned, does only *part* of the work of healthy kidneys. So, the more dialysis people get, the fewer limits they must have on what they can eat and drink.

In the U.S., most people on dialysis do standard in-center HD. Their diet needs to give them good nutrition *and* help to reduce the build-up of wastes between treatments. (NOTE: Those who do PD, nocturnal HD, or daily HD can eat and drink in a more normal way. This is something you can tell patients who complain about not being able to eat their favorite foods, or about being thirsty all the time.)

The diet is planned for each patient. Levels of protein, calories, fluid, minerals, and vitamins may change based on the patient's needs. Keeping these levels in balance can help patients feel better during and between treatments.

PROTEIN
All foods have *some* protein and there are two types:
1. *High biological value* (HBV) **animal** or **soy** protein (e.g., meat, fish, poultry, eggs, tofu, soy milk, and dairy products).
2. *Low biological value* (LBV) **plant** protein (e.g., breads, grains, vegetables, dried beans and peas, and fruits).

A balanced diet has both types. **In the body, proteins help maintain body muscle and tissue.** People on dialysis need twice as much protein each day (at least 1.2 grams per kilogram per day) as people with non-dialysis CKD, because they lose some protein at each treatment.[124]

When we eat protein, *nitrogenous wastes*, like urea and creatinine, are left in our bodies. Healthy kidneys remove these wastes, but damaged kidneys cannot.

Dialysis clinics test patients' blood levels of urea and creatinine each month. The results help us to see how well patients are doing. (See Blood Test chart on page 38.)

Calories and Malnutrition

Calories in food provide energy to run the body. People on dialysis must eat enough calories to meet their energy needs; if they do not, they will be malnourished, and their bodies will burn protein (i.e., cannibalize their own muscles) for fuel. If this happens, they will not have enough protein left to perform other key body functions and they can become weak and debilitated.

It is vital to note loss of "*real*" weight (muscle and fat) and *not* mistake it for water removal from treatment. If a patient loses real weight, it may not be seen right away. Signs that a patient has lost real weight, even if weight after treatment is the same, may include:

- Fluid build-up in the ankles and fingers
- Shortness of breath
- Not being able to lay flat in bed (ask the patient)

"I have NO appetite. And I never liked to cook. So now my dilemma is that I try to munch as often as possible, but most finger foods are on the restricted list or don't have high biological value."

Patients who are uremic often lose their appetites. Food may taste strange or metallic, and patients may feel sick to their stomachs or vomit. Watch your patients closely for weight loss. Pay special attention to new patients, since their appetite tends to be poor before their kidneys fail. Tell the dietitian if you think a patient is not eating well or s/he complains of having no appetite.

Protein malnutrition in people on dialysis is a risk factor for death.[124] A 3-year study looked at patients who lost 5% or more of their body weight *without meaning to* vs. those who kept a healthy weight. Those who lost the weight without trying were three times more likely to die.[125] Protein levels are checked with a blood test for serum *albumin*. This level should be 4.0 g/dL or higher. Lower levels raise the risk of death in people on PD or HD.[126] Low cholesterol levels in people on dialysis can also mean poor nutrition.[127]

Malnutrition can be treated. Often, the first step is to try to get the patient to eat more. If this does not work, protein drinks, powders, or bars may be tried. Many protein options are on the market, and some are made just for dialysis. They have calories and protein, with less sodium, potassium, and phosphorus. Only products the patient will eat or drink will help. If supplements do not work, there are other options, which may require medical justification for Medicare or other insurance coverage:

- A feeding tube placed in the stomach
- *Intradialytic parenteral nutrition* (IDPN) – IV feeding during dialysis of a fluid that may have carbohydrates, protein, fat, sugars, and amino acids
- *Total parenteral nutrition* (TPN) – IV feedings (similar to IDPN) that provide all or most of a patient's nutrition

Malnourished patients can be helped with a team approach. YOU are a key link between patients and the rest of the team. Keep a close eye on changes in target weight. Listen to what patients say about what they eat and drink, and share what you learn with the team. Finding and treating malnutrition early can help save your patients' lives.

How You Can Help Your Patients Eat Better

At each treatment, ask your patients how they are eating. Tell the dietitian and nurse if there is any change in appetite, how food tastes, or GI problems (feeling full after very little food, constipation, diarrhea, bloating, heartburn, nausea, or vomiting). Be mindful of the words you use and your body language. Share that you are asking because you care. No adult likes to be nagged or talked to as a child.

- Ask your patients how well they are eating.
- Tell the dietitian and social worker if a patient is missing meals due to treatment times or cannot pay for food, get to a grocery store to buy food, or cook.
- Tell the dietitian and nurse when a patient often comes in for a treatment below target weight. Any unplanned weight loss or loss of energy may suggest nutrition concerns.
- Tell the dietitian if patients with diabetes say they do not eat or cannot keep their blood sugar in control.
- Tell the nurse and dietitian if a patient gains a lot of water weight between treatments.
- Encourage patients to follow their prescribed meal plans.
- Remind patients to take their binders with meals and snacks, and other drugs and nutritional supplements as prescribed.
- Encourage patients to come for their treatments and stay for the whole time.
- Know your patients' meal plans.
  Not all patients have the same limits. Listen when the dietitian talks to the patient, read the chart notes, and look at the labs.

Obesity

In the U.S., 2 out of 3 adults are overweight with a body mass index (BMI) of 25–29.9. And, 1 out of 3 adults are obese, with a BMI > 30. Five percent of those are extremely obese with a BMI > 40.[128] While some studies suggest that a slightly higher BMI may improve survival in CKD patients, obesity is a risk factor for wound healing and poor overall outcomes with kidney transplant. For this reason, a BMI > 35 may keep a patient from qualifying for a transplant.[129] Patients with BMI > 40 can cause extra challenges in the clinic, especially if they cannot walk and need help to transfer into the dialysis chair. In some cases, larger chairs may be needed for the patient to have a comfortable treatment.

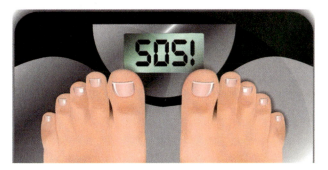

Figure 19: Patient Weight

Even obese patients may still be protein malnourished, and finding the right nutrition prescription can be challenging. The dietitian will work with the team and the patient to come up with a plan that will work best for that patient.

Fluid Intake and Water Weight

"My husband has steadily lost weight while on dialysis—maybe a kilo a month. When we notice that his blood pressure is "high" for him when he is coming off runs, and stays that way for a week or so, we know it is time to drop his target weight, so we set his goal for about .5 kilo less. If he does not feel any of the symptoms of low blood pressure, we know he needed to take it off."

NOTE: As you have learned, dialysis removes wastes and excess water. Patients may drink many kinds of liquids, or eat foods that contain liquid. For the purposes of the *Core Curriculum*, we call liquids that patients drink or eat "*fluids*," and liquid that we remove "*water*."

Most dialysis patients may make little or no urine, but some patients *do* make urine, especially when they first start treatment. Their kidneys are still removing some water. **Ask patients if they make urine**. If they do, tell the nurse. The amount of urine they make may need to be measured so their treatments can be adjusted to be safe and comfortable. Trying to remove too much water during dialysis can cause severe muscle cramps and blood pressure drops. These symptoms can make treatment so painful that people may want to stop doing dialysis. In fact, sudden death on dialysis peaks during the first month of treatment—and choosing to stop dialysis peaks in the second month.[130]

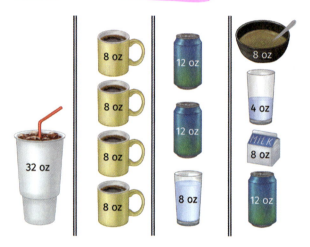

Figure 20: Examples of 4 Cups (32 oz) of Liquid

Patients who do not make urine must have much more water removed by dialysis. Most patients on standard in-center HD who do not make *much* urine must limit their fluid intake, often to the volume of urine output plus 1 liter (4 cups). Patients who make *no* urine may *only* be able to drink 4 cups of fluid per day (see Figure 20). *Foods* that are liquid at room temperature, like Jell-O, ice cream, or popsicles, count as fluids (see Figure 21). See Table 6 to see how much fluid is in some common foods and drinks.

Before each treatment, you will set an amount of water to remove on the dialysis machine. In a perfect world, each treatment removes just the amount of water the patient gained between treatments. As you will learn, knowing just how much to remove at each treatment is a fine art.

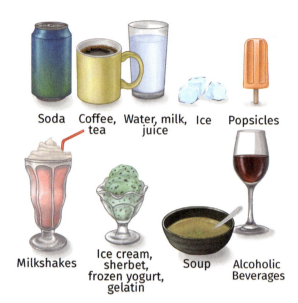

Figure 21: Examples of Different Types of Fluids

TARGET OR DRY WEIGHT

Target weight is a patient's weight after a treatment when all (or most) excess water is gone. In some clinics the term "dry weight" may be used instead. People at their true target weight should feel well, have no excess water or trouble breathing, and need few—if any—blood pressure pills. Each patient's target weight must be adjusted often, because people on dialysis tend to lose real weight (muscle) and replace it with water weight over time. Weight is measured in kilograms (kg); one kilogram is 2.2 pounds (lbs).

Patients on standard HD need to know what can happen if they drink or eat too much fluid:

- **In the short term, if a treatment removes too much water, or removes it too quickly, the patient's blood pressure will drop** (*hypotension*). Painful cramps can then occur in any muscle. The patient may feel dizzy, have a headache, and pass out or throw up. S/he may feel "washed out" and ill for hours after the treatment.

- **Removing a lot of water in a short time can cause *organ stunning*—tissue damage due to lack of blood flow and oxygen**. The heart is a muscle, too, and lack of blood will cause damage.

- **If not enough water can be removed during treatment**, the patient must try to be even more strict with his or her fluid intake until the next treatment. If this is over a weekend, the task is nearly impossible. Options to remove extra water include adding time to that treatment or adding another treatment that week.
- **In the long term, leaving too much water in the body** can worsen *left ventricular hypertrophy* (LVH), a leading cause of death on standard in-center HD.[38]

The body is used to *euvolemia* (normal water balance kept by the kidneys). Trying to recreate this balance without pulling off too much water too quickly or leaving too much in the blood may be the greatest challenge for people on in-center HD and the staff who care for them. Your clinic will have a policy for the ideal water weight gain between treatments (for example, 3% or less of their body weight) (see Table 5). Do not blame patients for gaining too much water weight: *work with them to find solutions*. Table 6, Measurement Conversions, may help you to show them how much fluid is in what they eat or drink.

SODIUM MODELING – A DYING PRACTICE
Sodium modeling was the practice of changing the amount of sodium in the dialysate during an HD treatment. This did help to remove more water, but also left high levels of sodium in the blood (far more than patients could ever possibly eat). High blood sodium levels (*hypernatremia*) then trigger the thirst drive in the brain, so patients *have* to drink—which starts a vicious cycle.[131] Most U.S. clinics have stopped using sodium modeling for this reason.

HOW YOU CAN HELP YOUR PATIENTS GAIN LESS WATER WEIGHT
How much weight each patient can gain between treatments will vary, but blood pressure checks and watching for signs of *edema* (swelling) in the feet, face, and hands are the same for all patients.
- Urge your patients to follow their fluid limits and teach them how to relate how much they drink to how they feel—such as shortness of breath, swelling, and cramps.
- Talk to your patients about limiting salt, which will make them thirsty. Ask if they know how to read food labels to look for sodium content by serving. No? Ask the dietitian to help.
- If patients have a scale at home, teach them to weigh themselves each day and know how much they can safely gain. Change kilograms to pounds for them.
- If a patient is not able to get to target weight at each treatment, document the reason why and talk to the nurse and dietitian to see what can be done to help. Remember, more hours of HD means slower, gentler water removal.
- Ask the dietitian to share tips to help manage fluids.
- Ask the doctor or nurse if any medicines the patient takes has the side effect of dry mouth or thirst.
- Avoid pulling so much water that you need to give saline to get blood pressure up. The extra sodium will make patients thirsty so they have to drink more after dialysis.

Table 5: Weight Gain by Body Weight

Target Weight (TW) in Kilograms (Kg)	3% TW (Kg)	5% TW (Kg)
45	1.4	2.3
50	1.5	2.5
55	1.7	2.8
60	1.8	3.0
65	2.0	3.3
70	2.1	3.5
75	2.3	3.8
80	2.4	4.0
85	2.6	4.3
90	2.7	4.5
95	2.9	4.8
100	3.0	5.0
105	3.2	5.3
110	3.3	5.5
115	3.5	5.8
120	3.6	6.0
125	3.8	6.3
130	3.9	6.5
135	4.1	6.8
140	4.2	7.0
145	4.4	7.3
150	4.5	7.5

Table 6: Measurement Conversions

Food/Drink	Ounces	mL	Household Measure
Quart (a bit less than 1 liter)	32	960	4 cups
Soda pop (1 can)	12	360	1 and 1/2 cups
Coffee, tea			
■ Large	16	480	2 cups
■ Medium	12	360	1 and 1/2 cups
■ Small	8	240	1 cup
Milk (1 small carton)	8	240	1 cup
Milkshake			
■ Large	16	480	2 cups
■ Medium	12	360	1 and 1/2 cups
■ Small	8	240	1 cup
Ice cream	4	120	1/2 cup
Sherbet	4	120	1/2 cup
Soup	8	240	1 cup
Wine	4	120	1/2 cup
Beer (1 can or bottle)	12	360	1 and 1/2 cups
Popsicle			
■ Single popsicle/fudgsicle®	1.65	49	3 tablespoons
■ Double Creamsicle	2.5	74	1/3 cup
Ice cube (household, 8 pieces)	4	120	1/2 cup
Ice chips	4	120	1/2 cup

Sodium

"Stay away from processed foods! I cook everything from scratch, so I have control over the sodium content of what I eat. For dinner I will marinate some boneless chicken and throw it on the grill, and have it with perhaps some green beans, and bread."

Sodium is a major part of table salt, and most Americans eat too much salt. In fact, U.S. Dietary Guidelines 2015 for the general public suggest a limit of less than 2,300 mg of sodium per day—less than 1 teaspoon.[132] This level can be reached if we avoid table salt, canned foods, packaged "helper" foods, pickled foods, or preserved meats such as cold cuts, sausages, and hot dogs. Encourage your patients to read food labels and try no-salt herbs and spices like basil, lemon pepper, Mrs. Dash®, Chef Paul Prudhomme's™ Magic Savory Blends, or Lawry's® Salt-free 17 seasoning. Since all foods have small amounts of sodium, it is impossible to avoid *all* salt in the diet. But, people on HD should avoid:

■ Table salt

■ Most salt substitutes (they may have potassium)

■ Sea salt—it is still salt

■ Salty processed foods. Foods in a can, bottle, box, or bag are processed; some more than others.

A long list of ingredients with chemical names is a good clue that a food is highly processed. Processed meats like bacon and lunch meat raise patients' blood pressure much more than fresh meats.[133]

Sodium causes thirst and, as you learned, plays a key role in high blood pressure and fluid weight gain. Sodium in the blood attracts water, which leads to swelling. When the kidneys fail, they stop removing excess sodium. Patients who limit sodium in their diet tend to be less thirsty. This makes it easier for them to drink less, too. Patients must take in less sodium *and* fluid if:

■ They have swelling (*edema*) in the face, hands, or feet

■ Their blood pressure rises

■ They gain water weight quickly

Potassium

Patients who get good dialysis should have a range of serum potassium (3.5–5.0 mEq/L) if they limit what they eat and drink.[70] They can learn to eat fewer high-potassium foods like avocados, mangos, bananas, oranges, dried fruit, melon, dried peas and beans, tomato sauce, potatoes, salt substitute, espresso, or cappuccino (see Figure 22). Chewing tobacco can have a lot of potassium. Patients who drink orange juice can switch to apple, cranberry, or Sunny D®, which are low in potassium. They might eat pasta or rice, not potatoes. But, these limits are still a big challenge for most.

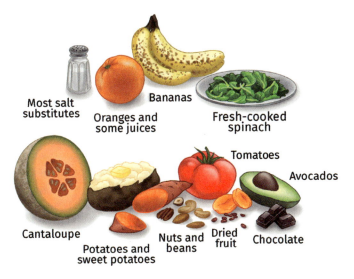

Figure 22: Examples of High-Potassium Foods

It is vital for patients to read food labels. By 2018, most food labels will have to list potassium, but, until then, some food labels must list it while others may not.[134] Not listing potassium on a label does not mean that a food or drink does not contain it. Many foods now have less salt—but more potassium. For example, Campbell's® Chunky Healthy Request® Chicken Noodle soup has 850 mg of potassium in just a 1-cup serving! Many energy, vitamin, and mineral drinks and waters have a lot of added potassium. Fresh meats or chicken may be injected with potassium to give them a longer shelf life.

Patients also need to learn portion sizes. One apple is okay—but eating three or four could cause a problem. Fruits and vegetables are most often limited to 4–5 servings a day. This is tailored for each patient and may change based on the monthly lab results.

The dialysate may have more or less potassium (K) to meet a patient's needs. Note your patients' prescriptions when you talk about potassium. Patients who have *low* potassium levels may dialyze with a higher K dialysate (K 3.0 mEq/L), and may *not* have a potassium limit in their diet.

> **Facts Patients Need to Know about Potassium**
> - Too much potassium can cause sudden death.
> - Symptoms of high potassium include muscle weakness— like trouble walking, skipped heartbeats, and cardiac arrest.
> - Most salt substitutes have potassium and should *not* be used.
> - Potassium is at its highest level after a weekend—the longest span between in-center HD treatments.
> - Patients who do not get enough HD are at a higher risk for *hyperkalemia* (high potassium).
> - A drug called kayexalate may be used for a short time in some patients to lower potassium levels between treatments. There is a black box warning from the U.S. Food and Drug Administration about possible digestive tract problems with this drug.
> - Veltassa® is a drug that can be mixed with water and taken by mouth to lower potassium. The FDA has a boxed warning to take this drug 6 hours apart from other drugs or it could absorb them so they do not work as well.
> - Patients need to know that foods labeled "low salt" may have a lot of potassium.

Calcium

When the kidneys fail, they become less able to convert vitamin D into its active form or to keep calcium and phosphorus (bone minerals) in balance. Too little active vitamin D and bone minerals that are out of balance lead to *mineral bone disorder* (MBD) (See page 33.)

To help prevent MBD, KDOQI™ guidelines say to keep the serum calcium levels of people with stage 5 CKD at the lower end of normal (8.4–9.5 mg/dL).[135] CMS rules say that calcium levels must be kept under 10.2 mg/dL.[136] A patient's albumin level can affect his or her serum calcium, so, if a patient has a low albumin level, s/he may need a change in the amount of calcium prescribed in the treatment plan. Patients' total calcium intake (diet and binders) should be ≤ 1,000 mg per day.[70]

Phosphorus

"I was having great difficulty paying for my meds. I hit the Medicare donut hole by March and spent the rest of the year playing a game I called "Begging for Binders!" Then, I switched to home hemo. Within 2 months my phosphorus levels were down below 4.0 and I was able to cut the number of binders I was taking to 3–4 a day instead of 12–14 a day."

Standard in-center HD removes *some* phosphorus—but not much. And, since many foods contain phosphorus, most patients who do standard in-center HD must limit foods that have a lot of phosphorus. These include dairy products, cola, dried beans or legumes, whole grains, nuts, and many processed foods (see Figure 23).

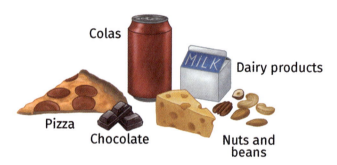

Figure 23: Examples of High-Phosphorus Foods

A common phosphorus diet limit is 800–1,000 mg/day.[70] Dietitians work with patients to make a meal plan that will meet their needs. Today, there is a lot more phosphorus in our food from additives, flavor enhancers, and preservatives. While 40% to 60% of phosphorus found in real foods like meat and dairy is absorbed, 100% of added phosphate may be absorbed.[137] And, since food makers are not required to list phosphorus on labels, patients need to learn to look for long words with "phosphate" in them and avoid these foods. Serum phosphorus levels should stay between 3.0–4.5 mg/dL.[70] Elevated phosphorus levels, called hyperphosphatemia, are linked to MBD—and a higher risk of death.[134]

Help Your Patients Manage Phosphorus

Share these tips with your patients:

- Never skip or shorten treatments—standard in-center HD does remove *some* phosphorus, so it helps to get every minute of treatment the doctor prescribes.
- Follow a low-phosphorus diet.
- Be aware of phosphorus on food labels. Look for words like "phosphate" or "phosphoric acid" and avoid or limit foods that have these.
- Avoid highly processed foods and fast foods that have the most added phosphorus.
- Take binders *with* meals and snacks. To work, they need to be in the gut at the same time as the food. If you are not taking them, work with the team to find a binder you will use.
- If you cannot afford the prescribed binder, the doctor may be able to prescribe a less costly one. Or, the social worker may be able to find help to pay for it.
- Do not like to take binders? Think about doing a type of treatment that removes more phosphorus so you do not need them.

Phosphate binders are medicines used to keep phosphorus from being absorbed. They work by bonding with phosphorus from food so it passes harmlessly out of the body in the stool. For this reason, binders must be taken *with* meals and snacks—they must be in the gut at the same time as the food. Since binders can cause constipation, the nephrologist may prescribe a stool softener. Other patients may have problems with diarrhea or trouble swallowing their binders. Tell the nurse or dietitian if the patient complains. A different binder may work better for that patient. Table 7 is provided so you can recognize the names of common binders in case your patients talk about them or report side effects.

Table 7: Common Phosphate Binders

Brand Name	Generic Name	Binder Form(s)
PhosLo®	Calcium acetate	Capsule, tablet
Tums®	Calcium carbonate	Liquid, tablet, chewable, capsule, gum
Renagel®	Sevelamer-HCl	Tablet
Renvela®	Sevelamer carbonate	Tablet, powder
Fosrenal®	Lanthanum carbonate	Wafer, chewable, powder
Velphoro®	Sucroferric oxyhydroxide	Chewable tablet
Auryxia®	Ferric citrate	Tablet

Vitamins

Dialysis removes some water-soluble vitamins, so patients may need to take supplements. But high doses of some vitamins are not safe for people on dialysis. See Table 8 for a list of water-soluble vitamins that may be removed by dialysis and fat-soluble vitamins that will not be. For example, patients may be asked to take:

- 60–100 mg of vitamin C
- 1–5 mg of folate
- 2 mg of vitamin B6
- 3 µg of vitamin B12

Patients need to talk to their doctor, dietitian, or pharmacist before they take *any* over-the-counter vitamins, herbs, folk, or home remedies. Healthy kidneys remove many products from the body. People on dialysis may build up toxic levels of these products in the blood.

Table 8: Water-Soluble and Fat-Soluble Vitamins

Water-Soluble Vitamins Dialysis May Remove These	Fat-Soluble Vitamins Dialysis Will Not Remove These
- Biotin - Folacin - Niacin - Pantothenic acid - Riboflavin (B2) - Thiamin - Vitamin B6 - Vitamin B12 - Vitamin C	- Vitamin A - Vitamin D - Vitamin E - Vitamin K

The Person with Kidney Failure

Helping Patients Cope

"When I found out about my kidneys, I had a breakdown and started drinking. They had given me such restrictions on food and everything, I snapped. I started partying and my husband left me. I lost custody of my daughter, started doing drugs, and had a rocky 5 years of total self-destruction. I quit drugs at 25 and have been clean since then. Twenty years ago, they told me I would have to start dialysis in 3 months, but I actually started last year. I am on PD now and at peace with dialysis, and working on my tests for transplant."

Dialysis can cause many problems for patients. Working, eating, sleeping—even planning daily life around dialysis—can be a huge challenge for patients and their families. People whose kidneys fail often have many serious questions, such as:

- Am I going to die?
- Will I lose my job?
- Will my life be worth living?
- Can I still work and take care of my family?
- How will this impact my sex life?
- Can I still have a baby?
- Will my partner leave me?
- Will I be able to pay for my treatment?
- Will I ever feel better?
- Why me?

It is common for patients to have strong feelings about dialysis. They may move from anger to depression to fear and back. In time, they may come to accept their new lives—or they may not. How each patient copes depends on factors like personality, support from family and friends, and other life events and health problems. All clinic staff will see patients who are under severe stress at some point. You and your fellow technicians will spend the most time with patients. So, you are key to helping them cope with their kidney disease and dialysis.

Patients who are just starting treatment tend to be very fearful, in part due to the unknown. When they learn what to expect and start to feel better, they may feel more hopeful again, and grateful that they are alive. This can be a sort of "honeymoon period." During this time, patients may keep up with things they liked to do and start to plan again for the future.

When the long-term nature of kidney failure and the ongoing demands of treatment sink in, patients may feel angry and depressed all over again. This may also happen if there are health setbacks or problems during a treatment. Patients react not only to their real losses but also to *possible* losses—what they believe their future would have been like if they had not become ill. They may resent having to depend on machines, the care team, and their families. You can ask the social worker to help you support and encourage patients who are having a hard time.

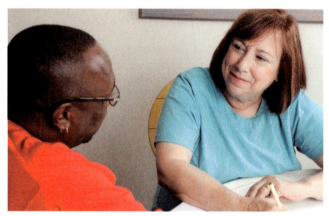

Figure 24: Social Worker

Life Changes and Empathy

In many ways, people on in-center HD may feel set apart from others. They may not be able to keep the same schedules that they used to, or spend time with family and friends as often as they would like. They may have to take many pills throughout the day, which reminds them that they are "sick" and may have side effects. They may have to severely limit the liquids they drink each day. They may not be able to eat pizza or French fries when out with their friends. The ethnic meals they used to share with their families may be off-limits. Having to learn totally new ways to eat and cook is a huge day-to-day burden. Almost all of us would have a very hard time dealing with major life changes like these!

Patients may react to the changes in their lives by withdrawing, leaving dialysis early, or missing treatments. They may act hostile, dependent, or demanding. Beneath these behaviors is a grieving process for the loss of the way things used to be. Try to keep this in mind when patients are rude or mean.

One important way to help patients adjust to the life changes of kidney disease and dialysis is to use *empathy*: put yourself in your patients' "shoes" and think about how you might react if your kidneys failed. Think about these questions:

- What would it feel like to be told that you need dialysis for the rest of your life (or a kidney transplant that could be years away or may never come?
- What adjustments would you need to make to your job and your routine?
- How would this news change your plans for your future?
- How would it feel to have to sit still for hours at a time three times a week to get in-center HD, and have to rely on dialysis technicians and the team for your care?
- What changes would dialysis make to your schedule, your activities, your friends and your family?
- Think about your favorite foods: how many would be off-limits or severely restricted?
- What would it be like to have to take many medicines every day?
- How much fluid do you drink every day? What would it feel like to have to drastically reduce that amount?
- How would you feel if you were told your access is your lifeline and the person caring for you infiltrated your access, and your arm was swollen, bruised, and painful?

Would you be sad, in shock, or angry, if you had to make these changes? Having empathy can help you to understand why patients may be coping as they are with kidney disease and dialysis. **Do not take patients' feelings personally**. They are not about you.

At times, the clinic may be the only safe place for patients to show that they feel sad or angry. Or, they may hide sadness or fear under anger or hostility. Anger—though it seems aimed at you—is most often about other things in their lives. **Never show anger to your patients**. You cannot control how you feel, but you *can* control how you act. As a caregiver, always act in a calm, accepting, and professional way. Never argue with a patient. If a patient confronts you, seek help from the charge nurse, social worker, or other staff. You will find that most people will act with respect when you treat them with respect. Treat your patients and fellow staff members the way you would like to be treated.

When you are having a tough day, remind yourself that patients must cope with many difficult things. Resist the urge to give advice and try to solve their problems. You go home to your own life at the end of the shift. Patients must take kidney failure, and the limits of their illness, home with them.

Money Concerns

"Financially it was devastating. We didn't have a huge income to begin with, but once I was on dialysis and could no longer go out to work at my job, things became tight! We knew things would change eventually, so we had put away a little money, but it wasn't enough. We learned to be even more frugal..."

Many people on dialysis have money problems. Their bills do not stop just because their kidneys did. Disability or retirement pays most people only about one third as much as a job. Patients also need to buy special foods, costly drugs, and get to and from the clinic three times a week if they choose in-center HD. Talk to your patients. If they cannot afford food or their medicines, tell the social worker. Food insecurity—not having enough to eat—can be common among people on dialysis.[138]

The social worker knows about local resources that may be able to help. However, these programs rely on donations and may have limits. Do not *promise* patients that the social worker can solve their financial problems. It is best if working-age patients work so they are more active and earn money. Care team members can encourage patients to work and be as active as possible. Vocational rehabilitation programs in your state may help patients who need to go back to school or change jobs due to dialysis.

Travel

"I recently went to Atlanta for my daughter's wedding and had to travel 45 minutes to a clinic across town when there were two right in the neighborhood where we stayed. It worked out but was not very convenient."

Some standard in-center HD patients do travel. As a dialysis technician, you can encourage your patients to take trips. The more active they are, the better they can feel. Most dialysis companies have a way to match patients with clinics when they travel. The social worker or charge nurse can give patients information about how to arrange for "transient" dialysis when they leave their home clinic.

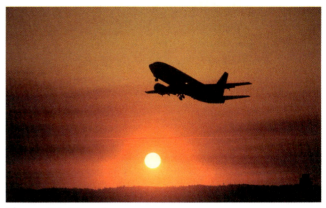

Figure 25: Travel

There can be challenges for HD patients who want to travel, though. Not all clinics have the space or staff to care for transient patients. The best way to assure space is to plan far in advance—so, encourage patients to talk to the social worker as soon as they are thinking about going somewhere. Some health plans or state Medicaid programs will not pay for out-of-network care. So, those patients will need to pay for part or all of their treatments away from home, *plus* their trip. If patients leave the country, they may have to pay for all of the costs of dialysis. Medicare does not cover in-center dialysis outside the U.S. and its territories, but other health plans may. One company, Dialysis at Sea, offers dialysis cruises. Some patients love them, but they can be very expensive.

Some patients are also afraid to travel, because they trust *you* to put in their needles—and they do not trust techs they do not know. If you teach your patients how to put in their *own* needles, you can give them back the world! When they always have their best cannulator with them, they are not afraid to take a vacation or go to a wedding or graduation. As a bonus, their accesses may last longer.

"Check everything: the type of dialyzer, dialysate being used, needle size, pump speed, time of run, amount of EPO, and so on. You need to be somewhat flexible. Most clinics do try hard to accommodate your schedule and requests. Sometimes changes are necessary, but LET THEM KNOW if something is not acceptable or dangerous to your health."

Patients who get transplants have a much easier time traveling, and just take their medicines with them. PD is portable and can be taken along for travel. Home HD with a small machine can also make travel easier. Patients who love to travel may want to think about these options.

"My husband is on nocturnal hemo 6 nights a week. We travel and love it. It just means we have to go to a clinic 3 times a week instead of being at home. We watch his diet very close while on vacation."

Body Image

"I feel self-conscious when I'm out in public, because being sick has left me looking frail and skinny, and no matter what I do I can't gain weight. Trust me on this one, my dietitian has tried! Feeling this way about myself has left me kind of antisocial."

Body image concerns are common for people on dialysis. They may worry about scars, skin problems, hair loss, and weak muscles. They may think that their fistulas, grafts, or PD catheters are ugly. Sometimes, HD patients may not even want a graft or fistula because of this.

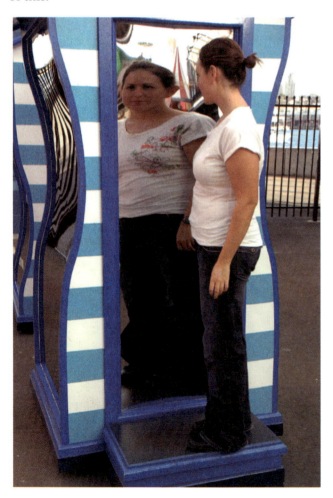

Figure 26: Body Image

"I have a very large fistula on my left arm. I work with young children and one day made the mistake of wearing a short-sleeved shirt and one of the kids got so scared he started to cry. There is nothing more damaging to your self image than to have a child cry just by looking at you. So now I wear long-sleeved shirts to work no matter what.

If your patients share body image concerns with you, you can let the social worker know. Also, you can tell your patients that it is normal to feel this way, and give them encouragement that no one is perfect: we *all* have scars, whether or not you can see them. Some of the best helpers can be other patients who have come to terms with the changes in their bodies. A patient who looks at his or her fistula as a "battle scar" and is proud of it can really help someone who is still hiding under long sleeves on a hot summer day.

Sexuality and Fertility

"Something worries me about dialysis. Who could possibly love me now? I know it sounds harsh, and I know there are lots of people who go through dialysis with support of loved ones. But I gotta be honest, I'm still young and I still want romance. Who'd want me?"

Patients of *all* ages may have issues about sexuality. Men and women who do standard in-center HD or PD may have problems with sexual function.[139] Medicines like blood pressure pills can cause changes in the level of desire and may cause erectile dysfunction in men. All care team members can remind patients that concerns about sexuality are very normal. The social workers can work with patients or refer them to a specialist who can address these worries. A transplant—or more dialysis—can help with all of these issues.

Younger women may want to have a child, and this can be a challenge. Women on dialysis are less likely to get pregnant. Many do not get their periods any more, and the uterus can *atrophy* (waste away) when women do standard in-center HD.[140] If women do get pregnant, their pregnancies are high-risk—and babies may be born early. Among those who have enough time to wait for a year after a kidney transplant, many have had healthy babies. But, it can take years to get a transplant.

There is hope for women who have always wanted to be mothers and cannot wait for a transplant: get a *lot* more HD. Pregnant women who got 36 or more hours of HD per week had an 85% chance of having a healthy baby; women who got 20 hours of HD or less had only a 48% chance.[141] Of course, it is easier to get this many hours of HD at night during sleep—at home or they may do nocturnal in-center dialysis 3–4 nights a week. But, some women do come in to the clinic five or six days a week to get treatment if they become pregnant. You can tell the nephrologist and dialysis team if patients are interested in having a baby, and work with the team to support and educate patients about this.

"My doctor told me about a patient of his who, against his wishes, had two or three kids while she was a dialysis patient. He said, amazingly, she had no major complications and eventually got a transplant and had MORE kids!!!"

Men may want to father a child. If they are having challenges with desire, erections, or a low sperm count, they may need to ask their doctors to test their hormone levels. Between 26% and 66% of men on dialysis may have too little testosterone, a problem that can be treated.[142]

Patients who do not want to risk a pregnancy should be advised to use birth control. While unwanted pregnancy on dialysis is rare, it does happen.

Pain

"I do suffer from a lot of pain. Tonight is one of those nights. I took two pain pills and three Benadryl® and my sleeping pill. I am still up and in pain at 4:07 am. My dialysis days are my worst pain days it seems and I do try SO hard not to take the pain meds, but at times I have no choice."

As many as 92% of patients on dialysis may be in pain, and, for many, that pain is severe.[143] Pain can come from surgeries, cramps, needle sticks, nerve damage, and bone disease. If patients tell you that they have pain, share this with the nurse, who can help them to get the treatment they need. All dialysis units need to assess patients for pain (see Figure 27), and create a plan for this pain.[73] Technicians can work with nurses and the care team to monitor patient pain and make sure that it is treated.

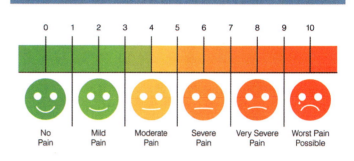

Figure 27: Pain Assessment Scale

Mood

"I was depressed and getting 'keep your chin up' from my doctor. So, I used my employee assistance program at work to find a wonderful counselor. She suggested that I may need an antidepressant. My doctor was much more responsive when I said that another professional recommended medication."

At any given moment, from 23% to 39% of those who receive dialysis may be depressed.[144] People on dialysis who are depressed may seem sad, irritable, or angry—or they may hide their feelings. They are less likely to follow their treatment plans, and far more likely to die.[145] Because depression is such a big problem, social workers must assess all dialysis patients for depression.[73] If you think a patient may be depressed, tell the social worker and nurse. Treatments for depression in dialysis patients include:

- **Antidepressant medicines**[146]
- **Counseling and family support**[147]
- **Exercise**[148]
- **A change of treatment options**[149]

Volunteering to help others, spending time in nature, and having a pet may help with depression, too.

You will not be surprised to learn that many people on dialysis are also anxious. In one small study, nearly half of those on dialysis had an anxiety disorder.[150] You may see patients who get very upset or panic if they or another patient have a problem. The social worker may be able to help patients ease anxiety.

Communication

"As a person with hearing loss, I have made it clear to the staff and my doctors that to ensure my rights to confidentially, I will not discuss any details of my treatment in the clinic. They have to speak louder, and I have NO concept of how far voice travels any more (theirs or mine). So, personal matters need to be discussed in a private office, before or after my treatment."

How you talk with your patients is vital to their care. What you say, do, and your body language are part of the care you provide and the messages you send. Patients see and talk to techs more than any other team member. You have a key role in helping patients cope.

The Health Insurance Portability and Accountability Act (HIPAA) and Patient Confidentiality

HIPAA, which became law in 1996 and took effect in 2003, created national rules about how to guard patient privacy. Your clinic has policies to meet the HIPAA standards, and you will need to learn and follow them. The penalties for those who violate HIPAA include fines and even prison time.

Patients need to feel safe in the clinic and know that their health and personal information is kept confidential. They see and hear everything that goes on around them, and talk to each other about what they hear. They need to know that their health information is taken seriously and not shared with others who do not need to know. Keep written and electronic patient records private, and *never*:

- Talk about a patient when someone else can overhear
- Talk to patients about *other* patients' problems or issues
- Talk about your patients to your own friends or family

Active Listening

Active listening is a way to give patients close attention and to be sure you know what they mean. *To listen actively, look the patient in the eye.* This may mean sitting down next to patients when they are in their chairs. Focus on his or her words, and ask questions. Short, open-ended questions are best. Open-ended questions *cannot be answered with "yes" or "no."* Here are a few examples:

- What does the pain in your feet feel like?
- Tell me more about what you ate yesterday.
- How did you feel when you learned you had to have another access surgery?
- You seem sad when you talk about having to take early retirement. Can you tell me about it?

Watch your patients' body language, facial expressions, and tone of voice. Team members use these clues to help patients share their feelings and to find more information. Asking open-ended questions and giving some time to answer can help patients tell you what is really going on. These types of questions also send a message that you care for and support them.

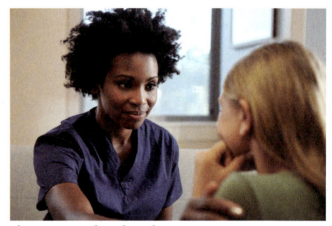

Figure 28: Active Listening

Do not think about what you want to say to the patient while s/he is talking. *Just listen*, and then form your response. Active listening is a skill that takes some time to master, but what you learn will help the whole team better care for each patient—and it will even help you in your own life with the people you care about. Using empathy will also help you to become an active listener.

When it is your turn to talk, try not to say "*You should*," or "*You have to.*" Few adults like being told what they must do, and the sorts of lifestyle changes patients have to make are difficult. Find something positive to say. Be a cheerleader: *"Mrs. H, it's great that you stayed for your whole treatment three times in a row! You can really be proud of that."*

It is *never okay* to yell or curse at a patient, even if someone yells or curses at you. You are a professional. *Listen* to patients, even when they are angry or frustrated. If someone becomes angry or yells, it is okay to say things like:

- *"You seem really angry right now. Is there something you could tell me about what is making you so angry?"*
- *"I am so sorry that ____ didn't go right today. This must be really hard for you."*
- *"I wish you could have (whatever you want), too!"*
- *"Is something bothering you? You seem kind of down today."*

Rehabilitation

When someone has an acute illness, like strep throat, the goal of healthcare is a cure. But a chronic disease like kidney disease will never go away—there *is* no cure. So, the goal of treatment is rehabilitation: helping patients live as normal a life as they can.

People do dialysis so they can feel their best and can keep doing things they enjoy. They may want to care for children or grandkids, stay active in their towns or churches, golf, play music, or keep a job. When patients are on the dialysis machine, it may seem as if they cannot do much. But when they are outside the clinic, they are living their lives—and you can help make that possible.

Self-Management—Not Compliance

You and the care team have a job—to give good care to patients. Patients also have a job: to *self-manage*. Self-management means patients learn to become their own experts and can:

- **Follow their treatment plans** – as partners with their care teams
- **Keep themselves safe** – by knowing how the treatment should be done
- **Recognize and report symptoms** – to avoid serious problems

In a dialysis clinic, a team takes care of patients. But, as you can see from Figure 29, most of the time patients are *not* in the clinic. And, they care for themselves with each bite of food, each drink, each pill they take (or forget to take), each symptom they report (or keep quiet about), and each treatment they go to (or miss). This is self-management in action. Patients need to learn a *lot* about kidney disease and its treatment to do a good job self-managing.

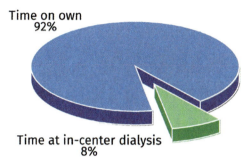

Figure 29: Patient Time In-Center vs. Time on Own in a Typical Week

Most adults like to feel in control, and helping kidney patients to be in control can help them live longer. A large study found that patients who chose their *own* treatment for kidney failure had a 39% lower risk of death than those who relied on the doctor or the care team to choose for them. They were also much more likely to get a transplant.[151]

Note that we have *not* said patients must *comply* or *adhere*. These terms mean that patients need to "take orders" and do what they are told. They also suggest that medical professionals are the experts and patients are the passive recipients of our expert knowledge who must do what we tell them. But, we need to remember that patients can (and should) be very active participants in their care—and CMS gives them that right.

In the clinic, *you* can help patients to feel more in control. When patients believe their families and caregivers—like you—think they can do well, they believe it, too—and they are even more likely to keep their jobs.[152] Your clinic staff can urge patients to do as much as they can. Patients may be able to:

- Track their blood test results in a notebook or on a computer
- Make good food choices
- Wash their fistula or graft
- Learn to put in their own needles
- Weigh themselves and write down the number
- Calculate how much fluid to remove at each treatment
- Check their dialyzer with a staff member
- Check their machine settings and dialysate

- Run their whole treatment
- Tell the staff about any symptoms they have
- Know what each of their pills is for and how to take them as prescribed

Patient Education: Creating Expert Patients

To feel their best, patients need to stay positive, learn all they can, and take action to follow their care plans. All of this can be summed up in three words:

1. **Attitude** – looking on the bright side, being grateful to be alive
2. **Answers** – learning what they need to know to care for themselves
3. **Action** – staying involved in the world and keeping physically fit

Attitude

"Scars, scars, and more scars, but I'm still me!! I have had 27 surgeries since the age of 10. I have scars on my arms, legs, belly, neck, you name it. Do not worry about them. They are who makes you, you! Call them war scars of life!!! They show how strong a person you are, and what makes you unique—your awesome one-of-a-kind self!!!"

Social workers and nurses play major roles in teaching new patients and helping to address their fears. You, too, are a key staff person who can help patients stay positive:

- **Be positive yourself**. As the saying goes, "Attitudes are contagious—is yours worth catching?" Be *excited* when patients tell you they have done something new. Praise their efforts, even if they do not succeed on the first try.
- ***Expect* patients to keep doing the things they love**. Some patients believe that since they are "sick" they can no longer sing in the choir, tend a garden, raise puppies, work, etc. Since kidney failure will not go away, we need to challenge these beliefs. Ask, "*Why not?*" when patients tell you they cannot do something.
- **Share success stories**. Give patients some examples (with no names) of what others with kidney failure have done. Maybe someone traveled to visit grandchildren, planned a family reunion, or started a business. A newsletter or bulletin board can highlight patient achievements and inspire others to try new things.
- **Teach patients to help with their treatments**. Self-care is a powerful tool to build hope. Chronic illness can make patients feel as if they have lost all control of their lives. Getting back some control by taking part in treatment, even if at first their role is very small, can build self-esteem. Small successes build confidence so patients feel they can take on bigger challenges.
- **Talk to patients and find out what they value most**. Use this to help motivate them to work harder toward a goal.
- **Be a "holder of hope."** Patients cannot always see the light at the end of the tunnel. They have never walked this path before. Staff can hold out the hope that the patient will begin to feel better in a month or two and share examples of others who have done so.

Answers

"It's very scary when you begin. It's all so new—the whole world of dialysis—and if you have good techs and nurses who empower you, then you can learn about the process and how you can make your life healthier and easier."

As someone who spends a lot of time with patients, you must be able to reinforce what patients are taught by other team members. So, you need to know about CKD and its treatments.

Patients will ask you questions. Be sure not to give answers or advice that are beyond your scope of practice. It is okay not to know an answer; no one knows everything. But, it is *not* okay to give a patient an answer that is not true. If you do not know an answer, refer the patient to the right member of the care team, as seen in Table 9.

To help you become a better "teacher," read on to learn some key points about how adults, including your patients, learn new information.

Table 9: Questions for the Care Team

For Questions About...	Ask the...
What to eat or drink, or blood test values	**Dietitian**
Keeping a job, coping with dialysis, relationship or body image concerns, Medicare, insurance, or local resources	**Social worker**
Dialysis side effects, other treatment options, symptoms, changes in health status	**Nurse**
Medicines (including how to take them and their side effects), dialysis prescription, transplant	**Nephrologist**

READINESS

Adults learn only when they are ready. They cannot take in what you tell them if they are afraid or in pain. For example, you might see that the dietitian does not try to talk to patients about what to eat while you are putting in needles.

Hope is the first step in learning. *Patients need to have hope that they can still have a good life.* In one study, patients who were more hopeful were less depressed and anxious, and did not feel their kidney disease was as much of a burden.[153] You can see why they might be better able to learn, too.

Patients who are afraid—who worry that they will die or have a poor quality of life—cannot learn. *When adrenaline from the "fight or flight" reflex kicks in, learning is impossible.*[154] They may also think that what you tell them does not matter, since they are just going to die anyway. But, some people live 20 or 30 years or more on dialysis—a fact you can share that may give patients hope.

When patients first start treatment, they may be too ill or scared to learn much. Watch for signs that patients may be ready to learn:
- They might show less fear.
- They might start to ask questions.

NEED

Adults learn only what they feel they *need* to know—what is relevant to them *right now*. The nurse will assess what patients want and need to know, and then write a teaching plan. For example, a nurse or doctor would not talk about transplant in detail at a patient's first dialysis treatment. Rather, they might focus on the machine, the steps of the treatment, the need to check vital signs, and the symptoms to watch for.

LANGUAGE LEVEL

All learning must be tailored to the learner. If Ms. Brown has a PhD in science, staff will explain how the dialyzer works quite differently than they would for Ms. Green, who did not finish high school. The only way for staff to know patients' educational background is to ask them—*never assume*.

The right level includes how patients see, read, hear, and understand the language. Sometimes we are so eager to get our message across that we forget about things like language and reading level. It does an 86-year-old woman who speaks only Polish little good to get a detailed pamphlet written in English.

As the staff person who talks most to patients, you can help ensure that they receive information in a way they can understand. Listen to patients' questions and how they answer your questions. If you can tell that there is a language, hearing, vision, or reading barrier, tell the nurse. Once they know of a problem, the team can work on a solution.

Even if someone has a lot of schooling, he or she may not know the meaning of complex medical terms. Think of some of the words we use each day in dialysis. They may sound like a foreign language: fistula, phosphorus, pruritus, cannulate, dialyze, nephrology, etc. Most patients do not know what *any* of these words mean. Explain medical terms when you use them and try to use plain, simple language as much as you can. Better yet, use pictures, brochures, or videos for patients.

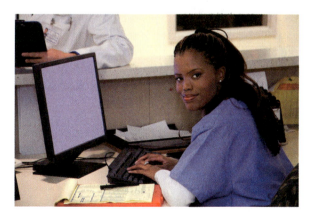

Figure 30: Dialysis Technician

REPEAT, REPEAT, REPEAT

Patients may be told so much at once that it can be hard for them to remember it all. Most people need to see a concept 5–8 times before they learn it. This means teaching must be *repeated* to be learned. It is common for patients to say that they "never heard that" when you know you told them. If they are uremic, they may not remember. Try not to get frustrated when this happens. Stay calm and keep trying.

BELIEF

To learn from the care team, patients must:

- Believe that what the staff is trying to teach them is true
- Believe that it will help them
- Believe that learning it will improve their lives

Bone disease is a good example of how patient beliefs can make a difference. Patients are at risk for a long-term complication they cannot yet feel—so they may not believe there is a problem. They are asked to take (and pay for) drugs that do not make them feel any better, and may even have side effects. So patients may not believe these drugs really work. You can see why they may not follow their treatment plans. Good communication about things like the meaning of blood tests can help people believe that they need to take good care of themselves, even when they cannot feel a change right now.

Beliefs are even more vital when you deal with patients from other cultures. Often they have very different "truths" about health, illness, and the effects of some remedies. If you think a patient's religion or culture affects his or her dialysis, talk to the nurse. The team, family, and clergy can be called upon to help find answers.

The team will assess patients to see if they are ready and able to learn, and make a plan to help them learn what they need. Share any clues or tips you learn from working with the patient with the other team members.

Think about how much you must learn to become a technician. Patients *also* need to know a lot to live well with kidney failure. All staff members can help patients learn. As a technician, you can help in these ways:

- **Talk about what you are doing as you do it.** Even if patients do not ask questions, you can tell them how the machine works, what the alarms are for, how the alarms protect them, what the dialyzer does, etc. Use simple, clear language when you do this.
- **Be "askable."** Take a moment to answer patients' questions or tell them when you can talk to them in more detail. If you do not know an answer, never guess. Refer the question to another staff person or learn the right answer.
- **Ask patients simple "quiz" questions.** If you have been telling a patient about the machine, you might ask what the dialyzer does. Say that you want to be sure you explained this well enough to them.
- **Share patient questions or misconceptions with the nurse or social worker.** If the team pools its knowledge about what patients ask about, and what they do and do not know, you will be able to help patients learn more.

Action

Staying active in life includes things like keeping a job, volunteering, or exercising. Work is a source of income, identity, and self-esteem. Those who work may have a health plan and paid vacation time. Patients who are just starting dialysis may suffer from uremic symptoms and not know that they can feel better in a few weeks. They may quit their jobs and go on disability, which can make it very hard to return to work later. If you get a sense that a patient is thinking about stopping work, encourage him or her to talk with social worker.

KEEPING A JOB

"I'm 49 and have worked 50-60 hour weeks most of my adult life. Part of me is dog tired physically, mentally and spiritually, and that part screams, 'Thank God, a chance to rest.' Another part says, 'Okay, but I don't want to sit in the recliner and watch TV and wait for my next Big D session.' And…could we make it financially with me on disability and my wife working?"

Fewer than 1 in 3 working-age, in-center HD patients keep a job.[155] But, keeping a job is much easier than finding a new one. Helping patients keep their jobs and health plans is a win-win for the patient and the clinic. Why? A clinic's "payer mix" is the blend of Medicare only, Medicare plus Medicaid, and employer group health plans (EGHPs) that pay for dialysis. *Clinics that support working patients have a payer mix with*

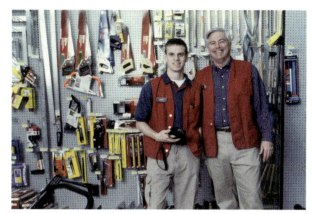

Figure 31: Working

more EGHP payers. These bring more money into the clinic than Medicare.

Clinic barriers, like schedule problems, can force patients to quit their jobs. Clinics can remove these barriers by:

- Adding evening or early morning shifts
- Offering home treatments or in-center nocturnal shifts
- Letting working patients "bump" other patients to get the shift they need

Urge patients who are working or in school to continue. Patients who are willing and able to work but do not have jobs will need help from the social worker and a vocational rehabilitation agency. Others who are too old, too ill, or cannot work may still be able to pursue hobbies, travel, or exercise.

STAYING FIT

In a study of more than 20,000 people on dialysis, those who exercised had better physical function and tended to live much longer than those who did not.[147] In this study, people were much more likely to exercise if their clinics had exercise programs. Those who did:

- Had better physical function
- Slept and ate better
- Had less pain
- Were in better moods and less depressed

Some patients can keep doing the same exercises they did before dialysis. Some may start a new plan. Patients with heart disease may need cardiac rehabilitation. Those who are very weak may need physical therapy. Some clinics offer fitness options during treatment.

Let patients do as much as they can for themselves. It is often faster to offer wheelchairs to frail elderly patients than wait for them to use walkers. But the body is a "use it or lose it" machine. Patients who stop walking will stop being able to walk. In this case, they may also lose their independence and their homes.

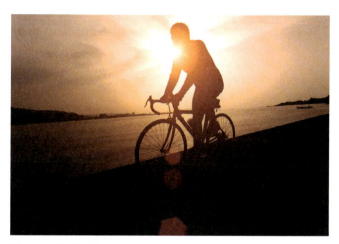

Figure 32: Biking

You can help patients stay fit—and active in life—if you:

- **Share success stories** (without sharing patient names).
- **Ask patients how they stay fit**. Sometimes just asking the question can help patients see that they do not have to stop being active because of their illness. They do not have to do jumping jacks or ride an exercise bike. People can stay fit in the garden, walking the dog, mowing the lawn, swimming, dancing, etc.
- **Urge patients to take part in your clinic's exercise program, if you have one**.
- **Suggest that patients with job concerns talk with the social worker**. The social worker has resources that can help patients keep their jobs. S/he can help an employer learn what job changes a patient needs. The employer needs to know that the patient is protected under the Americans with Disabilities Act, and the social worker can help. For example, a leave of absence may help a patient avoid disability.
- **Work with the care team to help patients understand their disease and its treatment**. Once they know what to expect, they can explain it to a boss.
- **Talk to patients about what they enjoy doing**. Help them brainstorm ideas for work or volunteer tasks that can help keep them involved in life.
- **Talk with retired patients to help them plan activities they will enjoy**.

69

Special Challenges

Some concerns can be very challenging in a dialysis clinic. You may not run into these often, but they can happen, and you will need to deal with patients in a sensitive way. If this is hard to do, imagine that the patient is someone in your own life that you care about. Treat them the way you would want your loved one to be treated.

Challenges and What You Can Do

HYGIENE
The patient has not bathed or has an odor.

- **Watch for clues as to *why* this is happening**. A patient may be depressed. S/he may have lost some sense of smell and not know there is an odor. Memory issues may mean that s/he forgets to shower. Or, s/he may worry about falling—if so, a shower chair and hand wand at home may help.
- **If you feel up to it, gently point out that s/he may not be aware of it, but there is an odor**. Share that we go "nose blind" when we smell odors that are around us all the time, so we may not notice them after a while.
- **Consider a clothes swap if your clinic has a washing machine**. If the patient brings in a change of clothes, s/he can wear the clean ones during treatment while the others are laundered. Offer this in a kind way as a service.
- **Tell the social worker**. S/he may need to involve the family or home healthcare services to help. Family members can try not taking the patient on non-urgent outings unless s/he washes up first.

INCONTINENCE
The patient loses bowel control.

- **Pull curtains around the chair and/or disconnect and help him or her to the bathroom to clean up**. Maintain your patient's dignity, and do *not* leave a patient sitting in a mess. This is humiliating and upsetting for *all* of the patients nearby, and can cause skin breakdown and bedsores. Tell him or her how sorry you are that this happened. Wear gloves and gather paper towels, damp washcloths, and towels to clean the patient's skin, and a biohazard bin. Find scrubs for the patient to wear and ask if s/he wants to keep the soiled clothes. If so, put them into a plastic bag for laundering. If not, throw them away in the bin.
- **Tell the nurse**. If this is a one-time event, it may be due to a medicine, illness, or a response to a drop in blood pressure. If it happens often, the patient needs to see a doctor. A patient who is incontinent at home, too, may need to make food changes, take medicine, wear adult diapers, start bowel training, or, rarely, may need surgery.

BEDBUGS
Apple seed sized, blood-sucking insects are brought into the clinic.

- **Tell the nurse right away if patients have bites**. The itchy bites may look like mosquito bites, but are hard. Several bites in a row are common, and they may be seen along a blood vessel. The sooner an infestation is dealt with, the better.[156]
- **Cover dialysis chairs with white paper so bedbugs can be easily seen**.[157]
- **Use an end of row chair to care for a patient who has bedbugs, to provide some separation**.[156]
- **If bedbugs have been sighted in the clinic, inspect the waiting room and equipment**. Check supply carts, wheelchairs, patient chairs, etc., often.[156]
- **Consider using bedbug monitors to detect them**.[156]
- **Do not talk about bedbugs on the patient floor**. To avoid upsetting other patients, one clinic refers to them as "blueberries."[156]
- **Give the patient paper scrubs to wear during a treatment**. His or her clothes can be put in a plastic tub while s/he is on dialysis.[156]
- **Limit personal belongings brought into the unit from affected homes**. Provide blankets that can be cleaned, and avoid purses, bags, etc.[156]
- **Use steam to clean bugs from chairs or in crevices**. If your clinic has a steam device, it can be used on a chair when the patient is *not* in it.
- **Consider a clothes swap if your clinic has a clothes dryer or clothing heater** (e.g., "Enviro Case"). If the patient brings in a change of clothes, s/he can wear the clean ones during treatment while the others are heated. Offer this in a kind way as a service.[156]
- **Consider an exterminator for the patient's home**.[156] Insecticides or heat treatment may be needed in the clinic.

SCREAMING

A patient cries out during a whole treatment.

- **Tell the social worker**. Patients who scream and do not seem to know where they are or what is happening may not be good candidates for dialysis. The social worker or nephrologist may need to talk to the family or even bring them in to see how hard the treatments are on their loved ones. It is very difficult for other patients to have someone in so much distress.

Coping with Patient Deaths

When a patient's heart or breathing stops in the dialysis clinic, the correct response is to take care of that patient. You will also need to think about the other patients in the treatment area or waiting room, who may be thinking:

- What happened?
- Was something wrong with the dialysis?
- Did someone do something wrong?
- What are the staff doing to help him/her?
- Is the patient going to live?
- Could the same thing happen to me?

Since 2008, patients have had the right to be told about advanced directives (ADs) and whether the clinic will honor them.[89] We do not know how many dialysis patients have ADs or do not resuscitate (DNR) orders. A recent 5-year study found that only 49% of patients in the general population had an AD.[158]

Dialysis staff or paramedics will do CPR if a patient's heart or breathing stops, unless a patient's DNR order or AD says not to. On television, most people who have CPR survive. In the real world, the outcome may not be as positive. A study of dialysis patients who had inpatient CPR for cardiac arrest showed that fewer than 22% lived to discharge.[159]

If CPR is *not* performed (following a patient's wishes) and he or she dies, other patients may wonder why "everything" was not done. They may think the staff did not like that patient, which could lead to anger at staff and fear that staff will not try to save them. Staff need to address these feelings with understanding, while honoring the deceased patient's privacy.

The social worker can help other patients while staff are in the midst of a crisis. Due to HIPAA law, staff cannot share health information about the patient

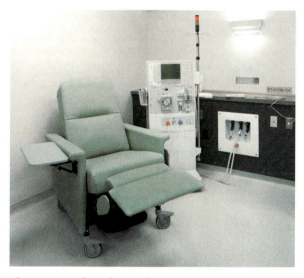

Figure 33: Dialysis Chair

they are working on without permission. The social worker can calm patients by helping them talk about what they are seeing, feeling, and worried about. It may help them to talk through how they are not the same as the person who died, even though they are on dialysis, too. If patients do not want to talk, the social worker can make sure they know that when they are ready, s/he is there, and cares about them, too.

After the crisis is over, you and the other staff may need someone to talk with, too. You may have some of the same questions as the patients. You may wonder if a warning was missed, if the treatment caused the problem, or if something more could have been done. If you are closer to some patients than to the one who died, you may feel guilty. You may have never seen or touched a deceased person. Moving the patient to an out-of-the way location in the clinic may make you feel sad and uncomfortable. Like patients, you may need a safe place and someone who listens to help you grieve. The social worker can be that resource for you, too.

If family members are present during the crisis, the social worker can sit with them. S/he can help them know what is happening and how the patient is doing. Your clinic should have a policy for who is to notify the patient's next of kin if they are not present, and how to do that in a way that shows caring and concern.

Due to HIPAA, some clinics wait for an obituary in the paper to let others know of a patient's death. Patients who were close to the deceased may feel bad that they did not get a chance to go to the funeral or send their sympathies to the family. Some clinics ask if patients would like to sign a HIPAA release to let the others know why they are not at the clinic. Staff may ask a patient with a DNR order if it is okay to share that with other patients if something happens. Having a release lets the social worker or other staff talk more freely about the death of a patient. The social worker can then explain why staff may not be doing CPR.

It can help patients and staff cope if the clinic recognizes the loss and celebrates the patient's life. People who work for years in dialysis will meet, get to know, and lose many patients. This may help you come to terms with your own mortality and the need to have an AD yourself. The Coalition for Supportive Care of Kidney Patients has resources to address end of life decisions and deaths at www.kidneysupportivecare.org.

Patient Resources

Many groups exist to help kidney patients. You can help your patients by knowing about these groups and how to reach them. You may want to visit their websites to learn more about kidney disease, or even join the groups. Besides the national programs listed here, there may also be local groups in your area.

Website Resources

DIALYSIS OUTCOMES AND PRACTICE PATTERNS STUDY (DOPPS)

In this module, we have shared data from the DOPPS, which is a long-term study of people on hemodialysis from more than 20 countries around the world. The more recent PDOPPS is studying peritoneal dialysis in 5 countries. You can keep up with DOPPS real-time on their website: www.dopps.org.

HOME DIALYSIS CENTRAL™

The nonprofit Medical Education Institute (MEI), which runs Life Options and Kidney School and develops this *Core Curriculum*, built a website to raise awareness and use of PD and home HD (see Figure 34). Home Dialysis Central lists all clinics in the U.S. that offer home treatments. It describes each option and offers patient stories, tools, information, links, and much more. Visit www.homedialysis.org and encourage patients to join the Facebook group at www.facebook.com/groups/HomeDialysisCentral/.

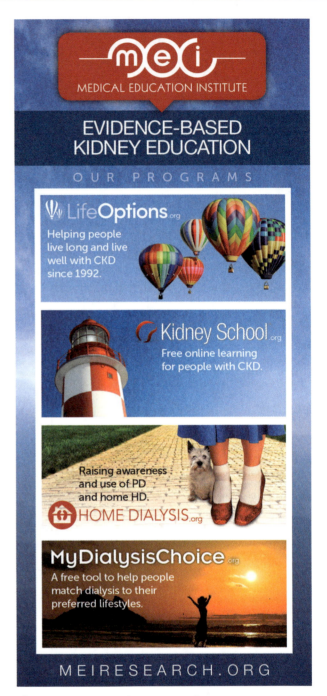

Figure 34: MEI Patient Education Programs

KIDNEY SCHOOL™

MEI offers a free online kidney learning center for patients and families. There are 16 modules, and each has a pre- and post-test, photos and graphics, a lesson, a completion certificate, and an action plan. Topics include kidneys and how they work, treatment options, coping, vascular access, sexuality and fertility, nutrition, staying active, long-term complications, and more. Users can go through the modules online, download PDFs to print and read (in English or Spanish), or listen to audio files. Kidney School helps patients learn how to self-manage their kidney disease. Visit www.kidneyschool.org. To obtain online continuing education credits for Kidney School modules, visit https://credits.meiresearch.org.

LIFE OPTIONS

MEI's Life Options program reaches more than 1.5 million unique visitors a year with free, research-based booklets and fact sheets for people with chronic kidney disease. There is also an "everything a patient needs to know" book called *Help, I Need Dialysis!* You can preview the book online. Free tools for professionals include *Let's Talk About...* movies and six sets of CKD patient education PowerPoint slides called *A Good Future with Kidney Disease.* Call (800) 468-7777, e-mail lifeoptions@meiresearch.org, or visit www.lifeoptions.org.

MY LIFE, MY DIALYSIS CHOICE

MEI's free online decision aid helps people match a type of dialysis to their lives by asking the key question: *What matters to you?* Users can choose between 25 lifestyle, health, and relationship values, and then see how the four types of dialysis will affect each one, rate their favorites with stars, and see what might fit their values best. Visit www.mydialysischoice.org.

Patient Organizations

AMERICAN ASSOCIATION OF KIDNEY PATIENTS (AAKP)

The AAKP is a voluntary patient organization that has been dedicated to improving the lives of fellow kidney patients and their families by helping them to deal with the physical, emotional, and social impact of kidney disease for more than 40 years. AAKP programs inform and inspire patients and their families to better understand their condition, adjust to their circumstances, and assume more normal, productive lives. Patients can join for free and can choose to attend their annual meeting. Visit www.aakp.org to learn more about AAKP or call the AAKP National Office at (800) 749-2257.

AMERICAN KIDNEY FUND (AKF)

The AKF fights kidney disease through direct financial support to patients in need, health education, and prevention. AKF also fights kidney disease through public awareness campaigns, free health screenings, health education materials and courses, online outreach, and a toll-free health information helpline at (866) 300-2900. Visit www.kidneyfund.org to learn more about the AKF. You can also find AKF on Facebook at www.facebook.com/AmericanKidneyFund.

DIALYSIS PATIENT CITIZENS (DPC)

DPC is a patient-led organization that is working to improve quality of life for dialysis patients through education and advocacy. Their goal is to provide patients with the education, access, and confidence to be their own advocates. DPC is committed to raising awareness of dialysis issues, advocating for dialysis patients, improving the partnership between patients and caregivers, and promoting favorable public policy. Members help choose DPC priorities. To contact DPC, call (866) 877-4242 or visit www.dialysispatients.org. Find DPC on Facebook at www.facebook.com/patientcitizens, or follow them on twitter (@PatientCitizen).

HOME DIALYZORS UNITED (HDU)

The non-profit HDU is the only dialysis patient organization dedicated to home dialysis (PD and home HD), with the mission to inspire, inform, and advocate for an extraordinary quality of life for the home dialyzor community. Membership is free, and the group has a quarterly e-newsletter, a buddy system, arranges special trips, and offers online support. Visit www.homedialyzorsunited.org. Find HDU on Facebook at www.facebook.com/groups/nxstageusers, or follow them on twitter (@hdunews).

NATIONAL KIDNEY FOUNDATION (NKF)

The NKF has been providing hope and help to kidney patients and their families since 1950. The NKF helps to meet the growing public health challenge of chronic kidney disease with a range of programs and services for the public, patients, and healthcare professionals. There is information about CKD, dialysis, and transplant on the NKF website, as well as free early detection screenings for those at risk for kidney disease, and research to prevent and treat CKD. **NKF Cares** is a toll-free patient helpline at 1-855-653-2273. The NKF does patient advocacy through public policy and legislative action, offers continuing education and membership for kidney professionals. Visit www.kidney.org or call (800) 622-9010.

PKD FOUNDATION

PKD, in most cases, is an inherited condition. It causes cysts to grow on the kidneys, which can reduce kidney function and may cause kidney failure. There is no cure for PKD, but the PKD Foundation is a 501(c)3 not-for-profit organization dedicated to promoting programs of research, education, support, advocacy, and awareness to find treatments and a cure for polycystic kidney disease and improve the lives of all the people affected by PKD. The PKD Foundation offers education and information about PKD on its website, www.pkdcure.org, or by calling (800) PKD-CURE.

RENAL SUPPORT NETWORK (RSN)

RSN was founded in 1993 by Lori Hartwell—a kidney disease survivor since 1968—to instill health, happiness, and hope into the lives of those with CKD. RSN is a nonprofit, patient-focused, patient-run organization that provides non-medical services to those affected by CKD. Through its many programs, RSN strives to help patients develop their personal coping skills, special talents, and employability by educating and empowering them (and their family members) to take control of the course and management of the disease. Find out more about RSN programs by calling toll-free (866) 903-1728 or visiting www.RSNhope.org.

Government Resources

CENTERS FOR DISEASE CONTROL AND PREVENTION

The CDC has a wealth of information about diseases, precautions, emergency preparedness and much more. Visit www.cdc.gov.

END-STAGE RENAL DISEASE (ESRD) NETWORKS

The 18 regional ESRD Networks are CMS contractors formed by Congress to improve quality of care and quality of life for ESRD patients. They help dialysis clinics troubleshoot patient issues, and gather and report data on ESRD. Networks handle grievances for patients that cannot be solved by the clinic. You can find your Network on the Forum of ESRD Networks' website at www.esrdnetworks.org.

HEALTHCARE.GOV

People who qualify for health insurance under the Affordable Care Act can find or change plans on the www.healthcare.gov site.

MEDICARE

Patients can sign up for Medicare Part D (drug) plans or change plans, find out costs and coverage, learn about Medigap supplements, and much more at www.medicare.gov. Patients can also sign up for a MyMedicare.gov account to review claims as far back as 3 years. Medicare's Dialysis Facility Compare website lets patients see the ratings of dialysis clinics at www.medicare.gov/dialysisfacilitycompare/.

Conclusion

The most challenging—and rewarding—aspect of being a dialysis technician is working with people whose kidneys have failed. Kidney failure is a blow to those who have it, but it doesn't have to be the end of their hopes and dreams. You have a key role to play in the care of these patients. You see them and talk to them more than anyone else on the care team. You may see them at their worst, but you have a chance to help them be their best. You can make a real difference in your patients' lives by giving them hope, helping teach them how to take care of themselves, and providing the best possible dialysis care.

References

1. Greco K, Mahon SM. The kidney in health and disease: Assessment of kidney structure and function. In C.S. Counts (Ed.), *Core Curriculum for Nephrology Nursing: Module 2. Physiologic and psychosocial basis for nephrology nursing practice* (6th ed., 2015. pp. 1-152). Pitman, NJ: American Nephrology Nurses' Association
2. *Definition of Hormone*. MedicineNet.com. Available at http://www.medicinenet.com/script/main/art.asp?articlekey=3783. Accessed October 2016
3. Wadei HM, Textor SC. The role of the kidney in regulating arterial blood pressure. *Nat Rev Nephrol*. 2012;8(10):602-9
4. Hamm LL, Nakhoul N, Hering-Smith KS. Acid-base homeostasis. *Clin J Am Soc Nephrol*. 2015;10(12):2232-42
5. UK Renal Association. *Clinical practice guidelines, acute kidney injury*. 2011, 5th Edition. http://www.renal.org/docs/default-source/guidelines-resources/5_-_Acute_Kidney_Injury_-_Current_version_-_08_April_2008_FINAL.pdf?sfvrsn=0. Accessed April 2017
6. Faulhaber-Walters R, Scholz S, Haller H, et al. Health status, renal function, and quality of life after multiorgan failure and acute kidney injury requiring renal replacement therapy. *Int J Neprhol Renovasc Dis*. 2016;9:119-28
7. Dalrymple LS, Katz R, Kestenbaum B, et al. Chronic kidney disease and the risk of end-stage renal disease versus death. *J Gen Intern Med*. 2011;26(4):379-85
8. Kidney Disease: Improving Global Outcomes (KDIGO) CKD Work Group. KDIGO 2012 clinical practice guideline for the evaluation and management of chronic kidney disease. *Kidney Inter Suppl*. 2013;3:1-150
9. Cooper BA, Branley P, Bulfone L, et al. IDEAL Study. A randomized controlled trial of early versus late initiation of dialysis. *N Engl J Med*. 2010;363(7):609-19
10. Thilly N, Boini S, Soudant M, et al. Outcomes of patients with delayed dialysis initiation: results from the AVENIR study. *Am J Nephrol*. 2011;33(1):76-83
11. Evans M, Tettamanti G, Nyren O, et al. No survival benefit from early-start dialysis in a population-based, inception cohort study of Swedish patients with chronic kidney disease. *J Intern Med*. 2011;270(1):85-6
12. Rosansky SJ, Eggers P, Jackson K, et al. Early start of hemodialysis may be harmful. *Arch Intern Med*. 2011;171(5):396-403
13. United States Renal Data System. *2016 USRDS Annual Data Report: Epidemiology of Kidney Disease in the United States.* National Institutes of Health, National Institute of Diabetes and Digestive and Kidney Diseases. Bethesda, MD, 2016 (Reference Tables, Volume 2, Table A.7). Available at https://www.usrds.org/reference.aspx. Accessed February 2017
14. U.S. Department of Health and Human Services. *Diabetes*. Available at https://www.niddk.nih.gov/research-funding/research-programs. Accessed October 2016
15. Center for Disease Control and Prevention. *National Diabetes Statistics Report: Estimates of Diabetes and Its Burden in the United States*. 2014. Atlanta, GA: U.S. Department of Health and Human Services; 2014. Available at https://stacks.cdc.gov/view/cdc/23442. Accessed October 2016
16. Cabassa LJ, Blanco C, Lopez-Castroman J, et al. Racial and ethnic differences in diabetes mellitus among people with and without psychiatric disorders: results from the National Epidemiologic Survey on Alcohol and Related Conditions. *Gen Hosp Psychiatry*. 2011;33(2):107-15
17. American Diabetes Association. *Pivotal diabetes prevention study reinforced*. Available at http://www.diabetes.org/newsroom/press-releases/2009/pivotal-diabetes-prevention-dppos.html. Accessed October 2016
18. American Heart Association. *Understand your risk for high blood pressure*. Available at https://www.empoweredtoserve.org/index.php/articles/understand-your-risk-for-high-blood-pressure/. Accessed October 2016
19. Beers MH, Berkow R (eds). *The Merck Manual of Diagnosis and Therapy, 17th ed*. Whitehouse Station, NJ. 1999
20. *Low sodium level*. Available at https://medlineplus.gov/ency/article/000394.htm. Accessed November 2016
21. Sterns RH, Gottlieb SS. *Hyponatremia in patients with heart failure*. Available at http://www.uptodate.com/contents/hyponatremia-in-patients-with-heart-failure. Accessed February 2017
22. *Low potassium level*. Available at https://medlineplus.gov/ency/article/000479.htm. Accessed November 2016
23. Tucker B, Moledina DG. We use dialysate potassium levels that are too low in hemodialysis. *Semin Dial*. 2016;29(4):300-2
24. *Hypercalcemia*. Available at https://medlineplus.gov/ency/article/000365.htm. Accessed November 2016
25. Lewis JL. *Hyperphosphatemia (High level of phosphate in the blood)*. 2016. Available at http://www.merckmanuals.com/home/hormonal-and-metabolic-disorders/electrolyte-balance/hyperphosphatemia-high-level-of-phosphate-in-the-blood. Accessed November 2016
26. Nigwekar SU, Sterns RH, Hix JK. Calciphylaxis from nonuremic causes: a systematic review. *Clin J Am Soc Nephrol*. 2008;3:1139-43
27. Schatell D, Ellstrom-Calder A, Alt PS, et al. Survey of CKD patients reveals significant gaps in knowledge about kidney disease. Part 2. *Nephrol News Issues*. 2003;17(6):17-9
28. MedlinePlus. *Glomerular filtration rate*. Available at https://medlineplus.gov/ency/article/007305.htm. Accessed October 2016
29. Personal communication with Dr. John Agar. September 16, 2016
30. Shepshelovich D, Rozen-Zvi B, Avni T, et al. Intravenous versus oral iron supplementation for the treatment of anemia in CKD: An updated systematic review and meta-analysis. *Am J Kidney Dis*. 2016;68(5):677-90
31. Rostoker G, Vaziri ND, Fishbane S. Iatrogenic iron overload in dialysis patients at the beginning of the 21st century. *Drugs*. 2016;76(7):741-57
32. Tolouian R, Mulla ZD, Diaz J, et al. Liver and cardiac iron deposition in patients on maintenance hemodialysis by magnetic resonance imaging T2. *Iran J Kidney Dis*. 2016;10(2):68-74
33. Rockwell Medical. *Anemia and kidney disease*. Available at www.rockwellmed.com/therapeutic-anemia-kidney-disease.htm. Accessed April 2017
34. U.S. Food & Drug Administration. *FDA drug safety communication: Modified dosing recommendations to improve the safe use of erythropoiesis-stimulating agents (ESAs) in chronic kidney disease*. Available at http://www.fda.gov/Drugs/DrugSafety/ucm259639.htm. Accessed October 2016
35. Wetmore JB, Tzivelekis S, Collins AJ, et al. Effects of the prospective payment system on anemia management in maintenance dialysis patients: implications for cost and site of care. *BMC Nephrol*. 2016;17(1):53
36. Mayo Clinic. *Left ventricular hypertrophy*. Available at https://www.mayoclinic.org/diseases-conditions/left-ventricular-hypertrophy/basics/definition/con-20026690. Accessed October 2016
37. Di Lullo L, Gorini A, Russo D, et al. Left ventricular hypertrophy in chronic kidney disease patients: from pathophysiology to treatment. *Cardiorenal Med*. 2015;5:254-66
38. Burton JO, Jefferies HJ, Selby NM, et al. Hemodialysis-induced cardiac injury: determinants and associated outcomes. *Clin J Am Soc Nephrol*. 2009;4:914-20
39. Cheung AK, Sarnak MJ, Yan G, et al. Cardiac diseases in maintenance hemodialysis patients: results of the HEMO study. *Kidney Int*. 2004;65:2380-9
40. Breidthardt T, Burton JO, Odudu A, et al. Troponin T for the detection of dialysis-induced myocardial stunning in hemodialysis patients. *Clin J Am*

Soc Nephrol. 2012;7(8):1285-92

41. Eldehni MT, Odudu A, McIntyre CW. Randomized clinical trial of dialysate cooling and effects on brain white matter. *J Am Soc Nephrol*. 2015;26:957-65
42. Flythe JE, Kimmel SE, Brunelli SM. Rapid fluid removal during dialysis is associated with cardiovascular morbidity and mortality. *Kidney Int*. 2011;79(2):250-7
43. Selby NM, McIntyre CW. Peritoneal dialysis is not associated with myocardial stunning. *Perit Dial Int*. 2011;31:27-33
44. Jefferies HJ, Virk B, Schiller B, et al. Frequent hemodialysis schedules are associated with reduced levels of dialysis-induced cardiac injury (myocardial stunning). *Clin J Am Soc Nephrol*. 2011;6:1326-32
45. Arbor Research Collaborative for Health and the University of Michigan Kidney Epidemiology and Cost Center. *End stage renal disease (ESRD) hemodialysis adequacy clinical technical expert panel summary report*. Contract No. 500-2008-000221, Task Order No. HHSM-500-T0001. Baltimore MD, 2013
46. Dad T, Sarnak MJ. Pericarditis and pericardial effusions in end-stage renal disease. *Semin Dial*. 2016 Sep;29(5):366-73
47. Landry CS, Ruppe MD, Grubbs EG. Vitamin D receptors and parathyroid glands. *Endo Pract*. 2011;17 Suppl 1:63-8
48. Cannata-Andia JB, Rodriguez-Garcia M, Carillo-López N, et al. Vascular calcifications: pathogenesis, management, and impact on clinical outcomes. *J Am Soc Nephrol*. 2006;17(12) Suppl 3:S267-73
49. Morten IJ, Gosal WS, Radford SE, et al. Investigation into the role of macrophages in the formation and degradation of β2-microglobulin amyloid fibrils. *J Biol Chem*. 2007;282(40);29691-700
50. Winchester JF, Salsberg JA, Levin NW. Beta-2 microglobulin in ESRD: an in-depth review. *Adv Renal Replace Ther*. 2003;10(4):279-309
51. Dember LM, Jaber BL. Dialysis-related amyloidosis: late finding or hidden epidemic? *Semin Dial*. 2006;19(2):105
52. Okuno S, Ishimura E, Kohno K, et al. Serum β2-microglobulin level is a significant predictor of mortality in maintenance haemodialysis patients. *Nephrol Dial Transplant*. 2009;24(4):571-7
53. Pan Y. Uremic neuropathy. *Medscape*. Dec. 28, 2015. Available at http://emedicine.medscape.com/article/1175425-overview#a5. Accessed October 2016
54. Krishnan AV, Keirnan MC. Uremic neuropathy: clinical features and new pathophysiological insights. *Muscle Nerv*. 2007;35(3):273-90
55. Ghazan-Shahi S, Koh TJ, Chan CT. Impact of nocturnal hemodialysis on peripheral uremic neuropathy. *BNC Nephrol*. 2015;16:134
56. Okada H, Moriwaki K, Kanno Y, et al. Vitamin B6 supplementation can improve peripheral polyneuropathy in patients with chronic renal failure on high-flux haemodialysis and human recombinant erythropoietin. *Nephrol Dial Transplant*. 2000;15(9):1410-3
57. Moriwaki K, Kanno Y, Nakamoto H, et al. Vitamin B6 deficiency in elderly patients on chronic peritoneal dialysis. *Adv Perit Dial*. 2000;16:308-12
58. Otte J, van Netten JJ, Woittiez AJ. The association of chronic kidney disease and dialysis treatment with foot ulceration and major amputation. *J Vasc Surg*. 2015;62(2):406-11
59. Han T, Bai J, Liu W, et al. A systematic review and meta-analysis of α-lipoic acid in the treatment of diabetic peripheral neuropathy. *Eur J Endorinol*. 2012;167(4):465-71
60. Ziegler D, Low PA, Litchy WJ, et al. Efficacy and safety of antioxidant treatment with α-lipoic acid over 4 years in diabetic polyneuropathy: the NATHAN 1 trial. *Diabetes Care*. 2011;34(9):2054-60
61. Pisoni RL, Wikström B, Elder SJ, et al. Pruritus in haemodialysis patients: International results from the Dialysis Outcomes and Practice Patterns Study (DOPPS). *Nephrol Dial Transplant*. 2006;21(12):3495
62. Tuohy CV, Montez-Rath ME, Turakhia M, et al. Sleep disordered breathing and cardiovascular risk in older patients initiating dialysis in the United States: a retrospective observational study using Medicare data. *BMC Nephrol*. 2016;17:16
63. La Manna G, Pizza F, Persici E, et al. Restless legs syndrome enhances cardiovascular risk and mortality in patients with end-stage kidney disease undergoing long-term haemodialysis treatment. *Nephrol Dial Transplant*. 2011;26(6):1976-83
64. Russcher M, Koch BCP, Nagtegaal JE, et al. Long-term effects of melatonin on quality of life and sleep in haemodialysis patients (Melody study): a randomized controlled trial. *Br J Clin Pharmacol*. 2013;76(5):668-679
65. Beecroft JM, Hoffstein V, Pierratos A, et al. Nocturnal haemodialysis increases pharyngeal size in patients with sleep apnoea and end-stage renal disease. *Nephrol Dial Transplant*. 2008;23(2):673-9
66. Koch BC, Hagen EC, Nagtegaal JE, et al. Effects of nocturnal hemodialysis on melatonin rhythm and sleep-wake behavior: an uncontrolled trial. *Am J Kidney Dis*. 2009;53(4):658-64
67. Kaw D, Malhotra D. Platelet dysfunction and end-stage renal disease. *Semin Dial*. 2006;19(4):317-22
68. Tentori F, Hunt WC, Rohrscheib M, et al. Which targets in clinical practice guidelines are associated with improved survival in a large dialysis organization? *J Am Soc Nephrol*. 2007;18(8):2377-84
69. Centers for Medicare & Medicaid Services. (2015). *Measures Assessment Tool (MAT), version 2.5*. Available at https://www.cms.gov/Medicare/Provider-Enrollment-and-Certification/GuidanceforLawsAndRegulations/Dialysis.html. Accessed October 2016
70. McCann L (ed). *Pocket guide to nutrition assessment of the patient with kidney disease (5th ed)*. New York, NY, National Kidney Foundation, 2015
71. National Kidney Foundation. KDOQI clinical practice guideline for hemodialysis adequacy: 2015 update. *Am J Kidney* Dis. 2015;66(5):884-930
72. National Kidney Foundation. KDIGO Clinical Practice Guideline Update on Diagnosis, Evaluation, Prevention, and Treatment of CKD-MBD: 2016 update
73. *Centers for Medicare & Medicaid Services End-Stage Renal Disease Quality Incentive Program Payment Year 2020 Final Measure Technical Specifications*. October 5, 2016. Available at https://www.cms.gov/Medicare/Quality-Initiatives-Patient-Assessment-Instruments/ESRDQIP/. Accessed April 2017
74. Kliger AS, Foley RN, Goldfarb DS, et al. KDOQI US Commentary on the 2012 KDIGO Clinical Practice Guidelines for Anemia in CKD. *Am J Kid Dis*. 62(5):849-59
75. Personal communication, Lesley McPhatter, RD on September 27, 2016
76. Matas AJ, Smith JM, Skeans MA, et al. OPTN/SRTR 2013 Annual Data Report: Kidney. *Am J Transplant*. 2015;15(Suppl 2):1-34
77. United States Renal Data System. *2016 USRDS Annual Data Report: Epidemiology of Kidney Disease in the United States*. National Institutes of Health, National Institute of Diabetes and Digestive and Kidney Diseases. Bethesda, MD, 2016 (Reference Tables, Volume 2, Table A.1). Available at https://www.usrds.org/reference.aspx. Accessed February 2017
78. Hart A, Smith JM, Skeans MA, et al. OPTN/SRTR Annual Data Report 2015: Kidney. *Am J Transplant*. 2017;17(Suppl 1):21-116
79. Mjoen G, Hallan S, Hartmann A, et al. Long-term risks for kidney donors. *Kidney Int*. 2014;86(1):162-7
80. Janki S, Klop KWJ, Kimenai HJAN, et al. Long-term follow-up after live kidney donation (LOVE) study: a longitudinal comparison study protocol. *BMC Nephrol*. 2016;17:14
81. Lerma EV. Kidney-pancreas transplantation. *Medscape*. August 3, 2015. Available at http://emedicine.medscape.com/article/1830202-overview. Accessed October 2016

82. United Network for Organ Sharing. *Questions and answers for transplant candidates about kidney allocation.* Available at https://unos.org/transplantation/matching-organs/. Accessed October 2016
83. Massie AB, Luo X, Lonze BE, et al. Early changes in kidney distribution under the new allocation system. *J Am Soc Nephrol.* 2016;27(8):2495-501
84. Wongsaro P, Kahwaji J, Vo A, et al. Modern approaches to incompatible kidney transplantation. *World J Nephrol.* 2015;4(3):354-62
85. Akkina SK, Muster H, Steffens E, et al. Donor exchange programs in kidney transplantation: rationale and operational details from the north central donor exchange cooperative. *Am J Kidney Dis.* 2011;57(1):152-8
86. United States Renal Data System. *2016 USRDS Annual Data Report: Epidemiology of Kidney Disease in the United States.* National Institutes of Health, National Institute of Diabetes and Digestive and Kidney Diseases. Bethesda, MD, 2016 (Reference Tables, Volume 2, Table D.6). Available at https://www.usrds.org/reference.aspx. Accessed October 2016
87. United States Renal Data System. *2016 USRDS Annual Data Report: Epidemiology of Kidney Disease in the United States.* National Institutes of Health, National Institute of Diabetes and Digestive and Kidney Diseases. Bethesda, MD, 2016 (Reference Tables, Volume 2, Table J.5). Available at https://www.usrds.org/reference.aspx. Accessed October 2016
88. Curtin RB, Johnson HK, Schatell D. The peritoneal dialysis experience: insights from long-term patients. *Nephrol Nurs J.* 2004;31(6):615-25
89. *Conditions for Coverage for End-Stage Renal Disease Facilities: Final Rule.* 73 *Federal Register* 73 (15 April 2008), pp. 20387, 20478-9
90. Zimmerman DG. Presternal catheter design—an opportunity to capitalize on catheter immobilization. *Adv Perit Dial.* 2010;26:91-5
91. National Kidney Foundation. KDOQI clinical practice guidelines and clinical practice recommendations for 2006 Updates: hemodialysis adequacy, peritoneal dialysis adequacy and vascular access. *Am J Kidney* Dis. 2006;48(1) Suppl:S96-146
92. United States Renal Data System. *2016 USRDS Annual Data Report: Epidemiology of Kidney Disease in the United States.* National Institutes of Health, National Institute of Diabetes and Digestive and Kidney Diseases. Bethesda, MD, 2016 (Reference Tables, Volume 2, Table I.23). Available at https://www.usrds.org/reference.aspx. Accessed April 2017
93. Home Dialysis Central database. Available at www.homedialysis.org/clinics/search. Accessed September 2017
94. United States Renal Data System. *2016 USRDS Annual Data Report: Epidemiology of Kidney Disease in the United States.* National Institutes of Health, National Institute of Diabetes and Digestive and Kidney Diseases. Bethesda, MD, 2016 (Reference Tables, Volume 2, Table D.1). Available at https://www.usrds.org/reference.aspx. Accessed February 2017
95. Tentori F, Zhang J, Li Y, et al. Longer dialysis session length is associated with better intermediate outcomes and survival among patients on in-center three times per week hemodialysis: results from the Dialysis Outcomes and Practice Patterns Study (DOPPS). *Nephrol Dial Transplant.* 2012;27:4180-88
96. Saran R, Bragg-Gresham JL, Levin NW, et al. Longer treatment time and slower ultrafiltration in hemodialysis: Associations with reduced mortality in the DOPPS. *Kidney Int.* 2006; 69:1222-8
97. United States Renal Data System. *2016 USRDS Annual Data Report: Epidemiology of Kidney Disease in the United States.* National Institutes of Health, National Institute of Diabetes and Digestive and Kidney Diseases. Bethesda, MD, 2016 (Reference Tables, Volume 2, Table I.17). Available at https://www.usrds.org/reference.aspx. Accessed April 2017
98. American Cancer Society. *Cancer Facts & Figures 2015.* Atlanta: American Cancer Society; 2015
99. Fadem SZ, Walker DR, Abbott G, et al. Satisfaction with renal replacement therapy and education: the American Association of Kidney Patients survey. *Clin J Am Soc Nephrol.* 2011;6(3):605-12
100. Schatell DR, Bragg-Gresham JL, Mehrotra R, et al. *A description of nephrologist training, beliefs, and practices from the National Nephrologist Dialysis Practice Survey (2010).* Abstract F-FC209 presented at the American Society of Nephrology meeting, Denver, CO, November 19, 2010. Available at http://www.asn-online.org/education/kidneyweek/archives/. Accessed October 2016
101. Zhang H, Schaubel DE, Kalbfleisch JD, et al. Dialysis outcomes and analysis of practice patterns suggests the dialysis schedule affects day-of-week mortality. *Kidney Int.* 2012;81:1108-15
102. Lacson E Jr, Wang W, Lester K, et al. Outcomes associated with in-center nocturnal hemodialysis from a large multicenter program. *Clin J Am Soc Nephrol.* 2010;5(2):220-6
103. Troidle L, Finkelstein F, Hotchkiss M, et al. Enhanced solute removal with intermittent, in-center, 8-hour nocturnal hemodialysis. *Hemodial Int.* 2009;13(4):487-91
104. Lacson E Jr., Xu J, Nesrallah G, et al. Survival with three-times weekly in-center nocturnal versus conventional hemodialysis. *J Am Soc Nephrol.* 2012;23(4):687-95
105. Ok E, Duman S, Asci G, et al., on behalf of the Long Dialysis Study Group. Comparison of 4- and 8-h dialysis sessions in thrice-weekly in-centre haemodialysis: a prospective, case-controlled study. *Nephrol Dial Transplant.* 2011;26(4):1287-96
106. Blagg CR. A brief history of home hemodialysis. *Adv Renal Repl Ther.* 1996;3(2):99-105
107. Jaber BL, Schiller B, Burkart JM, et al., on behalf of the FREEDOM Study Group. Impact of short daily hemodialysis on restless legs syndrome and sleep disturbances. *Clin J Am Soc Nephrol.* 2011;6(5):1049-56
108. The FHN Trial Group: Chertow GM, Levin NW, Beck GJ, et al. In-center hemodialysis six times per week versus three times per week. *N Engl J Med.* 2010;363(24):2287-300. Erratum in *N Engl J Med.* 2011;364(1):93
109. Kjellstrand C, Buoncristiani U, Ting G, et al. Survival with short-daily hemodialysis: association of time, site, and dose of dialysis. *Hemodial Int.* 2010;14(4):464-70
110. Schorr M, Manns BJ, Culleton B, et al. Alberta Kidney Disease Network: The effect of nocturnal and conventional hemodialysis on markers of nutritional status: results from a randomized trial. *J Ren Nutr.* 2011;21(3):271-6
111. Ipema KJR, Struijk S, van der Velden A, et al. Nutritional status in nocturnal hemodialysis patients – A systematic review with meta-analysis. *PLoS ONE.* 2016;11(6):e0157621. doi: 10.1371/journal.pone.0157621
112. Van Eps CL, Jeffries JK, Johnson DW, et al. Quality of life and alternate nightly nocturnal home hemodialysis. *Hemodial Int.* 2010;14(1):29-38
113. Chan CT, Li GH, Valaperti A, et al. Intensive hemodialysis preserved cardiac injury. *ASAIO J.* 2015;61(5):613-9
114. Pauly RP, Gill JS, Rose CL, et al. Survival among nocturnal home haemodialysis patients compared to kidney transplant recipients. *Nephrol Dial Transplant.* 2009;24(9):2915-9
115. Hussain JA, Mooney A, Russon L. Comparison of survival analysis and palliative care involvement in patients aged over 70 years choosing conservative management or renal replacement therapy in advanced chronic kidney disease. *Palliat Med.* 2013;27(9):829-39
116. Untas A, Thumma J, Rascle N, et al. The associations of social support and other psychosocial factors with mortality and quality of life in the Dialysis Outcomes and Practice Patterns Study. *Clin J Am Soc Nephrol.* 2011;6(1):142-152. doi:10.2215/CJN.02340310
117. Swaminathan S, Mor V. Monitoring the Kidney Care Partners' PEAK campaign to reduce the 1-year mortality rates of dialysis patients: Final Report.

August, 2013. Available at http://www.nephrologynews.com/ext/resources/files/documents/SpecialSectionsReports/PEAK-report.pdf. Accessed October 2016

118. Wingard RL, Chan KE, Lazaruz JM, et al. The "right" of passage: surviving the first year of dialysis. *Clin J Am Soc Nephrol.* 2009; 4 Suppl 1:S114-20
119. Lacson E Jr, Wang W, DeVries C, et al. Effects of a nationwide predialysis educational program on modality choice, vascular access, and patient outcomes. *Am J Kidney Dis.* 2011 Aug;58(2):235-42
120. Perry BD. Fear and learning: Trauma-related factors in the adult education process. *New Directions for Adult and Continuing Education.* 2006:21-27. doi:10.1002/ace.215
121. Almasri J, Alsawas M, Mainou M, et al. Outcomes of vascular access for hemodialysis: A systematic review and metaanalysis. *J Vasc Surg.* 2016;64(1):236-43
122. Chan M, Kelly J, Batterham M, et al. A high prevalence of abnormal nutrition parameters found in predialysis end-stage kidney disease: is it a result of uremia or poor eating habits? *J Ren Nutr.* 2014;24(5):292-302
123. Takahashi R, Ito Y, Takahashi H, et al. Combined values of serum albumin, C-reactive protein and body mass index at dialysis initiation accurately predicts long-term mortality. *Am J Nephrol.* 2012;36(2):136-43
124. Obi Y, Qader H, Kovesdy CP, et al. Latest consensus and update on protein energy-wasting in chronic kidney disease. *Curr Opin Clin Nutr Metab Care.* 2015;18(3):254-62
125. Campbell KL, MacLaughlin HL. Unintentional weight loss is an independent predictor of mortality in a hemodialysis population. *J Ren Nutr.* 2010;20(6):414-8
126. Mehrotra R, Duong U, Jiwakanon S, et al. Albumin as predictor of mortality in peritoneal dialysis: Comparisons with hemodialysis. *Am J Kidney Dis.* 2011;58(3):418-28
127. Kalantar-Zadeh K, Ikizler TA, Block G, et al. Malnutrition-inflammation complex syndrome in dialysis patients: causes and consequences. *Am J Kidney Dis.* 2003;42(5):864-81
128. National Institute of Diabetes and Digestive and Kidney Diseases. *Overweight & Obesity Statistics.* Available at https://www.niddk.nih.gov/health-information/health-statistics/overweight-obesity. Accessed April 2017
129. Gray-Byham L, Stover J, Wiesen K. *Clinical Guide to Nutrition Care in Kidney Disease.* Second Edition. Academy of Nutrition and Dietetics. Pp 28 and 88. June 1, 2013
130. Peer Kidney Care Initiative. *Peer Report: Dialysis care and outcomes in the United States, 2014.* Chronic Disease Research Group, Minneapolis, MN, 2014. Available at http://www.peerkidney.org/download-the-peer-report/. Accessed October 2016
131. Agar J. (2016 April 7) *Towards compassionate dialysis: Thirst and hemodialysis duration* [Web blog post]. Available at: http://homedialysis.org/news-and-research/blog/146-towards-i-compassionate-i-dialysis-thirst-and-hemoialysis-duration. Accessed October 2016
132. U.S. Department of Health and Human Services and U.S. Department of Agriculture. *2015–2020 Dietary Guidelines for Americans.* 8th Edition. December 2015. Available at http://health.gov/dietaryguidelines/2015/guidelines/. Accessed October 2016
133. Wu PY, Yang SH, Wong TC, et al. Association of processed meat intake with hypertension risk in hemodialysis patients: a cross-sectional study. *PLoS One.* 2015 Oct 30;10(10):e0141917. doi:10.1371/journal.pone.0141917
134. U.S. Food and Drug Administration. *Changes to the nutrition facts label.* 2016. Available at https://www.fda.gov/food/guidanceregulation/guidancedocumentsregulatoryinformation/labelingnutrition/ucm385663.htm. Accessed October 2016
135. Uhlig K, Berns JS, Kestenbaum B, et al. KDOQI US Commentary on the 2009 KDIGO Clinical Practice Guideline for the Diagnosis, Evaluation, and Treatment of CKD–Mineral and Bone Disorder (CKD-MBD). *Am J Kidney Dis.* 55(5):773-799
136. Medicare Program End Stage Renal Disease Prospective Payment System, 81 Fed Reg 77834. 42 CFR Parts 413, 414, and 494. January 2017
137. Noori N, Sims JJ, Kopple JD, et al. Organic and inorganic dietary phosphorus and its management in chronic kidney disease. *Iran J Kidney Dis.* 2010;4(2):89-100
138. Wilson G, Molaison EF, Pope J, et al. Nutrition status and food insecurity in hemodialysis patients. *J Ren Nutr.* 2006;16(1):54-8
139. Finkelstein FO, Finkelstein SH. Sexual inactivity among hemodialysis patients: The patients' perspective. *Clin J Am Soc Nephrol.* 2014;9(1):6-7. doi:10.2215/CJN.11831113
140. Matuszkiewicz-Rowinska J, Skorzewska K, Radowicki S, et al. Endometrial morphology and pituitary-gonadal axis dysfunction in women of reproductive age undergoing chronic haemodialysis—a multicentre study. *Nephrol Dial Transplant.* 2004;19(8):2074-7
141. Hladunewich MA, Hou S, Odutayo A, et al. Intensive hemodialysis associates with improved pregnancy outcomes: A Canadian and United States cohort comparison. *J Am Soc Nephrol.* 2014;25(5):1103-9
142. Iglesias P, Carerro JJ, Diez JJ. Gonadal dysfunction in men with chronic kidney disease: Clinical features, prognostic implications and therapeutic options. *J Nephrol.* 2012;25(1):31-42
143. Brkovic T, Burilovic E, Puljak L. Prevalence and severity of pain in adult end-stage renal disease patients on chronic intermittent hemodialysis: a systematic review. *Patient Prefer Adherence.* 2016;10:1131-50
144. King-Wing Ma T, Kam-Tao Li P. Depression in dialysis patients. *Nephrology (Carlton).* 2016;21(8):639-46
145. Bautovich A, Katz I, Loo CK, et al. Depression and chronic kidney disease: A review for clinicians. *Aust N Z J Psychiatry.* 2014;48(6):530-41
146. Palmer SC, Natale P, Ruospo M, et al. Antidepressants for treating depression in adults with end-stage kidney disease treated with dialysis. *Cochrane Database Syst Rev.* 2016;23(5):CD004541. doi: 10.1002/14651858.CD004541.pub3
147. Grigoriou SS, Karatzaferi C, Sakkas GK. Pharmacological and non-pharmacological treatment options for depression and depressive symptoms in hemodialysis patients. *Health Psychol Res.* 2015;3(1):1811. doi: 10.4081/hpr.2015.1811
148. Tentori F, Elder SJ, Thumma J, et al. Physical exercise among participants in the Dialysis Outcomes and Practice Patterns Study (DOPPS): Correlates and associated outcomes. *Nephrol Dial Transplant.* 2010;25(9):3050-62
149. Jaber BL, Lee Y, Collins AJ, et al., on behalf of the FREEDOM Study Group. Effect of daily dialysis on depressive symptoms and postdialysis recovery time: Interim report from the FREEDOM (Following Rehabilitation, Economics and Everyday-Dialysis Outcome Measurements) Study. *Am J Kidney Dis.* 2010;56:531-9
150. Cukor D, Coplan J, Brown C, et al. Anxiety disorders in adults treated by hemodialysis: a single-center study. *Am J Kidney Dis.* 2008;52(1):128-36
151. Stack AG, Martin DR. Association of patient autonomy with increased transplantation and survival among new dialysis patients in the United States. *Am J Kidney Dis.* 2005;45(4):730-42
152. Curtin RB, Oberley ET, Sacksteder P, et al. Differences between employed and nonemployed dialysis patients. *Am J Kidney Dis.* 1996;27(4):533-40
153. Billington E, Simpson J, Unwin J, et al. Does hope predict adjustment to end-stage renal failure and consequent dialysis? *Br J Health Psychol.* 2008;13(Pt. 4):683-99
154. Perry BD. Fear and learning: trauma-related factors in the adult education process. *New Directions Adult Cont Educ.* 2006;110:21-7
155. Kutner NG, Zhang R, Huang Y, et al. Depressed mood, usual activity level, and continued employment after starting dialysis. *Clin J Am Soc Nephrol.* 2010;5(11):2040-5

156 Bed Bugs and Blueberries. The Renal Network, Inc. Available at http://www.therenalnetwork.org/services/resources/BedBugs/Bedbugs_Blueberries.pdf. Accessed May 2016

157 Parker LK. Bed bugs: Who are you sleeping with?" Presentation. http://networkofnewengland.org/wp-content/uploads/2013/02/LPark.pdf. Accessed May 2016

158 Feely MA, Hildebrandt D, Edakkanambeth Varayil J, et al. Prevalence and Contents of Advance Directives of Patients with ESRD Receiving Dialysis. *Clin J Am Soc Nephrol*. 2016;(12):2204-2209

159 Wong SP, Kreuter W, Curtis JR, et al. Trends in in-hospital cardiopulmonary resuscitation and survival in adults receiving maintenance dialysis. *JAMA Intern Med*. 2015;175(6):1028-35

3 Principles of Dialysis

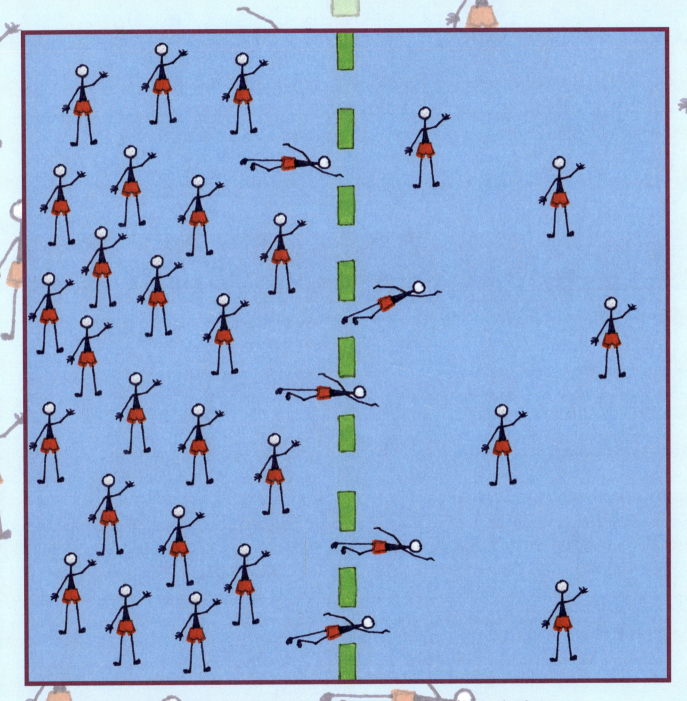

I've lived with kidney failure for 32 years. Some of those extra years of life are thanks to dialysis and some have been thanks to transplantation. We dialysis patients are so very grateful for the extra time we're allotted on this earth to enjoy our families, friends, jobs and life in general. And, we certainly rely on, and appreciate from the bottom of our hearts, all the folks who make our extended lives possible.

—Judith Gluck

"'I never saw anyone with chemistries this high still alive!' said everyone who walked into my room and picked up my chart. I didn't know anything about dialysis or what my problem was until a wonderful, good-looking guy came in and said, 'I'm Dr. Smith. I do kidneys.'"

Objectives

MODULE AUTHORS

Jim Curtis, CHT, CCHT

Nicole Griffiths, BSN, RN, CNN

Cindy Medina, RN, CDN

Michael Morales, MHA/Ed, CHT, CHBT, CDWS, CCHT-A

Lyle Smith, RN, CNN, CDPN

MODULE REVIEWERS

Nancy M. Gallagher, BS, RN, CNN

Susan K. Hansen, RN, CNN, CHT, MBA

Pam Havermann, RN

Darlene Rodgers, BSN, RN, CNN, CPHQ

John H. Sadler, MD

Dori Schatell, MS

Vern Taaffe, BS, CBNT, CDWS

Tamyra Warmack, RN

After you complete this module, you will be able to:

1. Define key principles used in dialysis, including solution and solubility, semipermeable membrane, diffusion, osmosis, adsorption, fluid dynamics, filtration, and ultrafiltration.

2. Describe two ways to remove wastes during dialysis and how they differ.

3. Explain what a safe ultrafiltration rate is, and why.

4. Name at least three forces that affect the flow of fluids (fluid dynamics) and how they relate to dialysis.

An acronym list can be found in the Glossary.

Practice Test Questions at:
www.meiresearch.org/cc6

Introduction

Dialysis seems complex, and it is. But, dialysis is driven by a handful of scientific principles that explain how two fluids behave when they are kept apart by a semi-permeable membrane. Dialysis uses these principles to help replace some of the functions of healthy kidneys:

1. Removing wastes from the blood
2. Removing excess water from the blood
3. Balancing *electrolytes* (electrically charged particles) in the blood
4. Restoring acid-base balance (the pH level) of blood

Basic Concepts and Principles

In this section, you will learn the basic principles behind:

- Solutions
- Solubility
- Semipermeable membranes
- Diffusion
- Convection
- Osmosis
- Adsorption
- Hydraulic pressure
- Fluid dynamics
- Filtration and ultrafiltration
- Fluid compartments in the human body

Solutions

A *solution* is a mixture of a *solvent* and a *solute*, where:

- A **solvent** is a fluid.
- A **solute** is a substance that can be dissolved.

Seawater, for example, is a solution where water is the solvent and salt is the solute.

Solubility

Solubility means how completely a solute will dissolve into a solvent. Four factors affect solubility:

1. Concentration
2. pH
3. Temperature of the solvent
4. Presence of other solutes

CONCENTRATION

Concentration tells you how *much* of a solute is fully dissolved in a solution. There are a number of measures of concentration (shaded box below). The simplest measure is to know how much of a solute is in a given volume of solvent. So, if you dissolve **500 milligrams** (mg) of sodium into **1 liter** (L) of water, your 1 L of solution will have a concentration of **500 mg/L** of sodium. (NOTE: See Appendix A for a brief review of the Metric system.)

Only so much solute can dissolve into a solvent before a solution is *saturated* (full). Once that level is reached, no more solute will dissolve. Some solutes, like sodium, can reach very high levels before a solution is saturated. Others, like calcium, will only fully dissolve in small amounts before a solution is saturated.

> **Measures of concentration:**
>
> - **mg/L**: milligrams per liter. Measures the amount of solute in a liter of solution. One mg per liter is equal to one part per million.
> - **PPM**: parts per million. One gram contains 1,000 mg, and one liter contains 1,000 mL of water. Since 1,000 x 1,000 = 1 million, ppm is the same as mg/L.
> - **mg/dL**: milligrams per deciliter. A deciliter is 1/10 of a liter. This measure is often used for blood test results. For example, normal fasting blood sugar is 70–105 mg/dL.[1]
> - **mEq/L**: milliEquivalents per liter. See definition of Equivalent on page 91.

pH

pH is a measure of how many *acid* (hydronium) or *base* (hydroxyl) ions are dissolved in a solution (see Figure 1). NOTE: Base is also called alkaline. A solution with:

- **An equal number of acid and base ions** is *neutral*, with a pH of 7.0
- **More acid than base ions** is *acidic*, with a pH of less than 7.0 (< 7.0)
- **More base than acid ions** is *alkaline*, with a pH that is greater than 7.0 (> 7.0)

The effect of pH on a solution depends on which solutes are present.

Module 3

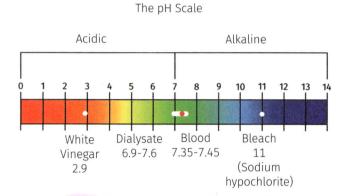

Figure 1: pH Values of Common Substances[2]

Dialysate must have a pH close to blood, so it does not change the blood pH

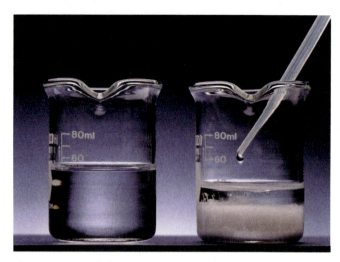

Figure 2: Precipitate

TEMPERATURE OF THE SOLVENT

More solutes will dissolve in a warm solvent than in a cold one. So, the concentration level of a solute can rise as the solvent gets warmer.

PRESENCE OF OTHER SOLUTES

The solutes in a solution can impact how well *other* solutes will dissolve when we add them. For example, a chemical reaction can make one or more solutes less soluble. Or, a change in temperature can affect whether or how much solutes will dissolve. When we add a new solute, some of the solutes may even "un-dissolve" and form **precipitate** (see Figure 2). For example, when blood levels of calcium and phosphorus are both too high at the same time, these minerals can be forced out of the blood. Sharp, calcium-phosphate crystals form, which can harm soft tissue and blood vessels. Called *calcific uremic arteriolopathy* or *calciphylaxis*, these crystals can lead to strokes, *gangrene* (tissue death), amputation, and death.[3]

Semipermeable Membranes

A *membrane* is a thin layer of living or synthetic tissue:
- A *permeable* membrane lets water and particles freely pass through it.
- A *semipermeable* membrane lets only *some* particles (smaller than a certain size) pass through it.

Think of a semipermeable membrane as a pasta strainer: water can drain out, but the noodles are too big to pass through the holes. The membrane's holes, or **pores**, let water and small wastes pass through quickly. Larger particles will take longer, and some are too large to pass through at all.

Diffusion

Diffusion explains how molecules spread out to occupy a space. Molecules have energy of their own. They bump into each other and move around rapidly, which is called *Brownian motion*. This movement will go on until **equilibrium** is reached—the molecules are distributed evenly (see Figure 3). You can smell this principle at work if you crack a rotten egg in one corner of a room: in a short time the odor will be constant all over the room.

Diffusion can occur with or without a membrane. A tea bag is an example of diffusion *with* a semipermeable membrane. When you put a tea bag into hot water, some of the water goes into the bag, and

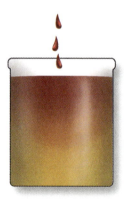

Figure 3: Diffusion

Diffusion is the movement of solutes from an area of higher concentration to an area of lower concentration.

becomes very concentrated with tea flavor, while the water outside the tea bag has less tea flavor. As the tea steeps for a few minutes, molecules from the tea leaves diffuse into *all* of the water until your tea is ready. At this point, the water inside and outside of the tea bag has the same concentration of tea (see Figure 4).

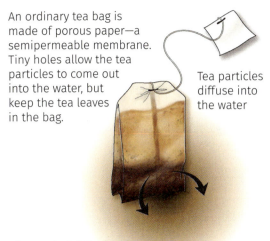

An ordinary tea bag is made of porous paper—a semipermeable membrane. Tiny holes allow the tea particles to come out into the water, but keep the tea leaves in the bag.

Tea particles diffuse into the water

Figure 4: Diffusion in Tea

SOLUTIONS AND DIFFUSION

When a membrane is used, three factors affect the rate and amount of diffusion:[4] (see Figure 5)

1. **Concentration level of the solutions**. Solutes *must* move through a membrane from a higher concentration level to a lower one. A difference between concentration levels is a **gradient**.

2. **Solute Size**. Small molecules diffuse more easily and quickly than large ones. We measure molecule size by *molecular weight* in *daltons* (Da). (See box on page 91.)

3. **Solution Temperature**. Warm molecules have more energy than cold ones, so they move faster—which speeds up diffusion. (You will get tea sooner with hot water than with cold.)

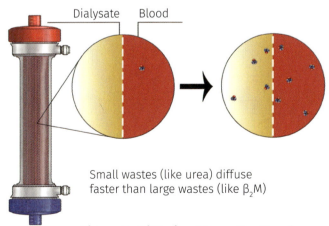

Small wastes (like urea) diffuse faster than large wastes (like $\beta_2 M$)

Figure 5: Diffusion Through a Membrane

Convection

Convection is the transfer of heat and solutes in a liquid or gas by physical circulation or movement.

In dialysis, convection moves solutes across the dialyzer membrane with the movement or "drag" of water. So, when more water is removed, more solutes are removed. This is secondary to diffusion, but still important. For this reason, 300 mL/hr may be used as a minimum ultrafiltration rate.

Osmosis

Osmosis is an action that works to reach balance between two solutions. But, there is an important difference from diffusion:

- In diffusion, **solutes** (*particles*) move across a membrane.
- In osmosis, a **solvent** (water) moves through a membrane (see Figure 6).

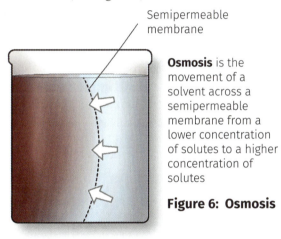

Osmosis is the movement of a solvent across a semipermeable membrane from a lower concentration of solutes to a higher concentration of solutes

Figure 6: Osmosis

In all of nature, water and solutes *must* move from higher concentration levels to lower ones. Imagine that you have a jar that is divided in two by a membrane that lets water—but not sugar—pass through. If you fill one side of the jar with water, you will find that half of the water will slowly pass through the membrane until the water level is the same on both sides of the jar.

Now, you can use sugar to create osmotic pressure. Dissolve sugar into the water on one side of the membrane. This creates an **osmotic pressure gradient** that will push *water* across the membrane to dilute the sugar water. In time, the water level on the sugar side will rise *above* the level on the plain water side. The more sugar you add, the higher the osmotic pressure will be, and the higher the sugar water level will rise (see Figure 7).

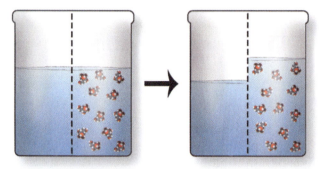

Osmosc gradient formed with glucose.

Figure 7: Osmotic Gradient

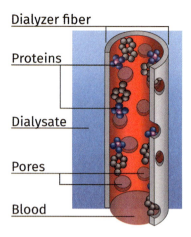

Figure 8: Adsorption

In a solution, the solutes take up space, so there is a bit less solvent when two solutions have the same volume—but different solute levels. If you fill one test tube with 10 cc of pure water, and a second one with 10 cc of salt water, the salt water tube would have less water—because salt takes up some of the space. A common misconception about osmosis is that the solute is pulling water across the membrane in an attempt to achieve solute equilibrium. In reality, the water is *pushing* across the membrane to achieve solvent equilibrium.

> **A Tip: Diffusion or Osmosis?**
> Some people find it hard to keep diffusion and osmosis straight. One trick that may help is to think "H_2Osmosis," to link water (a solvent) with osmosis—how solvents move.

Adsorption

Adsorption occurs when molecules *adhere* (stick) to a surface and form a film (see Figure 8). Adsorption is more likely with higher molecular weight substances, such as proteins. Plasma proteins from the blood can adsorb to a membrane in just seconds. Adsorption affects how molecules move across the membrane. A membrane with a coating of blood proteins may also be more biocompatible for a patient—which makes it less likely to cause a reaction.[5-7]

Hydraulic Pressure

Like osmotic pressure, *hydraulic pressure*, applied with gravity or a pump, can help move a solvent across a membrane. This type of pressure can reduce—or exceed—osmotic pressure.

Fluid Dynamics

A *fluid* is a liquid—or a gas—that changes shape at a steady rate when acted upon by a force (such as heat, cold, or pressure) and will take the shape of its container. *Dynamics* explains how fluids behave, so we can predict what happens to each of them. Three forces affect the flow of fluid through tubing:

1. **Flow rate**: how much fluid flows through a tube segment in a given time (e.g., 10 milliliters per minute, or mL/min).

2. **Flow velocity**: how fast a fluid moves through a given length of tubing. *Velocity* is based on the flow rate and the cross section size (based on the diameter) of the tube. So, if the flow rate stays the same, but the cross section of the tube is reduced by half (50%), flow velocity will double.

3. **Resistance**: slowing of the flow rate due to friction or a narrow spot in the tube.

FLOW IN ACTION

Imagine that one gallon of water must move through a tube that is 1-inch in diameter in 1 minute. If you reduce the tube diameter, the fluid must go faster to move the whole gallon in 1 minute. To keep the same flow rate, the flow velocity would need to increase.

However, if you add a piece of tubing with a ½-inch diameter to the end of a 1-inch tube, you will add *resistance*, which will *reduce* the flow rate. The narrowest part of a tube is the limiting factor for the flow rate. If all of the water must pass through the tube, it will take longer with a narrow spot, (i.e., the flow rate will be lower) and the pressure in the tube will be higher.

The pressure in any fluid system is always a matter of flow and resistance. The greater the flow or resistance, the higher the pressure.

Filtration and Ultrafiltration

Filtration is the process of trapping particles by passing a fluid through a filter. Ultrafiltration (UF) traps very small particles; in fact some ultrafilters can remove particles as small as .001 microns in size. In dialysis, we also use ultrafiltration to refer to removing water from the blood.

Fluid Compartments in the Human Body

The human body is mostly water that is contained inside cells, tissues, and blood vessels. Body water is in *compartments*, or spaces (see Figure 9):

- The **intracellular** space is *inside the cells* – about 60% of body water.[8]
- The **extracellular** space—about 40% of body water—is *outside* the cells, and includes:
  - **Interstitial** (water *between cells*) – about 20% of body water.[8]
  - **Vascular** (*blood in the blood vessels*) – about 7% of body water.[8]
  - **Other** (bone, fat, etc.) – 13% of body water.[8]

As you have learned, healthy kidneys help us to maintain *homeostasis*, a constant balance of water and chemicals in our bodies. One part of this process is maintaining *equilibrium*: the same level of water and solutes—in all of the fluid spaces—all the time. **Water and solutes shift back and forth from one space to the next until the levels are the same**—and they do not stay the same for long. Each time we eat or drink, move our muscles, take a medicine, etc., more shifting of water and wastes occurs between the spaces.

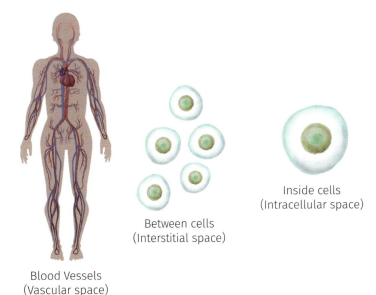

Figure 9: Fluid Compartments

Applying Scientific Principles to Hemodialysis (HD)

"I am grateful that dialysis keeps me alive for a transplant and for the time it gives me with my loved ones. If it weren't for dialysis I wouldn't be here."

Patients come to dialysis with wastes and extra water in their blood and electrolyte levels that are out of balance. One of the main tasks of dialysis is to remove as much of the wastes and water as we can. Another key task is to rebalance the electrolytes. All of the principles you just learned apply to each treatment. We use a semipermeable membrane to separate the patient's blood from the dialysis solution or dialysate.

In this section, you will learn about:

- Solutions in hemodialysis: blood and dialysate
- Dialyzers and diffusion in hemodialysis
- Osmosis, ultrafiltration, and organ stunning in hemodialysis
- Convection in hemodialysis
- Adsorption in hemodialysis
- Fluid dynamics in hemodialysis
- Hemodiafiltration

Solutions in Hemodialysis: Blood and Dialysate

In dialysis, there are two solutions, blood and dialysate. During a treatment, the patient's blood is on one side of a membrane, the dialysate is on the other side, and the two solutions interact through the membrane.

BLOOD

Whole blood contains cells *suspended* (floating) in a straw-colored solution called *plasma*. Plasma is a solvent (like water), with solutes, such as *electrolytes* (minerals that break up into ions in fluid) and chemicals (like hormones). Blood cells include red blood cells, white blood cells, and platelets (see Figure 10).

Blood Components

Normal Blood
- Plasma (~55%)
- White blood cells and platelets (<1%)
- Red blood cells (~45%)

Dialysis Patient Blood
- Plasma (~70%)
- White blood cells and platelets (<1%)
- Red blood cells (30%)

Figure 10: Composition of Blood

If our plasma does not contain the correct levels of electrolytes, our bodies will not work as they should. Electrolytes carry nerve signals to all of our muscles, including our hearts. Kidney failure disrupts electrolyte levels—and dialysis helps to restore the balance.

In dialysis, we often use terms that compare the concentration level of blood to other solutions. These are:

- **Hypotonic:** solute level is *lower* than in blood. E.g., pure water has less sodium than blood.
- **Isotonic:** solute level is the *same* as blood. E.g., normal saline has the same level of sodium as blood.
- **Hypertonic:** solute level is *higher* than blood. E.g., hypertonic saline has *more* sodium than blood.

Cells Found in Blood

Red blood cells

Red blood cells, or erythrocytes, contain hemoglobin, a red, iron-based pigment that carries oxygen. With each heartbeat, red blood cells bring oxygen from the lungs to every cell in the body. On the way back to the heart, red blood cells bring carbon dioxide to the lungs so it can be exhaled.

White blood cells

White blood cells, or leukocytes, are part of the body's immune system, which helps fight off infections.

Platelets

Platelets, or thrombocytes, are small, colorless cell fragments in the blood that work with clotting proteins to stop or prevent bleeding.

DIALYSATE

Dialysate, or dialysis fluid, is a solution made of:

- **A solvent** – water treated for purity
- **Solutes** – a precise mix of electrolytes prescribed by a doctor

Dialysate makes dialysis possible, because we use it to create the gradients we need to remove wastes and balance electrolytes. The doctor prescribes the *osmolality* (total solute level) of dialysate to closely match that of healthy blood. Dialysate has some of the solutes patients need, like calcium. It should contain little or none of the wastes that must be removed. You will learn more about dialysate in Module 4: *Hemodialysis Devices*. NOTE: You may hear dialysate called "bath," perhaps since it bathes the outside of the dialyzer membrane.

We make dialysate by mixing two concentrates with treated (ANSI/AAMI quality) water:

1. An **acid (low pH) concentrate** that has most of the electrolytes, such as calcium.
2. A **bicarbonate concentrate** that contains the buffer to maintain pH.

We dilute one of these concentrates with treated water to make a solution. Then, we mix that solution and the other concentrate to make dialysate. If we skip a step and mix the two concentrates, the calcium and magnesium will react with the bicarbonate to form solids. We always have *some* precipitate. So, we clean the machine with vinegar (5% acetic acid) or a citric acid product to dissolve what does form. You will learn more about how to mix dialysate in Module 4: *Hemodialysis Devices*.

Dialyzers and Diffusion in Hemodialysis

"This is what dialysis looks like: two needles in my arm, a set of lines, and the place where the blood goes to be cleaned is at the end of the dialysis machine, called a dialyzer."

In hemodialysis, we use a *dialyzer*, or artificial kidney, to remove wastes and water:

- The **blood compartment** (or blood side) is inside the hollow fibers of the dialyzer.
- The **dialysate compartment** (or dialysate side) is around the outside of the fibers.

When the kidneys fail, wastes and excess water build up inside cells, between cells, and in the bloodstream. We try to remove all of the wastes and excess water. **Yet, dialysis can only *directly* reach the blood**. And, since only about 7% of body water is in the blood, most of the wastes and excess water are *not* in the blood at any given moment. Thus, to be removed by dialysis, wastes that are not in the blood must:

1. Diffuse through each cell wall and into the interstitial space
2. Diffuse through the blood vessel walls and into the bloodstream
3. Flow into the blood compartment of the dialyzer
4. Pass through the hollow fiber dialyzer membrane (via diffusion or convection) and into the dialysate (see Figure 11)

Used dialysate is sent to a drain, and fresh dialysate flows in to keep a high concentration gradient. The slow rate of diffusion is why more than one pass of blood through the dialyzer is needed to clear wastes out of the blood—and why longer treatments remove more wastes. Each pass of the blood through the

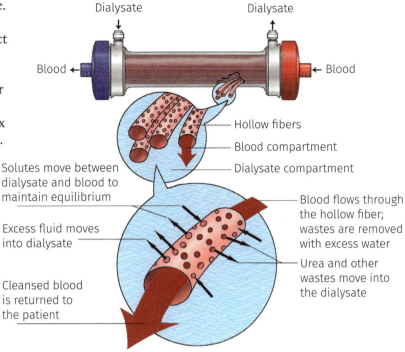

Figure 11: Diffusion Inside a Dialyzer

dialyzer removes more water and wastes. At a blood flow rate of 300 mL/min, blood only spends about 20 seconds in a dialyzer with each pass. Several factors affect the rate of diffusion in dialysis:

1. Number and size of membrane pores
2. Dialyzer surface area
3. Flow geometry
4. Dialysate temperature
5. Solute size

We use diffusion in dialysis to help balance electrolytes, too. Each electrolyte will move until its level is the same on both sides of the membrane. The doctor may prescribe:

- A **low level** of an electrolyte in the dialysate to **remove** any excess
- A **higher level** to help bring a patient's blood level back to normal

NUMBER AND SIZE OF MEMBRANE PORES

A dialyzer membrane with more pores allows faster diffusion. Larger pores let larger molecules through. A membrane's thickness and design also affect the diffusion rate (see Figure 12). You will learn more about pore size in Module 4: *Hemodialysis Devices*.

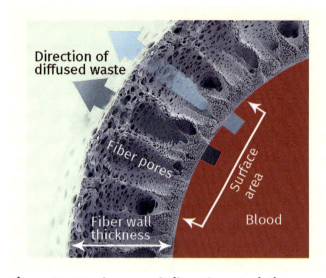

Figure 12: Membrane and Fiber Characteristics
Image adapted and used with permission from Baxter Healthcare Corporation

DIALYZER SURFACE AREA
Surface area is the amount of membrane that touches a fluid. Larger surface areas allow more diffusion.

FLOW GEOMETRY: DIRECTION OF FLOW
Blood flows through a dialyzer in one direction. Dialysate flows in the opposite direction (see Figure 13). We use this *countercurrent* flow on purpose: it aids diffusion by keeping high concentration gradients between the solutes in the blood and in the dialysate.

NOTE: A *concurrent* flow occurs when blood and dialysate flow the *same* direction. This makes a dialyzer about 20% less effective.[9]

DIALYSATE TEMPERATURE
To maintain patient safety, dialysate is kept in the temperature range of 34.5° C to 36.5° C.[10] Dialysate that is on the cooler side may make patients feel a bit cold during a treatment—but can help keep their blood pressure from dropping.[11] Dialysate that is too warm—over 45° C—can cause blood proteins to break down, and red blood cells to burst (*hemolysis*).[12]

SOLUTE SIZE
In the U.S., we use urea (a small molecule; 60 Da) to measure dialysis dose. However, at least 90 wastes have been found; 68 small (< 500 Da), 10 "middle" (500–12,000 Da) and 12 large (> 12,000 Da).[13] Middle and larger wastes may cause long-term problems for patients if they build up, but in the U.S., we rarely measure these. *This means that a patient whose* "adequacy" numbers are good may still have high levels of other wastes and need more treatment to avoid long-term complications.

The nephrologist factors in diffusion when prescribing a treatment. S/he will choose a large or small dialyzer, based on the patient's body size and the treatment length. The only thing that cannot be chosen is the size of the patient. To get enough treatment in a large patient, the doctor can increase treatment time, dialyzer size (clearance), or both to remove more wastes.

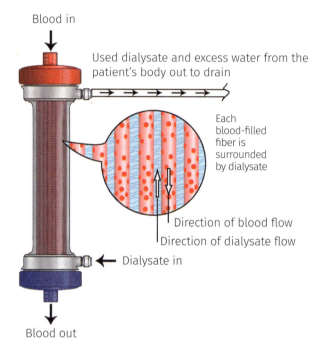

Figure 13: Blood and Dialysate Countercurrent Flow

Osmosis, Ultrafiltration, and Organ Stunning in Hemodialysis

"Normally my husband doesn't have any bad days. He felt bad this morning because the machine pulled off more than his target weight last night."

In our bodies, osmotic forces constantly shift water from one fluid compartment to the next. These forces go on even when the kidneys fail. So, in any type of dialysis, we use osmosis as one way to remove water from a patient's blood. In hemodialysis, we use osmosis *and* apply pressure with a pump to remove water through *ultrafiltration* (see Figure 14).

Principles of Dialysis

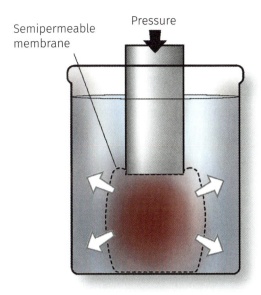

Ultrafiltration is the removal of extra fluid through the membrane using additional pressure.

Figure 14: Ultrafiltration

As with wastes, most excess body water is inside and between patients' cells—*not* in their bloodstreams. A patient who has swollen ankles or is short of breath, for example, has a water build-up in and between his or her cells. During a hemodialysis treatment, a series of events takes place, a bit like a waterfall in slow motion (see Figure 15):

1. We pull some excess water out of the blood.

2. As the water level of the blood drops, water shifts out of the extracellular space and through the capillary blood vessel walls to refill the blood vessels (intravascular space).

3. As the water level drops between the cells, water shifts out of the cells, through their membranes, to refill the extracellular water.

4. As dialysis continues to pull water out of the blood, water will keep shifting out of the extracellular space and cells to balance the fluid compartments. In this way, given enough time, we may be able to remove most or all of the excess water that has built up between treatments.

Measuring Solute Size

Some solutes are so small that we can only measure them by counting their atoms. Knowing the terms below and what they mean can give you a sense of the types of wastes we want to remove with dialysis and their relative size and help you understand some blood test results.

Dalton: A standard unit for atomic or molecular mass, also called atomic mass unit or amu. One dalton is *very tiny* (1/12 the mass of a carbon-12 nucleus, to be precise).[14]

Equivalent: One mole (see below) of charge—positive or negative. For example, sodium (Na^+) has one positively charged ion. So, 1 mole of Na^+ is 1 Equivalent. Calcium (Ca^{++}) has 2 positively charged ions. So, 1 mole of Calcium is 2 Equivalent. 1/1,000 Equivalent = 1 milliEquivalent = mEq.

Gram atomic weight: The weight in grams of one mole of a certain atom. For example, the gram atomic weight of sodium (Na) is 22.989770,[15] and the gram atomic weight of chloride (Cl) is 35.453.[15]

Gram molecular weight: The sum of the atomic weights of all of the atoms in a molecule. For example, sodium chloride (NaCl) is 58.4427 (22.989770 + 35.453).[15]

Mole: A chemistry shortcut that lets you count molecules by knowing the weight of a substance. A mole is 6.023×10^{23} molecules of any substance.[16]

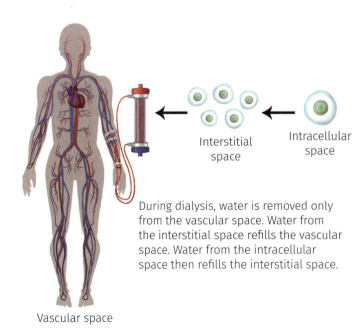

During dialysis, water is removed only from the vascular space. Water from the interstitial space refills the vascular space. Water from the intracellular space then refills the interstitial space.

Figure 15: Ultrafiltration in Hemodialysis

Dialysis Disequilibrium Syndrome (DDS)

In HD patients, DDS can occur when levels of wastes in the blood are very high—and drop rapidly during a treatment. DDS is rare these days, but may still occur in patients who are new to dialysis or have missed a number of treatments. The "blood–brain barrier" keeps solutes in the brain from shifting between fluid compartments as readily as they do in the rest of the body to protect the brain.[17] When we remove wastes from the blood, we form an osmotic gradient between the blood and cells in the brain. While solutes may not pass through, water moves into the brain through osmosis, causing swelling. The symptoms of DDS can be severe: headaches, nausea, vomiting, restlessness, or even seizures and coma—and death. Slowing the blood flow rate (and thus, the rate of diffusion) can help.[18]

TARGET WEIGHT

The dialysis prescription will include a target weight (TW) for the patient.* At target weight, a patient ideally has no excess water in his or her blood. When a patient comes into the clinic, you will subtract the target from his or her pre-dialysis weight. The difference *may* be the amount of water to remove during the treatment. However, a gain or loss in clothes or shoes, muscle, or fat will also show up on the scale. **Before you assume that all weight gained or lost is water weight,** *ask your patients.* Many patients get to know their bodies and can tell you if they have gained real weight, or if the excess weight really is water.

*NOTE: Some clinics call the target weight "dry weight" or "estimated dry weight" (EDW).

ULTRAFILTRATION RATE (UFR)

"I gained 6 kilos over the weekend a while back. Never, never again. I had major cramping, major BP drop, passed out. I did treatment Monday, Tuesday, and Wednesday. It kicked my butt. I felt bad all week."

In other fields, ultrafiltration (UF) removes very small particles. In dialysis, UF removes water from the blood. Once you choose a safe UF goal, enter that into the dialysis machine. The machine will divide the UF goal by the treatment time to set a UR rate (UFR in ML/hr) and remove the correct amount of water. (See Module 4: *Hemodialysis Devices* to learn more.) The "UF goal" for a treatment will include:

- **The water weight to remove**
- **The amount the patient will drink during the treatment.** (NOTE: When a patient drinks a cup of coffee during a treatment, the coffee is absorbed in the small intestine, and will pass into the bloodstream—but not right away. That coffee may be removed at the *next* treatment. But, we still add the amount to the UF goal.)
- **Saline or medicines used in the treatment**

When the UF control system is removing water from the blood it creates a pressure difference between the blood and dialysate compartments. This is called **trans** (across) membrane pressure (TMP).[19] The amount of pressure needed is determined by the dialyzer UF coefficient (KUF) and the patient's UFR. **TMP = UFR ÷ KUF**. (See Module 7: *Hemodialysis Procedures and Complications* to learn more.)

The machine may display TMP as a positive or a negative number:

- A machine that monitors TMP on the **blood** side will display it as a **positive** number.
- A machine that monitors TMP on the **dialysate** side will display it as a **negative** number.

We apply more pressure on the blood side of the membrane than on the dialysate side to pull water out of the blood and into the dialysate.

When a patient does gain a lot of water weight, the UFR needed to remove the water in one treatment may be too high for him or her to tolerate. In recent years, dialysis experts have learned that a too-high UFR can cause rapid blood pressure drops called *intradialytic hypotension, or IDH*. The patient may have painful muscle cramps, headaches, nausea, vomiting, and, in some cases, shock. In a large study, IDH occurred in 30.1% of U.S. standard in-center HD treatments—and patients with IDH were more likely to die.[20] Blood pressure drops can also harm the patient's access. Having patients cramp and drop their blood pressure is still common in many clinics. But, now we know how harmful this can be to our patients.

The **plasma refill rate** is the speed at which water and salts shift from the interstitial space (between cells) into the bloodstream. This rate has a finite maximum. The plasma refill rate can be influenced by many

Table 1: Risk of Symptomatic Blood Pressure Drop by UFR

HD (hrs)	Fluid gain in mL	Hourly UFR Volume	UFR: mL/kg/hr (based on 75 kg)	Rate of refill from interstitium	Change in blood volume	Chance of BP drop
Standard 4-hour Session						
4	800 mL	200 mL/hr	2.7 mL/kg/hr	200 /hr	0	0
4	1,600 mL	400 mL/hr	5.3 mL/kg/hr	400 /hr	0	0
4	2,400 mL	600 mL/hr	8 mL/kg/hr	400 /hr	-200 mL/hr	Small
4	4,000 mL	1,000 mL/hr	13.3 mL/kg/hr	400 /hr	-600 mL/hr	Major
4	4,800 mL	1,200 mL/hr	16 mL/kg/hr	400 /hr	-800 mL/hr	Definite
Nocturnal 8-hour Session						
8	800 mL	100 mL/hr	1.3 mL/kg/hr	100 /hr	0	0
8	1,600 mL	200 mL/hr	2.7 mL/kg/hr	200 /hr	0	0
8	2,400 mL	300 mL/hr	4 mL/kg/hr	300 /hr	0	0
8	3,200 mL	400 mL/hr	5.3 mL/kg/hr	400 /hr	0	0
8	4,800 mL	600 mL/hr	8 mL/kg/hr	400 /hr	-200 mL/hr	Small

Table adapted with permission from *Help, I Need Dialysis* (lifeoptions.org/resource-library/help-i-need-dialysis/).

factors, such as age, gender, serum albumin, inflammation, nutrition, and heart status. While the rate is very difficult to measure, most experts suggest that it is between 5 and 10 mL/kg/hour, and may be closer to 5 or 6 mL/kg/hour in stable patients.[21,22] If the UFR during dialysis is higher than the plasma refill rate, the patient's blood volume will shrink. If the patient cannot maintain a stable blood pressure, s/he may "crash"—with muscle cramps, headaches, nausea and vomiting—and it may take many hours to recover after a treatment. As you have learned, removing too much water or removing it too quickly can cause organ stunning.[23-26] In Table 1, you can see how the risk of a drop in blood pressure changes depending on the UFR.

AVOIDING ORGAN STUNNING

Organ stunning occurs when the blood flow and oxygen supply to the organs falls too low. Changing our practice to prevent this problem is a new focus in dialysis. So, you may find that clinics have not yet put protocols in place to prevent stunning. The nephrologist can prescribe dialysis in a way that will reduce patient risk. If your patients have symptoms of stunning, like cramps or long recovery time after treatments, advise them to ask their doctors about:

1. **A lower UFR**. A UFR of less than 10 mL per kilo of body weight, per hour (< 10 mL/kg/hr) reduces the risk of death from organ stunning.[27] A Medicare panel suggested 13 mL/kg/hr as an upper limit for UFR.[28] This rate is higher than what the evidence suggests, but is still less than current practice, and is a step in the right direction. Figure out a safe UFR for your patients by using this free calculator from www.homedialysis.org/ufr-calculator (see Figure 16).

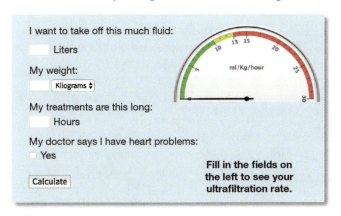

Figure 16: UFR Calculator

2. **Longer treatments**. More hemodialysis time takes off more water with a lower UFR. Most patients do not want to stay longer, transportation can be a challenge, and longer treatments can disrupt clinic schedules. But, longer treatments save lives. The U.S. has the shortest in-center hemodialysis (HD) time in the world: an average of 197–231 minutes. (Australia has the longest: 233–279 minutes.)[29] Yet, patients who get at least 4 hours of HD three times a week have a 30% higher survival rate than those who get less. *Each extra 30 minutes of HD further boosts survival by 7%.*[30]

3. **Cooler Dialysate**. Dialysate that is ½° C below core body temperature (measured with an ear thermometer) can prevent stunning.[10] While experts suggest a dialysate temperature range of 34.5° C to 36.5° C,[10] some clinics may still be using warmer dialysate. Most patients can handle a change to cooler dialysate, but some may feel cold. So, when lowering dialysate temperature, it may be wise to do so slowly, in steps.

4. **Oxygen**. Low-flow oxygen (by nasal tube) can increase blood oxygen and reduce the chance of blood pressure drops at dialysis.[31] With less hypotension, there may also be less risk of stunning, though there are few studies.[32] Oxygen must be used with caution in patients who have chronic obstructive pulmonary disease (COPD), like emphysema, or congestive heart failure (CHF). In these patients, breathing may slow down or even stop.[32]

Sodium Modeling – A Dying Practice

Some clinics still try to pull more water out of patients' blood by adding sodium to the dialysate to create an osmotic gradient. More sodium might be added at the start of a treatment, and less toward the end.

KDOQI Guidelines for dialysis recommend that we do *not use this type of sodium profiling*.[33] Adding sodium to the patient's blood triggers the thirst drive in the brain. The patient *must drink*—and then comes in for the next treatment even more overloaded.[34]

Instead, using a lower sodium level in the dialysate and following diet limits for salt can reduce thirst so the patient does not gain so much water weight in the first place.[34] It is the job of the nephrologist to prescribe the level of sodium in the dialysate.

Convection in Hemodialysis

"One thing is painfully clear to me. If I had known I was going to end up on dialysis I would have paid more attention in science class!"

In dialysis, convection boosts clearance by dragging some wastes through the membrane pores. The ease with which a solute can be dragged depends on its size: smaller solutes move easily while larger ones may be trapped by the membrane. Middle molecules do not diffuse easily, and convection can help remove them. In fact, in an experiment, a dialyzer designed to aid convection was able to remove twice as many middle molecules as one that was not.[35]

A *porous* membrane has many pores, large pores, or both, which boosts convection. In fact, highly porous membranes are *designed* to aid convective clearance. The sieving coefficient (SC) of a membrane is a measure of its porosity.[36] An SC of 1.0 means that, in most cases, a membrane could let 100% of a given solute through; an SC of 0.4 means that just 40% of a solute would pass.

Fresh dialysate that enters the dialyzer has no wastes. The water that is pulled out of the patient's blood at the arterial end of the dialyzer has the highest level of wastes. This part of the dialyzer is where larger, slower moving molecules will be "dragged" through the membrane by convection.

Adsorption in Hemodialysis

In dialysis, adsorption is a build-up of a thin film of protein that adheres to the dialyzer membrane. This process can both help and harm patients. On one hand, the film, made of the patient's own plasma proteins, makes the membrane more *biocompatible* (like the body) and less likely to cause harmful inflammation. And, more middle molecules, like beta-2 microglobulin, may be removed from the patient's blood by adsorption than by other means.[37] On the other hand, adsorption can slow diffusion and osmosis and make the treatment less efficient. Some types of membrane are more adsorptive than others. You will learn more about the protein film and membranes in Module 4: *Hemodialysis Devices*.

Fluid Dynamics in Hemodialysis

"Today I was 10 minutes from being done and got some of the worst cramps ever. When I was finished, my standing blood pressure dropped (54/27) and I was so dizzy I had to sit for a 1/2 hour and drink some water before I could walk out to my ride. Now, 4 hours later, I am again light headed and my back and stomach are cramping and I just feel so drained."

When you turn on the HD machine and start a treatment, a *blood pump* will control the rate of blood flow from the patient to the dialyzer. The pump *pulls* blood through the needle, which is a restriction that creates resistance to the blood flow. **Pre-pump pressure** is most often *negative*: less than zero. Then, the blood pump *pushes* blood through the tubing to the dialyzer. **Post-pump pressure** is *positive*: greater than zero. Both pulling and pushing occur at the same time as the pump turns (see Figure 17). The higher the blood flow rate or resistance, the more negative **the pre-pump** pressure will be.

Fluid dynamics change the pressure as blood is pumped through the *extracorporeal* (outside of the body) *circuit*. This circuit includes:

- The blood pump
- Blood tubing
- A *heparin* (anti-clotting drug) pump
- The dialyzer
- Monitors for air bubbles, blood pressure, and blood flow

You will learn more about the extracorporeal circuit in Module 4: *Hemodialysis Devices*.

The blood pump *pushes* the blood against the resistance of the tubing, the hollow fibers in the dialyzer, and the venous needle or catheter. This resistance creates *positive* pressure in the lines and dialyzer fibers. As blood passes through each of these, the pressures change:

- The highest positive pressure is in the *arterial header* of the dialyzer—where blood enters the hollow fibers.
- As blood flows through the hollow fibers, the pressure drops.
- The lowest positive pressure in the *blood path* (tubing) is after blood leaves the dialyzer.
- The average pressure of blood flowing into and out of the dialyzer fibers is the true amount of force (positive hydraulic pressure) that aids UF of water out of the blood.[38]

Dialysate also undergoes pressure changes as it passes through the dialyzer:

- Dialysate pressure is highest (most negative) at the *venous* end of the dialyzer (where the blood compartment pressure is lowest) and lowest (least negative) at the arterial end.
- This pressure gradient forces water out of the blood and into the dialysate.
- Less pressure loss occurs in the dialysate compartment, since water is not as thick as blood, *and* the dialysate flow path is much wider than the blood flow path.
- The dialysis machine controls the average pressure in the dialysate compartment. This assures that the prescribed amount of water is removed during the treatment.

Hemodiafiltration (HDF)

"I've been doing HDF at home for some time. I take my beta-2-microglobulin pre and post bloods now and again, and clearance does seem much better than normal HD. My hemoglobin stays high longer with less iron, and my BP is stable even if I am slightly under my dry weight."

HDF, is a way to fully use the convective capabilities of the dialyzer that is just starting in the U.S. During a treatment, the UFR in the dialyzer is kept very high, to remove more wastes and water through convection. To ensure good UF control, a sterile replacement fluid is infused into the patient's bloodstream during HDF.

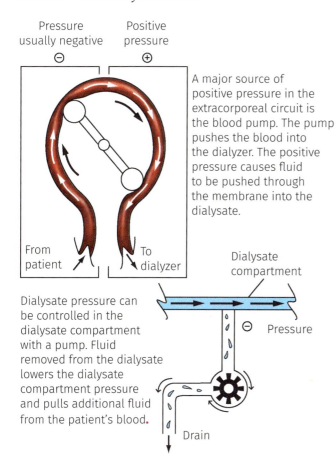

Figure 17: Actions of Positive and Negative Pressure in Dialysis

The added fluid also washes out more wastes. Less replacement fluid is added than is removed by UF, so the correct amount of water can be removed from the patient. The replacement fluid can be injected into the patient's bloodlines:

- *Before* the dialyzer: pre-dilution HDF (see Figure 18)
- *After* the dialyzer: post-dilution HDF
- *Within* the dialyzer: mid-dilution HDF

With pre-dilution HDF, we need to use more replacement fluid and UF to get good convective clearances, since blood is diluted when it goes into the dialyzer. We control fluid removal from the patient with the replacement fluid. So, if a patient needs to remove 2 liters during a treatment, the HDF system might remove *20 liters*—and replace 18 liters.

Hemodialysis dialysate is not sterile. Dialysate water must be treated, because it touches the patient's blood through the dialyzer membrane. But HDF replacement fluid *must* be sterile, because it is put directly into the patient's bloodstream. The fluid can be bagged or created online by the machine. Extra ultrafilters are often used to assure that the fluid is safe. Mid-dilution infuses fluid (made online by the machine) into the blood by *backfiltration*: forcing dialysate across the membrane into the blood compartment.

Applying Scientific Principles to Peritoneal Dialysis (PD)

"Last year I refused to wear a bikini because of my PD tube. This year I'm rocking one and doing so for all those other people who lack some sort of self-confidence because of imperfections! I may not have the perfect body, but I'm alive and that's all that matters!"

In hemodialysis, we bring the patient's blood outside the body to the dialyzer to filter out excess water, balance pH and electrolytes, and remove wastes. With PD, the cleansing takes place *inside* the body (see Figure 19). PD depends on four of the dialysis principles occurring at the same time: 1. Diffusion, 2. Osmosis, 3. Convection, and 4. Adsorption.

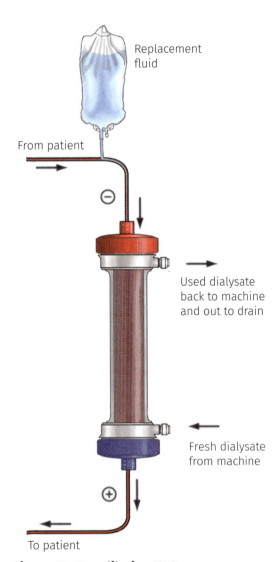

Figure 18: Pre-dilution HDF

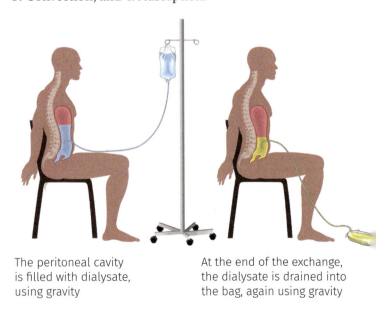

The peritoneal cavity is filled with dialysate, using gravity

At the end of the exchange, the dialysate is drained into the bag, again using gravity

Figure 19: Peritoneal Dialysis

The peritoneum is a one cell layer thick *living* membrane that lines the inside of the abdomen and the outside of all of the internal organs. Its capillary blood vessels are used as a membrane for PD. Total peritoneal blood flow ranges from 50–150 mL/min.[39] A PD catheter is placed into the patient's abdomen and gravity is used to fill the peritoneal space with sterile dialysate. In effect, this turns the patient's abdomen into a dialysate compartment, with blood on one side of the membrane and dialysate on the other.

Diffusion in Peritoneal Dialysis

"I chose PD as my first option and did it for 6 years until a leaky hernia made it impossible for me to continue. I would go back to it if I had the option."

In PD, diffusion is the main method of clearing the blood of wastes and electrolytes. We form a gradient between the patient's blood and the PD dialysate, which has few wastes. Wastes and electrolytes diffuse across the membrane into the dialysate. While the PD dialysate *dwells* (remains) in the patient's belly, the wastes and electrolytes approach equilibrium, and diffusion slows down. At this point, the "used" dialysate is drained and replaced with fresh dialysate. The concentration gradient is created again and diffusion will speed up once more. Draining and refilling is called an *exchange*. Patients do four exchanges each day by hand (manual), or use a cycler machine at night to do exchanges while they sleep. Cycler patients may also do one or two manual exchanges during the day.

The nephrologist prescribes:
- The number of exchanges
- Length of time for each exchange
- Volume of PD dialysate
- Concentration of solutes in the dialysate

Osmosis in Peritoneal Dialysis

"I did manuals for a few months before I got on the cycler. I finally decided to do the cycler because it was better for my lifestyle, but sometimes I do the manuals if I need to. I love the freedom PD gives me. I don't feel limited."

In PD, sugar (dextrose) in the bags of sterile dialysate is most often used to create an osmotic gradient. Water shifts out of the blood, which has less sugar, into the PD dialysate, which has more. There is no UF pump in PD; excess water is removed from the blood by osmosis. How much water is removed at each exchange depends on the osmotic concentration of the dialysate (see Table 2). Patients are taught to limit salt and water in their diets as needed to keep their blood pressure in a safe range and avoid gaining water weight. PD diet and fluid limits tend to be much less than they would be for standard in-center hemodialysis. However, failing to follow the limits or changes to the membrane over time may require the use of higher concentration dialysate.

Table 2: PD Dialysate

Concentration	Connector (bag) color	Manufacturer
1.5% Dextrose	Yellow	Baxter, Fresenius
2.5% Dextrose	Green	Baxter, Fresenius
4.25% Dextrose	Red	Baxter, Fresenius
7.5% Icodextrin (a non-sugar polymer)[40]	Purple	Baxter

It is best if PD patients use the lowest dextrose bags as often as they can. Patients may absorb nearly 20% of their daily calories from the dialysate.[41] Higher dextrose dialysate contains more calories. And, heating dextrose to make dialysate breaks down some of the sugars, which forms glucose degradation products (GDPs) that can harm the peritoneal membrane over time. Any remaining kidney function can be damaged as well. Research has found that using lower GDP dialysate can help protect the peritoneum and the kidneys.[42,43] Those who must often use high dextrose bags to remove water may be nearing the end of their time on PD.

Dextrose in PD dialysate can also be a challenge for patients with diabetes. A non-dextrose dialysate (icodextrin, called Extraneal) may be used for the long (nighttime) dwell. However, this option is more costly and not often used in the U.S. And, some blood sugar monitors and test strips will not be accurate when patients who use icodextrin test their blood. Patients may need to switch monitors or test strips.[44]

Convection in Peritoneal Dialysis

"I chose PD because I have a problem dealing with blood, and I wanted to live the rest of my life to the fullest since I have no hope for a transplant. It suits me just right, and I even stayed at work for nearly 2 years. You have to dedicate yourself to handle every detail, and that's good for me because I don't trust anybody but myself to do things."

Convection boosts PD clearance by dragging some wastes through the membrane pores. The number and size of the pores and thickness of the membrane varies from patient to patient. PD dialysate with more dextrose (or icodextrin) removes more water—and increases convective movement of small solutes.[45] In PD, convection may remove the most sodium.[46]

Adsorption in Peritoneal Dialysis

"Ugh, my albumin is only 2.9, and I don't know what to do to get that number up. I know it is so dangerously low. I can barely eat most days. I'm just so frustrated."

In PD, adsorption can help remove wastes that are bound to proteins. As used dialysate exits the body, some proteins will adhere to the inside of the catheter.[47] Unfortunately, PD can remove protein that patients need along with the wastes. *Fibrin*, a blood-clotting factor, can also clump and form long strings that block a PD catheter *lumen* (opening).

Conclusion

Dialysis that lets patients live life to the fullest is a complex mix of time and efficiency. Replacing the tasks of organs that clean blood 24-hours a day takes time. Once you understand the principles that make dialysis work, you can see how the doctor can tailor treatments to meet the needs of each patient. And, you can talk to your patients about why it is so vital to get all of the treatment the doctor prescribes—and even ask for more.

Appendix A: Metric System and Temperature Conversions

The metric system is commonly used for measurements in dialysis. Each day as you care for patients, you will need to make precise calculations to ensure that their treatments are safe.

COMMONLY USED METRIC UNITS

Quantity	Unit	Symbol	Relationship of Units
Volume	Milliliter	mL	1 mL = 0.001 L
	Deciliter	dL	1 dL = 0.01 L
	Liter	L	1000 mL = 1 L
Mass	Milligram	mg	1 mg = 0.001 g
	Gram	g	1 g = 1000 mg
	Kilogram	kg	1 kg = 1000 g
Length	Millimeter	mm	1 mm = 0.001 m
	Centimeter	cm	1 cm = 0.01 m
	Meter	m	1 m = 100 cm
	Kilometer	km	1 km = 1000 m

These common conversions may be helpful:

- 1 kilogram (kg) = 2.2 pounds (lb)
- 1 ounce (oz) = 28.35 grams (g)
- 1 fluid ounce (fl oz) = 29.57 milliliters (mL)
- 1 milliliter (mL) = 1 cubic centimeter (cc)
- 1 gallon (gal) = 3.785 liters (L)
- 1 liter (L) = 1.057 quarts (U.S.) (qt)
- 1 meter (m) = 39.37 inches (in)
- 1 inch (in) = 2.54 centimeters (cm)

You will see temperature conversions from Fahrenheit to Celsius in the dialysis setting. Online calculators make this easy, but to provide a sense of how the two measures differ, these conversions may be helpful.

Scale	Fahrenheit °F	Celsius °C
Freezing point of water	32° F	0° C
Body temperature (normal)	98.6° F	37° F
Boiling point of water	212° F	100° C

References

1. McCann L (ed). *Pocket guide to nutrition assessment of the patient with kidney disease* (5th ed). New York, NY, National Kidney Foundation, 2015
2. *Definition of Blood pH*. Medicinenet.com 13 May 2016. Available at http://www.medicinenet.com/script/main/art.asp?articlekey=10001. Accessed October 2016
3. McCarthy JT, El-Azhary RA, Patzelt MT, et al. Survival, risk factors, and effect of treatment in 101 patients with calciphylaxis. *Mayo Clinic Proc*. 2016;91(10):1384-94
4. Castner D. Hemodialysis: Principles of hemodialysis. In C.S. Counts (Ed.), *Core Curriculum for Nephrology Nursing: Module 3. Treatment options for patients with chronic kidney failure* (6th ed., pp. 69-166). Pitman, NJ: American Nephrology Nurses' Association, 2015
5. Clark W, Macias W, Molitoris B, et al. Plasma protein adsorption to highly permeable hemodialysis membranes. *Kidney Int*. 1995;48:481-88
6. Cheung A. Biocompatibility of hemodialysis membranes. *J Am Soc Nephrol*. 1990;1:150-161
7. Platelets.se. *Protein adsorption*. Available at http://platelets.se/protein-adsorption/. Accessed May 2017
8. Bhave G, Neilson E. Body Fluid Dynamics: Back to the future. *J Am Soc Nephrol*. 2011;22:2166-81
9. Baldwin I, Baldwin M, Fealy N, et al. Con-current versus counter-current dialysis flow during CVVHD. A comparative study for creatinine and urea removal. *Blood Purif*. 2016;41:171-76
10. Daugirdas JT. Chronic hemodialysis prescription, in Daugirdas JT, Blake PG, Ing TS (eds): *Handbook of Dialysis* (5th ed). Philadelphia, PA, Wolters Kluwer Health, 2015, pg 209
11. Eldehni MT, Odudu A, McIntyre CW. Randomized clinical trial of dialysate cooling and effects on brain white matter. *J Am Soc Nephrol*. 2015;26:957-65
12. Gershfeld NL, Murayama MJ. Thermal instability of red blood cell membrane bilayers: Temperature dependence of hemolysis. *J Membrane Biol*. 1988;101(1):67-72 doi:10.1007/BF01872821
13. Yavuz A, Tetta C, Ersoy FF, et al. Uremic toxins: a new focus on an old subject. *Semin Dial*. 2005;18(3):203-11
14. Senese, F. *What is a "dalton"?* Available at http://antoine.frostburg.edu/chem/senese/101/atoms/faq/what-is-a-dalton.shtml. Accessed November 2016
15. *Molecular weight of sodium chloride*. Available at http://www.convertunits.com/molarmass/Sodium+Chloride. Accessed November 2016

16   Senese, F. *Moles confuse me- why are they used?* Available at http://antoine.frostburg.edu/chem/senese/101/moles/faq/why-use-moles.shtml. Accessed May 2017
17   Johns Hopkins University. *Blood-brain barrier*. (working group) Available at http://bloodbrainbarrier.jhu.edu Accessed October 2016
18   Mah DY, Yia HJ, Cheong WS. Dialysis disequilibrium syndrome: A preventable fatal acute complication. *Med J Malaysia*. 2016;71(2):91-2
19   King B. Principles of hemodialysis, in Counts CS (ed): *Core Curriculum for Nephrology Nursing* (5th ed). Pitman, NJ, American Nephrology Nurses Association, 2008, pp. 662-81
20   Stefansson BV, Brunelli SM, Cabrera C, et al. Intradialytic hypotension and risk of cardiovascular disease. *Clin J Am Soc Nephrol*. 2014;9(12):2124-32
21   Kim KE, Neff M, Cohen B, et al. Blood volume changes and hypotension during hemodialysis. *Trans Am Soc Artif Intern Organs*. 1970;16:508-14
22   Chaignon M, Chen WT, Tarazi RC, et al. Blood pressure response to hemodialysis. *Hypertension*. 1981;3(3):333-9
23   McIntyre CW, Burton JO, Selby NM, et al. Hemodialysis-induced cardiac dysfunction is associated with an acute reduction in global and segmental myocardial blood flow. *Clin J Am Soc Nephrol*. 2008;3(1):19-26
24   Regolisti G, Maggiore U, Cademartiri C, et al. Cerebral blood flow decreases during intermittent hemodialysis in patients with acute kidney injury, but not in patients with end-stage renal disease. *Nephrol Dial Transplant*. 2013;28(1):79-85
25   McIntyre CW. Haemodialysis-induced myocardial stunning in chronic kidney disease – a new aspect of cardiovascular disease. *Blood Purif*. 2010;29(2):105-10
26   McIntyre CW, Harrison LE, Eldehni MT, et al. Circulating endotoxemia: a novel factor in systemic inflammation and cardiovascular disease in chronic kidney disease. *Clin J Am Soc Nephrol*. 2011;6(1):133-41
27   Flythe JE, Kimmel SE, Brunelli SM. Rapid fluid removal during dialysis is associated with cardiovascular morbidity and mortality. *Kidney Int*. 2011;79(2):250-7
28   Arbor Research Collaborative for Health and the University of Michigan Kidney Epidemiology and Cost Center. *End-stage renal disease quality measure development and maintenance hemodialysis adequacy clinical technical expert panel summary report*. Baltimore MD, 2013
29   Tentori F, Zhang J, Li Y, et al. Longer dialysis session length is associated with better intermediate outcomes and survival among patients on in-center three times per week hemodialysis: results from the Dialysis Outcomes and Practice Patterns Study (DOPPS). *Nephrol Dial Transplant*. 2012;27:4180-8
30   Saran R, Bragg-Gresham JL, Levin NW, et al. Longer treatment time and slower ultrafiltration in hemodialysis: associations with reduced mortality in the DOPPS. *Kidney Int*. 2006;69:1222-28
31   Diroll D. Oxygen as an adjunct to treat intradialytic hypotension during hemodialysis. *Neph Nursing J*. 2014;41(4):420-3
32   Meyring-Wösten A, Zhang H, Ye X, et al. Intradialytic hypoxemia and clinical outcomes in patients on hemodialysis. *Clin J Am Soc Nephrol*. 2016;11(4)616-25 doi: 10.2215/CJN.08510815
33   National Kidney Foundation. KDOQI clinical practice guideline for hemodialysis adequacy: 2015 update. *Am J Kidney Dis*. 2015;66(5):884-930
34   Jung ES, Lee J, Lee JW, et al. Increasing the dialysate sodium concentration based on serum sodium concentrations exacerbates weight gain and thirst in hemodialysis patients. *Tohoku J Exp Med*. 2013;230(2):117-21
35   Lee JC, Lee K, Kim HC. Mathematical analysis for internal filtration of convection-enhanced high-flux hemodialyzer. *Comput Methods Programs Biomed*. 2012;108(1):68-79
36   Kallenbach J, Gutch C, Stoner M, et al. *Review of Hemodialysis for Nurses and Dialysis Personnel* (7th ed). Philadelphia, PA, Elsevier, Inc., 2005, p. 66
37   Aucella F, Gesuete A, Vigilante M, et al. Adsorption dialysis: from physical principles to clinical applications. *Blood Purif*. 2013;35 Suppl 2:42-7
38   King B. Principles of hemodialysis, in Counts CS (ed): *Core Curriculum for Nephrology Nursing* (5th ed). Pitman, NJ, American Nephrology Nurses Association, 2008, pp. 662-81
39   Fresenius Medical Care. Advanced Renal Education Program. *Anatomy of the peritoneum*. Available at http://advancedrenaleducation.com/content/anatomy-peritoneum. Accessed November 2016
40   Frampton JE, Plosker GL. Icodextrin: A review of its use in peritoneal dialysis. *Drugs*. 2003;63(19):2079-105
41   Davies SJ, Russel L, Bryan J, et al. Impact of peritoneal absorption of glucose on appetite, protein catabolism and survival in CAPD patients. *Clin Nephrol*. 1996;45(3):194-8
42   Cho Y, Johnson DW, Craig JC, et al. Biocompatible dialysis fluids for peritoneal dialysis. *Cochrane Database Syst Rev*. 2014;(3):CD007554. doi: 10.1002/14651858.CD007554.pub2
43   Wang J, Zhu N, Yuan W. Effect of neutral pH and low-glucose degradation product-containing peritoneal dialysis solution on residual renal function in peritoneal dialysis patients: a meta-analysis. *Nephron*. 2015;129(3):155-63
44   Baxter Healthcare Corporation. 14 June 2016. Available at http://www.glucosesafety.com/us/index.html. Accessed November 2016
45   Asghar RB, Diskin AM, Spanel P, et al. Influence of convection on the diffusive transport and sieving of water and small solutes across the peritoneal membrane. *J Am Soc Nephrol*. 2005;16(2):437-43
46   Fischbach M, Schmitt CP, Shroff R, et al. Increasing sodium removal on peritoneal dialysis: applying dialysis mechanics to the peritoneal dialysis prescription. *Kidney Int*. 2016;89(4):761-6
47   Yanagisawa N, Li DQ, Ljungh A. Protein adsorption on ex vivo catheters and polymers exposed to peritoneal dialysis effluent. *Perit Dial Int*. 2004;24(3):264-73

4 Hemodialysis Devices

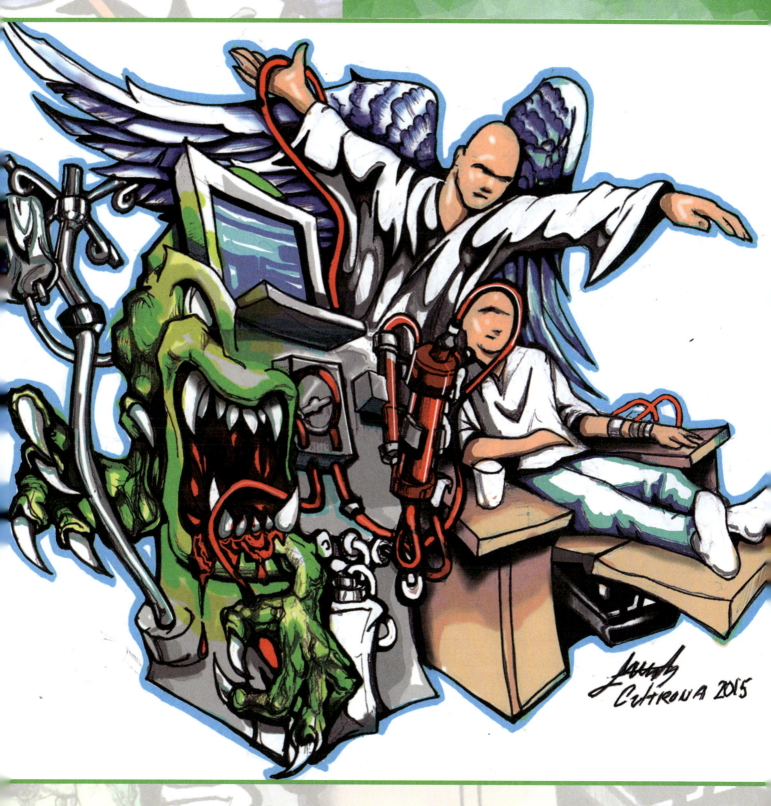

"When I drew this image, it meant to me that the machine seemed to be like an evil blood-sucking beast—but on the other hand, I know that it is also an angel keeping me alive."
—Mitchell J Cultrona

"The best thing a technician did for me...I was in-center because I could no longer do PD. He came and looked me in the eye, put his hand on my shoulder, and said, 'I know this isn't what you want, but we'll do everything we can to make it work for you.' It helped me so much to know that he understood."

Objectives

MODULE AUTHORS

Jeff Boyd, CHT

Emily Michalak

Michael Morales, MHA/Ed, CHT, CHBT, CCHT-A, CDWS

Kazim Naqvi, CHT, CBNT, CHBT

Dennis Shell, CHT, CHBT

MODULE REVIEWERS

Stanley Frinak

Nancy M. Gallagher, BS, RN, CNN

Susan K. Hansen, RN, CNN, MBA

Darlene Rodgers, BSN, RN, CNN, CPHQ

John H. Sadler, MD

Dori Schatell, MS

Vern Taaffe, BS, CBNT, CDWS

Tamyra Warmack, RN

Practice Test Questions at:
www.meiresearch.org/cc6

After you complete this module, you will be able to:

1. Describe how dialyzers are made.
2. Explain why two concentrates are used to make dialysate.
3. List three basic functions of the dialysis delivery system.
4. Explain how the air detector and blood leak detector work.
5. Name five parts of the extracorporeal blood circuit.
6. Explain the steps we take to protect patient safety during a hemodialysis (HD) treatment.

An acronym list can be found in the Glossary.

Introduction

"If we let dialysis get us down, and see it as a ball and chain that keeps us from enjoying life, we won't enjoy life. We'll be angry, depressed, bitter, and an emotional wreck. I choose to see dialysis as a blessing. Do I enjoy coming in three times a week? No. But for the most part I can come into my clinic with a smile, happy to see the people that are here, and able to give a kind word and hopefully be a blessing."

Healthy kidneys help to keep the constant climate inside the body that we call *homeostasis*. While dialysis cannot do all that healthy kidneys do, it can remove some wastes and excess water. And, dialysis can help keep electrolytes and pH at levels that keep patients alive.

This module covers the HD devices you will learn how to use and monitor:

- Dialyzers
- Dialysate
- Single Pass Hemodialysis Delivery Systems
- Monitoring Devices

The Role of the Biomedical Technician

Patients need safe equipment. If you like to work with machines, you may want to become a Biomedical Technician. In this role, you would make sure that all equipment meets the industry standards (CMS, OSHA, AAMI, state, and local). As members of the care team, you would work with:

- HD machines
- All medical equipment – from IV pumps to blood pressure cuffs
- Water treatment – all parts of the system
- Concentrate mixing systems
- Dialyzer reprocessing systems
- Physical plant
- Training and education

As a Biomedical Technician, you would take part in a Quality Assessment Performance Improvement program. This program gives you a chance to share what you do with the rest of the team.

Today's HD machines monitor each treatment and show you what is going on in real time. Better technology lets you focus more of your time on your patients. Trained staff who know how dialysis works, know the equipment, and follow procedures have the best chance of keeping patients safe.

Dialyzers and How They Work

"It's my second month using a different dialyzer, and my labs are better! Phosphorus 3.3! Potassium 4.9. I could not be more happy about the change!"

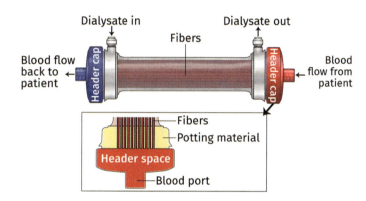

Figure 1: Dialyzer

The dialyzer replaces some of the functions of the patient's failed kidneys. <u>*Hollow fiber dialyzers*</u> are the most common ones in use today. These dialyzers fit a large surface area into a compact, sturdy, clear plastic case[1] (see Figure 1):

- Thousands of hair-thin hollow fibers are the semipermeable membrane. As you have learned, the volume inside of the fibers is the blood compartment of the dialyzer. (This volume does not change when the pressure in the blood compartment changes.) The dialysate compartment surrounds the outside of the fibers.

- At each end of the case, a plastic header connects the bloodlines securely to the dialyzer. Headers may be clear, or they may be color-coded red for arterial and blue for venous. Some headers are removable. This allows a Reuse Technician to remove the cap to clean the blood compartment end when a dialyzer is reprocessed.

- Just inside the header, a clay-like polyurethane "potting" material holds the fibers in place and keeps them open.
- Ports on the side of the dialyzer allow dialysate to flow in and out of the space around the fibers: the dialysate compartment.

During dialysis, blood enters the dialyzer at the top, flows through each fiber, and exits at the bottom. Dialysate flows around the fibers from bottom to top, in a countercurrent flow (see Figure 2).

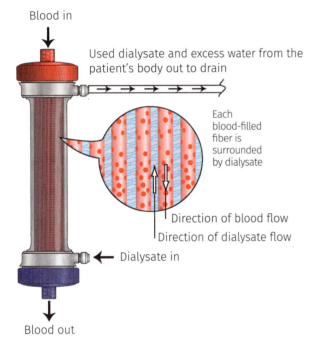

Figure 2: Blood and Dialysate Flow

How a dialyzer is made can affect the patient's comfort, safety, and how well a treatment removes wastes and excess water. In this section, you will learn about:
- *Membrane materials* – what membranes are made from
- *Biocompatibility* – how much the membranes are like the human body
- *Membrane surface area* – how large the membrane is
- *Membrane pore size* – the solute size that can pass through the membrane
- *Clearance* – the rate of solute removal
- *Mass transfer coefficient* – how well a solute will diffuse through the membrane
- *Ultrafiltration (UF) coefficient* – how much water will be removed
- *Testing dialyzer clearance* – how to tell the real clearance of a dialyzer vs. the manufacturer's specifications

The nephrologist prescribes the dialyzer. One of your tasks as a technician will be to match the dialyzer with each patient's prescription.

Membrane Materials

Like a nephron in a kidney, a dialyzer membrane is *selective*. Only water and waste solutes of a certain size can pass through. Large substances, like bacteria and blood cells, will not fit through the small pores. However, endotoxin fragments of the cell walls of bacteria *can* pass through the membrane, where they can cause fever and chills.

Several membrane factors affect how well a membrane will remove water and wastes. These include material, pore size and number, fiber diameter, and surface area (see Figure 3).

Biocompatibility

As you have learned, biocompatible means that a substance is so much like the body that the immune system does not react to it. *All* dialyzers are foreign to the body and will react to some degree with patients' immune cells:
- A reaction may be so subtle that patients do not notice it. Blood tests can detect changes to the white blood cells.[2]
- An immune reaction may cause symptoms like headaches or itching during a treatment.
- Rare but severe allergies (anaphylaxis) can occur that may even lead to death.[3]

The doctor prescribes the dialyzer. It is vital to use a membrane the patient can tolerate. Most *synthetic* (man-made) membranes are more biocompatible than *cellulose* (plant fiber) membranes. Synthetic fibers are *hydrophobic*: they repel water, so they are better able to adsorb blood proteins. The patient's blood touches the blood proteins and not the membrane.[4]

CELLULOSE MEMBRANES

Early dialyzer membranes made from cellulose—a plant fiber—were thin and strong, but caused immune reactions in some patients.[4] For this reason, unmodified cellulose membranes are rarely used in the U.S.

Table 1: Features of Synthetic Membranes[7]

Material	Features
Polyacrylonitrile (PAN)	- *Hydrophilic* surface attracts water to form a hydrogel with good diffusion and water permeability - May be coated to improve biocompatibility - Some types allow heparin-free dialysis
Polysulfone (PSf)	- Removes a broad range of wastes - High sieving capacity and permeability aid convection - Retains endotoxins
Polyethersulfone (PES)	- Excellent middle molecule removal without much albumin loss (all high flux membranes lose some albumin) - Retains endotoxins
Polymethylmethacrylate (PMMA)	- Highly adsorptive - Excellent middle molecule removal - Adsorbs PTH and improves itching
Polyester polymer Alloy (PEPA)	- Unique three-layer structure allows tight control of water and solute permeability and albumin loss - Can be used as an endotoxin filter
Ethylene vinyl alcohol copolymer (EVAL)	- Smooth, hydrophilic surface retains water - Few plasma proteins adsorbed; less inflammatory - May help patients maintain better blood flow to limbs

MODIFIED CELLULOSE MEMBRANES

Starting in the 1970s, cellulose membranes were chemically changed. The aim was to make them more biocompatible. This was done by:[4,5]

- Replacing some of the *hydroxyl* groups—atoms that form alcohol—with cellulose acetate, diacetate, or triacetate
- Adding an antioxidant coating, like vitamin E

SYNTHETIC MEMBRANES

Synthetic membranes are made from *polymers* (groups of plastic molecules). They remove wastes by diffusion, adsorption, and a bit of convection. Since they remove solutes up to 15,000 Da, they clear some $\beta_2 M$.

Biocompatibility of synthetic membranes is very good. They adsorb blood proteins quickly, which keeps blood from touching the membrane.[6] Each material also has features that can make it useful for a certain purpose (see Table 1).

Synthetic membranes have improved over time. The fibers and pore size are now more consistent, so we can better control diffusion to remove *wastes*. Clearance of *water* depends mainly on UF rates, so with better membranes, we have more precise UF control.

Patient Reactions to Dialyzers During HD

"Anyone else out there have an allergic reaction as soon as you get hooked up? I scratch until I bleed, and the reaction lasts until morning."

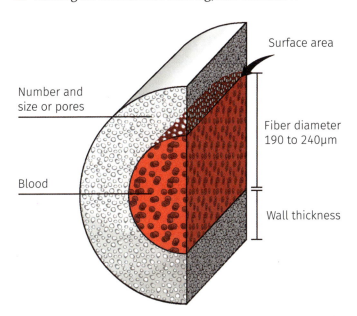

Figure 3: Membrane and Fiber Characteristics

Rarely, patients can be allergic to a dialyzer or the chemicals used to prepare it—but these allergies can be deadly. There are two types of reactions: Type A and Type B.[3]

TYPE A DIALYZER REACTIONS

Type A reactions may be due to *ethylene oxide*, a sterilant for new dialyzers. **Or, patients who take ACE inhibitors for blood pressure may react to PAN membranes, no matter how they are sterilized**. Type A reactions tend to occur *in the first few minutes of treatment*. These reactions may be seen in about one of every 25,000 treatments.

- **Mild Type A symptoms** may include:[3]
  - Itching or hives
  - Access site burning
  - Flushing, headache, fever, chills
  - Coughing, sneezing, or wheezing
  - Abdominal cramps, diarrhea, nausea, vomiting
  - Back and chest pain

- **Severe symptoms** may include *anaphylaxis*—a life-threatening allergy:
  - Trouble breathing
  - A feeling of impending doom
  - A drop in blood pressure that can lead to cardiac arrest and death

If a Type A reaction occurs, **stop the treatment and do not return the patient's blood**. The patient may need medications. Dialyzer reuse, rinsing with extra saline, a change of membrane, or giving an antihistamine or steroid drug to the patient may prevent future Type A problems.

TYPE B DIALYZER REACTIONS

Type B reactions are less severe than Type A, but more common. They occur in 3–5% of treatments with new modified cellulose membranes. The reaction tends to start in the first 15–30 minutes of treatment and decreases as treatment goes on. An immune response called *complement activation* may be the cause. Dialyzer reuse can help: the preprocessing cycle can flush out chemicals from manufacturing and/or reduce the immune response.

- **Symptoms** may include:
  - Chest and back pain
  - Trouble breathing
  - Nausea and vomiting
  - Drop in blood pressure

Toxins in Plastic

Any device used in dialysis can both help—and harm—patients. Since blood tubing, dialyzers, and bags of IV fluid are made of plastic, the contents of that plastic matters for patient safety. Two plastic additives are of special concern in dialysis:

- **DEHP**: A plasticizer is a chemical that lets plastic bend and change shapes. DEHP, di (2-ethylhexyl) phthalate, is a plasticizer that is often added to blood tubing sets, IV bags, and dialyzers and can cause health risks.[8]

- **Bisphenol A** (BPA): An endocrine (hormone) disrupter that can cause kidney and heart damage. BPA is found in plastic take-out food boxes, cash register receipts, in the linings of food cans—and in most dialyzers. Since the kidneys help remove BPA from the body, patients may have higher than normal levels anyway.[7,9]

The ELISIO–H single-use, high-flux dialyzer is, at the time of this *Core Curriculum*, the only one in the U.S. that is not made with DEHP or BPA. A clinical trial is looking at whether this matters to patient health.[10]

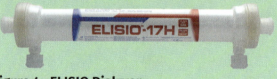

Figure 4: ELISIO Dialzyer
Image used with permission from NIPRO Medical Corporation.

Membrane Surface Area

"I'm so excited about this—my clinic manager finally ordered me a larger dialyzer! As far as I know, I'm the first in this area to use it!"

Surface area is how much area a membrane would take up if we unfolded all of the fibers and laid them out next to each other. When all else stays the same, a membrane with more surface area will expose more blood to dialysate, and remove more solutes. When a membrane with a smaller surface area is used, longer treatment times can allow for more solute removal. Total dialyzer surface area for adults tends to range from 0.5–2.5 square meters. Children or those with very high waste levels may be dialyzed with less surface area to help prevent brain swelling due to *dialysis disequilibrium syndrome*.[11]

Membrane Pores

Pore size matters when we want to remove wastes from patients' blood. Healthy kidneys clear the body of excess water and small, middle, and even large molecule wastes:

- **Small molecules**, like urea and creatinine, are less than 500 daltons.[7]
- **Middle molecules**, like β_2M, range from 500–15,000 daltons.[7]
- **Large molecules**, like albumin (which we do not want to remove) are 15,000 or more daltons.[7]

Dialyzers do not tend to do as thorough a job of removing middle or large wastes as kidneys do. Unfortunately, it is these middle and large wastes that can harm patients' hearts,[12] blood vessels,[13] and bones and joints[14] over the long term.

Molecular weight cutoff (given in daltons) is the solute size that a membrane retains by at least 90%. In other words, only 10% of a solute of this size will pass through the membrane (see Table 2). Doctors choose membranes that will remove certain molecules from the blood.

Table 2: Common Molecular Weights[15]

Molecule	Molecular Weight (Da)
Albumin ($C_{2936}H_{4624}N_{786}O_{889}S_{41}$)	66,500
Calcium (Ca^{++})	40
Creatinine $C_4H_7N_3O$	113
Nitric Oxide (NO_{3-})	62
Phosphate (PO_4^{2-})	95
Urea (CH_4N_2O)	60
Water (H_2O)	18
Zinc (Zn^{2+})	65

Flux is flow through a semipermeable membrane:

- **Conventional** or **low flux** membranes, rarely used in the U.S., have small pores that remove small wastes and not many middle or larger wastes. Water removal is also less, because these membranes have a KUF that is equal or less than 10 mL/hr/mmHg.[16] With smaller pores, low flux membranes are less prone to *backfiltration* which can allow endotoxin fragments to pass from non-sterile dialysate through the membrane and into the patient's blood.
- **High flux** membranes have a KUF of greater than 20 mL/hr/mmHg and larger pores than conventional membranes.[16] These membranes are more permeable (porous) and can remove protein-bound and middle molecule wastes. Due to their larger pores, high flux membranes are also more prone to backfiltration, which could lead to endotoxin reactions: fever and chills during dialysis.[16,17] Proper control of transmembrane pressure (TMP) prevents this problem. As you can see from Figure 5, urea is small *and* smooth, and can pass easily through the pores. Middle molecules, like β_2M, may be complex and twisted as well as larger—so they can be far more difficult to remove.
- **"High efficiency"** dialyzers may have a KUF between 10 and 19 mL/hr/mmHg.[16] Clearance of middle molecules may be high or low.[16]

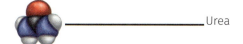

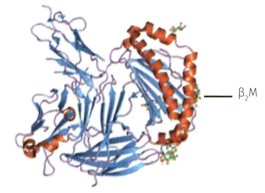

Figure 5: Urea and β_2M Molecules

Clearance

Clearance (K) is the amount of blood that can be cleared of a given solute in a given time.[5] Each dialyzer has a clearance rate for molecules at certain blood and dialysate flow rates. For example, a dialyzer with a urea clearance of **250 mL/min** will clear all of the urea from **250 mL of blood** *in one minute*. However, let us say:

- The blood flow rate on the dialysis machine is set to 400 mL/min.
- The dialysate flow rate is 500 mL/min.
- The dialyzer has a urea clearance of **308 mL/min**.

This dialyzer will clear all of the urea from **308 mL of blood out of the 400 mL of blood that flows through it *in one minute***.

During a treatment, the patient's blood goes through the dialyzer many times, and more urea is removed with each pass.

> ### Prescribing Dialysis to Remove More Wastes
>
> The nephrologist can boost clearance of solutes in a number of ways, which include:
>
> - **Prescribing a dialyzer with a larger surface area**. With more blood exposed to the membrane, more waste removal will occur during the same amount of treatment time.
> - **Prescribing a dialyzer with a higher clearance rating**. More clearance means more wastes removed during a treatment.
> - **Raising the blood flow rate (Qb)**. Qb limits clearance, since blood can only flow so quickly out of a patient's access. However, even if blood *could* flow at an infinite rate, clearance still levels off.[18] So, doubling the blood flow rate will not double the clearance (see KoA, on page 109 to learn more), and might harm a fistula or graft.[19]
> - **Raising the dialysate flow rate (Qd)**. If Qb is at least 350 mL/min, raising Qd to 800 mL/min will increase urea clearance by about 14%.[18] There may be no benefit of a Qd beyond 600 mL/min when a dialyzer with enhanced dialysate flow is used.[20]
> - **Extending the treatment time (T)**. More time allows more wastes to shift out of the *intracellular* (inside the cells) and *interstitial* (between the cells) fluid compartments into the bloodstream where we can remove them. Longer hemodialysis treatments remove more small and middle molecule solutes than shorter ones.[21,22]
>
> Your patients can ask their doctors to consider one or more of these options if they have uremic symptoms.

A dialyzer clears wastes from a patient's blood in three ways:*

1. Diffusion
2. Convection
3. Adsorption

*See the section on Ultrafiltration on page 110 to learn more about how a dialyzer removes excess water from a patient's blood.

DIFFUSION

In hemodialysis, diffusion removes the smallest—low molecular weight—solutes. The diffusion rate depends on factors that include:[23]

- Blood and dialysate flow rates
- Membrane surface area and thickness
- Size and number of pores
- Solution temperature
- Concentration gradient
- Size, weight, and charge of the solutes

> ### A Review of Diffusion in Dialysis
>
> Diffusion is movement of solutes across a semipermeable membrane from an area of greater concentration to a lesser one, until both sides are equal.

CONVECTION

Convection, or *solvent drag*, is the best way to remove middle and larger solutes.[24] Some solutes are dragged across the membrane in their solvent by UF. Hemodialysis uses only a small amount of convection.

As you may recall from Module 3: *Principles of Dialysis*, the **sieving coefficient** (SC) of a membrane is a measure of its porosity.[25] The SC is used to predict how much of a solute will be removed by convection (see Figure 6). A sieving coefficient of 0.5 for a solute means 50% of that solute in the blood will pass through the membrane. The rest will be adsorbed or rejected by the membrane. Convective clearance depends on:[24]

- Molecular weight cutoff of the membrane
- Membrane surface area
- Ultrafiltration rate (UFR)

> ### A Review of Convection in Dialysis
>
> When water crosses a semipermeable membrane, some solutes are pulled along with it. This is convection, or solvent drag.[24]

Hemodialysis Devices

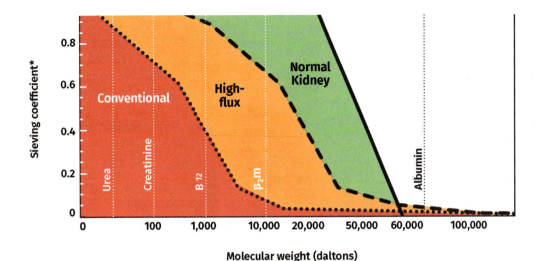

Figure 6: Comparison of Dialyzer Sieving Coefficients

ADSORPTION

All dialyzers *adsorb* (attract and hold) at least small proteins to some extent (see Figure 7). Synthetic membranes adsorb more protein than cellulose membranes. Adsorption has pros and cons. The protein protects the blood from the membrane, which helps "hide" the foreign material and avoid an immune response. First-use syndrome was one type of immune response we used to see with new, unmodified cellulose membranes. On the other hand, a build-up of protein on a membrane will block pores and prevent some diffusion (and convection).

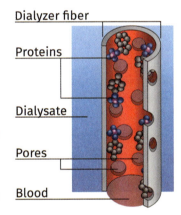

Figure 7: Adsorption

Some dialyzers are *reprocessed* (cleaned and reused by the same patient). Highly adsorptive membranes may not work as well when they are reused many times.

How well a dialyzer will adsorb depends on:
- Membrane material
- Surface area
- How much protein has been adsorbed

> **A Review of Adsorption in Dialysis**
>
> Dialyzers *adsorb* (attract and hold) blood proteins, which then form a coating on the membrane.

Mass Transfer Coefficient (KoA)

KoA is the highest possible clearance of a given solute through a membrane at a given blood and dialysate flow rate. A dialyzer membrane with a higher KoA is more permeable than a membrane with a lower KoA. We measure KoA as the dialyzer's diffusive clearance of a substance (Ko) times its surface area (A) in mL/min.[18] The *Handbook of Dialysis* rates a dialyzer's KoA as low, moderate, or high (see Table 3).[5]

The doctor will prescribe a dialyzer with a KoA to meet each patient's needs. The KoA can be used to estimate clearance of a certain solute at any blood flow and dialysate flow rate. The most common KoA we use in U.S. dialysis is for urea. To learn more about how and why we measure urea, read the section on Testing Dialyzer Effectiveness on page 110)

Table 3: Dialyzer KoA, Efficiency, and Use

KoA	Efficiency	Use
< 500 mL/min	Low	Small patients Low efficiency treatments
500–800 mL/min	Moderate	Routine treatment
800+ mL/min (may range up to 1,600 mL/min)	High	High efficiency dialysis

Ultrafiltration (UF) Coefficients

"They took three liters off of me once. I had cramps so bad I had to have help getting out to my car. Usually they take off two liters in 4 hours, and that works fine."

Dialyzers differ in how much water they can remove (UF), as well as how many wastes. We measure the UF rating of a dialyzer as a coefficient of ultrafiltration, called KUF. KUF tells you how many milliliters of water will pass through a membrane in one hour at a given transmembrane pressure (TMP). A dialyzer with a KUF of 10 mL/hr/mmHg will remove 10 mL of water per hour for each millimeter of mercury (mmHg) of TMP, stated as mL/hr/mmHg. Dialyzer manufacturers list a KUF for each model they offer.

KUF helps you predict how much water will be removed from the patient in a treatment. Here is an example:

- The patient is prescribed a dialyzer with a **KUF of 8 mL/hr/mmHg**.
- The TMP for the treatment is **100 mmHg**.
- The patient would lose **800 mL of water per hour of treatment** (8 mL/hr/mmHg x 100 mmHg = 800 mL/hr).

NOTE: Modern dialysis machines no longer rely on TMP to set the patient's fluid removal rate. Instead, the doctor will prescribe a patient's UFR which sets the fluid removal rate of a very accurate pump in the machine. This rate of removal by the pump may use far less than a dialyzer's full KUF. Thus, it may be best to think of a dialyzer's KUF as a *maximum*—rather than a fixed number.

A Review of Transmembrane Pressure (TMP)

The dialysis machine varies the pump pressure to control the ultrafiltration rate (UFR) and the UF amount. High pressure in the blood compartment forces water out of the blood. TMP is the average pressure difference *across* the membrane (blood side minus dialysate side pressure).

Testing Dialyzer Clearance

We measure how well a dialyzer works by testing its clearance (K). Manufacturers test dialyzers in a lab *in vitro* (in a controlled setting outside the body), using fluids that are much thinner than blood. Therefore, when we measure real clearance during real-life use on patients, the result can differ from the stated values by 5–30%.[5] Urea is most often used to test the dialyzer clearance.

Clearance of a given solute is checked by drawing two samples of a patient's blood, one going into the dialyzer, and one coming out. Once you know the solute levels in both samples, you can find the real clearance. The formula to determine this clearance (K) is:[5]

$$K_s = Q_b \frac{(C_{bi} - C_{bo})}{C_{bi}}$$

K_s = clearance of solutes (**s**)
C_{bi} = blood concentration of **s** at dialyzer inlet (arterial)
C_{bo} = blood concentration of **s** at dialyzer outlet (venous)
Q_b = blood flow rate

Some dialysis machines monitor how well the dialyzer removes wastes in real time during a treatment. This feedback lets a clinician adjust the treatment per the nephrologist's order to reach the patient's prescription. Three systems on the market as of press time can do this:

- The **Baxter (Gambro) Diascan** checks a dialyzer's sodium before and after the dialyzer. The difference in conductivity between the two levels is the sodium clearance. Since sodium clears from the blood at about the same rate as urea, this helps us to estimate clearance of urea.[26]
- The **B. Braun Adimea**™ uses a light-emitting diode (LED) to shine ultraviolet (UV) light through dialysate as it leaves the dialyzer. A sensor across from the LED measures the strength of the light. Wastes that cross the membrane scatter the UV light and make it weaker; a weaker light means more wastes in the dialysate.[27]
- The **Fresenius Medical Care Online Clearance Monitor®** This device briefly changes the dialysate sodium level before the dialyzer six times during a treatment. Then, dialysate conductivity is measured at the inlet and outlet of the dialyzer. The change in conductivity tells us the rate of sodium clearance.[28]

These measures may not be completely precise, but are a useful way to track clearance.

Dialysate

"I make sure that the correct bath is being used re: potassium level—K1,K2... Also, I make sure the blood flow and pump flow are running as prescribed by my Dr. I have had these changed for me at new centers, and if I hadn't had checked them myself I would not have had as good a dialysis."

Dialysate, dialysis fluid, or "bath," is a drug that is prescribed by a nephrologist for each patient. A mix of treated water, acid and bicarbonate, electrolytes, and glucose or (sometimes) iron lets us remove wastes from patients' blood. We can also replace some substances patients need. Calcium can be added back into the blood, as can bicarbonate to help keep the right pH level (see Table 4).

NOTE: Using the wrong dialysate can cause patient harm or death. Dialysate that fails one of three safety tests before or during a treatment will be sent to the drain. This is called **bypass mode,** and will occur if the dialysate:

- Has the wrong concentration of electrolytes
- Is too hot or too cold
- Contains blood

Dialysate Conductivity

"I just had the strangest thing happen. Everyone's treatment was going well, when suddenly, all of the alarms started going off within 30 seconds of each other. A nurse said it had to do with the conductivity."

Except for glucose and iron, all of the chemicals in dialysate are electrolytes. As you have learned, electrolytes break apart in water to form ions. **Dialysate electrolytes must be kept in strict limits to keep patients safe**. We test this with *conductivity* (how well a fluid will conduct an electrical current).

Table 4: Substances in Blood and Dialysate

Substance	Normal Blood Range[29]	Dialysate Range for Standard In-center HD[30,31] (Range for daily/nocturnal HD if different)
Acetate ($CH_3CO_2^-$)	0.025 +/- 0.002 mmol/L[32]	3–8 mmol/L
Bicarbonate (HCO_3^-)	22–28 mmol/L	25–35 mmol/L *(28–33 mmol/L)*
Calcium (Ca^{++})	9–10.5 mg/dL 2.2–2.6 mmol/L 4.8–5.6 mg/dL when ionized[33]	2.5–3.5 mEq/L 1.25–1.75 mmol/L *(3.0 for nocturnal HD)*
Chloride (Cl^-)	98–106 mEq/L 98–106 mmol/L	98–124 mEq/L
Citrate ($C_6H_5O_7^{3-}$)	67–400 (mean 161) µmol/L[34]	2.4–3.0 mEq/L *(0.8–1.0 mmol/L)*
Glucose ($C_6H_{12}O_6$)	Normal fasting: 70–105 mg/dL 3.5–5.8 mmol/L	0–11 mmol/L
Magnesium (Mg^{++})	0.62–0.99 mmol/L	0.25–0.375 mmol/L *(0.5 mmol/L)*
Phosphorus (P)	3.0–4.5 mg/dL (inorganic)	*(1–2 mg/dL for 30+ hours of dialysis /week)*
Potassium (K^+)	3.5–5.0 mmol/L	2.0–3.0 mmol/L *(2.0–3.5 mmol/L)*
Sodium (Na^+)	136–145 mmol/L	135–145 mmol/L *(135-140 mmol/L)*

Module 4

Mixing Dialysate Concentrates

The doctor prescribes the dialysate, which starts out as *two* salt concentrates: acid and bicarbonate.

1. **Acid concentrate** has an acidifier (often acetic or citric acid) to lower the pH of the final dialysate. You add the acidifier *before* you add the bicarbonate. These steps help keep bicarbonate and calcium from forming calcium carbonate precipitate. We use a vinegar rinse to remove deposits from dialysis machines for the same reason. The acid concentrate also contains precise amounts of:
   - Sodium chloride
   - Potassium chloride
   - Magnesium chloride
   - Calcium chloride
   - Glucose

2. **Bicarbonate concentrate** has sodium bicarbonate and, in some cases, sodium chloride.

To make dialysate, you will dilute each of the two concentrates with precise amounts of treated water. When the concentrates are mixed with the right amount of water, they will have the right level of electrolytes for the patient (see Table 4). Mixing will cause some bicarbonate to react with the acetic acid in the acid concentrate. Acetate ions and carbon dioxide (CO_2) will form.

This reaction helps to:
- Make the dialysate more stable
- Balance CO_2 in the dialysate with CO_2 in the patient's blood

Concentrates come in a number of formulas. **Take great care to match the right acid and bicarb concentrates together.** The Association for the Advancement of Medical Instrumentation (AAMI) has standard symbols to help you find and use the right concentrates. A machine set up for a 45X concentrate must use *only* that concentrate, which has a triangle and 45X on the label. You can see these symbols in Table 5.

Hemodialysis Machines

"I am from Sweden, and here the nurses want you to learn how to operate the machine. You are encouraged to do as much as possible to get a better understanding for the whole treatment."

The HD machine is one part of a larger system of devices, called a *delivery system*, that helps us to give safe treatments (see Figure 8). An HD machine will:
- Mix and deliver dialysate
- Pump blood through the dialyzer
- Monitor the treatment

Table 5: Concentrate Proportioning Ratios

Designation	35X (□)	36.83X (○)	45X (△)	36.1X (◇)	Other[a] (new)
Total Mix[bc]	1+1.23+32.77	1+1.83+34	1+1.72+42.28	1+1.1+34	TBD[a]
Acid mix[de]	1+34	1+35.83	1+44	1+35.1	TBD[a]
Bicarbonate Mix[fg]	1+27.46	1+19.13	1+25.16	1+31.8	TBD[a]
Symbol	Square □	Circle ○	Triangle △	Diamond ◇	TBD[a]

[a] Any new mix that does not fit the above matrix should be designated with a unique geometric symbol with the ratio contained in the symbol (to be determined).
[b] Acid concentrate + bicarbonate concentrate + water.
[c] There can be minor differences in mix proportions within each concentrate type; e.g. 1+1.18+32.82 and 1+1.26+32.74 can be used instead of 1+1.23+32.77 and 1+1.58+42.42 can be used instead of 1+1.72+42.28.
[d] Acid concentrate + bicarbonate concentrate + water
[e] The acid mix proportions may also be expressed as acid concentrate + (bicarbonate concentrate + water): Dilution Ratio 1:34 and 1:44 can be used instead of 1+34 and 1+44.
[f] The bicarbonate mix proportions may also be expressed as Bicarbonate concentrate + (acid concentrate + water)
[g] Bicarbonate mix ratios are based on 8.4% sodium bicarbonate solution (1,000 mmol/L). Other solutions may be used clinically and their use may result in a different mixing ratio.

Table used with permission from AAMI. Copyright 2008 Association for the Advancement for Medical Instrumentation, AAMI/ISO/CDV-1 23500-4. Symbols for Concentrate Container System: Concentrate Type. Table 3.

HD machines in use today are *single pass* (see Table 6). They use dialysate once and then send it to a drain.

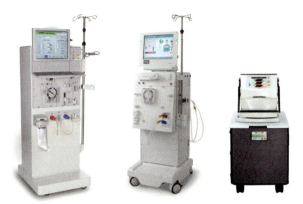

Figure 8: Examples of Hemodialysis Machines
Listing images from left to right. 2008T Hemodialysis Delivery System image used with permission from Fresenius Medical Care North America. Dialog+® Hemodialysis System image used with permission from B. Braun. NxStage System One™ with PureFlow™ SL image used with permission from NxStage.

HD machines check both patient and machine safety, including:
- Blood flow rate
- Blood leaks into the dialysate
- Dialysate flow rate
- Dialysate temperature
- Dialysate conductivity
- Venous pressure
- Arterial pressure
- Patient blood pressure
- Dialyzer clearance
- Ultrafiltration rate and amount
- Presence of pyrogens

Table 6: Single Pass HD Machines Used in U.S. Dialysis Clinics

Manufacturer	Website for Models and Specifications
B. Braun	www.bbraunusa.com
Fresenius	www.fmcna-hd.com
Gambro	www.baxter.com
Nikkiso	www.nikkiso.com
NxStage	www.nxstage.com
Tablo	www.outsetmedical.com/tablo

The delivery system has two major circuits that come together at the HD machine:[5]
1. The dialysate circuit
2. The extracorporeal blood circuit

Dialysate Circuit

The dialysate circuit has six subsystems that work together to make dialysate, bring it to the dialyzer, and monitor it for safety. One of these—water treatment—you will learn about in Module 8 of this *Core Curriculum*. The other five, we will cover below, including:
- Dialysate mixing
- Dialysate delivery
- Monitors and alarms
- Ultrafiltration (UF) control
- Advanced options

Dialysate Mixing

A **proportioning system** prepares dialysate by mixing the two fresh concentrates (bicarb and acid) with fixed amounts of treated water. Built-in pumps control the mixing, and the exact amount of water and concentrates is set on the machine. Your clinic's policies and procedures decide what the settings will be.

Proportioning systems can make dialysate using one of two kinds of pump. Both kinds of pump rely on a continuous supply of fresh concentrate and treated water:
- **Fixed ratio pumps.** Diaphragm or piston pumps bring set volumes of concentrate and water to a mixing chamber.
- **Servo-controlled pumps.** Conductivity sensors check the total ion level of the mixture. Electronic circuits compare the conductivity to what the doctor prescribed, and then the circuits adjust as needed. Once mixed, the dialysate is checked for conductivity, temperature, pressure, and flow rate.

Dialysate Delivery

The HD delivery system sends dialysate through the dialyzer. This can be done for one patient at a time (single patient) or for many patients at once (central delivery).

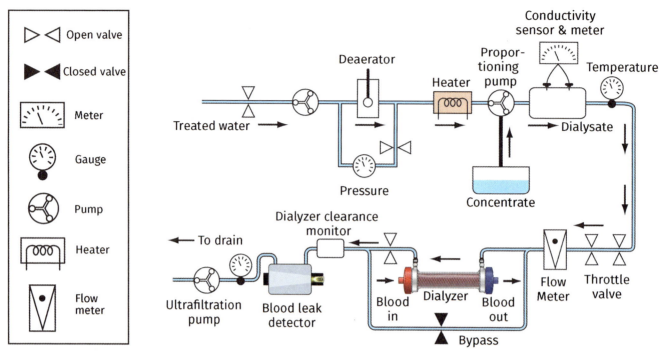

Figure 9: Single Patient Dialysate Delivery System Schematic

Single Patient Dialysate Delivery System

When dialysate is made for one patient at a time, it can be tailored to meet each person's needs. Of course, when each patient gets his or her own dialysate, there is a much higher chance of errors. It is always vital to double check that the right dialysate is used for the patient.

One way to bring dialysate to one patient at a time is to connect prepared liquid concentrate in a "carboy" jug to concentrate input lines on the machine (see Figure 9).

A second way to bring dialysate to one patient at a time is to use a powdered dialysate concentrate. You mount a container of powder on the machine next to the patient's chair. A hydraulic path then adds water into the powder to make a liquid and then draws off the new concentrate to be made into dialysate.

Central Concentrate Delivery System

Acid concentrate can be made up in large batches for all of the patients at once. An input line brings the concentrate to ports near each patient station. The machine then proportions the amount of acid concentrate and mixes it with the bicarbonate concentrate so each patient receives his or her prescribed dialysate.[35]

In this type of system, if there is a problem with the dialysate, it will affect everyone at the same time.

Monitors and Alarms

"Dialysis was exciting today. The power kept going out, and there is no generator for back-up electricity. Machines kept alarming!"

Dialysate must be checked throughout each treatment to make sure it is the right concentration (via conductivity), temperature, and flow rate. Some delivery systems also check the pH.

POWER OUTAGE

In a power failure, all of the machine lights will go out and a steady alarm will sound. To protect patients, a power failure will also:

- Stop the blood pump
- Close the venous clamp
- Stop the dialysate flow pump and heater

You will not be able to shut off this alarm with the mute button.

Hemodialysis Devices

Dry Bicarbonate Concentrate Options

Dry bicarbonate cartridges for use in the HD system can be a practical option instead of liquid bicarbonate or powder that needs to be mixed. There are two options on the market. Both attach to the machine to form online bicarbonate concentrate with less risk of bacterial growth:

- **bibag® Online dry bicarbonate concentrate**. The bibag attaches to a Fresenius 2008T machine with bibag module to mix concentrate at the machine. The way the bag is connected to the machine eliminates dripping when disconnected. bibag is available in 650 gram and 900 gram sizes, the recyclable bag reduces waste.[36]

- **BiCart® cartridge**. This lightweight cartridge has an RO water inlet so purified water can enter and mix with the acid concentrate. Bicarbonate concentrate exits out of an outlet port. The cartridge is chemically stable and requires less storage space than liquid concentrates.[37]

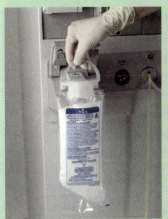 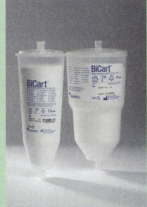

Figure 10: Bicarbonate Concentrates
bibag® Image used with permission from Fresenius Medical Care North America.
BiCart® Image used with permission from Baxter Healthcare Corporation.

WATER OUTAGE

Drops in water pressure may occur if there is a water main break, or a failure of the pump, plumbing, or a filter. If this happens, there will be visual and audible alarms, and:

- Loss of water to the RO will cause a low pressure alarm.
- The storage tanks will be empty.
- If the dialysis machine does not receive water, the conductivity and temperature alarms may alarm, and there may be flow alarms, too.

CONDUCTIVITY

The dialysate proportioning system tests the conductivity of the dialysate. A pair of electrodes or a sensor cell is placed in the dialysate. The machine applies a charge and measures the current. This tells us the total ion concentration level—mainly sodium—of the dialysate.

For safety, most HD machines have two or more conductivity alarms. Each has its own sensors and circuits to monitor the dialysate as it is made. One sensor tests the mixture of the first concentrate (most often acid) with water. A second one tests the final dialysate. This *redundant monitoring* is used so *two* sensors would have to fail before a patient could be harmed. Conductivity is most often checked at two points:

1. **Dialysate mixing**
2. **Before dialysate enters the dialyzer**

On the machines at your clinic, conductivity may be stated as one of these units:

- Micromhos/cm or μMho/cm – 1/1,000,000 of a Mho/cm
- Millimhos/cm or mMho/cm – 1/1,000 of a Mho/cm
- Microsiemens/cm or μS/cm – 1/1,000,000 of a siemens/cm
- Millisiemens/cm or mS/cm – 1/1,000 of a siemens/cm

The Mho is an American unit of measure. The siemen is an international unit. The two units have *unity* (the same value). So, a dialysate with 14.1 mMho/cm conductivity is equal to 14.1 mS/cm.

Most dialysate delivery systems have preset conductivity limits. Dialysate that is outside the limits triggers a conductivity monitoring circuit. The circuit *stops the flow of dialysate to the dialyzer and shunts it to the drain*. This is called **bypass**. Bypass keeps the wrong dialysate from reaching the patient. The circuit also sets off noise and light alarms to alert the staff:

- **Low conductivity alarms** are the most common. These often occur because an acid or bicarb jug runs out of solution. In central delivery systems, too little solution may reach the station due to low flow pressure.

- A **high conductivity alarm** is most often due to:
  - Poor water flow to the proportioning system
  - Untreated incoming water
  - Use of the wrong concentrate(s)

Before each treatment, check the conductivity alarm to verify that it is working. Check the machine readings against a separate meter as well. *You must always have enough of both concentrates in the system for a whole treatment.*

TEMPERATURE

"Some treatment days I had five blankets on me."

Dialysate is kept in the range of 34.5–36.5° C to maintain patient safety:[38]

- **Too-warm dialysate** can cause a patient's red blood cells to burst (*hemolysis*). When dialysate is over 47° C, protein can start to break down—including red blood cells. *Hyperthermia* (dangerous overheating) and even heat stroke can occur at temperatures over 39° C.[39]
- **Too-cool dialysate** can make patients feel cold, and less diffusion will occur. However, *slightly* cool dialysate—½° C below the patient's core body temperature (see Figure 11)—can help prevent deadly intradialytic hypotension and organ stunning. In most cases, this would mean a temperature of about 36.5° C (97.7° F).[40]

Your clinic's policies and the doctor's prescription will drive the dialysate temperature choice. Your job will be to ensure that the patient receives the prescribed treatment.

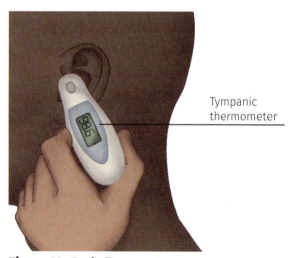

Figure 11: Body Temperature

Water must be heated before it is mixed with the concentrates. Some systems use a heat exchanger placed before the heater to save energy. Used dialysate transfers its heat to the incoming cold water, which warms the water before it enters the heater. Most systems connect a heater to a temperature regulation circuit, a type of thermostat.

To be sure the temperature is safe for the patient, a monitor is placed in the dialysate path before the dialyzer. This monitor is independent of the heater control thermistor. If the dialysate is too hot or cold, a circuit sets off noise and light alarms. The circuit also triggers bypass to shunt dialysate to a drain.

Check the dialysate temperature alarm before each treatment to be sure it works.

FLOW RATE

A flow pump controls the rate at which dialysate flows to the dialyzer. The patient's doctor prescribes the dialysate flow rate (Qd), which will range from 0–1,000 mL/min. Some systems have flow meters that display the flow rate on a gauge or digital display. Newer dialysis machines may have an option that allows the dialysate flow rate to be set automatically. Dialysate flow rate noise and light alarms may be set off by:

- Low water pressure
- Dialysate pump failure
- A blockage in the dialysate flow path
- A flow rate that is not what was requested

BLOOD LEAK DETECTOR

"There was a blood leak in my dialyzer today. We had to change my dialyzer and bloodlines (I lost about 250 mL of blood), but good thing my tech and nurse were on it! Shout out to the staff!"

Once dialysate leaves the dialyzer, it flows through a **blood leak detector** to check for blood (see Figure 12). The detector can sense very small amounts of blood, less than can be seen with the naked eye. Blood in the dialysate could mean a tear in the dialyzer membrane. So, blood leak detectors are often treated as *extracorporeal* (outside the body) alarms, even though the detector itself is in the dialysate circuit.

If blood and dialysate mix:
- The patient could have major blood loss.
- The patient could get *sepsis* (blood poisoning) if his or her blood is contaminated by non-sterile dialysate. This is unlikely, due to the pressure difference between the blood and dialysate compartments.

The blood leak detector shines a light through the used dialysate and onto a photocell or photoresistor. Since dialysate is clear, the light can pass through. Even a tiny amount of blood will break the light beam. The detector will sense such a break and trigger noise and light alarms.

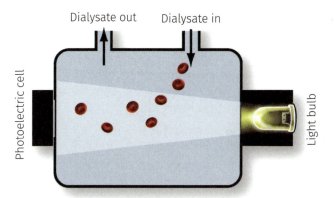

If the light beam is interrupted by blood, an alarm will sound and the blood pump will stop

Figure 12: Blood Leak Detector

When a blood leak alarm occurs, the blood pump stops. The venous line clamps to keep blood that could be contaminated with dialysate from reaching the patient. In some systems, **bypass mode** shunts dialysate to the drain. This reduces negative pressure to keep more blood from being pulled through a membrane tear and into the dialysate.

If a blood leak alarm occurs, use an FDA-approved dialysis blood leak test strip that reacts to blood to check the extent of the leak. Use the strip to test where the dialysate leaves the dialyzer:

- Blood or a pink color in the dialysate path means a *major* leak.
- Clear dialysate and a *positive* blood leak test strip result suggests a *minor* leak.
- Clear dialysate and a *negative* blood leak test strip result means a false alarm.

Follow your clinic's procedures for a blood leak to stop the treatment **without returning the patient's blood**. Since the blood could be contaminated, you do not want it to reach the patient: it could cause an infection. The blood leak detector is most often preset by the manufacturer. You may be able to override the alarm for a short time to troubleshoot the alarm.[41]

pH

The pH of blood is normally about 7.35–7.45, a weak base. Dialysate must have a pH close to that of the blood, so it does not change the blood pH. The range of dialysate pH is most often from 6.9–7.6.[42]

Some delivery systems monitor pH throughout the treatment. Whether or not there is a pH monitor, *at the start of each treatment, you must test to be sure the dialysate pH is in a safe range*:

- One way to test dialysate pH is to measure it using a pH meter with an electrode. The electrode releases a small voltage when placed in a solution. The voltage is then read by a detection circuit that converts the signal value into a pH value and displays it. If you use a meter, you must have test fluids with known pH levels on hand to check that the reading is correct.

- Test strips that change color are also frequently used to measure dialysate pH, and do not require the use of test fluids.

PYROGEN FILTERS

"Last week at dialysis I began to shiver violently every 30 seconds or so. I had no control over it! Staff took my temp and each time it went up. Next thing I know they are drawing blood, and patients on either side of me began having the same symptoms. I spent the next day in bed. My nephrologist told me I'd had a pyrogenic reaction."

Pyrogens are toxins bacteria release to protect themselves. If these reach the patient's bloodstream, they can cause fever and chills. Pyrogen filters are an option on some machines. After the proportioning system, dialysate flows through the filter, which helps keep out bacteria and most pyrogens. Small *endotoxin* particles, less that 20,000 Da may—rarely—pass through the membrane. Pyrogen filters are changed based on hours of use or per clinic policy.

Ultrafiltration Control

"I still urinate some, and my goal is usually under 1 kilo, so my UF rate is always low."

Taking excess water out of the blood (*ultrafiltration*, or UF) is a key part of dialysis. UF occurs when pressure on the blood side of the membrane is higher (more positive) than on the dialysate side. This pushes water in the blood across the membrane to the dialysate side.

The TMP governs how much water is forced across the membrane. In the past, you would have had to set a total water loss goal for each patient and calculate an hourly ultrafiltration rate (UFR) by hand with an equation.

Today, the UF control on the machine sets the UFR using its UF pump and a fluid balancing system. This system creates a dialysate pressure, which is used to calculate a TMP. The TMP is shown on a screen, so you can see what is going on in the dialyzer (see Figure 13). All you need to enter is the desired water removal amount (in mL) and the treatment time.

The dialysis machine removes water from the patient and measures it with either **volumetric** (the most common type) UF control, or **flow** control. Each of these is described below.

VOLUMETRIC UF CONTROL

Volumetric UF control systems have *balancing chambers* (see Figure 14). Here is how they work:

- Two chambers each have identical fixed volumes.
- Each chamber is divided in half by a flexible diaphragm.
- *Both* sides of *each* chamber have an inlet and an outlet.
- One side of each chamber is in the "*to* dialyzer" or fresh dialysate flow path.
- The other side is in the "*from* dialyzer" or used dialysate flow path.
- Valves on each inlet and outlet open and close. As fluid enters on one side of the chamber, it pushes on the diaphragm to force fluid out on the other side.
- One chamber is "on-line" with the dialyzer while the other, "off-line" chamber refills with fresh dialysate and purges spent dialysate to the drain.
- The two chambers take turns being on-line and off-line.
- The timing of the valves' opening and closing are synced for a continuous flow of dialysate to and from the dialyzer.

Safe Ultrafiltration

Safely removing water from your patients' blood during HD requires setting *two* things correctly:

- The **amount** of water to remove: goal weight or target weight
- The **speed** or **rate** at which we remove water to reach the goal: UFR

Not removing enough water leaves the patient *hypervolemic* (fluid overloaded), which can cause swelling and trouble breathing. Over time, fluid overload can cause heart failure.

Removing too much water—*or the right amount too quickly*—can make the patient *hypovolemic* (dehydrated). This can cause the patient's blood pressure to drop. The patient may have headaches, severe muscle cramps, vomit, or even pass out. Blood flow (and oxygen supply) to the patient's organs may fall dangerously. As you have learned, this is organ stunning, and it can cause permanent damage.

Research suggests that the safest UFR is no greater than 10mL/kg/hr.[43] Some dialysis companies and Medicare have set an upper limit of 13mL/kg/hr.[44] Be sure the UF amount and rate are set correctly for each patient. Patients who cannot tolerate removal of their goal weight at a safe UFR during a treatment may need more time or an extra treatment. Nocturnal HD in a clinic or at home can remove more water slowly and gently.

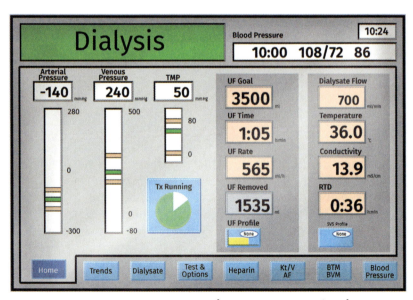

Figure 13: Screen Showing TMP

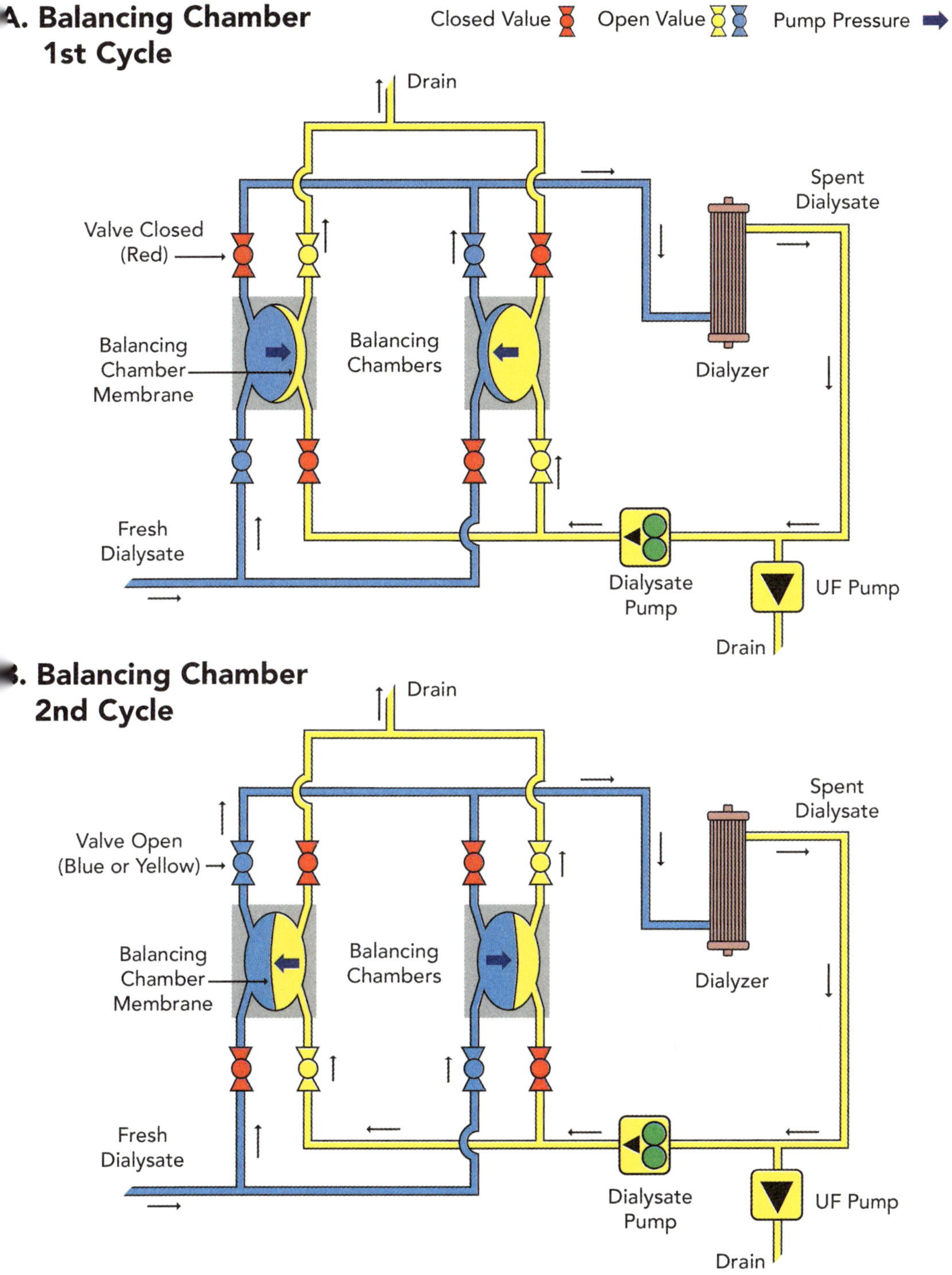

Hemodialysis Devices

A. Balancing Chamber 1st Cycle

B. Balancing Chamber 2nd Cycle

Figure 14: Volumetric UF Control System.

Image used with permission from Stan Frinak. This figure shows two cycles of the dialysis machine balancing chamber. Valves that are closed during a cycle are shown in red and open valves are shown in blue or yellow. In the first cycle (A) the left chamber is using fresh dialysate pump pressure to move the balancing chamber membrane to the right. This forces spent dialysate out to the drain. The right chamber is using spent dialysate pressure from the dialysate pump to push the balancing chamber membrane to the left. This forces fresh dialysate into the dialyzer. During the second balancing chamber cycle (B) the operation of the two chambers is reversed.

One flow pump pushes *fresh* dialysate to the balance chambers. A second flow pump pushes *used* dialysate to the balance chambers. Dialysate from the "on-line" chamber moves to and from the dialyzer in a closed loop. The same volume of dialysate comes in and goes out, since the volume on one side of the balance chamber displaces the same volume on the other side. So, the flow to and from the dialyzer is balanced.

A **UF pump** then removes water from the closed loop through the dialyzer membrane. Most UF pumps are diaphragms or pistons, and they are most often placed in the used dialysate flow path.

Removing water from the closed loop creates a relative negative pressure in the dialysate side of the dialyzer versus the blood side. This forms the pressure gradient

119

we need for UF. Each pump stroke removes a small, fixed amount of water (about 1 mL or less). This allows the machine to precisely remove the right amount of water from the patient.

A target UF goal will be set for each patient's treatment based on the patient's prescribed *target weight*. Informed patients may tell you how much water to remove, based on their weight gain and symptoms. Or, you or the nurse will set the goal for a patient. In either case, you will use the machine controls to enter the UF goal and the length of the treatment in hours. The machine's computer will calculate the UFR, which will then set the rate for the UF pump. **Double check that the correct UF goal has been set for each treatment**.

Other parts of the system control, monitor, and help assure safety:

- **Pressure sensors** control pump speeds, prevent over-pressurization, calculate TMP, and detect leaks.
- **Air separation chambers** remove any air that comes out when you prime a new (dry) dialyzer. Air separation chambers are important, because any air left in the closed loop system will lead to errors in water removal. Air that is removed from the separation chamber is sent to the drain.

FLOW CONTROL UF

Flow control UF systems have flow sensors on the inlet and outlet side of the dialyzer to control dialysate flow (see Figure 15). They use a post-dialyzer UF pump that removes water as a UFR set by the machine. The UF pump speed equals the UFR. Here is how it works:

- Inlet and outlet flow pumps are set so the flow is equal at the inlet and outlet flow sensors.
- Volume is removed by the UF pump *before* fluid reaches the outlet flow sensor. This sensor ensures that the outlet flow is equal to the inlet flow.
- The outlet flow pump will make up for the volume taken by the UF pump. This creates negative pressure to pull that UF volume across the dialyzer membrane.

Flow control UF systems use a post-dialyzer UF pump that removes water at a UFR set by the machine. The UF pump speed equals the UFR.

Hazards of Sodium Modeling

"This morning, about 30 minutes into my treatment, I started feeling bad, like my heart is coming out of my skin, and I was rushed into the ER!"

Dialysate machines can change the dialysate sodium level *during* a treatment, with a doctor's prescription. The intent of this *sodium modeling* is to remove more water without causing symptoms for the patient. In most cases, the sodium level would start out high, and be turned down as the treatment goes on. Most clinics no longer do sodium modeling, for two reasons:

- When dialysate sodium is high, sodium diffuses *into* the patient's blood. This forces water to shift out of the cells and interstitial space into the blood, where dialysis can remove it. But, sodium modeling *leaves* sodium in the blood. High blood sodium levels trigger the thirst drive in the brain so patients *must* drink, and then they gain even more water weight. So, the practice starts a vicious cycle.[45]
- Sodium modeling helps some patients handle more UF with fewer symptoms. But, if the UFR is higher than patients' *plasma refill rate*, their blood pressure will drop. The plasma refill rate is the time it takes for water between cells to refill the bloodstream, and is estimated to be about 5–10 mL/kg/hr.[46,47] So, if the UFR is higher than 10 mL/kg/hr, the patient's blood pressure may drop—which reduces blood flow and oxygen supply to the patient's organs and may cause organ stunning.

The Chief Medical Officers from *all* of the largest U.S. dialysis companies have publicly opposed the use of sodium modeling in routine HD. They noted that the practice could add as much as nine grams of sodium to patients' blood—4.5 times as much sodium as most patients can eat each day![48]

The pump speed is the time needed to fill a UF *burette* (small chamber of known volume). Filling and emptying a burette takes four steps:

- High- and low-level sensors in the UF burette signal a valve to open and close.
- When the UF burette is full, the valve opens.

Hemodialysis Devices

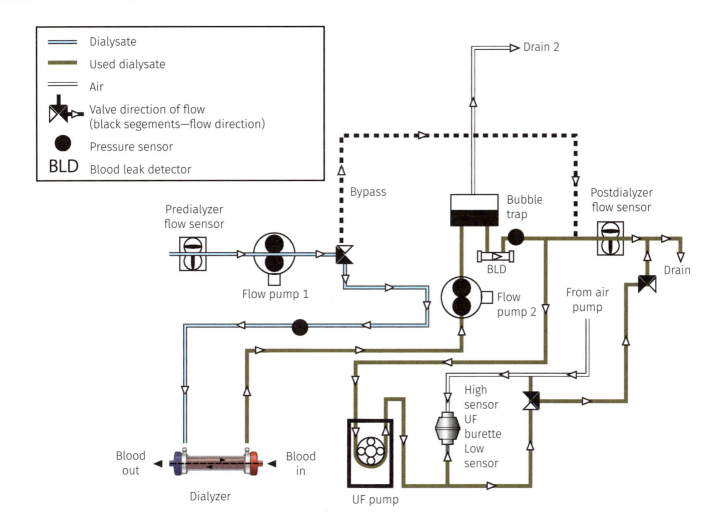

Figure 15: Flow Control UF System

- A pump empties the burette by forcing air into the top and the contents to the drain.
- When the UF burette is empty, the valve closes and the UF burette starts to refill.

These steps go on many times during the treatment. The outlet flow sensor does not measure the water removed by the UF pump. Flow control UF systems may use pressure sensors and air separation chambers to monitor and control dialysate flow and calculate TMP.

UF PROFILING

HD machines can run programs that control settings for UF, sodium, bicarbonate, temperature, and dialysate flow rates. Each of these is done per the patient's prescription and your clinic's policy. UF profiling lets you program the machine to vary the UFR during the treatment. The machine raises and lowers the TMP to make this happen. Unlike sodium modeling, UF profiling does not add sodium to the patient's blood.

Advanced Options

A number of standalone, or optional, parts can be connected to the dialysis machine. These collect, monitor, and analyze data from the patient and the delivery system during treatment. The care team can use the data to help improve treatment.

ADEQUACY MONITORING

All HD machines have options to measure the dose of HD that has been given during a treatment. Many machines can also test used dialysate to see how much urea has been removed from a patient's blood, but the results must be confirmed with blood tests.

Module 4

AUTOMATIC BLOOD PRESSURE MODULES

HD machines have cuffs built in to check blood pressure during treatment, with alarm limits that can be set for each patient. If you find that a blood pressure cuff does not work, unscrew the cuff connection from the line and let the cuff deflate. Then, screw the connector back into the line and restart the blood pressure check. NOTE: Never deflate the blood pressure cuff by hand; this will pop the internal module and cause the blood pressure pump to stop working.

BLOOD DETECTION SYSTEMS

Some HD machines have monitors that can tell when the bloodlines disconnect or a leak occurs at the patient's access.

BLOOD/DIALYSATE ANALYSIS DEVICES

A number of devices can check the patient's blood during treatment. Whether they are built into the extracorporeal circuit or the delivery system, they may:

- Measure the real blood flow rate
- Test the blood hemoglobin and/or oxygen levels
- Measure flow rate of blood through the access
- Measure the temperature of the blood in the arterial and venous lines
- Determine the amount of heat energy transferred to the patient during dialysis
- Check for access recirculation

HEALTH INFORMATION SYSTEMS (HIS)

Many HD machines connect to health information systems (HIS). These may collect machine settings and treatment readings. Or, data may be collected from standalone monitors.

Extracorporeal Circuit

"Had a very good treatment today! Just want to say thanks to the staff for always being on your 'A' game."

The *extracorporeal* (outside of the body) circuit carries blood from the patient's access to the dialyzer and back to the access (see Figure 16). It is the second

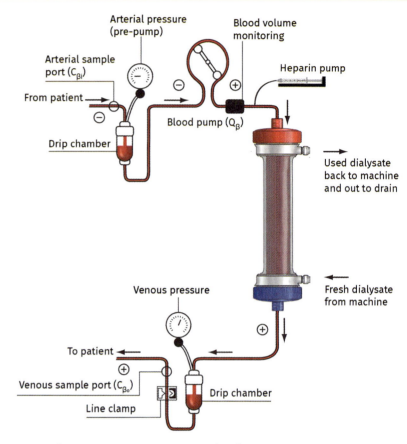

Figure 16: Extracorporeal Circuit

major subsystem of the HD delivery system and includes the:

- Arterial and venous blood tubing
- Blood pump
- Heparin pump
- Dialyzer
- Venous line clamp
- Safety monitors

Blood Tubing

"My husband told me that at dialysis he thought he had indigestion so he flagged someone down for a drink of water. When the tech came over he said, 'You need more than water, you're bleeding.' The tubing came apart at the connections and thank goodness the tech saw it when he asked for the water."

During HD, blood flows through tubing ("lines") from an arterial needle in the patient's access to the dialyzer. Blood flows back to the patient through the venous needle. The inner diameter of the blood tubing is small, so only about 100–250 mL of blood is outside the patient's body at a time. Blood tubing has two parts:

- **Arterial**—most often color-coded red
- **Venous**—most often color-coded blue

Bloodlines are smooth on the inside to reduce the chance of blood clots and air bubbles. Custom blood tubing is made for some types of equipment and patients. Each set of blood tubing has special parts. The order in which those parts are placed varies with the system's design, prescribed treatment, and the monitoring desired. Parts of blood tubing include:

- **Patient connectors** – a tip, or Luer lock connector, at one end of the arterial and venous blood tubing segments links the tubing to the patient's needles or catheter ports (see Figure 17).
- **Dialyzer connectors** – connectors at the other end of the tubing link to the dialyzer. The arterial blood tubing segment connects to the arterial end of the dialyzer. The venous blood tubing segment connects to the venous end of the dialyzer.
- **Drip chamber or bubble trap** – a monitoring line checks arterial or venous pressure in the blood circuit and traps any air. The drip chamber may contain a fine mesh screen to keep blood clots from reaching the patient. This type of drip chamber goes on the venous blood tubing segment, after the dialyzer and before the patient's access. Flexible membranes have replaced drip chambers in some newer bloodlines.
- **Blood pump segment** – a durable, pliable, larger diameter part of the arterial blood tubing. It is installed in the blood pump.
- **Heparin infusion line** – a very small tube that extends out of the blood tubing to give *heparin* (an *anticoagulant*, or blood thinner) to the patient. This line is most often placed on the arterial blood tubing segment just before the dialyzer.
- **Saline infusion line** – allows saline to be given to the patient during dialysis. This line is most often placed on the arterial blood tubing segment just before the blood pump, so saline can be pulled into the circuit. If the line is not clamped during treatment, too much fluid or air can enter the extracorporeal circuit.

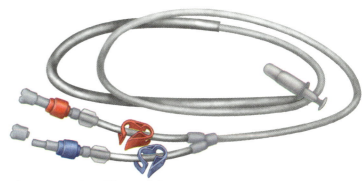

Figure 17: Bloodlines with Connectors

Transducer Protectors

A *transducer* is a device in the machine that turns air pressure into an electronic signal. This signal displays venous pressure, arterial pressure, and TMP. Moisture will harm electronics. A *transducer protector* is a cap with a filter that goes between blood in the tubing and each transducer to keep it dry. Since dry transducers are so vital, there may be both external protectors—as part of the blood tubing set—*and* internal protectors as a back up.

External transducer protectors connect to the machine's venous and/or arterial pressure ports via a small tubing segment on top of the drip chamber. Transducer port lines have a small line clamp in the middle. The protectors connect to the ends of these lines, and are the link between the machine and the blood tubing set (drip chambers).

Membrane filters with a small pore size (0.2 microns)[35] inside transducer protectors are *hydrophobic* (water repellent), so blood cannot pass all the way through. If the filters get wet, they prevent air flow.[35] For this reason, wet or clamped transducer protectors can cause pressure reading errors and TMP problems. A loose or damaged transducer protector on a pre-pump arterial drip chamber port could let air into the bloodlines, too.

The biggest risk of wet transducer protectors is infection. The Centers for Disease Control and Prevention (CDC) has tips to reduce this risk. If transducer protectors become wet, clinics must:[49]

- Change them right away.
- Inspect the machine side of the protector for contamination or wetting.

- Have the machine's internal transducer protector inspected or replaced by a qualified technician.
- Clean and disinfect the path between the external and internal transducer protectors if fluid breaks through the external transducer protector.

Newer bloodlines may have a flexible membrane instead of a drip chamber. In this case, the membrane goes between the bloodline and the internal pressure transducer.

Blood Pump

"Too fast of a blood flow rate is a burden to our hearts. The chambers of our hearts must fill to a certain volume before they can pump blood out to other organs. Hemo forces 350 to 450 mLs of blood a minute to the dialyzer to be cleaned. That is way faster than what a normal heart can pump in a minute."

The blood pump (see Figure 18) moves blood from the patient's arterial needle through the tubing to the dialyzer, and then back to the venous needle. Most often, the blood pump uses a monitor that turns a roller head. This type of pump is called a *peristaltic* pump, because it moves the blood in waves. The speed of the roller head controls the blood flow rate, which is prescribed by the doctor and set by the staff person.

Here is how it works:
- The blood pump segment of the blood tubing is threaded between the rollers and the pump head.
- The rollers turn, blocking the tubing and pushing blood out of the pump segment.
- Once the roller passes, the pump segment resumes its shape and blood is drawn in to refill it.
- In this way, blood is pulled into and pushed out of the segment at the same time.

A blood pump is, in essence, a rotating clamp with several safety features built in to protect patients:
- On the venous end, the venous line clamp should automatically clamp the venous line if there are blood handling alarms or a power failure.
- Stopping the blood pump is a "fail-safe" feature that protects the patient even when the power goes out.

In case of emergency, all blood pumps have a way to allow hand cranking. Most often, the pump will have a handle to crank. Crank the handle just fast enough to keep the venous pressure at the pre-alarm level (see Figure 19). *You must remove the line from the venous line clamp before you hand crank, so the extracorporeal circuit will be open and blood can be returned to the patient.*

PUMP OCCLUSION

Pump occlusion is the amount of space between the rollers and the pump housing. The blood pump rollers must press against the blood pump segment hard enough to pull and push the blood through the circuit:

- **Too-tight rollers** may crack the blood pump segment, or *hemolyze* (destroy) red blood cells by crushing them under the rollers.
- **Too-loose rollers** may allow blood to escape back across the rollers, so the blood flow is less than the prescribed rate. Red blood cells can be hemolyzed, too.

Modern rollers use springs to create a constant force between the roller and the occlusion wall. *You MUST*

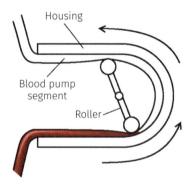
Step one — Blood enters the pump

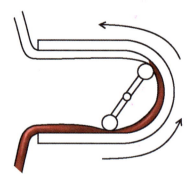
Step two — Blood is pushed along by the rollers

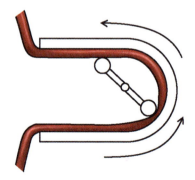
Step three — A constant blood flow rate is created

Figure 18: Blood Pump

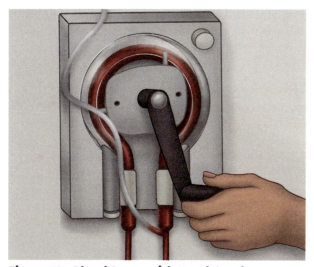

Figure 19: Blood Pump with Hand Crank

Some machines count blood pump turns and calculate the *number of liters processed* in a treatment. When you know the number of liters *prescribed* to be processed, you can calculate the blood flow rate: divide liters processed by minutes of treatment. This value can be used as a quality assurance tool. *The result should be the same as the blood flow rate on the machine.* The blood flow rate must be correct *and* must match the patient's prescription. You must assure that the rate on the readout is correct.

Heparin Pump

"My past few treatments I have had a bleeding problem. The top site is never an issue. The bottom site, I hold for 10 minutes and stand up and feel a rush and start to leak. Could lowering the heparin help?"

mount the pump tubing segment in the pump correctly. If you pull down on the ends of the pump segment in the housing, tension on the tubing segment can compress the springs and slow the effective blood flow rate.

Pump occlusion must be checked on each machine. Adjust the occlusion per the manufacturer's instructions. If your clinic changes tubing size or manufacturer, recheck the pump occlusion.

BLOOD FLOW RATE

"Do you feel awful after leaving in-center treatment and can't bounce back after? Do you feel your heart racing? It's my understanding that the 450 flow rate is sort of standard, but after I talked to my doctor and had them lower it to 400, I cannot tell you how much better I feel, even though I have to run 20 minutes longer."

We change the blood pump roller speed to set the machine to the patient's prescription. A typical blood flow rate (Qb) may be about 350 mL/min.[5]

The machine will display the blood pump setting, which is based on the number of pump turns per minute and the volume inside the blood pump segment of the tubing. Pressure before the dialyzer is always negative, since the blood pump pulls blood into the circuit. However, negative pressure *flattens* the blood pump segment—which then holds less volume—so the calculated Qb is higher than the actual.[35] When the arterial pressure is -150 mmHg or less, the difference can be enough to create a less efficient treatment. Very low arterial pressures can also mean a problem with the vascular access that should be checked.[35]

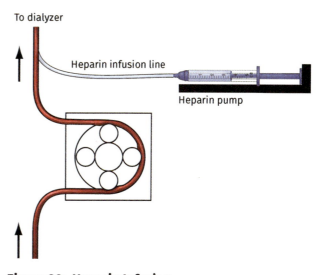

Figure 20: Heparin Infusion

When the patient's blood touches the lines and dialyzer, it tends to clot. Heparin, an anti-clotting drug, or *anticoagulant*, is used to prevent clotting in the extracorporeal blood circuit. Heparin can be given in one of three ways:

- **Intermittently** (on and off) during dialysis. A prescribed amount is injected into the arterial bloodline at prescribed times.
- **By bolus** (the full amount all at once) just before the treatment.
- **By continuous infusion** (a prescribed rate throughout the treatment). A syringe filled with heparin, a heparin infusion line, and an infusion pump are used (see Figure 20). The pump slowly injects heparin into the extracorporeal circuit. A small

starting dose may be given to the patient before treatment. Heparin pumps have variable speeds that can be set to the doctor's prescription. A continuous infusion heparin pump has four parts:

1. A syringe holder
2. A piston to drive the plunger of the syringe
3. A motor to drive the plunger and infuse the heparin
4. A way to set the prescribed rate

Heparin is infused into the heparin line on the arterial blood tubing. The heparin line is after the blood pump segment and before the dialyzer. The positive pressure in this part of the bloodlines is a safety feature. With negative pressure, air could be pulled into the circuit through the heparin line. Or, enough heparin could be pulled into the bloodline if the syringe came loose to cause an overdose.

For most patients who have fistulas or grafts, heparin is stopped *before the end of the treatment* so normal blood clotting can resume.

Venous Line Clamp

The venous line clamp is the patient's last line of defense against a blood leak, air in the bloodlines, or a power outage. Placed on the venous line after the venous drip chamber, during a treatment the clamp is held "open" by a spring-loaded electromagnet. If an adverse event is detected, the magnet is released, the line clamps shut, and blood return to the patient will stop. *You must be sure the venous line clamp works before you start a treatment.*

Safety Monitors

"My graft doesn't want to run, and my arterial pressure keeps going up. I hate being a problem child. Back to the vascular surgeon for me!"

A number of extracorporeal circuit monitors check the patient's blood for pressure and air to help maintain safety. You must set and check these so they work properly. Even with these devices, mistakes can occur, and patients can be harmed. When you get to know your patients and how they react to the treatment, you can help protect their safety by watching for changes. YOU are the most important safety monitor.

EXTRACORPOREAL PRESSURE MONITORS

Pressure in the extracorporeal circuit depends on blood flow rate and resistance to the flow. There is resistance in most of the circuit from the needles (or catheters), tubing, and dialyzer. The blood pump helps overcome resistance. Pressures are shown in millimeters of mercury (mmHg) on a gauge, meter, or screen.

We monitor extracorporeal pressure to calculate TMP and ensure patient safety. In some systems, pressure monitors have high and low limits that can be set. Others have a preset range, and staff can choose a midpoint. When pressure is too high or low, the system will trigger noise and light alarms, stop the blood pump, and clamp the venous line (see Table 7 and Table 8).

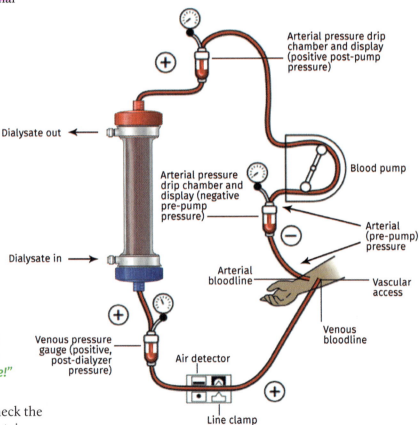

Figure 21: Pressure Monitoring Devices

Table 7: Types of Pressure in the Extracorporeal Circuit

Pressure	Location	Level
Arterial (or pre-pump)	From the patient's access to the blood pump	< 0 (-)
Pre-dialyzer (post-pump or post-pump arterial)	From the blood pump to the dialyzer	> 0 (+)
Venous (or post-dialyzer)	Monitoring site to the venous return	> 0 (+)

Any of the pressures in Table 7 may be monitored, depending on the machine. The arterial bloodline may have a pre- or a post-pump drip chamber. The venous bloodline will have a drip chamber after the dialyzer and before the venous line clamp. Each drip chamber checks pressure in the extracorporeal circuit with a monitoring line or a pressure gauge (see Figure 21).

Pressure monitors must be engaged at all times when the blood pump is on. Common causes of high and low pressure alarms are shown in Table 8.

Before each treatment, you must check the extracorporeal blood pressure alarms to be sure they work.

MACHINE TROUBLESHOOTING

Machine test failures – if air is present in the machine, it will fail the pressure tests. Run through a 3-minute rinse and retest the machine. Most machines may take about 15 minutes to stabilize. This time *cannot* be shortened by rushing the set-up or forcing a machine to go into test mode before it is ready.

Leak on acid and or bicarb wall box connection – pull the connector back out and verify that the o-ring is still in place.

Table 8: Pressure Alarm Triggers[41]

LOW PRESSURE ALARM	HIGH PRESSURE ALARM
Arterial pressure (-) (pre-pump)	
• Arterial blood flow from the patient's access is blocked • Compression or a kink in the arterial bloodline • Wrong position or infiltration of the arterial needle • Blood pump set at a rate higher than the vascular access can supply • Hypotension • *Vasoconstriction* (tightening of the patient's blood vessels) • Poorly working central venous catheter	• A bloodline separation (if the upper limit is set below zero) • A leak between the patient and the monitoring site • A drop in the blood pump speed • Infusion of saline or medications
Pre-dialyzer pressure (+) (post-pump)	
• Poor blood flow or drop in blood flow rate (Qb)	• Pressure difference from one side of the dialyzer to the other • Poor placement or infiltration of the venous needle or HD catheter • A rise in the blood flow rate (Qb) • A kink in the blood tubing between the dialyzer and the monitoring site
Venous pressure (+)	
• Blood tubing separation from the venous needle or catheter • A drop in the blood flow rate • Blockage in the blood tubing before the monitoring site • A badly clotted dialyzer	• Blood tubing is blocked between the monitoring site and the venous needle • Poor position or infiltration of venous needle • Poorly working central catheter • Clotting in the access

Stop Preventable Bleeding at Dialysis

"I was having a flow study, fell asleep, and woke up with blood soaked through my pants. The blood filled up the spaces in the chair before it hit the floor. Now everyone is extra careful about tightening the lines back up."

When dialysis needles come out or bloodlines come apart, it takes just moments for a patient to lose enough blood to die. Each year, an estimated 400 U.S. patients bleed to death *during dialysis—with the staff there*.[50]

Since blood is the same temperature as the body, blood loss may not be felt by the patient, who may quietly lose consciousness. The blood may be soaked up by clothing or blankets, or may pool on the floor where you or other patients may see it.

Always tape needles and connect blood tubing securely. Get in the habit of glancing often at patients' access sites, clothing, blankets, and the floor to watch for blood.

Machine alarms may not detect venous needle dislodgement or line separation. (Resistance in the venous needle may read as pressure so the alarm does not sound.[51]) Some clinics use venous bloodline alarms, like RedSense® or bedwetting alarms to detect moisture.

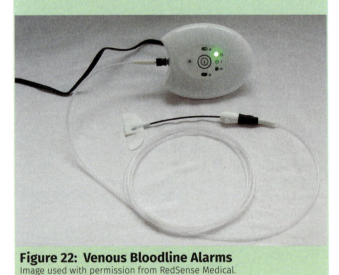

Figure 22: Venous Bloodline Alarms
Image used with permission from RedSense Medical.

AIR DETECTORS

"Just a few small bubbles at the end of the line where they connect it to the venous won't do any harm, but if I see that, I make them bleed the line a little more because I can feel the bubbles going in me and I don't like it."

Tiny amounts of air in the bloodstream (microbubbles) may act like blood clots in patients' organs.[52] In a small randomized study, keeping a high level of blood in the venous drip chamber (and wet-storing dialyzers between uses) reduced the number of microbubbles.[53] Larger amounts of air can cause death. Air/foam detectors check all of the blood in the venous tubing segment for air and foam. The system may check for air at the venous drip chamber or at the blood tubing just below it.

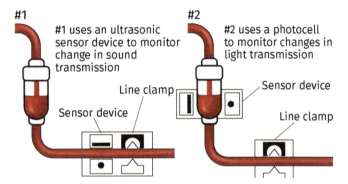

Figure 23: Air Detectors

There are two types of air detectors (see Figure 23):

- **Ultrasonic.** When the air detector is on, a transmitter sends a *sound* wave across a drip chamber or bloodline to a receiver on the other side. The detector will alarm if there is a change in the sound wave.
- **Photocell.** When a photocell is armed, a *light* beam is shot across the tubing. A sensor on the opposite side detects voids where there are no blood cells (due to air) as blood moves past the sensor.

The detector checks the signal throughout the treatment for any change. If the blood level in the drip chamber drops or air shows up in the bloodline, the sound level will drop. A drop in the sound level will set off noise and light alarms, stop the blood pump, and clamp the venous line to keep air out of the patient's bloodstream.

An air detector's alarm limits are most often preset by the manufacturer. They can be calibrated by qualified technicians.

Check the air detector to be sure it is working properly before each treatment, following the manufacturer's instructions. **Be sure the drip chamber or bloodline is properly seated in the sensor before you start a treatment.** The air detector must *always* be used during the treatment and the venous line clamps engaged with the tubing segment.

BLOOD VOLUME MONITORING (BVM)

"Trying to manage target weight without a monitor is a guessing game. It's a moving target, and how much sodium we have on board determines how easily we give up fluid. We can also gain or lose real weight, and that can be mistaken for water weight."

BVM is done to measure the volume of a patient's blood *during* a treatment. BVM devices can provide real-time feedback on:

- **Percent change in blood volume** – how much blood is left when you pull water out.
- **Hematocrit** – percent of the blood made up of red blood cells.
- **Oxygen saturation** – how much oxygen is in the blood.
- **Vascular refill** – water shifts from inside and between the cells into the blood.

If the patient's blood volume drops too much—or too quickly—his or her blood pressure will fall which can stun the organs. Having BVM lets you adjust the UFR during the treatment to match each patient's ability to give up water. The result is a safer, gentler treatment with fewer hypotensive "crashes."

Two devices are approved by the FDA and used for BVM in the U.S., Crit-Line® by Fresenius Medical Care and CVInsight®, by InteloMed.

Crit-Line Technology (Crit-Line III Monitor, Crit-Line IV Monitor, and Sensor Clip)

Crit-Line Technology (see Figure 24) measures changes in a patient's hematocrit (percent of the blood that is made up of red blood cells) by shining light through the blood to a sensor. Red blood cells absorb light differently than other parts of blood. A rising hematocrit shows blood volume falling as water is removed, so UF can be done safely. The Crit-Line monitor also measures oxygen saturation. To use the device, you clip a sensor onto the bloodline at the arterial port of the dialyzer.

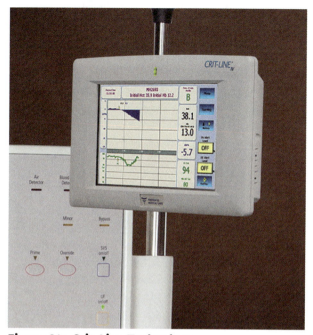

Figure 24: Crit-Line Technology
Image used with permission from Fresenius Medical Care North America.

CVInsight

This device uses a forehead sensor to measure **pulse amplitude**—the degree of change in a patient's heart rate. The result is shown on a monitor as *pulse strength* (percent change from baseline). Pulse strength is unique to each patient. The device (see Figure 25) also collects changes in the pulse rate and other key markers such as:

- Pulse irregularity
- Oxygen saturation

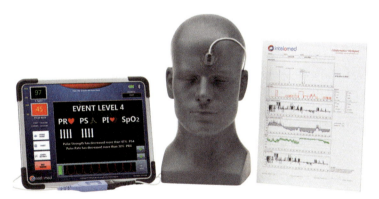

Figure 25: CVInsight® System
Image used with permission from InteloMed.

Waste Disposal and "Green" Dialysis

"I live in an area that prides itself on living "green" and recycling. So it was a shock to see all that went into the landfill with every treatment. Don't get me wrong, I totally appreciate dialysis. But, it does make me sad to think that our dialysis cartridges with all their plastic will probably outlive us buried in the landfill."

A new focus that is starting to gain some traction in dialysis is how to handle the waste that is formed at each treatment. Besides trash, such as empty boxes and wrappers and used dialysate jugs, HD creates two other types of waste:

- **Medical**. This may include used dialyzers, blood tubing, syringes, glass vials, dressings, and more.
- **Water**. This includes used dialysate and "reject" water made by the reverse osmosis (RO) device. (To learn more about RO, see Module 8: Water Treatment.)

Medical Waste

A single HD treatment produces 2.5 kg of solid medical waste, of which 38% is plastic.[54] Dialysis medical waste may be incinerated or processed on- or off-site. Or, the waste may be bagged and sent to a landfill—which can pollute the air or take up limited landfill space. Dialyzer reuse reduces the amount of waste per HD treatment. (Learn more in Module 5: *Dialyzer Reuse*.)

A number of researchers are working on new ways to handle waste plastic. In India, plastic is being recycled into roads,[55] and a company in the Netherlands is working on this as well.[56] The U.S. uses recycled plastic as a road binding material, and a Texas business turns used plastic soda bottles into road repair pins.[57] While *medical* waste is a bigger challenge, some pioneers are taking this on, too. In Pennsylvania, for example, mixed medical plastic is being sterilized, shredded, and turned into plastic lumber.[58] One large dialysis company has a pilot project to turn medical plastic into new plastic containers, which could keep up to 350,000 pounds of waste out of landfills.[59] Ideas like these may turn problem waste materials into assets.

Dialysis Water

Each HD treatment with a single pass machine may also use 500 liters of water—2/3 of which is RO "reject" water, which never comes in contact with patients. RO reject water is pure enough to drink, but is sent to the drain. In Australia, reject water is heated to make steam to sterilize equipment; used in parks and gardens; and used for home laundry and toilets.[60] A 173-patient clinic in France saves 1.2 million liters of water each year by using RO reject water for building maintenance—and made back its plumbing investment in 5 years.[61]

Conclusion

"I look at every nurse and tech as our angels, they listen to our complaints, they have seen us cry, smile in good days and bad, we really need to thank them."

As you have read in this module, the delivery system plays a key role in the safety of dialysis. During each treatment, the machine checks almost every part of the patient's care except one: YOU.

You are the most important monitor of all to keep patients safe. Alarms are of no use if they are ignored. Devices must be maintained. Many systems require tests before we use them for a patient's treatment.

The patient can be in great danger if you connect the wrong dialysate to the machine. Dialyzers and delivery systems are not just machines, monitors, and dialysate. They are the working parts of a treatment that allows people with kidney failure to lead full and active lives. Your attention to detail and skill at solving problems will help patients have better outcomes. When you understand the machine systems, you can use them safely.

References

1. King B. Principles of hemodialysis, in Counts CS (ed): *Core Curriculum for Nephrology Nursing* (5th ed). Pitman, NJ, American Nephrology Nurses Association, 2008, pp. 662-81
2. Aljadi Z, Mansouri L, Nopp A, et al. Activation of basophils is a new and sensitive marker of biocompatibility in hemodialysis. *Artif Organs.* 2014;38(11):945-53
3. Bellucci A. *Reactions to the hemodialysis membrane*. Available from UpToDate: https://www.uptodate.com/contents/reactions-to-the-hemodialysis-membrane. Accessed May 2017
4. Ford LL, Ward RA, Cheung AK. Choice of the hemodialysis membrane, in Henrich WL (ed): *Principles and Practice of Dialysis* (4th ed). Philadephia, Lippincott Williams & Wilkins, 2009, pp. 1-11
5. Ahmad S, Misra M, Hoenich N, et al. Hemodialysis apparatus, in Daugirdas JT, Blake PG, & Ing TS, *Handbook of Dialysis,* (5th ed). Philadelphia, Wolters Kluwer Health, 2015
6. Chanard J. Membrane biocompatibility in dialysis: the role of adsorption. *Nephrologie.* 2003:24(7):359-65
7. National Kidney Foundation. *A clinical Update on dialyzer membranes: State-of-the-art considerations for optimal care in hemodialysis*. Available from https://www.kidney.org/sites/default/files/02-10-6050_FBD_Clinical_bulletin.pdf. Accessed May 2017
8. Hoenich NA, Levin R, Pearce C. Clinical waste generation from renal units: implications and solutions. *Semin Dial.* 2005;18(5):396-400
9. Bacle A, Thevenot S, Grignon C, et al. Determination of bisphenol A in water and the medical devices used in hemodialysis treatment. *Int J Pharm.* 2016;505(1-2):115-21 doi: 10.1016/j.ijpharm.2016.03.003
10. Potential effect of dialyzer leaching of BPA from the Fresenius Optiflux 160NR compared to the Nipro ELISIO-15H (bisphenol-A). NCT02627118. Available from ClinicalTrials.gov, https://clinicaltrials.gov/ct2/show/NCT02627118. Accessed November 2016
11. Sahani MM, Daoud TM, Sare R, et al. Dialysis disequilibrium syndrome revisited. *Hemodial Int.* 2001;5(1):92-6
12. Lin CJ, Wu V, Wu CJ. Meta-analysis of the associations of p-Cresyl Sulfate (PCS) and Indoxyl Sulfate (IS) with cardiovascular events and all-cause mortality in patients with chronic renal failure. *PLoS One.* 2015;10(7):e0132589. Doi: 10.1371/journal.pone.0132589
13. Zumrutdal A. Role of β2-microglobulin in uremic patients may be greater than originally suspected. *World J Nephrol.* 2015;4(1):98-104
14. Yamamoto S, Kazama JJ, Narita I, et al. Recent progress in understanding dialysis-related amyloidosis. *Bone.* 2009;45(Suppl 1):S39-42
15. Available at http://www.convertunits.com. Accessed May 2017
16. Ambalavanan S, Rabetoy G, Cheung AK. High-efficiency and high-flux hemodialysis, In Schrier RW (ed): *Atlas of Diseases of the Kidney*, Vol 5. Hoboken, NJ, Blackwell Science, 1999
17. Schiffl H. High-flux dialyzers, backfiltration, and dialysis fluid quality. *Semin Dial.* 2011;24(1):1-4
18. Daugirdas JT. Physiologic principles and urea kinetic modeling, in Daugirdas JT, Blake PG, & Ing TS, *Handbook of Dialysis,* (5th ed). Philadelphia, Wolters Kluwer Health, 2015
19. Agar J. *Don't flog the fistulas: slow hemodialysis blood flow!* Available from http://homedialysis.org/news-and-research/blog/38-dont-flog-fistulas-slow-hemodialysis-blood-flow. Accessed October 2016
20. Ward RA, Idoux JW, Hamdan H, et al. Dialysate flow rate and delivered Kt/V urea for dialyzers with enhanced dialysate flow distribution. *Clin J Am Soc Nephrol.* 2011;6(9):2235-9
21. Cornelis T, van der Sande FM, Eloot S, et al. Acute hemodynamic response and uremic toxin removal in conventional and extended hemodialysis and hemodiafiltration: a randomized crossover study. *Am J Kidney Dis.* 2014;64(2):247-56
22. Cornelis T, Eloot S, Vanholder R, et al. Protein-bound uraemic toxins, dicarbonyl stress and advanced glycation end products in conventional and extended haemodialysis and haemodiafiltration. *Nephrol Dial Transplant.* 2015;30(8):1395-402
23. Castner D. Principles of hemodialysis. In Counts CS (ed.), *Core Curriculum for Nephrology Nursing: Module 3 Treatment options for patients with chronic kidney failure* (6th ed.). Pitman, NJ. American Nephrology Nurses' Association, 2015, pp. 69-166
24. Khosla N, Mehta RL. Continuous dialysis therapeutic techniques, in Henrich WL (ed): *Principles and Practice of Dialysis* (4th ed). Philadelphia, Lippincott Williams and Wilkins, 2009, pp. 196-218
25. Kallenbach JZ, Gutch CF, Stoner M, et al. *Review of Hemodialysis for Nurses and Dialysis Personnel* (7th ed.). Philadelphia, Elsevier Mosby, 2005, p. 217
26. Baxter. *Diascan monitoring system: a quality assurance tool*. Available from https://www.baxter.com/assets/downloads/products_expertise/renal_therapies/Diascan_Brochure.pdf. Accessed May 2017
27. Adimea™ *A unique technology for monitoring dialysis dose*. B.Braun, Bethlehem, PA, 2010. Available at www.bbraunusa.com. Accessed May 2017
28. *Online clearance monitoring: assuring the desired dose of dialysis*. Fresenius Medical Care, Deutschland GmbH, 2007. http://fmc-au.com/pdf/machines/OnLine%20Clearance%20Monitor-5008.pdf. Accessed November 2016
29. Wians, FH, Jr. *Blood Tests: Normal Values – Appendixes*. Merck Sharp & Cohme Corp., a subsidiary of Merck & Co., Kenilworth, NJ. Available from: http://www.merckmanuals.com/professional/appendixes/normal-laboratory-values/blood-tests-normal-values. Accessed May 2017
30. Ward RA, Ing TS. Dialysis water and dialysate, in Daugirdas JT, Blake PG, & Ing TS, *Handbook of Dialysis,* (5th ed). Philadelphia, Wolters Kluwer Health, 2015
31. Nesrallah GE, Suri RS, Lindsay RM, et al. Home and intensive hemodialysis, in Daugirdas JT, Blake PG, & Ing TS, *Handbook of Dialysis,* (5th ed). Philadelphia, Wolters Kluwer Health, 2015
32. Richards RH, Dowling JA, Vreman HJ, et al. Acetate levels in human plasma. *Proc Clin Dial Transplant Forum.* 1976;6:73-9
33. MedlinePlus [Internet]. Bethesda, MD: National Library of Medicine (US). *Calcium – ionized*; [updated 2015 May 5]. Available from: https://medlineplus.gov/ency/article/003486.htm. Accessed May 2017
34. Welshman SG, McCambridge H. Estimation of citrate in serum and urine using a citrate lyase technique. *Clin Chim Acta.* 1973;46(3):243-6
35. Mitra S, Mitsides N. Technical aspects of hemodialysis, in Magee CC, Tucker JK, Singh AK (eds.) *Core Concepts in Dialysis and Continuous Therapies.* New York, Springer, 2016. DOI 10.1007/978-1-4899-7657-4_2
36. Fresenius Medical Care North America. bibag® *On-line dry bicarbonate concentrate*. Available from: www.fmcna-bibag.com. Accessed June 2016
37. Baxter International Inc. *BiCart Cartridge*. Available from: https://www.baxter.com/assets/downloads/products_expertise/renal_therapies/BiCart_Brochure_FINAL.pdf. Accessed October 2016
38. Daugirdas JT. Chronic hemodialysis prescription, in Daugirdas JT, Blake PG, & Ing TS, *Handbook of Dialysis,* (5th ed). Philadelphia, Wolters Kluwer Health, 2015
39. Jepson R, Alonso E. Overheated dialysate: a case study and review. *Nephrol Nurs J.* 2009;36(5):551-3

40. Eldehni MT, Odudu A, McIntyre CW. Randomized clinical trial of dialysate cooling and effects on brain white matter. *J Am Soc Nephrol*. 2015;26(4):957-65
41. Fresenius USA, Inc. *2008K Hemodialysis machine operator's manual*. 2009. Available from: https://www.manualslib.com/manual/439583/Fresenius-Medical-Care-2008k.html. Accessed November 2016
42. Association for the Advancement of Medical Instrumentation. AAMI Recommended Practice, *Dialysate for hemodialysis* (ANSI/AAMI RD52:2004). Arlington, VA, American National Standard
43. Flythe JE, Kimmel SE, Brunelli SM. Rapid fluid removal during dialysis is associated with cardiovascular morbidity and mortality. *Kidney Int*. 2011;79(2):250-7
44. Arbor Research Collaborative for Health and the University of Michigan Kidney Epidemiology and Cost Center. *End Stage Renal Disease (ESRD) quality measure development and maintenance hemodialysis adequacy clinical technical expert panel summary report*. April 16-17, 2013 in Baltimore, MD. Sent to CMS on June 28, 2013. Available from: https://www.cms.gov/Medicare/Quality-Initiatives-Patient-Assessment-Instruments/MMS/Downloads/Hemodialysis-Adequacy-TEP-Summary-Report-and-Addendum.pdf Accessed June 2017
45. Raimann JG, Thijssen S, Usvyat LA, et al. Sodium alignment in clinical practice—implementation and implications. *Semin Dial*. 2011;24(5):587-92
46. Chaignon M, Chen WT, Tarazi RC, et al. Blood pressure response to hemodialysis. *Hypertension*. 1981;3(3):333-9
47. Kim KE, Neff M, Cohen B, et al. Blood volume changes and hypotension during hemodialysis. *Trans Am Soc Artif Intern Organs*. 1970;16:508-14
48. Weiner DE, Brunelli SM, Hunt A, et al. Improving clinical outcomes among hemodialysis patients: a proposal for a "Volume First" approach from the Chief Medical Officers of US dialysis providers. *Am J Kidney Dis*. 2014;64(5):685-95
49. Centers for Disease Control and Prevention. *Recommendations for preventing transmission of infections among chronic hemodialysis patients* April 27, 2001 / 50(RR05);1-43. Available from: http://www.cdc.gov/mmwr/preview/mmwrhtml/rr5005a1.htm Accessed November 2016
50. Sandroni S, Sherockman T, Hayes-Leight K. Catastrophic hemorrhage from venous needle dislodgement during hemodialysis: continued risk of avoidable death and progress toward a solution. 2008; *J Am Soc Nephrol*. 19(891A)
51. Axley B, Speranza-Reid J, Williams H. Venous needle dislodgement in patients on hemodialysis. *Nephrol Nurs J*. 2012;39(6):435-45
52. Stegmayr B, Brännström T, Forsberg U, et al. Microbubbles of air may occur in the organs of hemodialysis patients. *ASAIO J*. 2012;58(2):177-9
53. Forsberg U, Jonsson P, Stegmayr C, et al. A high blood level in the venous chamber and a wet-stored dialyzer help to reduce exposure for microemboli during hemodialysis. *Hemodial Int*. 2013;17(4):612-7
54. Hoenich NA, Levin R, Pearce C. Clinical waste generation from renal units: implications and solutions. *Semin Dial*. 2005;18(5):396-400
55. Kapur A. *India's 'Plastic Man' turns litter into paved roads*. July 11, 2014. Bloomberg. Available from: https://www.bloomberg.com/news/articles/2014-07-10/indias-plastic-man-chemist-turns-litter-into-paved-roads. Accessed November 2016
56. Building Design and Construction. Caulfield J (ed.) *Must see: Dutch company to test using plastic waste for road construction*. July 27, 2015. Available from: https://www.bdcnetwork.com/must-see-dutch-company-test-using-plastic-waste-road-construction. Accessed November 2016
57. Dykes Paving. *Texas roads made from plastic*. Available from: http://www.dykespaving.com/blog/texas-roads-made-from-plastic/. Accessed November 2016
58. Johnson J. *Alternative uses for processed regulated medical waste*. Available from: http://www.plasticsnews.com/article/20151230/NEWS/151239990/finding-new-life-for-medical-waste. Accessed November 2016
59. DaVita. *DaVita to launch dialyzer recycling pilot project through collaboration with waste management and BD*. July 27, 2011. Available from: https://www.wm.com/documents/pdfs-for-services-section/DaVita%20Recycling%20Pilot.pdf. Accessed November 2016
60. Agar JW. Green dialysis: the environmental challenges ahead. *Semin Dial*. 2015;28(2):186-92
61. Ponson L, Arkouche W, Laville M. Toward green dialysis: focus on water savings. Hemodial Int. 2014; 18(1):7-14

5 Dialyzer Reprocessing

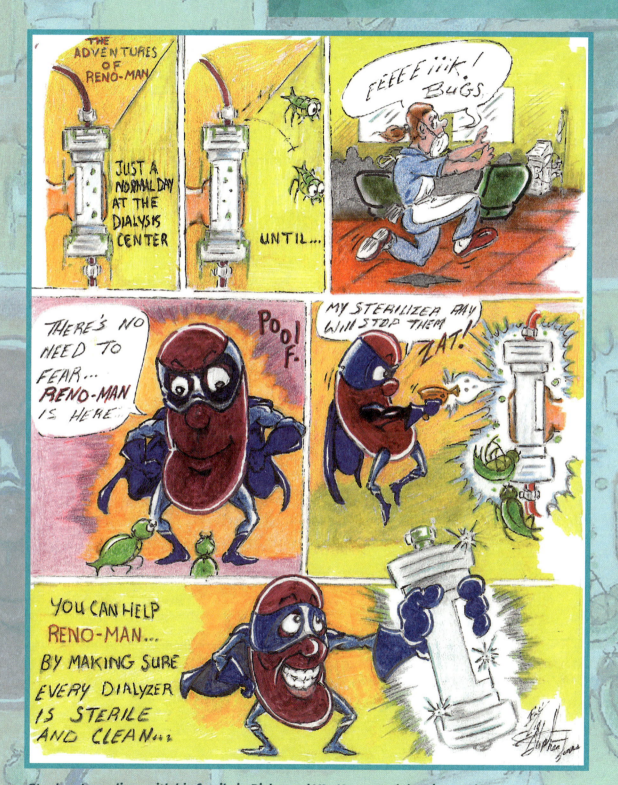

Stephen Jones lives with his family in Richmond VA. He started drawing at the age of 7. Art has been his passion for many years. He loves to draw and feels through his artwork he can escape to many places. Stephen can frequently be found drawing while at dialysis, and loves to share his artwork with others. He considers this a blessing and honor to share these drawings.

"I have been on reuse for about 3 years. I have had no side-effects. Prior to each dialysis run, the RN or technician runs a test in front of me, and we both have to agree that the test comes out clear. If not, the dialyzer is rinsed for another 15 minutes and re-tested."

Objectives

MODULE AUTHORS

James W. Bates
Charles H. Johnson, CHT
Suzanne E. Kuester, RN, CNN
Tia Sabin, CHT
Philip Varughese, CHT, CCNT

MODULE REVIEWERS

Nancy M. Gallagher, BS, RN, CNN
Darlene Rodgers, BSN, RN, CNN, CPHQ
John H. Sadler, MD
Dori Schatell, MS
Vern Taaffe, BS, CBNT, CDWS
Tamyra Warmack, RN

After you complete this module, you will be able to:

1. Discuss the history of dialyzer reprocessing.
2. Explain why dialysis clinics may reprocess dialyzers.
3. List the steps, in order, for dialyzer reprocessing.
4. Discuss the hazards to patients and staff that can occur with dialyzer reprocessing.
5. Describe the documentation needed when dialyzers are reprocessed.

An acronym list can be found in the Glossary.

Practice Test Questions at:
www.meiresearch.org/cc6

Introduction

The hollow fiber dialyzer, or artificial kidney, is a feat of modern engineering. It is complex enough to do some of the work of a human kidney. Yet, a dialyzer is reliable enough to use many times. Dialyzers can be *reprocessed*: cleaned, tested, and disinfected to be used again by the same patient, instead of being thrown out after one treatment. This is called *reuse*.

Federal and some state laws and rules cover dialyzer reprocessing. The rules state what clinics must do to make reuse as safe and effective as it can be for both patients and staff. A reprocessing technician has the key job of reducing the risks of reuse. This is done by carefully following all of the laws, rules, and clinic procedures.

This module covers the history of reprocessing, the role of rules and guidelines, and the steps used to reprocess dialyzers.

History of Dialyzer Reprocessing

Dialyzer reprocessing has been around since the late 1960s. At first, it was done manually. Today, reprocessing is most often done with an automated system. As dialyzer technology evolved, reuse equipment evolved as well.

In the mid-1960s, most patients were treated with Kiil dialyzers (see Figure 1). A Kiil was a "sandwich" made of layers of membrane sheets held apart by grooved plastic boards. Rubber gaskets and metal clamps held the sandwich together. The Kiil had to be assembled and pressure tested before each use—a slow and complex process. About 10%–20% of the time the Kiil would fail the pressure test and the whole process would have to start over with fresh sheets of membrane.

In 1967, Dr. Belding Scribner (who helped devise the arteriovenous fistula) reported that reuse of a Kiil was possible. The blood side of a Kiil could be filled with a *germicide* (germ killer), rinsed—and used again. This meant that a Kiil did *not* have to be taken apart and rebuilt for each use, which saved Dr. Scribner's home patients some of the need to "tear down" and rebuild the Kiil. At the time, most of his Seattle patients were doing home HD.[1]

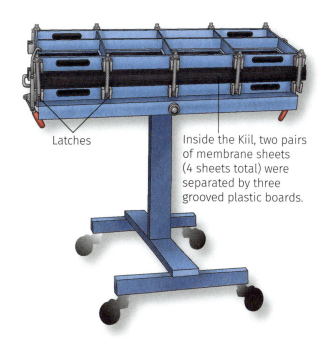

Figure 1: Kiil Dialyzer

By the late 1960s, coil dialyzers were preferred for reuse. Coils were easier to set up and prime (fill and rinse with normal saline) than Kiils. But, coils were too costly for many hospitals to use just once, as their manufacturers suggested. Before reuse, they were filled with a germicide and kept in a refrigerator.[2]

By the late 1970s, parallel plate dialyzers were in use and able to be reused. The dialyzer could be sealed off with germicide in the blood and dialysate sides, which reduced the chances that germs could grow inside.

Hollow Fiber Dialyzers and Reuse

When hollow fiber dialyzers came on the market in 1970, they proved to be well-suited for reuse. They were strong, easy to rinse, and high water pressure could be used to wash fibrin and blood out of the fibers. *Total cell volume** (TCV), the total fluid volume of the blood compartment, was easy to measure, and when a dialyzer lost 20% of the baseline TCV, it was discarded. For these reasons, hollow fiber dialyzers became the leading choice for reuse.

* For most hollow fiber dialyzers, a 20% loss of TCV is approximately a 10% loss of clearance.

Over time, dialyzer reuse evolved. It was studied, tested, and practiced. Researchers looked at how dialyzers differed in how well they cleared small solutes. They tried a number of different germicides, dwell times, concentrations, and temperatures. In time, they found the best ways to kill and prevent the growth of bacteria. Companies began to build automated systems for reprocessing. Some systems would process one dialyzer at a time, while others made multi-station systems.

Dialyzer Reuse Numbers

In 1976, about 18% of U.S. HD patients were dialyzing with reused dialyzers.[3] In the 1980s, many studies reported that reuse with proper quality control was safe.[3] Automated reprocessing systems aided the growth of the practice.

In 1983, Medicare changed the way it paid for dialysis. Instead of fee for service, clinics were paid a fixed sum (a *composite rate*) per treatment to cover all of the equipment, labor, lab tests, and supplies.[4] This change may have been the largest reason for the fast growth of reuse—which peaked in 1997, with 82% of clinics using it.[3]

By 2002, reuse dropped to 63%,[3] because in 2001, the largest U.S. dialysis provider stopped the reuse of dialyzers in their clinics—since they also manufactured dialyzers.[5] Today, only 4 of the 10 largest dialysis providers reuse some of their dialyzers. Reuse data from 2010 to 2015 show that reuse of dialyzers in these companies dropped from 28% to just under 12%.[6]

Why Dialyzers are Reused

Reasons for dialyzer reuse have changed over time. During HD treatments with a cellulose dialyzer, the inner membrane surface was coated with blood proteins. Reprocessing with some non-bleach germicides left these proteins in the dialyzer, which made it more biocompatible. This coating reduced the rate of *first-use syndrome*: symptoms of chest and back pain with new dialyzers.[7] Since newer synthetic membranes used in hollow fiber dialyzers tend to be more biocompatible, most patients do not have first-use syndrome.

Today, reuse is largely done to save money. Most clinicians believe it does not harm patients when it is done safely. In fact, preprocessing a dialyzer before the first use can rinse out plasticizers and manufacturing agents that could be lethal. In one case, 53 patients who were treated on new dialyzers died due to a chemical called PF-5070 used by a manufacturer.[8]

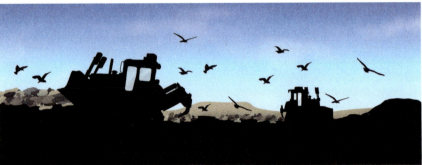

Figure 2: Reuse Reduces Medical Waste in Landfills

Saving Dollars and Reducing Medical Waste

Dialyzer reuse may reduce the cost per dialysis treatment—or it may not when *all* of the costs are considered. If a dialyzer costs $9.00 and can be used 15 times, its per-treatment cost is $0.60, which would seem to be a savings of $8.40 per treatment. However, reprocessing itself may cost $3.00 to $5.50 per treatment, there is staff time as well, and extra saline must be used to rinse the dialyzer for the next treatment. Calculations like these may be why fewer clinics each year reprocess dialyzers.

Using dialyzers just once does have an impact on the planet. Each year, the U.S. generates an estimated 2.6 million tons of medical waste.[9] One large dialysis company notes that reuse could mean using 46 million fewer dialyzers a year—and keeping 62 million pounds of waste (31,000 tons) out of landfills (see Figure 2).[10] Reuse also lowers the costs of disposing of medical waste. Used dialyzers may be incinerated, and this can affect air quality as well.

Safety of Reuse

How safe is dialyzer reuse? In a 2012 paper, researchers analyzed 14 studies that had both a reuse and a non-reuse group. They found about the same survival rates for both groups.[11] However, reuse may expose patients to pathogens or germicides if it is not done correctly. NOTE: CMS does not require written patient consent for reuse, but patient groups (AAKP and NKF) suggest it. CMS rules do state that patients must be told about reuse and how the process is done.[12] Patients have the right to have a new dialyzer for each treatment—but a less costly dialyzer may be used.[13,14]

Reuse and Exposure to Pathogens

Germs can enter a dialyzer from the water used to make dialysate. After a treatment, germs in the dialysate side may then stay in a dialyzer. If these germs multiply and enter the patient's blood, they could potentially cause lethal:

- **Pyrogenic reactions** (fever, chills, nausea, vomiting, low blood pressure, muscle pain)
- **Sepsis** (life-threatening blood infection)

A 2016 study tested to see if bacteria would grow after dialyzers were reprocessed—and they *did*.[15] Bacteria or endotoxin may survive reprocessing if:

- Dialysate water quality is poor
- The germicide is outdated, not mixed correctly, or not enough was used
- There was too little contact time between the dialyzer and germicide
- The dialyzer was not stored properly after reprocessing

Any bacteria or endotoxin in the reprocessed dialyzer could pose a risk to patients. It is important to check and record a patient's temperature at *least* pre- and post-treatment. This will give you baseline data just in case the patient develops any symptoms, such as chills, during treatment. A doctor will need to decide if the symptoms might be due to an adverse reaction to the dialyzer. If a patient has sudden symptoms, the team needs to take blood and dialysate cultures and assess for:

- Use of contaminated water
- Errors in treatment delivery
- Errors in dialyzer reprocessing

If a cluster of patients has pyrogenic reactions or sepsis *at the same time* due to reuse, the clinic must stop doing reuse. They may not restart until the whole reprocessing system has been checked.[16]

Never reuse a dialyzer from a patient who tests positive for hepatitis B surface antigen (HBV+). Both the Association for the Advancement of Medical Instrumentation (AAMI)[17] and the CMS *Conditions for Coverage*[18] state this rule. We discard these dialyzers after use to keep staff and other patients safe.

Reuse and Exposure to Germicides

Germicides are toxic if they enter the patient's blood, even in small amounts (see Figure 3). If *all* of the germicide is not rinsed out before the treatment begins, the patient may:

- Have burning in the access limb
- Feel numbness in the lips
- Lose vision or hearing
- Die

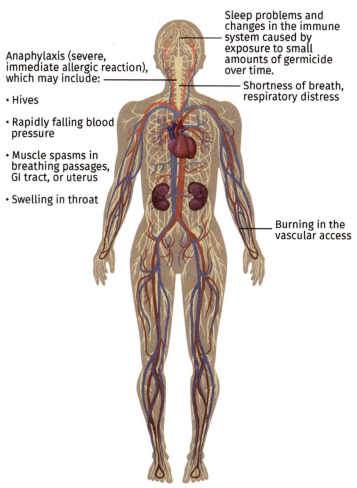

Figure 3: Medical Risks of Incorrect Dialyzer Reprocessing

Acute (sudden) toxicity can occur if dialysis does not start right after the germicide test is done. This may occur because there may be residual germicide in the dialysate side of the dialyzer. Waiting can let some of the germicide move to the blood side—where it can mix with the patient's blood.

Small amounts of some germicides may not cause acute symptoms, but may cause long-term problems, such as trouble sleeping and changes in the immune system.

Follow your clinic's policies and procedures for chemical use to avoid or minimize the risk of exposure. **Test every dialyzer before use to make sure all of the chemical has been removed**.

Reuse and Dialyzer Efficiency

Each reuse and reprocessing changes the dialyzer membrane and may reduce the TCV. The TCV tells us how well a dialyzer may work to remove solutes and water. Over time, a lower TCV can affect solute transport and ultrafiltration (UF). If this occurs, the patient does not receive the full dialysis dose, because:

- **Cleaning agents and germicide can harm the membrane**. Leaks and reduced clearance can occur.
- **Each time a dialyzer is used, fibers can clog with blood or other material**. These clogs reduce the surface area of the dialyzer. Having a smaller surface area reduces both clearance and the UF rate.

For most dialyzers, a 20% drop in TCV equals a 10% loss of urea clearance—and less waste removal for the patient.[19] When some fibers clot, the rest get a higher blood flow, so there is a higher diffusion rate in each unclotted fiber. This is why when TCV is 80% of baseline, urea, sodium, or ionic clearance only drops by about 10% and not the full 20%.

Rules for Dialyzer Reprocessing

Dialyzers must be reprocessed using the ANSI/AAMI standards. Medicare adopted the ANSI/AAMI *Reuse of Hemodialyzers*, third edition, as a *Condition for Coverage* and as federal rules.[20]

The ANSI/AAMI standard covers:
- Equipment
- Cleaning and disinfecting
- Labeling and the reprocessing procedure
- Record keeping
- Reprocessing supplies
- Physical plant and environmental safety
- Patient considerations and staff qualifications
- Training
- Preparation for dialysis
- Testing for germicides
- Monitoring
- Quality assurance

As we cover the reprocessing steps (see Figure 4), we will tell you what the rules require you to do.

Dialyzer Labeling for Reuse

Dialyzers must be FDA-cleared for reuse. In 1996, the FDA said that each dialyzer's label must say if it is for "single" or "multiple" use,[21] and this guidance is still in place today.[22] **We can only reuse dialyzers that say "multiple use" on the label.** Companies that sell dialyzers to clinics that reuse must include:[21]

- A method to reprocess the dialyzer
- *A list of approved cleaning agents and germicides.* (Not all dialyzers can be reprocessed with all germicides.)
- Scientific proof that reuse of the dialyzer is safe and effective.

Each dialyzer will have a manufacturer's "Directions for Use." Read this *before* you start to prepare it for reprocessing. Your clinic must set maximum use limits for dialyzers you reprocess.

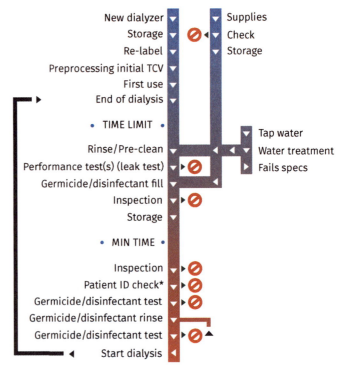

Figure 4: Systems Diagram for Reprocessing Dialyzers

Dialyzer Reprocessing

Automated Versus Manual Reprocessing

Dialyzers *can* be reprocessed manually. But, using an automated system (see Figure 5):[23]

- Is more efficient
- Is more consistent
- Tracks the process
- May be safer

Since reprocessing tasks are repetitive, it can be easy to become bored and make errors that could harm patients. And, automated systems use consistent standards, print proper labels, and keep records.

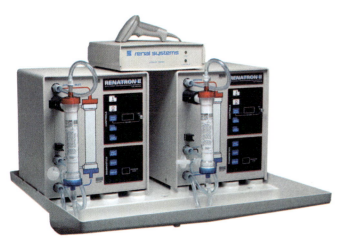

Figure 5: Automated Reprocessing System
Photo used with permission from Medivators Inc.

Automated systems can self-test the dialyzer. Follow the manufacturer's instructions to use them. If you reprocess dialyzers manually, you must test the tools you are using to be sure they are working. You will follow your clinic's procedures, and use:

- A graduated cylinder to collect and measure the fluid from the blood compartment of the dialyzer to find the TCV
- A stopwatch and a hand-held pressure bulb and manometer so you can apply pressure to the blood compartment to determine the timed pressure drop across the membrane

These tests can show whether the TCV measurement of a dialyzer is within 80% of its initial volume and the membrane is intact.

Preparing a Dialyzer for First Use

The CMS *Conditions for Coverage* state the rules for dialyzer labeling:[24]

- ***The dialyzer must be labeled and have the patient's name on it before the first use.***
- ***If patients have the same (or similar) last names, the dialyzer must have a warning or alert*** (see Figure 6). The label should also have extra information to prevent mix-ups, such as:
  - The patient's first name and middle initial
  - A color code
  - Medical record number
- ***The label will need space for***:
  - The number of uses
  - Date and time the dialyzer was last reprocessed
  - An identifier for the reprocessing staff member
  - Results of tests done on the dialyzer

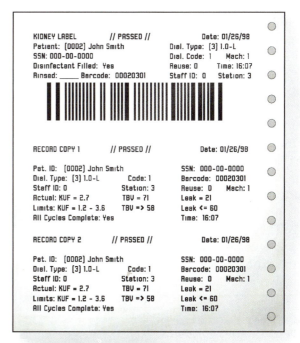

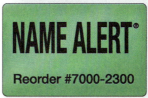

Figure 6: Example of a Reprocessing Label and Same Name Alert

CMS also says that you still need to be able to *read* the labels after reprocessing. The label should *not* cover up:
- The model or lot numbers
- Arrows for blood and/or dialysate flow
- Other key data

On dialyzers with clear casings, place labels so you can see some of the fibers all the way from one end of the dialyzer to the other.

Preprocessing

Before you use a new dialyzer for the first time, you will *preprocess* it. This means that you complete all of the reprocessing steps, which tells you the baseline TCV. Then, *after* each use, you will recheck a dialyzer against its *own* TCV value. **If the TCV is less than 80% of the baseline, it is time to discard the dialyzer.**

Clinics must preprocess *all* new dialyzers that will be reused.[19] If a "dry pack" (a dialyzer right out of the box) is used without preprocessing, you must throw it out after a treatment. Some manufacturers make dialyzers that cannot be preprocessed. These are single use only.

After Dialysis

At the end of a treatment, blood in the dialyzer is *rinsed back* (returned to the patient). Rinse as much blood as you can back to the patient to reduce blood loss. A rinseback that is fair or poor leaves too much blood in the dialyzer. Any blood left may clot in the fibers, so the dialyzer is harder to clean and does not perform as well (see Figure 7). After rinseback:
- *Recirculate* (send through the loop) the saline in the extracorporeal circuit before you remove the dialyzer from the machine. To do this, you will connect the bloodlines together and turn on the blood pump. The continuous saline movement will decrease clotting.
- Disconnect the bloodlines from the dialyzer. Place disinfected caps—made for dialyzer reuse—on each of the ports.
- Bring the capped dialyzer to the reprocessing room. Or, bag the dialyzer to prevent cross-contamination and place it in a tub with others to be moved to the reprocessing room.

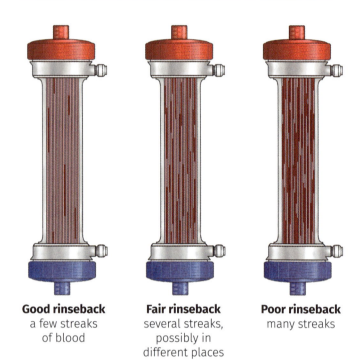

All water used to rinse, preprocess, reprocess dialyzers, and dilute germicide must meet ANSI/AAMI standards.[25]

Good rinseback
a few streaks of blood

Fair rinseback
several streaks, possibly in different places

Poor rinseback
many streaks

Figure 7: Good, Fair, and Poor Rinsebacks

Dialyzers that will not be reprocessed within 2 hours must be refrigerated—but not frozen. Keeping dialyzers cold slows the growth of bacteria. Dialyzers that are reprocessed off-site must be kept cold during transport. The temperature range and maximum refrigeration time will be set by your clinic.

Pre-clean the Dialyzer

Pre-cleaning is optional. A clinic may choose to pre-clean all, some, or none of the dialyzers before reprocessing. When pre-cleaning is done, it removes some blood from the blood compartment. **You must use ANSI/AAMI-quality water.***[26]

All product water used to make dialysate or concentrates or for reuse, must have a total viable microbe count lower than 200 CFU/mL. The endotoxin level must be lower than 2 EU/mL.
- The action level for the total viable microbial count in the product water is 50 CFU/mL.
- The action level for the endotoxin concentration shall be 1 EU/mL.[27]

Dialyzer Reprocessing

*ANSI/AAMI RD47 standard is used as accepted practice for dialyzer reuse. Much of the RD47:2008 standard has been adopted by CMS as a requirement in the *Conditions for Coverage*.

Pre-cleaning may use *reverse ultrafiltration (UF)*. If so, you will:[28]

- Purge all air from the dialysate compartment. Air left in the dialyzer will be forced across the membrane.
- Place a cap on one of the dialysate ports.
- Send a supply of ANSI/AAMI-quality water into the other dialysate port at a pressure (*maximum transmembrane pressure*, or max TMP) suggested by the manufacturer.
- Monitor the pressure if you use a manual system. Too-high pressures may break fibers and cause blood leaks. Automated systems monitor and regulate internal pressure.

Clean and Disinfect the Header

Dialyzer housings, supports, and membranes can adsorb endotoxin. If this occurs, they may be released into the blood at the next treatment. Endotoxin is very hard to rinse out. This is why bacteria levels in water used to make dialysate and to dilute germicide must be kept as low as possible.[25] Cleaning and disinfecting the header can also help reduce the level of endotoxin. For some dialyzers, you may need to take off the header caps to remove clotted blood from the headers (see Figure 8). If so, learn and follow your clinic's policy for removing dialyzer header caps. Once the caps are off:[29]

- Use *only* a free-flowing stream of ANSI/AAMI-quality water to clean the header, header cap and O-ring—not a paper clip, 4x4, or rag.
- Once the header, header cap, and O-ring are clean, dip them in disinfectant before you put them back on the dialyzer.
- **Keep the header caps and O-rings with the dialyzer they came from**. Putting the wrong part on a dialyzer could expose a patient to someone else's blood. For this reason, it is safest to clean one dialyzer at a time.

Test Dialyzer Performance

After you rinse and clean a dialyzer, you will need to test it. NOTE: dialyzer testing is a built-in process in automated systems.

- Since dialyzer performance is linked to TCV, federal and state rules require you to check TCV after each reuse.
- You will also need to do a leak test. This measures how well the dialyzer can withstand a pressure load and protects the patient from a blood leak.
- Inspect the dialyzer for cracks, chips, or defects in the plastic housing.

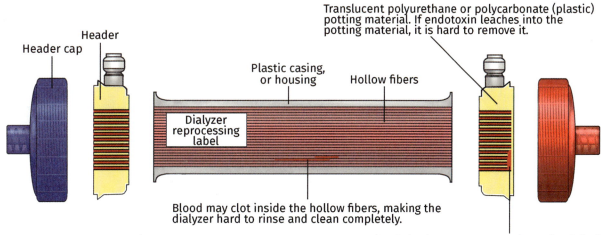

Figure 8: Parts of a Hollow Fiber Dialyzer

Module 5

Rejecting a Dialyzer

Before you go any further in reprocessing, discard dialyzers that:[30]

- Have reached their maximum number of uses (per your clinic's policy)
- Fail performance tests
- Have cracks or leaks in the plastic housing
- Have been exposed to more than one germicide
- Have large clots or other deposits in the headers
- Have more than a "few" discolored fibers - the dialyzer needs to look good to patients and staff
- Have labels that cannot be read
- Have less than 80% of the baseline TCV[19]

Disinfect the Dialyzer

Dialyzers that pass inspection will next need to be disinfected. Automated systems will fill dialyzers with a germicide when you connect them. **Medicare allows dialyzers to be exposed to only *one* reprocessing germicide**.[31] So, if your clinic switches to a new germicide, all dialyzers must be discarded before the new one is used.

Each germicide has pros and cons (see Table 1). The four main types of germicides that have been used in the U.S. are:

- **Peracetic acid**
- **Heat and citric acid**
- **Formaldehyde**
- **Glutaraldehyde**

When you use an automated system that mixes germicide on-line, you need to check it at least once a month.[17] Some germicides come premixed at their dialyzer use concentration. These are verified by the manufacturer, but it is good practice to check them before you use them.

Germicide must stay in a dialyzer for a certain amount of time to kill germs. This *contact time* differs for each germicide. Your clinic will have a policy for the contact time, based on what the manufacturer says. CMS requires your clinic to keep detailed records of all of this information.

Handling Hazardous Materials

Used dialyzers are *hazardous materials*. They contain blood. Handle them with Standard Precautions, until the inside and outside are disinfected. Wear personal protective equipment (PPE) to touch used dialyzers.[32]

Germicides kill germs, but **they can also harm you and your patients**. The use of germicides requires protective gear and routine monitoring of vapors in and around the reprocessing area.

OSHA standards require clinics to tell staff about all hazardous chemicals in the workplace. OSHA has also set exposure limits for germicides used in reprocessing. See Table 2 for OHSA environment exposure limits. Clinics must keep a file of results of the health exams of reuse staff who are exposed to hazardous chemicals.[33]

Table 1: Germicide Pros and Cons[23]

Germicide	Pros	Cons
Peracetic acid	When diluted, breaks down into biodegradable acetic acid (vinegar), oxygen, and water	- Higher cost
Heat and citric acid	Safe for staff and the environment	- Not all dialyzers can be heat disinfected
Formaldehyde*	Low cost	- Technician must wear a respirator - Clinic must have a quick drench shower - May cause cancer - Higher disposal costs
Glutaraldehyde*	Low cost	- Linked with skin and breathing problems - Higher disposal costs

*Used only with manual reprocessing and rarely seen in current practice

Dialyzer Reprocessing

Your clinic must provide a list of all chemicals and keep it up to date:

- One copy of the Safety Data Sheet (SDS) for each substance must be kept in a file that staff can access.[34]
- One copy must be posted near where a chemical is used, so you can find it quickly in an emergency.
- All containers must be clearly labeled, to avoid mix-ups.

Safety Training

Your clinic must train you in its procedures for handling hazardous materials.[35] They must have spill kits for the chemicals you will use and train you in their use. The clinic must encourage you to read its written policies. You should know where to find policies, emergency procedures, and training materials. A clinic with more than 10 staff must also keep records of occupational illnesses and injuries. It is the employer's job to comply with safety practices and rules.

Procedures alone cannot keep you safe from toxic substances. YOU must learn the steps and follow them. Taking shortcuts does not save time if it causes an accident. *Protect yourself, your coworkers, and your patients: learn how to handle hazardous materials safely.*

Peracetic Acid Safety

Air quality is tested for acetic acid and hydrogen peroxide to ensure safety.

Formaldehyde Safety

Formaldehyde is a strong irritant of the eyes, nose, and throat.[36] Because of this, it can:

- Cause coughing or wheezing
- Trigger severe allergic reactions of the skin, eyes, and breathing tract
- Possibly cause cancer

Table 2: OSHA Environmental Exposure Limits

Substance	Permissible Exposure Limit (PEL)
Acetic Acid	10 ppm TWA*
Chlorine Dioxide (syn.: chlorine oxide)	0.1 ppm TWA 0.3 STEL**
Citric Acid	None set
Formaldehyde	0.75 ppm TWA 2 ppm STEL (15 min) 0.5 ppm action level
Glutaraldehyde	0.2 ppm ceiling NIOSH/OSHA
Hydrogen Peroxide	1 ppm TWA
Peracetic Acid	See limits for acetic acid and hydrogen peroxide, the two main ingredients
Phenol (may be used to disinfect the inside of header caps or the casing)	5 ppm TWA

ppm = parts per million
NIOSH = National Institute for Occupational Safety and Health
OSHA = Occupational Safety and Health Administration
PEL – can be TWAs or STELs (below)
*Time-weighted average – how much an employee can be exposed to in an 8-hour period
**Short-term exposure limit – how much you can be exposed to in any 15-minute period

Table adapted and used with permission from AAMI. Copyright 2008, Association for the Advancement of Medical Instrumentation, ANSI/AAMI RD47:2008 Reprocessing of Hemodialyzers. Table 1.

Glutaraldehyde Safety

Glutaraldehyde is also a strong irritant. It can:[37]

- Irritate or burn eyes and skin
- Cause itching or rash
- Irritate the nose or throat, causing coughing, wheezing, or sudden asthma attacks
- Lead to headaches, feeling drowsy or dizzy, or nosebleeds

Storage of Reprocessed Dialyzers

Store dialyzers so they do not deteriorate, become contaminated, or break. Wall racks or carts can be used, as long as they are easy to clean. Your clinic should follow the germicide maker's guidance for the maximum storage time for a reprocessed dialyzer. After that time, a dialyzer must be reprocessed or discarded. Follow your clinic's policies and procedures to store dialyzers. These may include:

- Before storage, wipe off the outside of a dialyzer or soak it with a disinfectant.
- Before you label a dialyzer, look to see if it is clean and the ports are capped tightly.
- **Never store reprocessed dialyzers with new ones or dirty dialyzers with clean ones**.[38]

Prepare for the Next Use

Inspect the Dialyzer

The first step in getting a dialyzer ready for its next use is to look at it (see Figure 9) to be sure that:

- It is labeled properly.
- No structural damage or tampering has occurred.
- The ports are capped, and there is no leakage from the ports or other parts of the dialyzer.
- It was stored long enough for the germicide to work—but not so long that it exceeds the shelf life.
- The cosmetic appearance is good— it *looks* clean with no visible damage.

After you look at the dialyzer, use a potency test strip or ampule to confirm that germicide is present and strong enough to work. Just looking at the dialyzer cannot tell you how strong the germicide is. Some germicides, like peracetic acid, are clear. A dialyzer may accidentally be filled only with water. Germicides can also degrade over time. You *must* test the fluid to confirm the presence and strength of germicide.[39] How you test will depend on which germicide your clinic uses.

Remove the Germicide

The next step is to **thoroughly rinse the germicide out of the dialyzer before use**, following your clinic's procedure. Germicide can "hide" in a dialyzer. The steps in Table 3 can help you ensure that it is *all* out so the patient is safe.

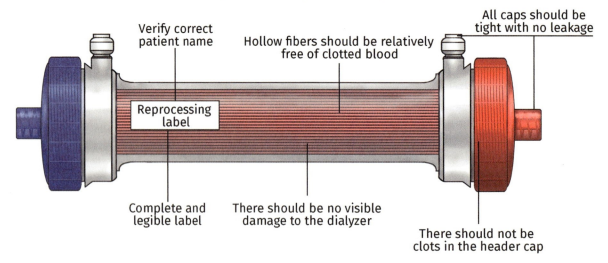

Figure 9: Reprocessed Dialyzer

Table 3: How to Rinse a Reprocessed Dialyzer[17]

Problem	Solution
Air bubbles in fibers can trap germicide inside.	**Fully prime the arterial line before you connect it to the dialyzer**. Flush the blood side before you start dialysate flow if you use a peracetic acid germicide.
Air in the dialysate side can trap germicide.	**Rotate the dialyzer while you rinse it** to release trapped air.
Germicide may back up into the heparin or monitor lines.	**Clamp the heparin line** so fluid cannot be forced in.
Germicide may back up into the saline bag.	**Do not force fluid from the dialysis circuit into the saline bag**. Follow your clinic's procedures.
Sampling too quickly after rinsing may lead to a false negative germicide test.	**Flush the dialyzer before testing**. Follow your clinic's procedure for the amount of time to continue flushing or rinsing.
The saline prime could contain some germicide.	**Always replace the saline prime with fresh saline** before you start blood flow to the dialyzer.

Rinse/prime and recirculate the extracorporeal circuit per your clinic's procedure.

- Priming forces air and germicide out of the dialyzer and bloodlines.
- Recirculation helps the germicide move from the blood side of the dialyzer to the dialysate side, and then down the drain.

Just before you start a treatment, **test the dialysis circuit for residual germicide**. Make sure the germicide is at or below the manufacturer's and clinic's accepted levels.[40]

If you do not rinse the dialyzer well, the germicide could be infused into the patient.

Check the Dialyzer Prior to Treatment

Staff members must ensure that the dialyzer has been prepared for use. **Doing dialyzer reprocessing incorrectly can harm patients**. The dialyzer must be labeled correctly, structurally sound (no cracks or leaks, all caps in place, etc.), free of germicide, and clean.

Just before the start of a treatment, **two people must check the dialyzer label to be sure it matches the patient**. It is best if the patient can be one of these two people. Record this step on the reprocessing record or dialysis flow sheet, and sign it to show who did the check.

Documentation

Reuse is part of a medical treatment. But, reprocessing is a type of manufacturing process. Clinics that reuse should follow the same "good manufacturing practice" standards used by companies that make dialyzers. Keep a record of all complaints and reactions to reused dialyzers in a Complaint Investigation File. Log blood leaks, changes in dialyzer performance, and other issues into the file. Include any corrective action. Review the file for trends to help make your clinic safer for staff and patients.

A large amount of documentation is required (see Table 4) for dialyzer reprocessing.[41] The staff person who completes the forms must be diligent, precise, and thorough.

Quality Assurance (QA) and Quality Control (QC)

A clinic must prove it can safely and effectively reprocess dialyzers. Federal (CMS) rules require clinics that reuse dialyzers to have a program to check their systems.[20] QA and QC are the two parts of the program.

QA shows that a clinic has written, used, and tested its reuse policies and procedures. All standards as well as state and federal rules must be included. Each person who reprocesses dialyzers must pass the clinic's training course, prove competence, and be certified by the

Module 5

Table 4: Dialyzer Reprocessing Documents

Document	Description
Dialyzer Reprocessing Manual	A summary of all reuse specifications, policies, procedures, training materials, manuals, methods, and samples of forms and labels
Reprocessing Log	Record of each step in dialyzer use—from entry in the clinic, to all testing, to disposal
Water Quality	Record of water treatment system maintenance and operation to meet ANSI/AAMI standards and the clinic's policies and procedures. Includes cultures, endotoxin, and chemical analysis.
Complaint Investigation Files and Special Incident Report	Record of all complaints by patients and staff about dialyzer failures or possible harmful reactions. Include results from complaints and actions taken to fix a problem. Complaints should be reviewed for trends.
Environmental Testing	Record of testing required by regulatory agencies on germicides or cleaning agents used in dialyzer reprocessing
Equipment Maintenance	Log of the dates of preventive maintenance, repairs, and results of scheduled testing on all reprocessing and safety equipment
Incoming Materials Log/Material Quality Records	Log of incoming materials such as dialyzers, port caps, disinfectants, other supplies, results of any quality control tests, first-in/first-out inventory control, and expiration dates
Personnel Health Monitoring Records	Record of staff medical exam results to monitor exposure to substances that may be toxic, as required by regulatory agencies
Training Records	Record of staff's completion of a training course in dialyzer reprocessing, proven ability to do reuse correctly, and certification by the Medical Director
Quality Assurance and Quality Control	Record of the dates and results of all quality assurance and quality control evaluations

Table 5: Quality Assurance Audit Schedule

	Monthly	Quarterly	Semi-annually	Annually
Patient information policy (14.3)				✓
Equipment manuals and procedures (14.4)				✓
Equipment maintenance and repair policies (14.4)				✓
Environmental safety (8.1)				✓
Environmental safety (8.2)		✓		
Environmental safety (8.4)		✓		
Reprocessing supplies (9)			✓	
Water treatment* (11.4.1.5)	✓			
Hemodialyzer labeling (10)		✓		
Reprocessing procedures** (14.8)	✓		✓	
Procedures for preparation for dialysis (14.9)			✓	

*More frequent monitoring may be required at first as described in 11.4.1.5
**These functions may allow for the less frequent review period indicated according to the circumstances specified in their respective sections
(Numbers in parentheses refer to AAMI sections)

Table adapted and used with permission from AAMI. Copyright 2008, Association for the Advancement of Medical Instrumentation, ANSI/AAMI RD47:2008 Reprocessing of Hemodialyzers. Table 2.

Medical Director. Each must pass a competency review once a year. The clinic should review all procedures and manuals each year *and* any time problems occur that could be due to equipment failure. ANSI/AAMI RD47:2008[17] has details on all parts of a reuse QA program (see Table 5).

QC shows that the materials, processes, and final product meet set standards. QC for reprocessing includes TCV, tests for bacteria and endotoxin, and tests for germicide.

Conclusion

Dialyzer reprocessing, performed properly, can be safe for patients. However, done incorrectly, it can pose a hazard to patients *and* staff. As a dialysis technician, your role is to follow the clinic's policies and procedures to ensure patient and staff safety.

References

1. Pollard TL, Barnett BMS, Eschbach JW, et al. A technique for storage and multiple re-use of the Kiil dialyzer and blood tubing. *Trans Amer Soc Artif Int Organs*. 1967;13:24-8
2. Deane N, Wineman RJ, Bemis JA (eds): *Guide to Reprocessing of Hemodialyzers*. Norwell, MA, Martinus Nijhoff Publishing, 1986, p. 4
3. Finelli L, Miller JT, Tokars JI, et al. National surveillance of dialysis-associated diseases in the United States, 2002. *Semin Dial*. 2005;18(1):52-61
4. Lockridge RS. The direction of end-stage renal disease reimbursement in the United States. *Semin Dial*. 2004;17(2):125-30
5. Fresenius phasing out reuse at its dialysis clinics. *Nephrol News Issues*. 2001;15(5):8
6. Neumann ME. The largest dialysis providers in 2016: Poised for change. *Nephrol News Issues*. Post. Available at: http://www.nephrologynews.com/largest-dialysis-providers-2016-poised-change/. July 11, 2016.
7. Charoenpanich R, Pollak VE, Kant KS, et al. Effect of first and subsequent use of hemodialyzers on patient well-being: the rise and fall of a syndrome associated with new dialyzer use. *Artif Organs*. 1987;11(2):123-7
8. Shaldon S, Koch KM. Understanding the epidemic of deaths associated with the use of the Althane dialyzer. *Artif Organs*. 2002;26(10):894-5
9. Homer A. *Syringes and sandcastles: a history of healthcare waste*. http://www.psna.org/a-history-of-healthcare-waste/. Accessed January 2017
10. DaVita. *Dialyzer reuse for dialysis*. https://www.davita.com/kidney-disease/dialysis/treatment-options/dialyzer-reuse-for-dialysis/e/5272. Accessed January 2017
11. Galvao TF, Silva MT, Araujo ME, et al. Dialyzer reuse and mortality risk in patients with end-stage renal disease: a systematic review. *Am J Nephrol*. 2012;35(3):249-58
12. Centers for Medicare and Medicaid Services, HHS. End Stage Renal Disease (ESRD) Program Interpretive Guidance Version 1.1, Part 494 *Conditions for Coverage for ESRD Facilities*. (V Tag 312) October 3, 2008
13. HealthInsight. ESRD Alliance/Network 18. *Patients' rights & responsibilities*. Available at: http://www.esrdnetwork18.org/patients/patient-rights/. Accessed on June 2017
14. National Kidney Foundation. *What you should know about dialyzer reuse: A guide for hemodialysis patients and their families*. Available from https://www.kidney.org/sites/default/files/docs/dialyzer_reuse.pdf. Accessed January 2017
15. Toniolo Ado R, Ribeiro MM, Ishii M, et al. Evaluation of the effectiveness of manual and automated dialyzers reprocessing after multiple reuses. *Am J Infect Control*. 2016;44(6):719-20
16. Centers for Medicare and Medicaid Services, HHS. End Stage Renal Disease (ESRD) Program Interpretive Guidance Version 1.1, Part 494 *Conditions for Coverage for ESRD Facilities*. (V Tag 382) October 3, 2008
17. Association for the Advancement of Medical Instrumentation. Reprocessing of hemodialyzers [ANSI/AAMI RD47:2008 (R2013)]. Arlington, VA, American National Standard
18. Centers for Medicare and Medicaid Services, HHS. End Stage Renal Disease (ESRD) Program Interpretive Guidance Version 1.1, Part 494 *Conditions for Coverage for ESRD Facilities*. (V Tag 301) October 3, 2008
19. Centers for Medicare and Medicaid Services, HHS. End Stage Renal Disease (ESRD) Program Interpretive Guidance Version 1.1, Part 494 *Conditions for Coverage for ESRD Facilities*. (V Tag 336) October 3, 2008
20. Centers for Medicare and Medicaid Services, HHS. End Stage Renal Disease (ESRD) Program Interpretive Guidance Version 1.1, Part 494 *Conditions for Coverage for ESRD Facilities*. (V Tag 300) October 3, 2008
21. U.S. Food and Drug Administration. *Guidance for hemodialyzer reuse labeling* (October 6, 1995). Available at https://www.fda.gov/downloads/MedicalDevices/DeviceRegulationandGuidance/GuidanceDocuments/UCM078470.pdf. Accessed January 2017
22. Code of Federal Regulations, Title 21, Volume 8. Revised as of April 1, 2016. *Food and Drugs*, Chapter 1, Subchapter H, Part 876. (21CFR876) Available from https://www.accessdata.fda.gov/scripts/cdrh/cfdocs/cfcfr/CFRSearch.cfm?CFRPart=876&showFR=1&subpartNode=21:8.0.1.1.25.6. Accessed January 2017
23. Parks MS. Reuse: Is it right for your facility? (Part 2.) *Nephrol News Issues*. 2003;17(7):30-4
24. Centers for Medicare and Medicaid Services. *Conditions for Coverage for End-Stage Renal Disease Facilities; Final Rule*, 73 *Federal Register* 73 (15 April 2008), p. 20484. Available at www.cms.gov/Regulations-and-Guidance/Legislation/CFCsAndCoPs/downloads/esrdfinalrule0415.pdf. Accessed January 2017
25. Centers for Medicare and Medicaid Services, HHS. End Stage Renal Disease (ESRD) Program Interpretive Guidance Version 1.1, Part 494 *Conditions for Coverage for ESRD Facilities*. (V Tag 178) October 3, 2008
26. Centers for Medicare and Medicaid Services, HHS. End Stage Renal Disease (ESRD) Program Interpretive Guidance Version 1.1, Part 494 *Conditions for Coverage for ESRD Facilities*. (V Tag 175) October 3, 2008
27. Centers for Medicare and Medicaid Services, HHS. End Stage Renal Disease (ESRD) Program Interpretive Guidance Version 1.1, Part 494 *Conditions for Coverage for ESRD Facilities*. (V Tag 180) October 3, 2008

28. Centers for Medicare and Medicaid Services, HHS. End Stage Renal Disease (ESRD) Program Interpretive Guidance Version 1.1, Part 494 *Conditions for Coverage for ESRD Facilities*. (V Tag 332) October 3, 2008
29. Centers for Medicare and Medicaid Services, HHS. End Stage Renal Disease (ESRD) Program Interpretive Guidance Version 1.1, Part 494 *Conditions for Coverage for ESRD Facilities*. (V Tag 334) October 3, 2008
30. Centers for Medicare and Medicaid Services, HHS. End Stage Renal Disease (ESRD) Program Interpretive Guidance Version 1.1, Part 494 *Conditions for Coverage for ESRD Facilities*. (V Tag 343) October 3, 2008
31. Centers for Medicare and Medicaid Services, HHS. End Stage Renal Disease (ESRD) Program Interpretive Guidance Version 1.1, Part 494 *Conditions for Coverage for ESRD Facilities*. (V Tag 379) October 3, 2008
32. Centers for Medicare and Medicaid Services, HHS. End Stage Renal Disease (ESRD) Program Interpretive Guidance Version 1.1, Part 494 *Conditions for Coverage for ESRD Facilities*. (V Tag 331) October 3, 2008
33. Centers for Medicare and Medicaid Services, HHS. End Stage Renal Disease (ESRD) Program Interpretive Guidance Version 1.1, Part 494 *Conditions for Coverage for ESRD Facilities*. (V Tag 310) October 3, 2008
34. OSHA Quickcard – Hazard Communication Safety Data Sheets. OSHA 3493-12R 2013. Available from https://www.osha.gov/Publications/HazComm_QuickCard_SafetyData.html. Accessed January 2017
35. Centers for Medicare and Medicaid Services, HHS. End Stage Renal Disease (ESRD) Program Interpretive Guidance Version 1.1, Part 494 *Conditions for Coverage for ESRD Facilities*. (V Tag 308) October 3, 2008
36. OSHA. OSHA FactSheet – *Formaldehyde*. 2011. Available at https://www.osha.gov/OshDoc/data_General_Facts/formaldehyde-factsheet.pdf. Accessed June 2017
37. OSHA. Healthcare Wide Hazards. *Gluteraldehyde*. Available from: https://www.osha.gov/SLTC/etools/hospital/hazards/glutaraldehyde/glut.html. Accessed June 2017
38. Centers for Medicare and Medicaid Services, HHS. End Stage Renal Disease (ESRD) Program Interpretive Guidance Version 1.1, Part 494 *Conditions for Coverage for ESRD Facilities*. (V Tag 321) October 3, 2008
39. Centers for Medicare and Medicaid Services, HHS. End Stage Renal Disease (ESRD) Program Interpretive Guidance Version 1.1, Part 494 *Conditions for Coverage for ESRD Facilities*. (V Tag 325) October 3, 2008
40. Centers for Medicare and Medicaid Services, HHS. End Stage Renal Disease (ESRD) Program Interpretive Guidance Version 1.1, Part 494 *Conditions for Coverage for ESRD Facilities*. (V Tag 353) October 3, 2008
41. Taaffe VS. Quality assurance for hemodialyzer reprocessing: Minimizing risks. *Nephrol News Issues*. 2001;15(7):36-39, 41-2

6 Vascular Access

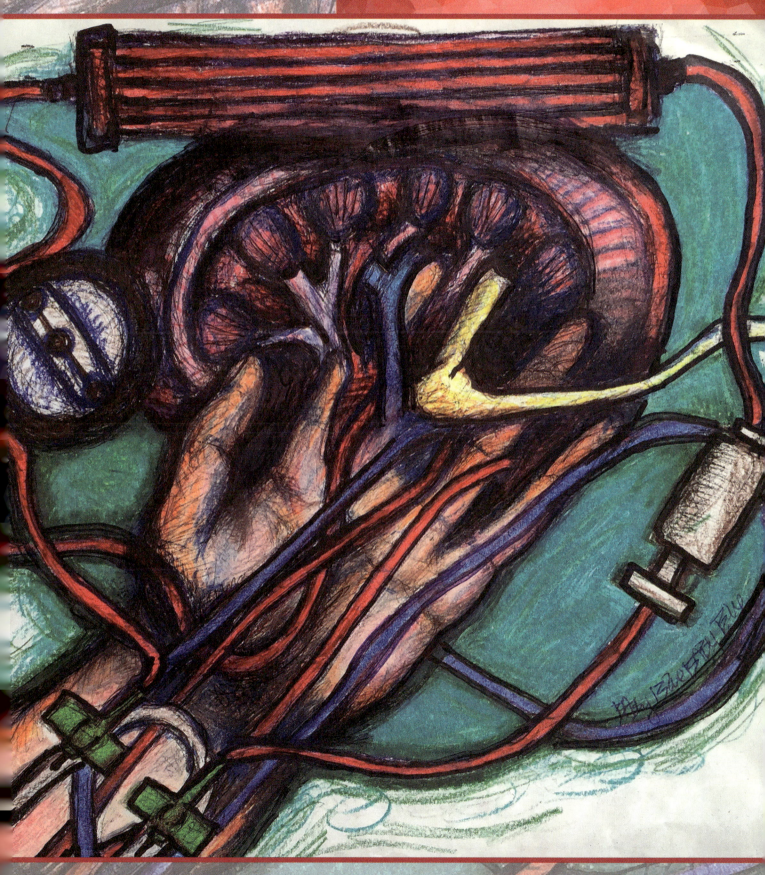

Cover art by Rebecca Schirmer

"My fistula is huge, but it is my lifeline, and I have grown to love it. It is part of me. I love me."

Objectives

MODULE AUTHORS

Lynda Ball, MSN, RN, CNN
Janet Holland, RN, CNN
Vickie Peters, MSN, MAEd, RN, CPHQ
Lynn Poole, FNP-BC, CNN
Lyle Smith, RN, BSN, CNN

MODULE REVIEWERS

Deborah Brouwer-Maier, RN, CNN
Gary W. Lemmon, MD, FACS
Nancy M. Gallagher, BS, RN, CNN
Nicole Gualandi, MS/MPH, RN, CIC
Christi Lines, MPH
Priti Patel, MD, MPH
Darlene Rodgers, BSN, RN, CNN, CPHQ
John H. Sadler, MD
Dori Schatell, MS
Vern Taaffe, BS, CBNT, CDWS
Tamyra Warmack, RN

Practice Test Questions at:
www.meiresearch.org/cc6

After you complete this module, you will be able to:

1. Describe the pros and cons of the three main types of vascular access.
2. Outline the steps for observing a fistula or graft before a hemodialysis treatment.
3. Identify the signs of infection, clotting, and stenosis, and state how to prevent each problem.
4. Explain how to place needles in a fistula or graft.
5. List the steps for using a hemodialysis catheter.

An acronym list can be found in the Glossary.

Introduction

Vascular access makes chronic hemodialysis (HD) possible. It is the pathway that lets the care team "access" the patient's blood for dialysis. Imagine an astronaut tethered to a spaceship with a lifeline. If the lifeline breaks, the astronaut will float off into space and die. *For a dialysis patient, the HD access is a lifeline.* Each HD patient will have one or more vascular accesses in place. A trouble-free, working access is a treatment goal for any patient on HD.

When the first fistula was created in 1966,[1] vascular access was one of the biggest challenges to the success of HD. It still is. Access problems can lead to surgery, illness, limb loss, and death. In fact, 27% of HD patient hospital stays are due to access problems.[2]

There are a limited number of sites on the body where an HD access can be made (see Figure 1). Each site is precious and must be cared for as if it is the last access a patient can have. **Each year, some people must stop HD because they run out of access sites**. If they cannot do PD or get a transplant, they die. You can help prevent this by learning to assess, monitor, and *cannulate* (put needles into) your patients' access sites safely and with great care.

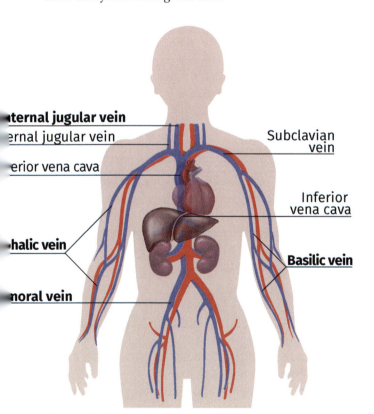

Figure 1: HD Access Sites

Types of Access

"I tell people I am a warrior and these are my battle scars. I have surgical scars on my left wrist to my shoulder from fistula surgeries."

An ideal HD access will:

- Permit blood flow rates that will allow the prescribed dose of HD to be given
- Be large enough in diameter to insert HD needles
- Be made of a substance that is not likely to cause allergies or infections
- Work well over a (long) period of time without needing lots of repairs
- Be located in a site that can be reached by the staff and is comfortable for the patient

The three main types of HD access are:
1. **Arteriovenous (AV) fistula**
2. **Arteriovenous (AV) graft**
3. **Hemodialysis catheters**

Fistula Basics

"I have scars all up and down my arm. People stare and I stare back. These are my warrior scars!"

An **AV fistula** may be called a *permanent* or *venous* (using the veins) *access*. To make an **arteriovenous** (artery + vein) *fistula*, a surgeon sews an artery and a vein together under the skin. Here is why:

- **Arteries** carry oxygen-rich blood from the heart and lungs to the rest of the body. Arteries used for a fistula must be large and have good blood flow. However, most arteries are deep below the skin and difficult to reach with needles.
- **Veins** bring oxygen-poor blood back to the heart and lungs. Some veins may be easy to reach—but many are too small for HD.

The site where the artery and vein connect is an **anastomosis** (uh-NAS-ta-mo-sis) (see Figure 2).

When surgery succeeds, a fistula will combine the strong blood flow of an artery with an easy-to-reach vein. For this to work, the patient's blood vessels must be healthy. The chosen veins must be healthy, straight, big enough for large-gauge needles, and long enough to allow room for a number of *cannulation* (needle insertion) sites. The surgeon must also assure enough blood supply to the *distal* (far) area of the patient's access *extremity* (e.g., hand or foot) so the patient will not have pain and signs of Steal Syndrome. (Learn about Steal Syndrome on page 178).

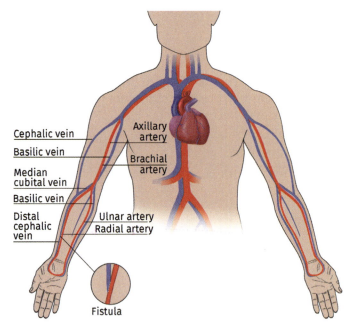

Figure 2: Arteries and Veins

Fistulas are most often placed in an arm. When a patient's surface veins are too small, a surgeon can *transpose* (move) a deep vein closer to the surface of the skin.[3] Transposition may mean a second surgery for the patient, with a long incision or a series of smaller ones from the armpit to the elbow. Rather than raise the vein, surgeons may do a *lipectomy*—remove fat between the vein and the skin so a fistula can be reached with the needles.[4] In patients who do not have arm access sites that will work, a leg access may be used.

In a successful fistula, within 4–6 weeks after surgery high-pressure blood flow from the artery will *arterialize* (thicken) the vein wall. The vein will *dilate* (enlarge)—so it is *mature*: large enough for HD needles. A mature fistula will carry the blood flow rates needed to do HD.

FISTULA PROS AND CONS
Since a fistula is made from only a patient's own tissue, it is biocompatible, and a fistula is beneath the skin, so it is protected from harm. (NOTE: Germs can enter the bloodstream from the dialysis needles if mistakes are made in technique.) It is the least likely type of HD access to become infected or clotted. A good fistula that works may last for more than 5 years, on average;[5] some have lasted for one or more decades.[6] New technology, surgical techniques, and ways to assess and preserve blood vessels have made fistulas an option for more patients. For these reasons, a working fistula is the "gold standard."

However:

- **Fistulas take 4–6 weeks to mature**—so they cannot be used for HD right away.
- **About 23% of the time, new fistulas clot or fail to grow**, a problem called *primary fistula failure*.[7] This can be devastating to patients. Tell your patients that this is not their fault, and they did nothing wrong. It may take more than one try to get a working fistula.
- **In elderly patients, more than half of fistulas (53.6%) had primary failure**.[8] For this reason, and because older patients may not have as long to live, some nephrologists suggest that grafts are a better choice for patients over age 80. However, others disagree. A study of 507,791 U.S. patients found that those with fistulas lived longer than those with other types of access even into their late 80s.[9]

Graft Basics

"I have a Gore-Tex® tube. It has worked very well since being placed in August. I have had to have it declotted only two or three times in 9 months."

An **AV graft** is also a permanent or venous access. To make a graft, a surgeon connects an artery to a vein **with a piece of artificial (man-made) or biologic (from a living source) blood vessel**. As with a fistula, the two sites where the vein connects to the graft are called *anastomoses*. In most cases, a graft is placed in an arm, or, when a patient runs out of access sites, a leg may be used (see Figure 3).

GRAFT PROS AND CONS
Like a fistula, a graft allows access to a large volume of blood for HD. It is beneath the skin, but germs can enter the body through the needles. Most grafts can be used as soon as they heal, in just 2–3 weeks after placement, and they come in many sizes and shapes. "Early cannulation" grafts can even be used within 3 days of placement.[10] No maturation is needed, and

there will be a long area to cannulate. A graft may be the best choice for a patient who does not have blood vessels that are large or strong enough for a fistula, such as those who are smaller or who have diabetes or other vascular disease.

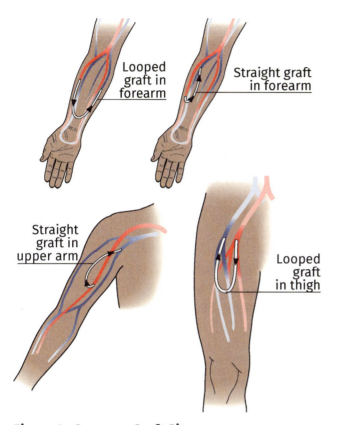

Figure 3: Common Graft Sites

However, grafts:

- **Are prone to *stenosis*** (narrowing) at the venous anastomosis. The smooth *intimal* cells that line the patient's vein and artery may be harmed by high blood flow rates as blood returns to the arm. The body tries to repair the damage by growing new cells. As more cells line the vessel, the diameter shrinks. Less blood can pass through, and *thrombosis* (blood clot) can occur. So, grafts tend to need far more "tune ups" than fistulas to remove clots, or balloon *angioplasty* (blood vessel repair) to open up a narrow spot. Patients who spend 3 days a week at HD must then also spend time in an intervention suite or vascular surgeon's office to have procedures.
- **Have a higher risk of infection**, because the graft material is foreign to the patient's body.
- **Have a shorter useful lifespan than fistulas** (about 2 years on average)[5]

Catheter Basics

"I hate catheters because they keep coming out, keep getting infections, and my clinic won't let me take a bath or a shower! That has about killed me!"

An **HD catheter** is a Y-shaped hollow plastic tube placed into a large, central vein, preferably the *internal jugular* (IJ) vein. In most cases, an HD catheter is tunneled under the skin of the chest wall until it reaches the vein. The catheter tip is in the right atrium of the heart, and the two "limbs" come out of the skin through an *exit site* on the chest wall—which can also be an entry point for germs (see Figure 4).

Other catheter sites are less common. Femoral catheters are placed in a large vein in the leg (*femoral*), which can be uncomfortable. These have a higher risk of infection, since they are close to the groin. Even more rarely, a catheter may be placed in a deep vein (the *inferior vena cava*) near the spine (*translumbar*) or liver (*transhepatic*). These placements are used only when patients have no other options.

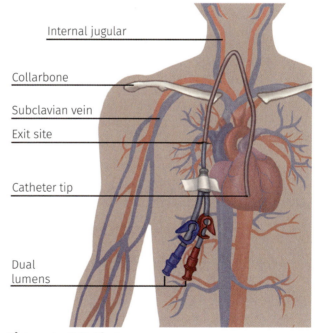

Figure 4: IJ Catheter

There are two main types of HD catheter:

- **Cuffed, tunneled catheters**. The surgeon forms a tunnel under the skin to reach the central veins. A cuff under the skin helps hold the catheter in place, as the patient's tissue will eventually grow into the cuff. The cuff also prevents migration of bacteria into the heart. Cuffed, tunneled catheters may be called "permanent," but it is always best to use a venous access if possible.

- **Non-tunneled catheters** (see Figure 5). These catheters are placed directly into a central vein through a small cut in the skin, and held in place with stitches. They are just 8–10 inches long, and are meant to be used for only a short time. The Centers for Disease Control and Prevention (CDC) suggest that if an HD catheter will be needed for more than 3 weeks, a tunneled-cuffed catheter be used instead.[11] There are no randomized studies that compare infection rates between tunneled and non-tunneled catheters. However, the studies we do have suggest that the rate of infection may be 2–3 times higher in non-tunneled catheters.[12]

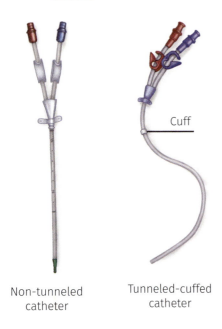

Non-tunneled catheter   Tunneled-cuffed catheter

Figure 5: Tunneled vs. Non-Tunneled Catheters

HD catheters are used for patients who:
- Are waiting for a fistula or graft to be placed or ready to use
- Cannot have a fistula or graft, due to small or diseased vessels, or no remaining sites
- Have acute kidney injury and may soon recover kidney function
- Are waiting for a peritoneal dialysis (PD) catheter to heal
- Are waiting for a scheduled, live donor kidney transplant

CATHETER PROS AND CONS

Catheters allow short- or longer-term access to patients' blood. They can be used the day they are placed, without needles. HD catheters can be hidden under clothing, so others cannot see them. During HD, patients with catheters may be able to freely move both arms and/or legs. However, catheters:

- **Are partly under and partly *outside of* the skin**, forming an entry for germs to get into the blood. Patients with catheters were more likely to get infections than those with fistulas or grafts, and were 53% more likely to die.[13]
- **Are foreign to the body**
- **Can cause *stenosis* (narrowing) of the central veins**, which can lead to blood clots and make future vascular accesses more difficult
- **May be *positional*** – blood flow may only be enough for dialysis if patients sit or turn their heads a certain way, which can be hard to do and may lead to poor treatment
- **May have poor blood flow rates**
- **Keep the patient from swimming**
- **Can shorten the lifespan of fistulas and grafts**. In a study of 314 patients, the survival of grafts and fistulas was 2 to 2 ½ times shorter when a catheter had been on the same side first.[14]
- **May damage the vessel they are placed in**. Rarely (0.4–1% of the time), HD catheters can *erode* (wear away) the vessels in which they are placed[15]—or even puncture the heart.[16]

Due to these problems, catheters must often be removed and then placed again, in the same vein or in a new one. HD catheters are no safer for home HD than they are for in-center HD.[17]

Access Planning

"I had a fistula put in last summer knowing I would need it, and used it for the first time just 3 months ago. I truly believe that it was the wisest choice I could have made. I did not need a catheter because I took this step before my kidneys failed and emergency measures had to be taken."

No access type is perfect for every patient. Patients have made it clear that they want to hear the facts and be fully informed so they can work with their care team to make a choice. Engaging patients to create an

Vascular Access

Table 1: Care Team and Patient Access Planning Roles

Care Team Roles	Patient Roles
Develop an access plan with the patient.	Take part in access planning.
Refer the patient for vessel mapping.	Obtain vessel mapping to find the best vessels.
Coordinate a surgeon visit with the patient.	Keep surgeon appointment(s).
Encourage the patient to get access surgery and follow-up.	Get a fistula or graft placed.
Assess fistula maturation or graft healing and readiness.	Wait for the fistula to mature or the graft to heal.
Have an expert cannulate the new fistula or graft with great care.	Allow the fistula or graft to be cannulated—or ask to learn how to self-cannulate.
Arrange to have the HD catheter removed when the fistula or graft is working.	Get the catheter removed.
Continue to monitor the access.	Care for the access outside of dialysis.

access plan before—or as soon as—they start dialysis can help prevent problems and improve outcomes. Staff can work with patients at every step (see Table 1).

Fistulas in Detail

How Fistulas are Made

"My fistula surgery was this morning. My arm aches. The site only hurts when I move my arm, but my hand keeps starting to fall asleep, so I have to keep moving my arm. I am very tired."

A fistula is *native* or *autogenous:* made from the patient's own blood vessels with no man-made tissue or plastic. Most often a scar marks the anastomosis site. It may take 4–6 weeks for a fistula to become strong enough for large-gauge needles, so it is best to create one well before HD is needed.

As soon as the surgery is done, strong, fast arterial blood flow starts to enlarge the fistula and make it tougher. When all goes well, this arterialization leads to the fistula maturing. About a week after the surgery, patients can start to do exercises, like squeezing a rubber ball or lifting light weights. Small, randomized studies show that these tasks may help fistulas mature more quickly.[18,19] The patient's surgeon may or may not want the patient to do these types of exercise.

If possible, a first access should be placed close to the patient's wrist. A common fistula type links the radial artery with the cephalic vein (between the wrist and

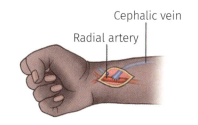
Radiocephalic fistula

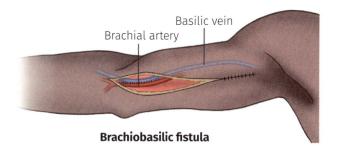
Brachiobasilic fistula

Figure 6: Common Fistula Sites

the elbow). This is a **radiocephalic** fistula (see Figure 6). If needed later, a fistula can be placed higher on the arm. A failed access may damage lower arm vessels so they may not be able to be used for other accesses.

A **brachiocephalic** (brachial artery + cephalic vein) fistula is the most common upper arm option. The cephalic vein lies along the thumb side of the arm, and may be easy to see and feel. If these vessels will not work, the brachial artery and basilic vein may be used (**brachiobasilic**) (see Figure 6). The basilic vein lies along the little finger side of the arm. Since this vein tends to be deep and on the inner arm, it can be challenging to cannulate. The surgeon may lift and transpose the vessel to the outer part of the upper arm. To do this, the surgeon may make a long cut or a series of smaller cuts on the inner arm. If you see these scars, you may be looking at a transposed flat brachiobasilic versus a brachiocephalic fistula.

Although a fistula is the best type of access in general, not all patients can have one, due to:

- **Damage to arm veins**. This may be caused by:
  - Needles used in the past for lab draws or IVs
  - Use of *peripherally inserted central catheters* (PICC lines)
  - Inflammation from drugs or blood vessel disease
- **Damage to central veins**. This may be caused by:
  - HD catheter use – stenosis, clot, or *fibrin* (blood protein) sheaths (build-up)
  - Inflammation from drugs or blood vessel disease
- **Past surgeries on the blood vessels**
- **Atherosclerosis** – plaque or waxy cholesterol that blocks blood vessels (most often arteries)
- **Poor arteries** due to blood vessel disease or diabetes
- **Only one working artery** that brings blood to the hand

Even when a fistula can be created, it may fail to mature, due to:

- **An anastomosis that is too small and limits blood flow**
- **A *juxta-anastomotic*** (next to the anastomosis) **stenosis** (JAS) that limits blood flow. You may be able to feel this as a flat spot within three inches of the anastomosis.
- **Too-small (< 2 mm) arteries or veins** that cannot enlarge
- **Veins that have been damaged** by too many blood draws, IVs, or PICC lines

Patients must be able to handle a 10% or more increase in *cardiac output* (the volume of blood passing through the heart) to have a fistula. Why? Arterial blood is re-routed *quickly* through a fistula—instead of passing *slowly* through tiny capillary blood vessels. So, a fistula can cause or worsen *high output cardiac failure,* also known as *congestive heart failure* (CHF).

Body Image and Patient Resistance to Fistulas

"Two weeks ago I got my fistula. I still have my arm, yet I feel like I lost it somehow. It's not the pain or even the scar. It's something more...mortal than that. I feel like I've lost a part of me—like my best friend—that is gone forever. I'll just never be the same again."

Fistulas can be seen by others when patients wear short sleeves. Fear of being disfigured by a large or unattractive fistula keeps some patients from agreeing to have the surgery.[20] Fear of needles (see Needle Fear, page 169) may keep patients from agreeing to *use* a fistula.

Dialysis clinics are expected to urge patients to have and use a fistula, when it is possible. This can put pressure on patients who have not yet made up their minds. Do not pressure your patients; talk to them. Learning *why* someone is afraid can help you and the care team to help each patient get the best and safest access. If you can, find patients who are positive about their fistulas and view them as lifelines to talk to new patients and help them get past their fears.

Vessel Mapping and Fistula Surgery

"My vessel mapping was very simple and totally relaxing. I just laid there on the radiologist's bed and they slid an ultrasound thingy over my arms and chest. Like a mini massage."

Before fistula surgery, patients should have *vessel mapping* done. This painless ultrasound test may improve the chance that a surgeon will find vessels that will work for a fistula.[21] Medicare pays for vessel mapping.

At the time of the surgery, the chosen blood vessel sites are marked on the skin. An incision is made in the skin over the blood vessels that will be used, then the vessels are sewn together. Whether the surgeon will make an anastomosis that uses the ends or sides of the vessels will depend on the patient's anatomy (see Figure 7).

Vascular Access

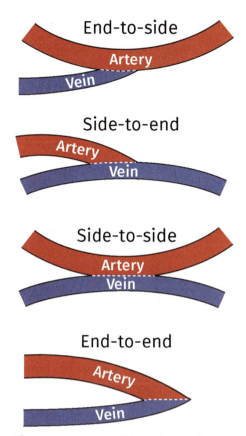

Figure 7: Types of Anastomosis

THRILL, PULSE, AND BRUIT

A thrill, bruit, and the pulse are ways to *validate* (prove) that a new fistula is *patent* (PAY-tent) or open:

- After the incision is closed, there should be a **thrill**—a vibration or buzz—over the new fistula. The thrill is strongest at the anastomosis and gets softer along the length of the fistula.
- You should be able feel a **pulse** that is like a heartbeat when you place your fingers lightly on the fistula. Your fingers will rise and fall slightly with each beat.
- With a stethoscope, you should be able to hear a **bruit**—a whoosh, or, for some, a constant, *low*-pitched sound like the beating of a snare drum—along the vein.

Assessing Fistula Maturity

"My first fistula failed immediately. My second one developed slowly (9 months) and needed ballooning to open it up, even though I used gripper exercisers. Then my surgeon decided I needed a transposition to bring it up near the surface."

As a new dialysis technician, you will not be putting needles into *new* fistulas. New staff should *never* cannulate brand new fistulas—they are delicate and require an expert.[22] Only the most skilled staff in your clinic should cannulate new fistulas.

An expert nurse will need to check all new fistulas at each treatment to see if they are maturing.[23] You can be watchful for signs to tell the nurse. If a new fistula has not grown after 2–3 weeks, the nephrologist and surgeon need to be told. All patients with new fistulas should have a post-op visit with the surgeon 4–6 weeks after the fistula is created.[24] The surgeon may use ultrasound to look at the diameter of the inside of the new fistula, as well as the blood flow. To check a new fistula, the nurse will:

Look for:

- A hand that looks the same as it did before surgery.
- A surgery site that is clean and dry.
- Skin over the fistula that is all one color and looks like the skin around it. Blue or pale skin could mean *steal syndrome*—a fistula that steals too much blood away from the hand. This problem may need surgical repair.
- No bruising or swelling of the skin over the access.
- No redness or drainage.
- A vessel wall thick enough to cannulate. How can someone tell how thick a fistula vessel wall is? An ultrasound device can show this, and the vessel wall should be at least 0.13mm thick.[25] Most clinics do not yet have these devices, but they may become more common soon.

Feel for:

- **A thrill** – the thrill will grow stronger as the fistula matures.
- **Pulse** – a slight beating that makes your fingers rise and fall slightly with each beat.
- **Vessel growth** – the new fistula should start to grow larger right after surgery, and growth should be clear within 2 weeks. Make a note of any flat spots.
- **A cannulation zone where needles can be safely placed** – a zone that is 3 or more inches long will allow needle placement without access damage. *Palpating* (feeling) along the whole length of the fistula will help to find the zone. The nurse will start at the anastomosis and measure out 2 inches. This is the first site where needles can be placed. A change in the vessel—it is too deep, or there is

How to Perform an Arm Elevation Test*

An expert nurse will perform this test for new fistulas. You will learn to use this with patients who have established fistulas. Here are the steps:

1. Have the patient hold his or her access arm down and open and close that fist a few times to engorge the fistula.

2. Raise the patient's arm above the level of his or her heart while you *look at the fistula to see if it collapses* (see Figure 8):

   ➢ A **full collapse** means the venous system is *free from stenosis*.

   ➢ A **partial collapse** means a stenosis is *within* the fistula

   ➢ **No collapse** typically means a stenosis *beyond* the fistula (i.e., in a central vein).

3. Have the patient return his/her arm to the normal position within 10 seconds.

4. **Report a partial or no collapse to the nurse**, so the patient can be referred for intervention.

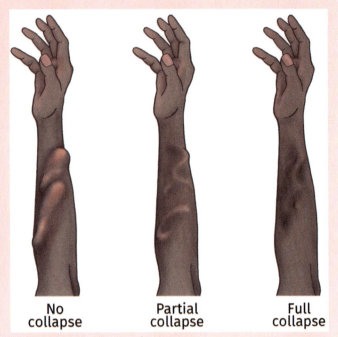

Figure 8: Arm Elevation Test

*NOTE: This test is used *ONLY* for a fistula, as a graft will not collapse.

rebound that does not feel as firm—is the end of the zone.

- **Steal syndrome** – *hypoxia* (lack of oxygen to tissue and nerves) due to low blood flow to the hand (see page 178)

  ➢ Is the patient's access hand colder or paler than his or her other hand?

  ➢ When the patient squeezes both of the nurse's or your hands, is his or her access hand weaker than the other one?

  ➢ Do the nail beds have a bluish tinge?

  ➢ Are there any ulcers or black spots (*necrosis*) on the fingers?

  ➢ Does the patient say s/he has pain in the access hand, particularly when you increase the blood flow rate?

  ➢ Does the patient report feeling numbness, tingling, etc. in the access hand?

Listen for:

- **A bruit**. The pitch of this sound should be low and continuous; one sound should connect to the next. The bruit should be audible along the whole cannulation segment, and most strongly at the anastomosis.

Once the fistula has grown and is firm, the care team will receive cannulation orders. Your clinic should have a written policy and procedures for new fistulas. Follow these carefully. For example, a sample protocol for new fistula cannulation[22] calls for small needles (17-gauge) and low blood flow rates (200–250 mL/min) for the first week. These steps help prevent *infiltration* (blood leaking out of the fistula into the tissues, causing swelling, pain, and bruising) (see page 175). If no infiltration occurs, needle size and blood pump speeds can go up, per treatment orders. Only an expert with good assessment skills should be cannulating new fistulas, to avoid infiltrations.

Starting HD with a Mature Fistula

"Even staff who have been there a while have trouble cannulating me. When people who know my access are on vacation, I am scared to go to dialysis."

At every treatment, before you place a dialysis needle you need to plan your needle placement approach. You have a chance to teach your patients about their fistulas *and* to deliver a safe, effective, HD treatment. **Every needle counts**, and safe cannulation starts with good planning (see Figure 9).

Before you touch a patient's fistula, *think* about what you will be doing and why:

- Which way will the needles go?
- What gauge and length of needles will make sense for this patient's fistula?
- Where will the needles be placed relative to where they were at the last few treatments?
- Can you teach the patient to self-cannulate?
- How will you handle your patient's needle pain and/or fear?

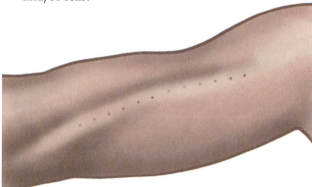

Figure 9: Mature Fistula

Plan where you will place **both** needles. You will need to leave 1–1.5 inches between the tips of the arterial and venous needles to prevent recirculation. If possible, try to leave space beyond the venous needle for another needle in case the first try does not work or it infiltrates. The arterial needle is always placed closer to the arterial anastomosis. NOTE: Never attempt to place more than two needles. If another needle is needed, ask someone else to insert it. No more than three needle sticks should be tried to prevent trauma to the patient and the access. Keep in mind how much is at stake for your patient, and how vital it is for you to preserve their lifelines.

Wash Your Hands

"I watch what my center does, and we have been told to police the techs and nurses ourselves. If we see a safety infraction, we are to tell them to wash their hands and get fresh gloves. If they drop a roll of tape on the floor, tell them to throw it away and not use it on anyone. I have to say I have only had to ask one tech to wash her hands and get new gloves."

The first step before you touch *any* access is *always* to clean your hands. Clean hands and new gloves prevent transfer of bacteria from your skin to an access. *Hand hygiene* is the CDC's term for either washing your hands with soap and water or using an alcohol-based hand sanitizer. If your hands are visibly soiled, you must wash them. If not, you can wash them or use hand sanitizer for your hand hygiene. Part of the preparation to cannulate is to:

- **Follow your clinic's policy.** The CDC recommends the use of alcohol-based hand sanitizer or soap and water before and after you put on and take off gloves. The CDC also directs when you must change your gloves to protect yourself and your patients.
- **Wear personal protective equipment (PPE).** The *Conditions for Coverage*[26] require HD clinics to follow the CDC rules for infection control. These rules are in force any time blood could splash. So, you will wear gloves, a gown, eye protection, and a face mask when you place or remove needles.

See Module 7: *Hemodialysis Procedures and Complications*, to learn more about hand hygiene and infection control.

Examine the Fistula

Over the last few months a bump grew on my fistula, and 2 weeks ago when I took the bandage off, one side was discolored. It was infected, so they took it out and it's healing and I now have a catheter till they decide what to do."

Do a 1-minute vascular access check at each treatment before you place needles: Look, listen, *palpate* (feel) the fistula, and do an arm elevation test.[27] Report any changes or problems you find to your charge nurse before you start to cannulate. When you alert the nurse to any changes in the fistula, you can help save a failing access so it can be fixed before it is too late.

Look for:

- **Signs of infection** – redness, drainage, pus, abscesses, open skin, fever, or pain. **Never put needles into a fistula that looks infected.** The needle can push skin bacteria into the patient's bloodstream which can cause *sepsis*, a serious blood infection that can be fatal. Tell the nurse right away if you see signs of infection so he or she can call the nephrologist.

- **Steal syndrome** – not enough blood flow to the access extremity: pale, or bluish skin or nail beds. In severe cases, the fingertips may turn black.
- **Stenosis** – narrowing of a blood vessel that causes a swollen access arm, pale skin, and enlarged blue or purple veins on the chest wall or neck area where the arm meets the body.
- **Cannulation site problems** – curves, flat spots, or *aneurysms* (ballooning of the blood vessels). If you see aneurysms, note their width, height, and appearance. Notify your charge nurse. Do not cannulate any of these areas: they could bleed for a long time—or rupture.

Listen for:

- **Bruit** – learn how each patient's access sounds and note any changes. A higher or louder than normal pitch may mean stenosis. Place a stethoscope along the whole length of the fistula and listen for the bruit. Then, move the stethoscope from side to side and listen for the bruit to stop. Taking this step will help you to outline the fistula, and is especially helpful with a deeper access.
- **Direction of blood flow** – compress the center of the access with your finger and listen to each end with a stethoscope. You should hear blood flow sounds on the *arterial* side.

Feel for:

- **Skin temperature** – increased warmth could be a sign of infection; cold spots could mean less blood flow.
- **Thrill** – should be present and constant, purring or vibration, not a strong or bounding pulse. A fistula should have a strong flow of blood, so you may be able to feel a stronger thrill at the anastomosis. A fistula should have only one thrill.
- **Pulse** – should feel the same as your own pulse. A *bounding* (throbbing) pulse that causes a big rise and fall when you lay your fingers on the anastomosis could mean stenosis.
- **Stenosis** – since stenosis narrows a vessel, you should be able to feel for any flat spots in the access and check them for changes to the thrill or bruit.
- **Vein diameter** – start at the anastomosis and run your thumb and forefinger along both sides of the fistula. You should be able to feel the walls of the fistula. The width will vary by individual, but as a general rule, a mature access should be at least as big around as your little finger (about 6 mm).

Ask yourself:

➤ **Is the fistula diameter the same along the whole length?**
➤ **If there are aneurysms, how wide are they?**
➤ **Are there any flat spots?**
➤ **Is the vessel wider than the gauge of the needle?**
➤ **How deep is the access?** This will affect your angle of needle entry.

Prepare the Access Skin

You can encourage patients to wash their access arm or leg before treatment. Washing some of the skin debris and germs off the skin before placing needles may help reduce the risk of infection. Soap and water or an alcohol-based gel can be used. If a patient cannot wash his or her own arm, you will need to wash off the access area with soap and water or another skin cleanser, and then gently pat it dry with clean paper towels.

Before each treatment, you will apply a skin antiseptic to the patient's access site and let it dry. This step will help keep bacteria from getting into the bloodstream when you place the dialysis needles. Infection is a leading cause of death in HD patients, because:

- Kidney disease weakens their immune system.
- Many patients have diabetes, which makes them more prone to infection.
- Hospital stays and surgeries put patients in contact with many germs.
- Other patients and staff can carry germs.
- **Staff do not always wash their hands or follow other infection control practices**. This deadly mistake can be prevented with *your* help.

Before needles are placed, clean and prep the patient's skin with one of the products in Table 2. Do not touch the patient's skin after the access site has been prepped.

Never Re-Touch a Needle Site

Exam gloves that come in bulk packages are clean—*not* sterile. They can be used as PPE, but do not protect against skin contaminants. If you touch the patient's skin at the point of needle entry, or touch the needle bore, you will contaminate the needle, and risk infecting the patient. **After you prep the skin with antiseptic, NEVER retouch it**. Only gloves labeled as sterile would let you retouch the skin at the needle site.

Vascular Access

Table 2: Access Skin Prep Options

Product and General Tips for Use (Check manufacturer's instructions for specifics)
Liquid: 2% chlorhexidine gluconate/70% isopropyl alcohol (ChloraPrep®)[27]
Saturate a sterile gauze pad with the product. Wet one needle site for 30 seconds, using a back and forth friction scrub. Repeat with the other site, using a fresh gauze pad. Allow to dry.
Swabs: 2% chlorhexidine gluconate/70% isopropyl alcohol (ChloraPrep®)[28]
Tear pouch at side notch to reach applicator handle. Twist and remove the packaging tip. Do not touch the foam tip. Place the foam tip flat side down on one needle site. Wet the site with gentle back and forth strokes for 30 seconds. Let dry for 30 seconds. Do not wipe or blot. Repeat with the other site.
Sodium hypochlorite (ExSept® Plus)[29]
Open two sterile 2x2 gauze pads, keeping each in its wrapper, and saturate both with ExSept Plus. Put on clean, non-sterile gloves. Use one pad to clean one needle site in a spiral from the center outward to 2 inches with the product and repeat for the other site with the other pad. Let the skin dry before you move onto the next step. Open a fresh alcohol prep pad and clean one site for 15 seconds, using a scrubbing motion. Repeat for the other site with another fresh alcohol prep pad. Allow skin to air dry.
70% alcohol[30]
Use a 60-second circular rub with a fresh pad on each site. Allow skin to air dry.
10% povidone iodine[30]
Apply to each site and then wait 2–3 minutes to place the needles.

Apply a Tourniquet

"The tech used a tourniquet on my fistula today and the needles went right in no problem! I hardly even felt them! No bleeding, no bruises, no swelling!"

Using a tourniquet when you place needles in a fistula—even when it is large—can:

- Help you see the fistula better
- Help you find the right angle for the needle
- Give you a better "feel" for cannulation
- Reduce the risk that you will *infiltrate* (puncture) the back wall
- Promote a "cleaner" entry
- Distend the vessel, so there may be less pain when the needles are inserted

Apply the tourniquet in the *axilla* area (just below the armpit). This helps distribute pressure evenly to reduce the risk of infiltration in a forearm access).

Never tighten a tourniquet to the point that it causes pain, tingling, or cuts off blood flow to the patient's fingers. The tourniquet should lay flat on the surface of the skin: tourniquets that roll up cause patients more discomfort. Another option is to have patients press on the vessel in the axilla area in place of using a tourniquet. NOTE: Use a tourniquet only to *access* and *place* the needles. Take the tourniquet off as soon as the needles are in place and discard it. Tourniquets are for single-use only.

Place the Needles

"I have the same fistula in use since I started. I'm living proof that if you keep your access site clean and pay attention to your doctors you can enjoy your life as an ESRD patient!"

Since HD is done at least three times a week, the fistula is used repeatedly. To let the vessel heal between treatments, you will use a pattern:

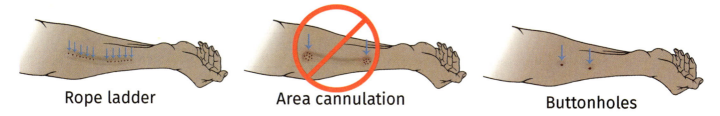

Rope ladder — Area cannulation — Buttonholes

Figure 10: Cannulation Techniques

Module 6

- **Rope ladder technique**. You choose new sites at each treatment, creating a pattern on the fistula that looks like knots on a rope ladder.
- **Buttonhole technique**. You reuse the same two sites until scar tissue tracts form, much like pierced earring holes. The two sites look like a button.

AVOID "area puncture"—cannulating in the same small areas over and over (see Figure 10). This approach quickly damages a fistula. Weak spots can form that can lead to loss of the access—or, if they rupture, the patient can die. In a study of more than 7,000 people on dialysis from nine countries, area cannulation was the most likely to cause access failure.[31]

Rope Ladder Technique

"My arm is so bruised and sore it was hard to find a place to cannulate without me crying in pain. The tech who hurt me should have stopped the moment I started screaming, but he didn't. He just kept on digging, saying he couldn't find the vein."

When a patient comes in for a treatment, look for the scabs from the last few treatments and choose sites that are at least ¼ inch away from the last sites. If the cannulation zone is large enough to allow it, keep the arterial and venous needles 1.5 inches apart (about two finger widths) from each other, or as far apart as

About Dialysis Needles

"Those hemo needles are huge! Like roofing nails!"

Two needles are needed for most treatments:

- The **arterial** needle pulls blood from the patient to the dialyzer
- The **venous** needle returns blood to the patient's body.

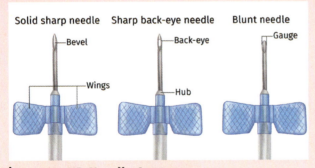

Figure 11: HD Needle Anatomy

Recently, a new single needle dialysis needle has been created that is a needle in a needle, with Y-shaped tubing. You may not see this in your clinic, but these are now in use in some home HD patients, especially those who do nocturnal HD. Single needle dialysis is not efficient enough for standard in-center HD, and is not approved for that use. See page 168 to learn more.

Needle Gauge
To handle a large volume of blood, *large* diameter needles are used. In the U.S., HD needles are made of thin-walled steel and come in gauge sizes from 17 to 14 for adults; *the smaller the gauge, the larger the needle diameter*. So, a 14-gauge needle is larger than a 17-gauge. The 17-gauge needles are used in new (or small) accesses due to small vessel size, low pressure, and/or lower blood flow rates.

Sharp vs. Blunt Needle Tips
Most needle tips have a sharp cutting edge to get through the skin. The Buttonhole technique (see page 165) uses sharp needles until a permanent tunnel forms, then *blunt* needles are used. (Sharp needles could risk cutting the tunnel and causing trauma or infection.) Blunt needles come in all of the needle gauge sizes and should match the sharp needle gauge size used to form the Buttonholes.

Needle Length
Needles come in three lengths: 3/5, 1, and 1.25 inch. The standard, 1-inch needle is used when the access is within 6 mm of the surface of the skin. Use shorter needles for superficial accesses to reduce the risk of infiltration. Use longer needles for deeper accesses.

Back-Eyes
Back-eye needles let blood flow into the needle even if the needle is near a blood vessel wall. Use a back-eye needle—a needle with a hole in the back side—for the arterial needle. Use a solid needle (with no back-eye) only as a *venous* needle. If you perform access flow testing, you will need to use two needles with back-eyes to get an accurate reading.

possible. Do not return to the old sites for at least 2 weeks, so they can heal. *Use the whole length of the fistula—the top* and *sides to help a fistula last as long as possible* (see Figure 12).

Rotating cannulation sites by using the Rope Ladder technique helps to prevent *aneurysms* (weak spots in a vessel wall that balloon out). Patients may *ask* you to cannulate an aneurysm because it hurts less. Tell them that aneurysms are damaged areas, and no one should put needles in those areas. Aneurysms can *rupture* (burst) if needles are placed into them, which can cause massive blood loss or death.

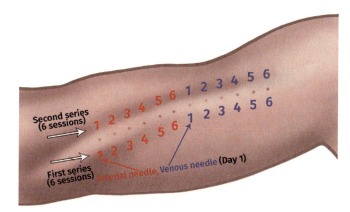

Figure 12: Rope Ladder Technique

Which Way Should the Needles Go?

Place the arterial needle first. This needle brings blood from the patient to the dialyzer, and you will place it closest to the anastomosis, or *distal* to (furthest from) the heart. To be sure you know which end of the access is the arterial end, before you place the needles, compress the center of the access for a few seconds with one finger:

- The **arterial** end will dilate and *grow firm*, with a strong pulse and a loud bruit.
- The **venous** end will *collapse*, due to reduced flow.

When there is space on an access, place the **arterial** needle **antegrade** (in the direction of blood flow, or toward the heart). *Retrograde* (against the flow) placement does not change the adequacy of a treatment.[32] However, it may cause harm to a fistula:

- Each HD needle cuts a flap in the vessel wall. When an antegrade needle comes out, the blood flow holds the flap *closed*. When a retrograde needle comes out, the blood flow holds the flap *open*. An autopsy study found much more vessel scarring with retrograde needles.[33]
- A study of more than 7,000 people found that fistulas were *much* more likely to fail when needles were placed retrograde with the bevel down.[31] **The safest placement was antegrade with the needle bevel up**. If retrograde placement must be used, bevel up may be a better choice.

You will place the **venous** needle second. A venous needle is *always* placed **antegrade**. This placement helps prevent turbulence when blood returns from the dialyzer to the patient. This needle is the one *proximal* (closest to) the heart. When HD patients put their own needles in, they use **antegrade** placement for both needles.

Two rules will help prevent cannulation problems so patients get a good HD treatment:

- Keep needle tips at least 1.5 inches apart.
- Stay at least 1.5–2 inches away from the anastomosis.

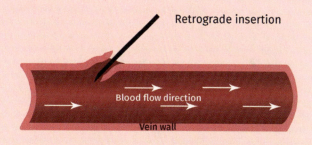
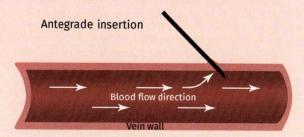

Figure 13: Needle Placement

Module 6

INSERTING SHARP NEEDLES IN A FISTULA

Some patients will use a *topical* (on the skin) *anesthetic* (numbing) product before you place the needles. Learn more on page 169.

Your clinic should have a written training program with a checklist to be sure that you learn all of the steps of cannulation. Patients' lifelines are not for practice. **Learn these skills on a practice arm before you try to cannulate a patient**. It takes a *lot* of practice to be a good cannulator. If it is possible in your clinic, sit down to cannulate. While no studies have been done on sitting vs. standing, you might have more control over the needle if you sit.

There are two ways to cannulate. Which one you use will depend on your clinic's policies and on the patient's access:

- **Dry cannulation** is the most often used technique. You will place the needles and watch for the flashback of blood into the tubing. Place a piece of tape over the needle wings to secure the needle in the vessel. Allow the needle lines to fill with blood before you attach the bloodline, or clamp the needle lines and attach an empty syringe to each. Unclamp the needle and check the blood flow by gently pulling and pushing the blood into and out of the syringe to be certain the needle is in the center of the vessel. Pull back quickly, but do not pull the plunger out. A well-placed needle will let the blood chase the plunger in the syringe. If you feel the plunger chug-chugging as you pull the blood, it is a good sign that your needle is *not* in the center of the blood vessel and needs to be adjusted before you apply any more tape. When the needles are correct, you should not have alarm issues once you start dialysis.
- **Wet cannulation** may be done for a new fistula, a difficult placement, or patients who clot quickly. Just before cannulation, draw up 10 cc of sterile normal saline into a sterile syringe, using aseptic technique, or use a pre-filled syringe. Attach the syringe to the dialysis needle and flush the tubing until saline drips out of the tip of the needle. You are now ready to cannulate.

The angle of needle entry will vary based on the depth of the access. You will use a steeper angle (45 degrees) for deeper accesses, and/or a longer needle. For accesses created within 6 mm (1/4 inch) of the surface of the skin, use an angle from 20 to 35 degrees. Some accesses may be too deep to safely cannulate and require surgery to raise them to aid cannulation.

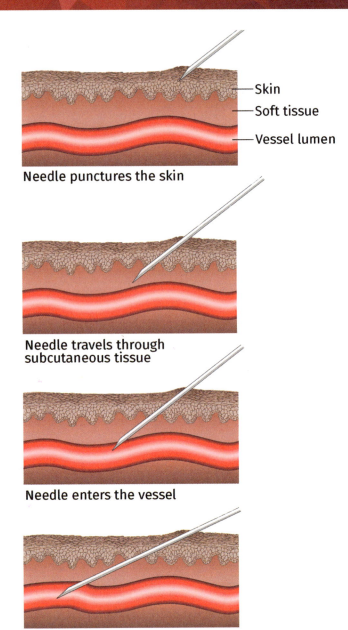

Needle punctures the skin

Needle travels through subcutaneous tissue

Needle enters the vessel

Needle is leveled out and threaded into vessel lumen

Figure 14: Needle Insertion

Cannulation is a *gentle* technique (see Figure 14). Do these steps as a *fluid* motion, with *no jabbing, digging, or probing with the needle*:

1. Clean the access site with soap and water if the patient has not.
2. Perform hand hygiene.
3. Put on new, clean gloves.
4. Choose your angle.

5. Apply skin antiseptic, per the manufacturer's instructions and let it dry. Do not touch the access site after you have prepped the skin.

6. Grasping the needle wings with the bevel up, smoothly guide the needle through the skin and tissue until you feel a release of pressure.

7. Check that you get a *flashback* (blood in the tubing).

8. Flatten the angle of the needle.

9. Advance the needle (push it forward into the vessel), keeping the wings parallel to the fistula.

10. Connect to the bloodlines using aseptic technique.

11. Secure the needles in place (see page 167).

12. Take off your gloves and repeat your hand hygiene.

NOTE: If you have trouble placing a needle, find another staff person to do it. Most patients can tell you who has most success with their fistulas.

Avoid Needle Stick Injuries

Sharp fistula needles have a needle protector (see Figure 15) to reduce the chance that you will accidentally stick yourself with a needle, which could expose you to germs in the patient's blood, including HIV or hepatitis. **When you remove a sharp needle, use the needle protector**. Buttonhole needles have been FDA-approved without needle protectors. However, these blunt needles could still break your skin. Handle them with care and place them in a sharps box as soon as possible.

Buttonhole Technique

"My fistula is 23 years old and in use for 21 years. I do home HD, nocturnal, and have been home for 9 years. I self-cannulate and my buttonholes are 10 years old."

The Buttonhole technique, first used on an access that had a small cannulation zone, has been used in Europe since 1977. Some studies have found less needle pain and fewer aneurysms with this technique.[34] Patients who use Buttonholes may then have less fear of needles or a disfiguring fistula. Others studies have not had these findings. Bloodstream and tunnel infections have been found to be a risk when the Buttonhole technique is used.[35,36] However, a study in Belgium that followed patients for 8 years or more did not find a difference in infection between the rope ladder and Buttonhole techniques.[37] Home HD patients are more likely to use the Buttonhole technique.

To form Buttonholes, you place sharp needles into the same two sites at each treatment, at the *same angle*. In 3–4 weeks (about 9–12 treatments), a scar tunnel forms, like a pierced earring hole.[38] The technique works best if the same person places the needles until the Buttonholes form. *It is best if this person is the patient.* The Buttonhole technique can be used *only* for fistulas—not grafts. Fistula walls have muscle fibers that will close the holes after the needles are removed.

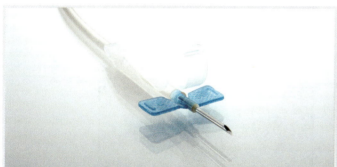
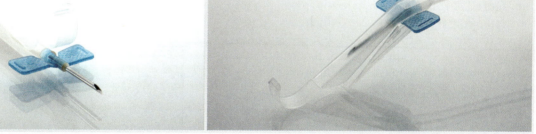

Figure 15: Needle Protector

MasterGuard® images used with permission from NxStage.

Three-Point Cannulation Can Ease Needle Pain

HD needles need to be large to allow enough blood flow for dialysis. So, needle placement can hurt. The goal is to insert the needles easily, with as little pain and trauma to the access as you can. This **three-point technique** may help you reduce needle pain and aid cannulation:[39]

1. After you apply the tourniquet, place the thumb and forefinger of your *non*-needle hand on either side of the fistula, just above where the needle will go.

2. With the pinky or ring finger of your *needle* hand, pull the skin tight and press down to keep the vein from rolling. This compresses the nerve endings, which will reduce pain.

3. Place the needles.

Pressing on the skin will block pain-to-brain sensation for up to 20 seconds—long enough to place a needle with less pain.

Learn more about how to reduce needle fear and pain on page 169.

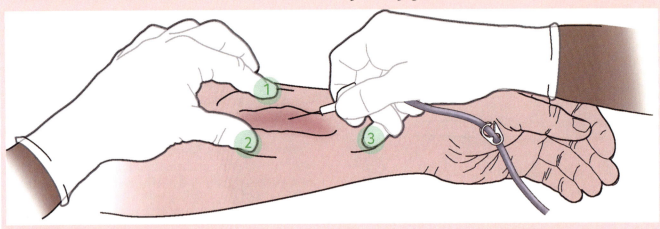

Figure 16: Three Point Cannulation
Image used and adapted with permission from Lynda Ball.

Once Buttonhole tunnels form, you use a sterile pick to remove the scab before each treatment. Cannulate with blunt needles to follow the tunnel. Using sharp needles in Buttonholes may increase the risk of causing an aneurysm.[40] *Do not push the needle hub against the skin.* Pressure from "hubbing" can cause the tissue to collapse, forming a cave-like Buttonhole[41] (see Figure 17). This makes it hard to remove the scab completely and it is hard to clean, which raises the chance of infection—the biggest risk of the Buttonhole technique. Some clinics reserve the technique for self-care patients (who may be in-center or at home), due to the risk.[42]

Buttonhole tracts—like all other places—can grow pathogens, like staph. When a needle pushes germs into the bloodstream, they can cause deadly blood infections. Use of careful technique to clean the skin and *completely* remove the scabs before treatment has been shown to help reduce the risk of infection.[43] Have patients wash their hands and access arm before treatment. Your clinic may use a two-step protocol after that, like this one:[44]

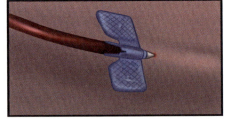

The hub of the needle should not enter the tunnel.

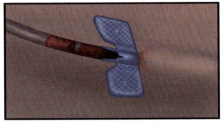

Hubbing is too-deep insertion of the needle. The needle hub becomes buried in the tunnel entrance and cannot be seen.

Figure 17: Hubbing

Vascular Access

Using a sharp AV fistula needle, grasp the needle wings and remove the tip protector. Align the needle cannula with the bevel facing up, over the cannulation site and pull the skin taut.

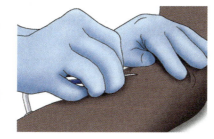

Cannulate the site. It is important to cannulate the developing constant-site in the exact same place, using the same insertion angle and depth of penetration each time. This requires that a single cannulator perform all cannulations until the sites are well established.

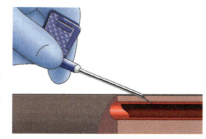

A flashback of blood indicates the needle is in the access. Lower the angle of insertion. Continue to advance the needle into the AV fistula until it is appropriately positioned with the vessel.

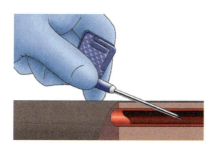

Securely tape the AV fistula needle and proceed with dialysis treatment per clinic protocol.

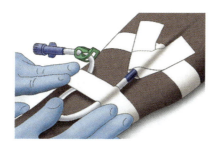

Figure 18: Forming Buttonholes
Image adapted and used with permission from NxStage.

1. **Apply skin antiseptic to clean the scab and needle site area, then remove the scab.** Scabs contain skin bacteria that we do not want to push into the bloodstream. Patients may tape an alcohol-soaked swab over their scabs at home to kill germs and moisten the scabs at the same time. Follow your clinic protocol to remove scabs. Options include:

   ➤ **Sterile tweezers.** *Never use fingernails or the tip of the fistula needle being inserted.*

   ➤ **A *sterile* scab-lifting device that comes on or in the cap of the blunt needles.** Do *not* remove this device from the packaging or lay it down on the protective pad. This will contaminate the scab-lifting device before it is used on the patient's arm.

2. **After the scabs are completely off, reapply skin antiseptic and let the buttonhole sites air dry. Do not touch the buttonhole sites after you apply the skin antiseptic. Place the needles per your clinic's policy.**

When the sites are dry, blunt needles can be inserted (see Figure 18). If your clinic's policy includes the use of *Touch Cannulation*, you will hold the needle tubing a bit *behind* the needle wings.[45] With this technique, you can use far less pressure to guide the needles into the Buttonholes and reduce the chance of breaking through the tunnel. Damaged tunnels are at a higher risk of infection.[39] See Appendix A to learn more about Touch Cannulation.

The Buttonhole technique is not a good option for every patient with a fistula. Common sense would say that some patients may be at higher risk for infection, such as those with:

- A history of endocarditis or heart valve disease
- Artificial implanted devices (like pacemakers or hip replacements)
- Poor hygiene
- A tendency to pick at scabs

Tape the Needles After Insertion

"After about 15 minutes on the machine, I had a horrible arterial pressure spike. It popped the tape off!"

After you place the needles, you must secure them so the needles do not move or pull out. Follow your clinic's policy and procedures. The **Butterfly Tape Technique** is a safe and effective way to do this (see Figure 19):

1. Place a 1-inch wide, 5–6 inch long piece of tape over the butterfly wings to anchor the needle. This keeps the needle from moving inside the access.

2. Place a ½-inch wide, 6-inch long piece of tape under the blood tubing just behind the wings, *sticky side up*.

3. Take the right end of this second piece of tape and

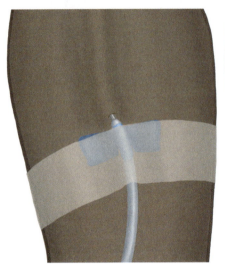 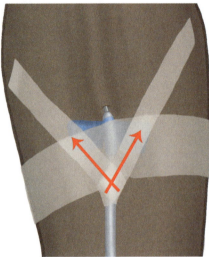 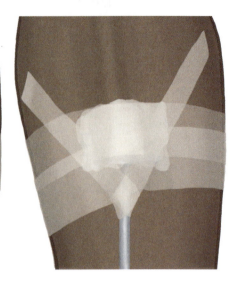

Figure 19: Butterfly Tape Technique
Image adapted and used with permission from Lynda Ball.

cross it over the left needle wing, then take the left end of the tape and cross it over the right needle wing. This crossover (or chevron) may keep the needles from dislodging.

4. Place one of the following on top of the venipuncture site to keep bacteria from migrating down the needle into the sterile bloodstream:

   ➤ Band-Aid®
   ➤ Gauze and tape
   ➤ Clean tape on a sheet
   ➤ Single-use roll tape torn after the wings are stabilized

Monitor Arterial Pressure

As a fistula grows and higher blood flow rates are used, you will need to monitor arterial pressures. Hemolysis (destruction of blood cells) increases as the pressure becomes more negative. Arterial pressure should not become more negative than -250 mmHg (see Figure 21). Pressure that is too negative may be one sign of a need to increase needle size. Check your clinic's policies about when to change needle size. The charge nurse will tell you what needle gauge and blood flow rate the patient needs to get adequate dialysis.

A Single Needle Option for Nocturnal Home Hemodialysis

OneSite™ Dual Lumen Needle

The OneSite™ is a dual-lumen needle designed for use with the NxStage System One machine for *low-flow HD*, especially nocturnal. At low blood flow rates, one needle can do the job of both the arterial and venous needles. The Buttonhole technique is used for cannulation. Since just one needle is required, the device cuts the work of self-cannulation in half. The OneSite is approved for home use only, so you will not see this in a clinic. If your job involves working with home HD patients, you may see it there.

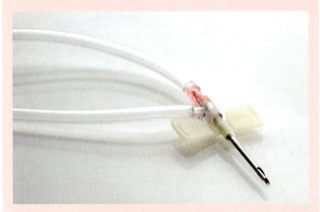

Figure 20: OneSite Single Needle
Image used with permission from NxStage.

Vascular Access

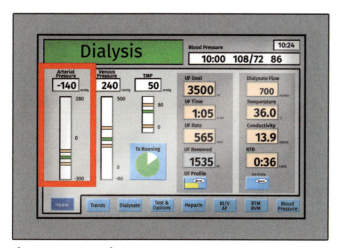

Figure 21: Arterial Pressure

Help Patients with Needle Fear

"I used to lie in bed the night before each treatment, rigid with fear. I was so afraid of cannulation. It was a battle each dialysis day just to get up the nerve to go. My fistula infiltrated many times, and I would find myself shaking all over even after the needles were in. Now, I take Paxil, and it helps some."

In the general public, 3–4% of people are afraid of needles. This problem is called "Blood, Injury, Injection Phobia," and it can make people avoid needed health and dental care. In those with a chronic disease, the rate is even higher: from about 6–17% of men and about 16–32% of women.[46] People with this fear may have an involuntary *vasovagal* (feeling faint) response to needles, the sight of blood, surgery, etc.:[46]

- First, the patient's pulse speeds up and blood pressure rises.
- Then, the pulse slows and blood pressure drops. Stress hormones are released, and heart rhythms may change (which can be fatal).
- Patients may become pale, sweaty, nauseated, or dizzy. About half may pass out.

Since dialysis needles are so large, they can terrify even those who do not otherwise have needle fear. Some fearful patients choose peritoneal dialysis (PD) to avoid needles. Medicare or insurance may pay for needle phobia treatment. Patients with needle fear may also be able to prevent the vasovagal response. Some of these tips may help:

- **Lay the chair flat** to keep blood in the brain so the patient does not pass out.
- **Have the patient tense the muscles** of his or her non-access limbs for 10 or 20 seconds, relax, and then re-tense them until the needles are in. (Get the doctor's okay first). The squeezing can briefly raise blood pressure and prevent the vasovagal response.[47]
- **Reduce needle pain**. Pain can cause part of the fear. Use the techniques in the next section.
- **Teach patients how to put in their own needles**. This distracts them from the pain and replaces it with control.
- **Use an imaging device to guide cannulation**.[48] When you can *see* the vessel under the skin, you may be less likely to miscannulate and infiltrate the patient[49]—which may reduce fear. It is not known how many U.S. dialysis clinics are using these new devices.

Reduce Pain from Needle Insertion

"I have never forgotten my first needles with EMLA. I turned my head aside to pray it would go well. It seemed it was taking a little longer than it should, so I turned back to look and found that both needles were in and I had felt nothing...not one thing!"

A patient who does HD three times a week will be on the sharp end of more than 300 large-gauge needles each year. Easing the pain of needle placement can go a long way toward improving the quality of life for your patients. Slow, deep breathing, guided imagery (perhaps with a headset and podcast or video), music, or other distractions may help. Or, *local anesthetics* numb the skin to reduce needle pain. Options include:

- *Topical* (applied to the skin's surface) lidocaine creams or gels
- *Intradermal* (injected just under the surface of the skin) lidocaine
- Ethyl chloride "skin freezing" spray

NOTE: As with any medicine, patients can develop an allergy to these products at any time. If a rash or blisters occur, stop use and seek a different approach. In some cases, patients may use these products for a short time and then choose to forego them. This choice must be theirs.

Module 6

Teach Patients to Put in Their Own Needles

"I had problems with needles. My arterial graft was very deep, and I had to use a 1–1/4 inch needle to reach it. It was a real hit or miss deal. Placing my own needles has stopped a lot of emotional distress. I no longer worry about who will be poking me. It's easier than I thought."

Medicare gives patients certain rights, and one of these is to be as active in their own care as they want to be. This right includes putting in their own needles. The tool Medicare surveyors use when they inspect clinics says:

"Patients have the right to know about and participate in their care and treatment to the extent they desire. Self-cannulation may be performed by the patient in any facility upon receiving appropriate training and demonstrating competence, should they so choose."[50]

Clinics do *not* need to have special approval to teach patients how to put in their own needles.[26]

See Appendix A for a step-by-step guide to teaching your patients how to put in their needles. Patients must also be taught the vital infection control practices for self-cannulation, such as hand hygiene and aseptic technique.

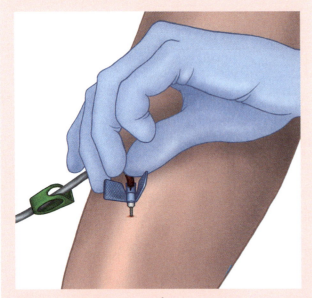

Figure 22: Self-cannulation

TOPICAL LIDOCAINE CREAMS OR GELS

Lidocaine is a numbing agent that can slowly absorb into the skin. In a randomized, controlled trial, a lidocaine-based cream (EMLA) worked best of all of the options to reduce pain from HD needles.[51] Since the cream or gel must be applied 1–2 hours *before a treatment*, the patient must put it on at home. The timing of the cream depends on how deep the access is:

- To numb the top 3 mm of tissue, apply the cream 1 hour before treatment.
- To numb the top 5 mm of tissue (for a deeper access), apply 2 hours before treatment.[52]

To use EMLA or other topical lidocaine creams or gels, patients will:

1. Wash the access arm to remove skin oils.
2. Apply a dime-sized blob of cream 1/8 inch thick to intact skin over each needle site (not on sores or rashes). Remind patients to wash their hands *after* putting on the cream and keep their hands away from their eyes to prevent damage to mucous membranes.
3. Cover the cream with an occlusive dressing to hold it in place. The dressing can be a Tegaderm™ bandage—or just kitchen plastic wrap.
4. Wash the cream off before treatment. The numbing action will go on for another hour.

A few examples of lidocaine creams (there are others) include:

- Prescription EMLA™ cream (2.5% lidocaine/2.5% prilocaine)
- Over-the-counter L.M.X.® (4% or 5% lidocaine)
- Over-the-counter Topicaine® (4% or 5% lidocaine)

LIDOCAINE INJECTION

An injection of 1% *intradermal* (under the surface of the skin) lidocaine can be used to numb the needle sites. NOTE: Since needles are used—and the injection burns—this form of lidocaine will *not* help patients who have needle *fear*.

- Apply skin antiseptic to the needle sites first, and allow to dry.
- Use a separate 1 mL or tuberculin syringe and needle for each site (see Figure 23).
- Inject the lidocaine just below the skin into the tissue above the graft or fistula at a 15-degree angle. *Never inject lidocaine into the patient's fistula or graft; it could enter the bloodstream.*[53] The lidocaine

will form a bubble or "wheal" just under the skin. Lidocaine burns, so use only a small amount.[53]
- Some of the lidocaine may leak out and/or oozing may occur at the injection site. Use a sterile gauze pad to wipe away any leakage or blood.
- Insert dialysis needles into the sites you have numbed.

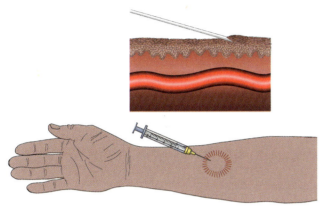

Figure 23: Intradermal Lidocaine

Injected lidocaine is a *vasoconstrictor* that can make the fistula smaller and pull it a little deeper under the skin. While there are no studies on this, some believe it may cause fibrosis over time that can make cannulation harder. Patients with shallow fistulas may have less pain *without* lidocaine. The patient can compare the amount of pain if you use lidocaine with one needle and not the other. Per your clinic's policy, let the patient choose which method he or she prefers.

VAPO-COOLANT SPRAY

A vapo-coolant spray, such as ethyl chloride, is a refrigerant that "freezes" the skin and can be used to reduce needle pain. In a randomized study, no patient who used a spray had severe needle pain. However, the spray did not numb the sites as well as a lidocaine cream did.[51] The spray can cause frostbite if too much is used or it is sprayed too close to the skin. It is highly flammable and must be kept away from heat or open flames. Vapo-coolant spray does not numb the tissue *under* the skin, so a patient with a deep access will still feel pain when the needle enters the vessel. Follow your dialysis clinic policy, and:
- Read the product label for how far away from the skin to hold the spray can, and how many seconds to spray—e.g., 2.5 inches for 2 seconds.[51]
- Apply **non-sterile** spray *before* you clean the needle sites with skin antiseptics.
- Apply **sterile** spray *after* you clean the skin.
- Clean the skin with skin antiseptic again before placing the needles.

Fistula Care After a Treatment

"I have a nurse at my clinic that is the sweetest ever, but, EVERY time she pulls my needles out, she presses so HARD that all weekend my fistula is swollen and VERY SORE. I know you need to firmly press, but she is the only one that I hurt for 2–3 days after she takes the needles out."

At the end of a treatment, you will untape and remove the needles and apply gauze dressing per your clinic's policy. Then, you or the patient must apply enough firm pressure to the needle sites to stop bleeding but not *occlude* (stop) the blood flow in the access:

- **Remove a needle all the way *before* you press on the skin.** The needle bevel is sharp, and you could cut the inside of the patient's access if you press too soon.
- **Apply the right amount of pressure to the puncture sites**. The goal is to stop bleeding from the needle puncture in the skin and the needle puncture in the access vessel. But, you do not want to damage the access or stop blood flow through it, which could raise the risk of a blood clot. The same amount of pressure you use to check a pulse is the right amount of pressure to push the tissues back together so a clot can form from needle punctures.
- **Teach your patients how to hold their own sites after a treatment**. They should hold one site at a time (the task takes two fingers). Proper site holding will allow a complete clot to form over each site, which can help prevent breakthrough bleeding after patients leave.
- **If the needle sites do not stop bleeding after 20 minutes for each needle, tell the nurse**. Prolonged bleeding from needle sites may be a sign of an access problem that needs to be fixed, such as stenosis.
- **Patients who take blood thinners may require a pressure dressing to stop bleeding**. Applying a safe pressure dressing is a nursing task.

Module 6

Tips to Help Increase Fistula Life

"I am truly blessed. My fistula was created 20 years ago. The connection was raised an inch 6 years later. I use the same vein today that I used at my first dialysis. I have self-cannulated for 19 years."

- Rotate needle sites or use the Buttonhole technique as prescribed at each treatment. **Avoid "area cannulation."** This could cause an aneurysm to form.
- Teach your patients not to allow IVs, routine blood draws, or blood pressure checks on their access arms. "Save the Vein" cards or wristbands can be helpful for when blood draws are needed.
- Keep accurate and detailed records of each treatment. If you see any problems with the patient's access, tell the nurse or the doctor.

How Grafts are Placed

A graft is inserted under the skin through a tunnel made by a surgeon, and looks like a "bridge" between an artery and a vein (see Figure 24). A fistula has *one* anastomosis where the vein connects to the artery. A graft will have *two*:

- An **arterial anastomosis** where the graft connects to the patient's artery.
- A **venous anastomosis** where the graft connects to the patient's vein.

When you cannulate a graft, you will need to *avoid both* anastomoses. Since the anastomoses are where the vessels were cut and the graft material sewn to them, they are the most fragile parts of the graft. Also, the pressure of blood returning to the venous anastomosis can harm the *neointimal* lining of the vessel wall. Then, this tissue can grow so many new cells that the diameter of the vessel is reduced. This problem, *neointimal hyperplasia*, can lead to stenosis. Stenosis is a leading reason for graft procedures.

Grafts in Detail

Grafts may be straight, curved, or looped. Some designs provide a larger surface area for needle insertion. The forearm loop graft is preferred, according to KDOQI because it provides the largest surface area for needle insertion.[54]

How Grafts for HD Access are Made

Grafts are tubes made of *biologic* (from a living creature) or *bioengineered* (synthetic) materials:

- **Biologic materials** – Some grafts may be made from a vein from the patient's leg. Some are made from human vessels donated after a donor's death (CryoPreserved™). *Bovine* (cow) arteries and veins can be used for grafts after treatment to remove proteins that would cause the human body to reject them. Some early bovine grafts had high rates of infection and aneurysm. Today, there are two bovine grafts on the market. They may be used for patients who are not fistula candidates or who have failed synthetic grafts.
- **Bioengineered materials** – Now used for nearly all grafts, the most common one today is expanded polytetrafluoroethylene, or ePTFE. Other new AV graft options are in testing.

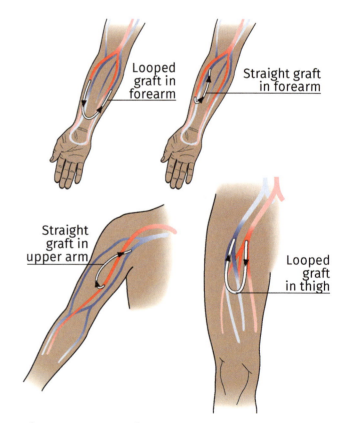

Figure 24: Graft Sites

Vascular Access

Ideally, a graft should be placed at least 2–3 weeks before use.[54] If a patient needs HD right away, "early-use" grafts can be cannulated with special care as soon as 24 hours after placement to avoid the need for an HD catheter.

Most grafts should be healed within about 2 weeks after placement. Swelling of the tissue should be gone, and the patient's own tissue will have grown into the graft.

HeRO® Graft

"Good news! I get to start at a new clinic next week! Hoping I'll have better experiences and a more proactive nephrologist. The clinic I'm at now doesn't seem to understand that I'm trying to preserve my HeRO graft, my lifeline, so I do not want new people sticking me."

Patients who have exhausted most of their access options may receive a *hemodialysis reliable outflow* (HeRO) graft, a two-part device:[55]

- The HeRO is a graft on one end, with a 6 mm inner diameter
- On the other end, the HeRO has a 5 mm silicone outflow component surrounded by a metal sleeve to prevent crushing of the central vein.
- The tip of the HeRO is in the right atrium of the heart.
- The HeRO is completely under the skin, thus infection rates may be lower than in catheters.
- It is FDA approved as a graft, and needles are placed in it just like any other graft.

A Super HeRO® version has a connector where the graft material and outflow component are joined. This allows surgeons to use any brand of graft they prefer.

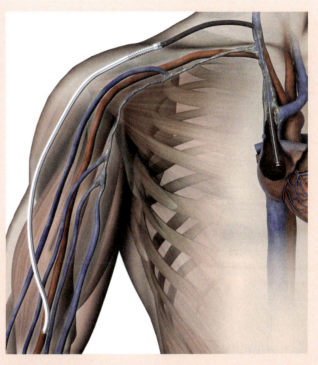

Figure 25: HeRO Graft
Graphic used with permission from Merit Medical.

NOTE: A HeRO has an all-arterial blood flow, which makes it hard to hear a bruit and feel a thrill. Lightly applying a tourniquet in the axilla area slows the flow of blood. This creates a mixture of high and slow flow, so you can feel a thrill and hear a bruit to verify patency. It may be possible to salvage a fistula by connecting it to a HeRO graft.

Starting HD with a Graft

"My husband has a Gore-Tex® graft. When it works, it works well—he clots off easily and has now had five revisions. Grafts do not last—generally—as long as fistulas."

Unlike a fistula, grafts do not need to mature, but they do need to heal. Cannulation can start as soon as the swelling has gone down. When you cannulate a graft, you will not use a tourniquet, as you do with a native fistula. The graft material will not expand under pressure. There are two exceptions to this, however, where placing a light tourniquet can help you feel the graft better:

- A *biologic* graft, made from a bovine or preserved human vessel
- A HeRO® graft

If the patient has an HD catheter, it should be removed as soon as possible after the graft has been successfully cannulated.

173

Prepare the Access Skin

Patients should wash their access sites before cannulation to remove skin debris and germs before the needles are placed. If patients cannot do this themselves, you will need to take this step.

Wash Your Hands

You will perform hand hygiene and put on personal protective equipment.

Examine the Graft

You must check over a graft before each treatment. Like fistulas, grafts also have a bruit and a thrill, since they are venous accesses.

Look for:

- Swelling and redness
- Pain and tenderness
- Drainage from puncture sites or from the skin around the graft
- Bruises
- Healing at the needle sites from the last treatment
- Local warmth or fever
- Skin erosion (stretching or thinning) of the skin especially in patients with diabetes

Listen for:

- **Bruit** – it should be low-pitched and constant. Use a stethoscope to listen along the graft. The sound should be strong and steady. Learn how each patient's access normally sounds. Like the thrill, the bruit should fade over the venous part of the graft.

Feel for:

- **Pulse** – there should be a soft pulse that you can stop by pressing down on the access
- **Thrill** – constant vibration or buzzing (feel it *without* pressing down on it)
- **Skin temperature** – should be normal, not hot
- **Hardness** – could be a sign that the graft is clotted
- **Pain or tenderness** – may mean that an infection is starting

Alert a nurse to a change in the thrill, bruit or other access changes. You may be able to help save a failing graft.

Find the Direction of Blood Flow

To find which way the blood flows, feel the entire length of the graft. Press the center of the graft with your finger. Feel for the pulse and/or thrill on both sides of the spot where you are pressing. You will feel the strongest pulse on the arterial side. The pulse or thrill will be faint or not palpable at the venous end.[53] This information will help you to place the needles the right way.

OBSERVE BLOOD FLOW

As with a fistula, a graft should have a strong blood flow from the artery through the access and into the vein. The thrill of a graft feels like a strong vibration or buzzing with each heartbeat. You should be able to feel it over the full length of the access, but it should fade over the venous part of the graft. The pulse should be soft and not bounding.

> **Patient Teaching**
>
> *"My graft is clotted again. I had dialysis yesterday and it clotted after I held my sites. I noticed I didn't have a thrill and with a stethoscope I couldn't hear anything. So I called the vascular surgeon's office and they scheduled me for surgery Monday."*
>
> Teach your patients to feel the thrill in their graft at least once a day and alert the nurse and/or nephrologist right away if there are any changes. Be sure your patients know that a change in the thrill (or in the volume of the bruit) can mean blood flow through the access is slowing down. The graft may be clotting, and quick action could help save it. If you notice this at a treatment, tell the nurse, so he or she can assess it before needles are placed.

Inserting Sharp Needles in a Graft

"Yesterday I called our local access center because my graft is starting to feel like it needs some attention. My graft gets hard, it pulses a lot, and when my needles go in blood likes to shoot everywhere. That's how I know I need to go."

The steps to prepare access skin and place the needles are the same for grafts as for fistulas (see page 160).

You can *only* use a Rope Ladder pattern in a graft (see Figure 26). Buttonholes are *not* safe, as graft material will not seal after the needles are removed. Area puncture is *never* safe. With a graft, this mistake can cause a dangerous pseudoaneurysm (see page 179).

Each graft material may have unique instructions for use. Read the graft maker's instructions for care and use. NOTE: You do not need to use small needles or lower blood flow rates with most new grafts. Per physician's orders you may use the standard gauge needles and prescribed blood flow rate right away.

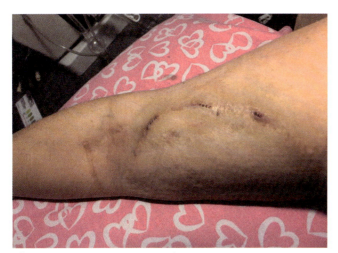

Figure 26: Graft Cannulation

CHOOSE CANNULATION SITES
Choose the sites for both needles before you place them:
- Divide the graft into equal halves at the middle.
- Look for sites at least 1/4 inch away from the last needle sites.
- Stay at least 1.5 inches away from an anastomosis.
- Try to keep the needle tips at least 2 inches apart. The only (small) study that looked at how far apart dialysis needles should be found that keeping them about 1 inch apart (2.5 centimeters) did not cause more recirculation.[56]

Be aware of where the tip of the needle will be when it is fully inserted so you do not infiltrate the graft. Grafts bend; steel needles do not!

NEEDLE DIRECTION
- As with fistulas, there are no data to support retrograde **arterial** needle placement. A large study found that **antegrade** placement with the needle bevel up was least likely to harm a graft.[31]
- A **venous** needle is inserted **antegrade** in a graft to prevent turbulence that could damage blood cells.

Graft Care After an HD Treatment

"What a day! I took my bandages off of my arm and left the house. A little later my arm felt wet. Look down, I'm bleeding? I put Band-Aids on and bled thru those. Thankfully, I had tape in the car. I put some tissue folded up with tape. That helped..."

Graft care after an HD treatment is the same as fistula care after a treatment (see page 171).

Complications of Fistulas and Grafts During Use

Infiltration

"I'm so frustrated. I only ran a little over an hour. My arm hurts so bad, it was infiltrated three times. I can hardly lift it and it hurts from my bicep to my neck. I'm, like, 4.3 kilos over my dry weight and look swollen in my face. I totally wanted dialysis today."

An *infiltration* occurs when the tip of the needle goes into the fistula or graft *and* punctures the back wall of the access (see Figure 27). Blood leaks out of the back wall into the patient's tissue, causing painful bruising (see Figure 28). Another needle must be placed to do the treatment, and the patient is likely to lose trust in the staff. Infiltration is the most common problem of needle placement. It occurs less often when staff have more practice placing needles.

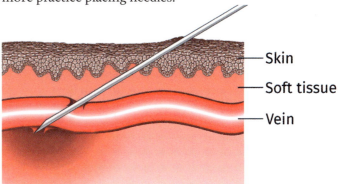

Figure 27: Infiltration

Even one infiltration can harm an access. The *hematoma* (pocket of blood under the skin) makes the arm swollen, hard, discolored, and painful. A hematoma can also squeeze the access, which slows blood flow and could lead to clotting.

If there is an infiltration, machine alarms may go off:
- An infiltrated *arterial* needle will make the arterial pressure more negative. This will set off the arterial pressure alarm and stop the blood pump.
- An infiltrated *venous* needle should raise the venous pressure. This will set off the venous pressure alarm and stop the blood pump.

Tips to Prevent Infiltration

"They poked me four times today and that was the fourth infiltration I've had the past 2 weeks. It was horrible. My arm is crazy sore and I have been so emotional all day today."

Closely follow the needle placement technique used at your clinic, and:
- Be gentle.
- Never rush.
- Develop a feel for the *least* bit of resistance in the vessel.
- Level the needle to the surface of the skin. Advance the needle slowly up to the hub as soon as you feel a pressure change and can see a flashback of blood in the tubing.
- **Never flip a needle** (turn it 180° when it is in the vessel).[57,58] Besides risking infiltration, flipping a needle can:
  - Stretch the *skin* hole, so blood oozes during treatment after the patient gets heparin.
  - Stretch the *blood vessel* hole, so bleeding around the needle may occur during HD.
  - Scoop out and damage or tear the lining of the vessel.

Flush the needles with saline after insertion to check for good placement (no pain, swelling, or resistance to the saline flush).

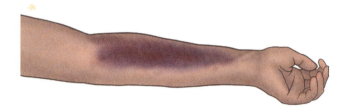

Figure 28: Arm with Infiltration

WHAT TO DO IF AN INFILTRATION OCCURS

If an infiltration occurs, you will need to place a new needle and help the patient with the pain and swelling:

- **Tell the patient you are sorry.** Infiltrations *hurt*, and they are scary for patients, who risk loss of their access. The bruising can hurt for weeks—and they still need dialysis.
- **Remove a needle that infiltrates *before* heparin is used.**[53] Have the patient apply pressure to the site, just as he or she would at the end of a treatment.
- **Leave in a needle that infiltrates *after* heparin is used**, unless the patient is in severe pain. Then place a second needle beyond the infiltration site (most often above).[53]
- **Use an ice pack for the first 24 hours.** If a *hematoma* (collection of blood forms, give the patient an ice pack wrapped in a washcloth right away to help reduce swelling. The patient should keep ice on for 20 minutes, off for 20 minutes, etc.[59]
- **Apply dry heat after 24 hours.** After the first day, the patient can apply dry heat or a warm compress to help reduce pain and absorb the blood.
- **Document the cause and outcome of the infiltration.**
- **Do *not* reduce the patient's HD run time.** Do not subtract the time you spend taking care of an infiltration from the patient's treatment. Lost minutes mean not enough dialysis. Add the lost time to be sure the patient gets the prescribed dose.
- **Give the patient a written handout for how to safely apply ice on and off for the next 24 hours.**
- **Teach the patient how to self-cannulate.** S/he is the only one who can feel both ends of the needle, and self-cannulation can prevent most infiltrations.

Bleeding During HD

Bleeding around the needles during a treatment may be a minor problem. Flipping needles or digging with a needle to find the vessel may be reasons for oozing. Frequent loss of small amounts of blood during HD adds to the risk of anemia.

Bleeding during dialysis can also be a life-threatening emergency. For example, a needle may come out when the blood pump is running, or an access may rupture. **Serious—even fatal—blood loss can occur in just minutes if a needle comes out or the lines come apart.** In one 6-year period, *1,654* fatal vascular access hemorrhages occurred in the U.S.[60] This should *never* happen. To prevent this:

- **Follow your clinic's procedures for taping the needles** (see Tape the Needles After Insertion on page 167).
- **Connect bloodlines securely**.
- **Set arterial and venous pressure monitor limits**. These alarms can help prevent severe blood loss if they are armed and working. NOTE: A *slow* blood leak may not cause a big enough drop in venous pressure to set off the alarm—but can still cause a lot of blood loss. And, you may not see the blood if the patient's arm is under a blanket. This is why patients must keep their accesses in plain view at all times during a treatment.[61]

Some clinics use blood leak-sensing devices. Placed over the venous needle, these will alarm if blood leaks out around a needle or the lines separate. The cost of disposables can be high. But, the cost of a lawsuit brought by the loved ones of someone who *exsanguinates* (bleeds to death) to death at dialysis is even higher. Nocturnal home HD patients routinely use these alarms for safety while sleeping. The only such device that is approved by the U.S. Food and Drug Administration for use in dialysis is Redsense™. A sensor patch is placed on the patient's arm over the access, and an alarm unit sends infrared light through an optical fiber to a sensor. If blood leaks, it disrupts the signal and triggers an alarm—but does not stop the blood pump.[62] U.S. Veterans Health Administration clinics have required the use of this device for all hemodialysis patients since 2010.[63]

If a patient is losing blood through the tubing, **turn off the blood pump and clamp the bloodlines.** Press on the needle site if the needles were pulled out. Call for help.

Bleeding After HD

Sometimes, long after an access has clotted, it may start to bleed again. Teach patients to try to stay calm, apply firm, even pressure to the bleeding site and call 911 if this happens. Patients should tell the 911 operator that they have an actively bleeding dialysis access. They should never try to drive themselves to the hospital or the dialysis clinic.

Patient Teaching: First Aid for Access Ruptures

"Wow was I lucky!! Last night after I went to sleep, something wet woke me up, I was horrified to be laying in a pool of blood! My access sprung a leak and I was lucky to wake up to stop the bleeding. A surgeon is going to operate tomorrow to repair my graft I've had for 13 years!"

A burst access is a life and death medical emergency. When a fistula or graft carries 600+ mL/min of blood, a patient can lose enough blood to die in about 3 minutes. If an access ruptures in the clinic:

- **Inflate a blood pressure cuff** over the rupture to keep pressure on it. Keep the cuff inflated.
- *Do NOT use towels or gauze*—these will wick even more blood out of the vessel.
- *Do NOT apply a tourniquet*. The patient could lose an arm (or leg).
- Call for help.

At home, where no blood pressure cuff is on hand, patients should apply direct pressure with their other hand, yell for help, and call 911.[64] Teach patients these steps and help them save their own lives if they are outside of the clinic when a fistula or graft ruptures. Learn more about access ruptures on page 243.

Report all bleeding to the charge nurse as an "adverse event" for the clinic's quality reporting.

> **Watch all Patients' Needles During Treatment**
>
> Get in the habit of looking at patient's clothes and blankets and under each chair often for pooling blood. The CMS *Conditions for Coverage* require access sites to be visible at all times during treatment. Teach your patients to always keep their accesses in plain view. You need to be able to see as soon as possible if a needle comes loose. A needle that pulls out or lines that come apart could lead to severe blood loss or death.

Recirculation

Recirculation means that blood coming back into the venous needle mixes with blood going into the arterial needle. If this happens, a small amount of the *same* blood gets cleaned over and over. This blood may turn dark from a lack of oxygen (*Black Blood Syndrome*). However, the rest of the patient's blood is *not* cleaned well so, recirculation means a poor treatment. Over time, poor HD can lead to symptoms of uremia. A blood draw for recirculation can be ordered. The blood is drawn 30 minutes into an HD treatment if adequacy drops or you suspect stenosis. Check your clinic policy to learn how to correctly draw blood for recirculation studies.

Steal Syndrome

"My new fistula is buzzing, but has left my hand with such painful severe steal syndrome and numbness that I can't use it, even to tie my shoe or cut my food."

A fistula or graft can "steal" too much blood from the hand, so it does not get enough oxygen and the tissue dies.[65] Patients with steal syndrome have hand pain that can range from minor to severe. In most patients, this pain lessens over time as new blood vessels grow and bring blood to the area (called *collateral circulation*).

However, patients with *neuropathy* (nerve damage) due to diabetes or blood vessel disease must be watched closely. Their symptoms may get worse, and they may need surgery to fix the blood flow[65] or risk loss of a finger, hand, or arm (see Figure 29). Watch for and ask your patients about:

- Pain, tingling, or feeling cold in the access limb
- A change in motor skills in the hand
- Nail beds that are blue in color
- Necrotic (dead, black) spots on the skin
- Loss of feeling in the access limb

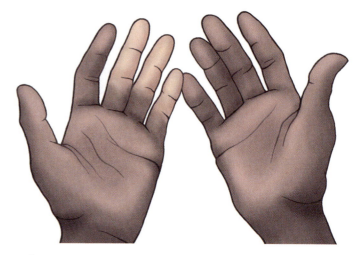

Figure 29: Steal Syndrome

Tell the nurse if you suspect steal syndrome so s/he can call the vascular access surgeon right away. In the meantime, try to keep the patient's hand warm during HD. A mitten or tube sock on the hand may help. Ask the patient if moving the access arm to a different position (to bring more blood to the hand) makes it feel any better. Be careful not to infiltrate the access when you move the arm. You can also have the patient squeeze a ball during treatment—this will increase blood flow and bring more oxygen to the hand, which may reduce or relieve the pain.

Longer Term Complications of Fistulas and Grafts

Some problems with fistulas and grafts may develop over time. You need to be aware of the signs and symptoms of these complications, so you can report possible problems to the nurses or physicians right away. Doing so could help save your patients' lifelines.

Aneurysms

"My surgeon says she may have to do yet another revision on my left arm fistula. An aneurysm has formed from over-using the space for the venous needle, just behind my bicep."

Aneurysms are thin, weak spots in a **fistula** wall that balloon out. Weak spots are more likely when there is high pressure in a fistula due to a *stenosis* (narrow spot) or uncontrolled high blood pressure (see Figure 30).

When you put needles into the same two small areas of a fistula over and over (*area cannulation*), the wall will quickly weaken and start to bulge. Due to poor cannulation technique, as many as 60% of patients with fistulas may have at least one aneurysm.[66] This number makes sense, since a large study found that 65.8% of patients had their needles placed using area cannulation.[31] **Rotate needle puncture sites or use the Buttonhole technique to help prevent aneurysms**.

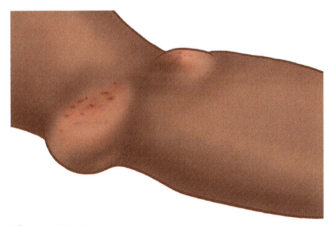

Figure 30: Aneurysms

Cannulation must always be done into full-thickness vessel wall. **Do not place needles into an aneurysm**.[54] Unfortunately, when there *is* an aneurysm, there is less surface area left to place needles. Blood clots can form in the "dome" of an aneurysm. These clots are a good hiding place for bacteria that could break free and cause sepsis. Aneurysm surgery is needed when:[66]

- **The aneurysm grows quickly** (more than 10% per year)
- **Skin over the aneurysm is thin or shiny or has a blister or sore** (see Figure 31)
- **Patients are upset about the appearance of large aneurysms**

It may be possible to cut out the aneurysm and change the anastomosis so the fistula can still be used. Or, a new fistula may be needed. In some cases, the patient may need a graft.[66]

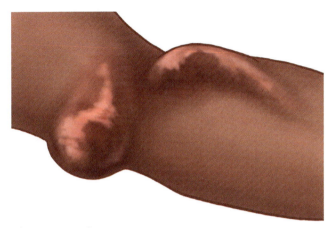

Figure 31: Risky Aneurysm

Pseudoaneurysms (False Aneurysms)

"I went to my access center because about a week ago I found a lump in my graft under my armpit. Today they said it is a very large pseudoaneurysm. My surgeon is going to rearrange his schedule to fit me in for surgery."

One of the biggest disadvantages of grafts is that they wear out. In most grafts, each needle puncture forms a permanent hole. Infiltrations form even larger holes. These holes allow blood to seep out into a capsule and form a big bump over the graft—a result we call *one-site-itis* (see Figure 32). This damage slows healing, can be a site for infection, and thins the skin above it so the graft is at risk for rupture. A *pseudoaneurysm* (false aneurysm on top of a graft that contains a large blood clot) can form (see Figure 33). If the clot dislodges after dialysis, the patient can bleed to death very quickly. NOTE: Fistulas can have pseudoaneurysms, too, when there is an infiltration. Blood can leak out of the fistula and pool under the skin.)

When you observe a graft before each treatment, look for thinning, shiny skin and unhealed needle sites in these enlarged areas.[54] Report any abnormality to the nurse. **Enlarging pseudoaneurysms should not be cannulated due to the risk of bleeding, rupture, and death.**[67]

Module 6

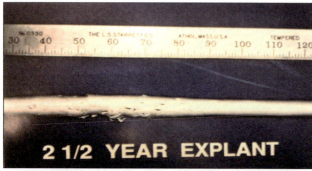

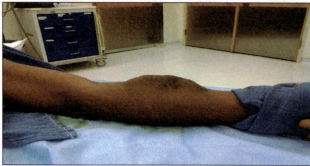

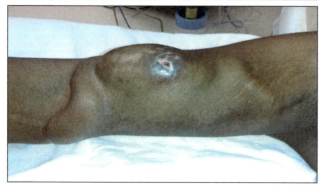

Figure 32: One-site-itis
Photos used with permission from Dr. Gary Lemmon.

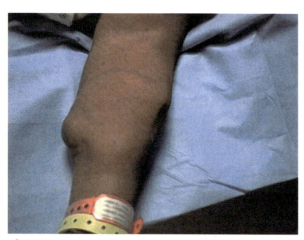

Figure 33: Pseudoaneurysms
Photo used with permission from Deborah Brouwer-Maier.

Stenosis (Narrowing)

"I had my graft placed 2 weeks ago and we have not used it yet. Today at dialysis when they went to listen to it they couldn't hear anything, and they did before. It also feels pretty hard. They are thinking there is a stenosis and it may have clotted off. Now I feel so sad and don't know what happens next."

Stenosis is a narrowing of the blood vessel that slows blood flow in a fistula or graft.

STENOSIS IN A FISTULA

In fistulas, stenosis is most often due to an injury to the blood vessel lining. An injury will cause flow turbulence, which leads to an overgrowth of cells (see Figure 34).

There are three major sites where stenosis is likely to develop in a fistula:

1. **Inflow stenosis** – occurs on the arterial side of a fistula. The most common type is called a *juxta-anastomotic* (next to the anastomosis) *stenosis* (JAS). A JAS will keep a fistula from maturing in the first place, because it does not let enough blood enter. A JAS may be caused by stretching, twisting, or other trauma during the surgery.[68] You may be able to feel a JAS as a flat spot just past the anastomosis.

2. **Outflow stenosis** – can occur anywhere along the venous side of a fistula. A spot where the patient has had a past IV or an infiltration may be damaged and become stenotic. The section of fistula past the stenosis is likely to be smaller, which can make needle placement harder. It can be easier to infiltrate a fistula again in this spot.

3. **Central venous stenosis** – occurs in a central vein. The patient's arm, leg, or breast on the same side may be much larger due to swelling.[69] Or, veins in the neck may be *distended* (swollen). If the doctor believes a stenosis is present, the patient's venous system should be checked from the fistula to the heart. This problem is most likely due to prior placement of an HD catheter in the subclavian vein. It can also be caused by pacemaker and defibrillator wires, or by the placement of PICC lines in an arm or leg.[69]

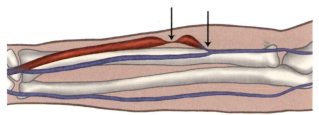

Two narrow areas in this mature wrist fistula

Figure 34: Stenosis

STENOSIS IN A GRAFT

Graft material is not alive, so it cannot grow cells. In grafts, stenosis is most likely to occur at the venous anastomosis, where the artificial graft material meets the patient's tissue. The graft at this spot is under stress from the returning blood flow. When blood rushes back into the graft, it causes trauma to the lining of the vein it is attached to. The patient's vein reacts by laying down new cells that build up and reduce blood flow. Since this trauma occurs 24/7, with each heartbeat, it can cause *neointimal hyperplasia*:

- *Neo* = new
- *Intimal* = blood vessel lining
- *Hyper* = too many
- *Plasia* = cells

The narrow spot causes the venous pressure to be higher (more negative) during HD, if the needle is placed close to the stenosis. Stenosis can also occur at any point along the length of a graft, for example, if there is a pseudoaneurysm.

SIGNS OF STENOSIS IN FISTULAS AND GRAFTS

The KDOQI guidelines say that fistulas and grafts should be checked for stenosis at least once a month by checking venous pressure or access flow.[54] All patient care staff need to watch for and report these symptoms of stenosis:

- A high-pitched or louder bruit
- Pounding or "water-hammer" pulse
- A bruit where each sound is separate—(whoosh… whoosh…whoosh)
- Less thrill in any part of the access
- Low blood pressure
- A pulse that is stronger than a normal pulse. When you place your fingers on the fistula, they rise and fall with each beat.
- Trouble inserting or threading the HD needles
- Swelling of the patient's access arm or leg
- Higher venous pressure during treatment, so you must turn the blood pump down
- Recirculation
- Extracorporeal system clotting during treatment
- More bleeding after needles are removed after HD
- Not being able to get the prescribed blood flow rate
- Prolonged or more than usual bleeding after treatment—bleeding may restart when the patient is out of the clinic
- "Black Blood" Syndrome

DIAGNOSING AND TREATING STENOSIS

To find stenosis, a doctor injects dye into the vessel. Any narrow spot will show up on an X-ray (*fistulogram or venogram*). Stenosis may also be found by color Doppler ultrasound.[66] These methods let the doctor pinpoint the site of the narrow spot.

Some cases of stenosis can be treated with *angioplasty*. The doctor threads a catheter with an inflatable balloon tip into the vessel. Once the balloon is in place, he or she inflates it to expand the *lumen* (diameter) of the vessel. This is an outpatient procedure. A *stent* (mesh tube) may be placed to hold the vessel open. Once placed, a stent can never be removed, and cannot be cannulated through. Or, surgery may be needed to try to repair the access. Stenosis can recur.

Thrombosis (Blood Clots)

"I'm going to the ER. My graft clotted and the access clinic wasn't able to declot it. I've had many grafts, so the pickings are slim. They are considering a leg loop graft, and I'm not sure how I feel about that."

Blood clots are a serious problem that can occur in both fistulas and grafts—and in catheters as well. Clots occur about 2.5 times more often in grafts than in fistulas.[70] Blood has a number of ways to stop a wound from bleeding by forming a clot. These include clotting proteins and *platelets* — cells that clump together to seal off damage.

Platelets clump when they are *activated* by contact with turbulence or rough walls inside a blood vessel. Activated platelets and rough spots that should be smooth signal the clotting proteins to form a strong net of fibers (fibrin). This net traps *more* platelets and red blood cells, so the clot grows bigger and gets more solid (see Figure 35).

A clot can start to form any time there is low blood flow. Blood flow can be low due to a blood pressure drop at treatment, dehydration, or something that squeezes the access, like a bracelet, a watch—or a hematoma. When blood flow is low, blood pools at a damaged surface—like a needle site. Blood flow through a fistula stenosis may cause enough turbulence to activate platelets, so they stick to the vessel wall and form clots.

Suspect a clot if you feel no pulse or thrill and hear no bruit along the outflow vein. Do not cannulate an access if you think there is a clot. Tell the team if you suspect stenosis or thrombosis so the nephrologist and/or vascular surgeon can be called. Early detection and repair may help save the access. When you use proper technique to place needles and apply the right amount of pressure to the needle sites after treatment, you help reduce the risk of thrombosis.

Access Monitoring and Surveillance

A patient's vascular access is often referred to as his or her "lifeline." Routine access monitoring and surveillance can help identify patients who are at risk for thrombosis and get them treatment early.

- **Monitoring** is the physical examination of the access: look, listen, and feel.
- **Surveillance** is periodic evaluation of vascular access with tests that may involve special instruments. The KDOQI guidelines say that clinics should have a program to do this.[54]

Several techniques and methods in use in the U.S. for access surveillance include:

- **Dynamic and static venous pressure measures** – venous pressure is monitored at a specified pump speed or while the pump is off and the lines are clamped.
- **Access flow measures** – this is done by reversing bloodlines on the dialysis machine and measuring access flow, or by using a device.
- **Online clearance** – some dialysis machines have a sensitive conductivity meter added to monitor solute clearance, during treatment. This meter also checks for dialysis adequacy.
- **Duplex ultrasound** – a non-invasive test uses sound waves to create a picture and record access flow.
- **Data analysis** – the treatment record is analyzed to evaluate the trends in intra-access pressure.

Technology that may be used can be seen in Table 3.

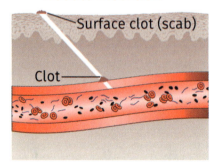 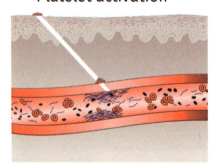 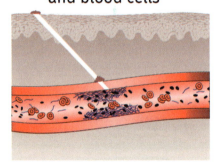

Figure 35: Blood Clotting at a Needle Puncture Site

Table 3: Vascular Access Surveillance Approaches

Access Type	Measures	How it Works	Staff Time	Disposables	What the Results Mean
ON-LINE CLEARANCE – FRESENIUS MEDICAL CARE NORTH AMERICA					
Fistula or Graft	**Access Flow:** volume of flow in a fistula or graft in mL/min. The OLC access flow range is 0–2,000 mL/min.	OLC is used to estimate the effectiveness of a dialysis treatment. Sodium is used as a close substitute as measured in OLC for urea to measure clearance. The dialysate sodium level is adjusted slightly for a short time. This changes the conductivity, which is then tested before and after the dialyzer. (Some sodium diffuses through the membrane, which changes the post dialyzer reading.) No saline is needed to check for clearance. Two on-line clearance tests are performed. One with the bloodlines connected in the normal position and one with the lines in the reversed position which causes recirculation.	1–2 min	A special bloodline (Twister ™ blood reversal device) eliminates the need to disconnect the bloodlines from the access during treatment. Or the lines can be manually reversed from the needle-Luer lock connection.	**Normal Range:** **Fistula:** > 400 mL/min **Graft:** > 600 mL/min > 2,000 mL/min is a "high flow" access. May indicate the presence of high cardiac output syndrome. Another test may be needed.
TRANSONIC HD MONITOR					
Fistula or Graft	**Access Flow:** volume of flow in a fistula or graft in mL/min. The Transonic flow range is 0–4,000 mL/min.	Ultrasound (U/S) dilution: Two sensors on the bloodlines measure flow. *Reverse the bloodlines to create recirculation.* Release saline from the bag into the venous bloodline. Sensors measure blood dilution and time for diluted blood to reach the arterial bloodline. The monitor displays flow.	2–3 min	A special bloodline or tubing insert can be used to reverse bloodlines. Or, bloodlines can be manually reversed at the needle-Luer connection.	**Normal Range:** **Fistula:** > 500 mL/min **Graft:** > 600 mL/min > 2,000 mL/min is a "high flow" access that can place the patient at risk for Steal Syndrome, hand ischemia, and/or high output cardiac failure.
	Recirculation: % recirculation in a fistula or graft.	U/S dilution: Keep bloodlines in the normal positions. Release saline from the bag into the venous bloodline. The arterial sensor measures blood dilution and displays % recirculation.	2 min	None	**Normal Range:** 0–10% > 10% is recirculation. Or, the needles are reversed. The test can be repeated with the lines reversed. If the reading is lower, the arterial and venous could be opposite from the current cannulation. Confirm by checking the bruit and thrill to find the access blood flow direction.

Table 3: Continued

Access Type	Measures	How it Works	Staff Time	Disposables	What the Results Mean
TRANSONIC HD MONITOR					
Catheter	**Recirculation**: % recirculation in a catheter.	U/S dilution: same as for fistula/graft recirculation. Keep the bloodlines in the *normal* catheter positions (Red/Red, Blue/Blue). Release saline from the bag into the venous bloodline. The arterial sensor measures the diluted blood and % recirculation is displayed.	2 min	None	**Normal Range:** 0–10% > 10% is recirculation. If clinic protocol allows, reverse the catheter to bloodline connections (red to blue, blue to red) and retest for recirculation.
Fistula, Graft, or Catheter	**Delivered Blood Flow**: true flow vs. the dialysis machine blood pump reading.	Transit-time U/S: Two sensors placed on the bloodlines measure flow. The bloodlines are in the normal positions (Red/Red, Blue/Blue). The monitor displays blood flow in mL/min.	1 min	None	**Normal Range:** Within 10% of the blood pump setting. **Abnormal Range:** > 10% difference (lower flow than set on the blood pump) can mean mismatch of the needle gauge to the blood pump setting, poor needle placement, blood pump out of calibration.
Fistula or Graft	**Cardiac Output**: measurements a doctor can use to assess how well a patient's heart is pumping. This can help the doctor see if the access has too-high flow (i.e., >2,000 mL/min) that can cause high out-output cardiac failure.	A special tubing set is connected to the bloodline prior to priming of the circuit. The tubing set connects to the fistula needles when the dialysis treatment is started. Two sensors are placed on a tubing set. Keep bloodlines in the normal positions. Inject a small amount of saline into the injection port of the tubing set. The sensors display results.	2 min	A special tubing set is needed to allow an injection of saline close to the venous needle.	**Normal range:** 5–8 L/min. Cardiac output changes with fluid volume status. Measurements are taken at the start and end of the treatment. Cardiac output may improve at the end of the treatment when extra fluid has been removed.

Table 3: Continued

Access Type	Measures	How it Works	Staff Time	Disposables	What the Results Mean
VASCALERT					
Fistula or Graft	**Intra-access Pressure**: Determines pressure at the needle tip by calculating the derived static pressure. This is a marker for stenosis. These data-driven results are shown and trended for each treatment.	Treatment data are securely sent weekly (or daily) to Vasc-Alert. Along with other factors (hematocrit, needle type, etc.) the data are used to produce individual patient reports. When derived static pressure exceeds the FDA threshold for three treatments in a row, an alert in the patient's report says the patient is at risk for complications. Reports can be viewed online at any time. Downloadable reports are produced weekly.	None No staff time is required to "test" the access.	None Vasc-Alert is a medical device, but there is no physical device or time for clinicians to test. Results use treatment data that are already collected.	The FDA threshold was set to help identify most patients with hemodynamically significant (> 50%) stenosis. Continuous trending informs the staff about the rate of stenosis growth. I.e., rising pressure over time suggests that stenosis is getting worse. Trending drives better clinical decisions.

Infection

Fistulas and grafts can become infected, which is serious, because germs in the access can spread throughout the body. They can attack the patient's joints or heart, or can cause *sepsis*—a serious blood infection—and death. In fact, infection is the second leading cause of death in people on dialysis, whose immune systems do not work as well as those of healthy people.

As you have learned, signs of infection in a fistula or graft include redness, drainage, pus, abscesses, open skin, and fever. The patient in Figure 36 gave permission to use the image so technicians like you can see what can happen when a fistula becomes infected and must be removed. The wound was left open to drain so it would heal, which was upsetting and can leave large scars. This patient lost a precious access site.

Staff failure to use good infection control techniques is a main cause of infection. Always follow your clinic's policies and procedures to prepare the needle site with aseptic technique. Tell the nurse right away if you see any signs of infection so s/he can call the nephrologist. Document what you see in the patient's medical record.

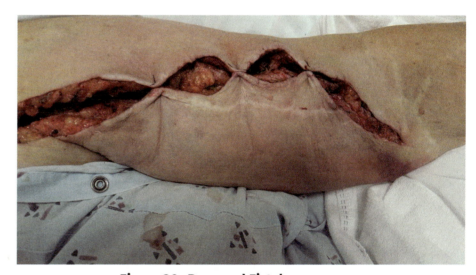

Figure 36: Removed Fistula

The CDC has many tools and resources to help staff prevent access infections. All of the tools can be downloaded for free at the CDC Dialysis Safety website: www.cdc.gov/dialysis.

Module 6

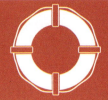

It only takes a minute to save your patient's lifeline.

 GO

STOP

Look

GO: The skin over the access is all one color and looks like the skin around it.

STOP: There is redness, swelling or drainage. There are skin bulges with shiny, bleeding, or peeling skin.

Listen
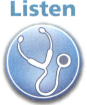

GO: Bruit - the hum or buzz should sound like a "whoosh," or for some may sound like a drum beat. The sound should be the same along the access.

STOP: There is no sound, decreased sound or a change in sound. Sound is different from what a normal Bruit should sound like.

Feel
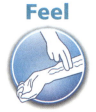

GO: Thrill: a vibration or buzz in the full length of the access.
Pulse: slight beating like a heartbeat. Fingers placed lightly on the access should move slightly.

STOP: Pulsatile: The beat is stronger than a normal pulse. Fingers placed lightly on the access will rise and fall with each beat.

Arm Elevation
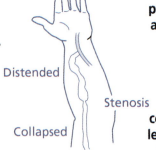
Distended
Stenosis
Collapsed

GO — Upper Arm AVF
The AVF outflow vein partially collapses when the arm is raised above the level of the heart. It may feel "flabby" when palpated.

GO — Lower Arm AVF
The AVF outflow vein collapses when arm is raised above the level of the heart.

STOP — Upper Arm AVF
The AVF outflow vein does not partially collapse or become "flabby" after being raised above the level of the heart. This finding should be reported to an expert clinician.

STOP — Lower Arm AVF
The AVF outflow vein does not collapse after being raised above the level of the heart. This finding should be reported to an expert clinician.

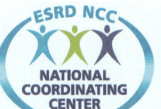

www.esrdncc.org

This material was prepared by the End Stage Renal Disease (ESRD) National Coordinating Center (NCC) contractor, under contract with the Centers for Medicare & Medicaid Services (CMS), an agency of the U.S. Department of Health and Human Services under CMS contract HHSM-500-2013-NW002C; and was adapted by the contractor under CMS contract #: HHSM-500-2016-00007C. The contents presented do not necessarily reflect CMS policy nor imply endorsement by the U.S. Government.
Publication Number: FL-ESRD NCC-7N1T02-10032016-10

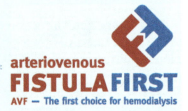
arteriovenous **FISTULA FIRST**
AVF — The first choice for hemodialysis

Figure 37: Fistula First Catheter Last Resource

Vascular Access

Teach Patients How to Monitor and Protect their Fistulas or Grafts

"Last night the scab on my fistula ripped open. Blood was EVERYWHERE! I kept telling my boyfriend to call 911, and he did that very calmly, but I know he was scared for my life."

Patients should look, listen, and feel their access *at least once a day* and tell a member of the care team right away if they find any changes.[71]

- **Look for** signs of infection like redness, swelling, or a sore.
- **Watch for** a blister on the access or a tight or shiny aneurysm (even a small one), loss of skin pigment, or scabs that stick up can be signs that a fistula or graft will rupture. The patient could bleed to death if this happens.
- **Listen to** the bruit by placing the fistula next to their ear. A higher pitched or quieter bruit can mean stenosis or a blood clot. A trip to the access center could save their access.
- **Feel** the thrill. A change can mean blood flow through the access is slowing down. The fistula may be clotting, and quick action could help save it.
- **Stop staff** from using the access or even the access arm or leg for routine blood draws, IVs, or blood pressure checks.

Encourage patients to self-cannulate to reduce the risk of mispuncture. Teach patients *not to*:

- Sleep on the access arm
- Put too much pressure on the puncture site after removing the dialysis needles
- Wear tight-fitting clothing or jewelry that squeeze the access arm
- Carry heavy objects across the arms that compress the access, such as a purse or grocery bags
- Use the access for IV drugs
- Wear a watch on an arm with a lower arm fistula

You can find many tools (including Figure 36) from Fistula First Catheter Last to help you teach your patients. http://esrdncc.org/en/resources/patients/

HD Catheters in Detail

"A catheter is the 'white hose of death.' It's a way for infection to go straight to your heart. Yes, fistulas don't look pretty and the needles hurt. Learn about buttonholes and learn to put in your own needles. Your access is your lifeline. But catheters are bad!"

Far too many patients still start HD with a catheter instead of a fistula or graft. Patients may have an urgent need for treatment and no venous access due to:

- Acute kidney injury
- Peritonitis from peritoneal dialysis
- Uremia with no matured fistula
- A scheduled living donor transplant
- Refusal of fistula or graft surgery
- Access failure or infection
- Central venous stenosis

Catheter Placement

Catheters must be placed using sterile technique. This may be done in an operating room, radiology, or a vascular access center. Checking the placement with an X-ray can ensure that the catheter is in the right place. The risks of catheter placement can include:

- *Bleeding or hematoma*
- *Air embolism* (air in a blood vessel that acts like a clot)
- *Pneumothorax* (air between the lungs and chest wall, that can cause lung collapse)
- *Hemothorax* (blood in the lungs)

How HD Catheters Work

HD removes and returns blood at the same time, so HD catheters have two side-by-side limbs, or chambers called *lumens*:

- The end of the catheter that enters the patient's bloodstream is the "tip." The tip has holes for blood entry and exit (see Figure 38).
- The other end, or *limb,* is outside the body with the two lumens apart (see Figure 39).
- Each lumen has a connector (hub) on the end to attach to the bloodlines.
- In most cases, the *exit site* where the catheter comes out through the skin is covered by a sterile dressing.

Module 6

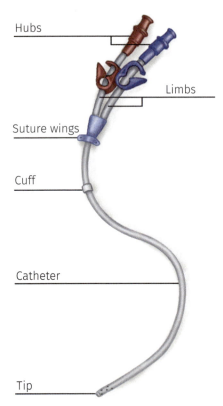

Figure 38: HD Catheter

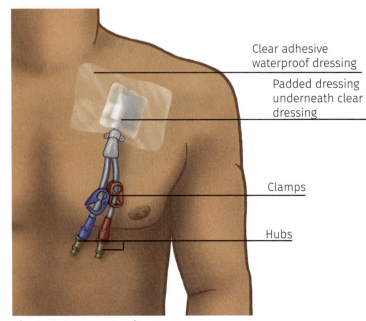

Figure 39: Catheter in Place

Veins Used for Catheters

Catheters are placed in veins that can handle the high blood flows needed for HD. The large veins in the neck and chest that empty into the right atrium of the heart are well suited for this. The **right internal jugular (RIJ)** vein is the best entry vein for a catheter because:

- In most people, the RIJ is the largest vessel that can be reached.
- The RIJ is the shortest and straightest path to the right atrium of the heart.

The **left internal jugular (LIJ)** is the second choice. It is longer than the RIJ and has two large curves to go through, which could reduce blood flow. Stenosis of the IJ does not prevent return blood flow from a future fistula or graft in the arm. NOTE: A catheter should not be placed on the same side as a working fistula or graft.

Catheters placed in **subclavian** veins are more likely to cause stenosis that could make it impossible to place an access in the arm on that side of the body. Therefore, these veins should *not* be used for a catheter unless:[54]

- There is a life-threatening emergency.
- It is known that no venous access can ever be placed in the *ipsilateral* (same side) arm.

The **femoral veins** in the groin can be used for catheter access (see Figure 40) when:

1. Short-term access is needed for urgent HD and the RIJ cannot be used.
2. Long-term catheter access is needed and none of the upper central veins can be used.

The tip of a femoral catheter should be well up into the inferior vena cava (IVC). Most femoral catheters are placed in a hospital. Patients who use these tend to be on bed rest, or the catheter is removed after each treatment. If a patient has no upper body vessels left for access, a cuffed tunneled catheter can be placed in the thigh. Infection risk is higher because the catheter could be contaminated by stool, so good hygiene is vital. When a femoral catheter is in use, you will need to protect the patient's privacy with a curtain or screen.

There are other catheter sites, such as translumbar or transhepatic for patients who no longer have any other sites left.

Vascular Access

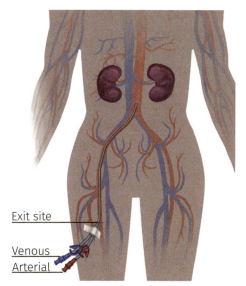

Figure 40: Femoral Catheter Placement

Care of Hemodialysis Catheters

State laws restrict who can care for and handle HD catheters. In many states, catheter care must be done by a registered nurse. You will need to learn the laws of the state in which you practice. Refer to your clinic's protocol for care instructions.

Starting HD with a Catheter

"Tomorrow is my third successful two needle run! Then we'll be moving up to a bigger size needle. I can't wait to be able to have this catheter taken out already!"

If your state's law allows you to handle HD catheters, you will need to follow your clinic's policies and procedures. These may include the steps below.

LOOK AT THE CATHETER BEFORE A TREATMENT

Remove your gloves, wash your hands, and put on new, clean gloves before you touch the patient and his or her equipment. Always use aseptic technique if you open, touch, or clean a catheter and dressing.

- Ask the patient about any problems with the catheter during treatments or at home.
- Any time the exit site is exposed or the catheter is open, the KDOQI Guidelines and CMS suggest that you *and* the patient wear a mask that covers your nose and mouth.[54]
- Remove the dressing and note any changes in the catheter position, such as being able to see the cuff at the exit site.
- Look for any skin redness or drainage (fluid or pus coming out around the catheter). Is the catheter cuff crusty? Is there any pain or tenderness at the catheter exit site? These can be signs of infection—tell the nurse right away and document the symptoms in the patient's medical record.

CLEAN THE CATHETER BEFORE USE

Exit Sites

Before you touch a catheter, you will gather your supplies, put on a mask, perform hand hygiene, and put on new, clean gloves. Remove the dressing. The CDC then provides the following guidance:[72]

1. Clean skin with a > 0.5% chlorhexidine solution with alcohol. Some patients may react to skin antiseptics. If a patient cannot use chlorhexidine, use tincture of iodine, an *iodophor* (water-soluble iodine), or 70% alcohol.
2. Let the skin dry and do not touch it again after it has been cleaned.

Connection Steps

The CDC's eight-step Scrub-the-Hub protocol[73] outlines a suggested way to prepare catheter hubs before and after a catheter is used for HD.

> **Definitions:**
>
> **Catheter** – a central venous catheter (CVC) or a central line
>
> **Hub** – the end of the CVC that connects to the bloodlines or cap
>
> **Cap** – a device that screws on to and occludes the hub
>
> **Limb** – the catheter portion that extends from the patient's body to the hub
>
> **Bloodlines** – the arterial and venous tubes that connect the patient's catheter to the dialyzer

Catheter Connection Steps:

1. **Perform hand hygiene and put on new, clean gloves.**
2. **Clamp the catheter.** (NOTE: **Always** clamp a catheter limb before your take off a cap. **Never** leave an uncapped catheter unattended.)
3. **Disinfect the hub** using an appropriate antiseptic:
   a. (*Optional*) Before you take off the caps, disinfect each cap and the part of the hub that you can reach with an antiseptic pad. Discard the pad after use.
   b. Remove one cap and disinfect its hub, using a new antiseptic pad. Scrub the sides (threads) and end of the hub thoroughly, using friction, and remove any residue (e.g., blood).
   c. Use the same antiseptic pad as you did for the hub to clean that catheter limb with friction, moving from the hub at least several centimeters up toward the patient's body. Hold up the catheter limb so it does not touch anything while you let the antiseptic dry.
   d. Repeat steps a–c to clean the other hub and limb. Leave each hub "open" (i.e., uncapped and disconnected) for the shortest time possible.
4. **Always handle catheter hubs aseptically**. Once you disinfect them, do not let the catheter hubs touch nonsterile surfaces.
5. **Attach a sterile syringe, unclamp the catheter, withdraw blood, and flush, per clinic protocol.**
6. **Repeat for the other limb** (this might occur in parallel).
7. **Connect the ends of the bloodlines to the catheter aseptically.**
8. **Remove your gloves and perform hand hygiene.**

Line Reversals

Sometimes a patient may need to be disconnected during treatment. This may occur if s/he needs to use the restroom, or if the bloodlines must be reversed to improve blood flow. If the bloodlines must be disconnected, disinfect the hub and end of the bloodlines again.[72] Minimize the number of times a patient's catheter is disconnected from the bloodlines as much as possible.

Patient Catheter Teaching

Patients may be at home when a problem occurs with their catheter. Your clinic staff should teach patients and their families:

- **How to protect a catheter and keep it clean**. Most clinics change the dressing at each treatment, so patients should not need to do so. But, if the dressing gets wet, it is best for the patient to remove it, dry carefully around the exit site, and bandage the site. Some clinics will provide emergency dressing supplies for patients to have at home.

- **How to recognize and report signs of infection**. Patients and their families need to know that redness, swelling, pus, or fever must be reported right away to the care team. If these occur on days or times when the clinic is closed, the patient needs to go to an ER.

- **What activities to avoid**. To keep the dressing dry, most clinics suggest no showers or swimming for patients with catheters. But, there are devices made to keep catheters dry in the shower. Check your clinic's catheter care protocol. Patients need to know not to pull or tug on the catheter or let anyone else do so. The tip of the catheter is in the patient's heart. Pulling on the catheter could move the catheter from where it needs to be.

- **Why to keep sharp objects like pins or scissors away from their catheters**. Holes put the patient at risk for infection and require the catheter to be changed before the next treatment. *Accidentally cutting the catheter can cause severe blood loss or air embolism (air in the bloodstream).* Show the patient how to pinch off the catheter and seek medical help right away if a cut occurs in the tubing.

- **What to do if a catheter comes out**. First aid for an HD catheter that comes out is for the patient to lie flat, put pressure on the site with a hand, and call 911.[74]

Vascular Access

Catheter Disconnection Steps:[72]

1. **Perform hand hygiene and put on new, clean gloves**.
2. **Clamp the catheter**. (NOTE: **Always** clamp a catheter limb before your take off a cap. **Never** leave an uncapped catheter unattended.)
3. **Disinfect the hub** before putting on a new cap, using an appropriate antiseptic:
   - (*Optional*) Disinfect the connection before disconnecting the bloodlines.
   - Disconnect the bloodline from the catheter and disinfect the hub with a new antiseptic pad. Scrub the sides (threads) and end of the hub thoroughly, using friction, and remove any residue (e.g., blood).
   - Use a separate pad for each hub. Leave each hub "open" (i.e., uncapped and disconnected) for the shortest time possible.
4. **Always handle catheter hubs aseptically**. Once disinfected, do not let the catheter hubs touch nonsterile surfaces. Hold the catheter until the antiseptic has dried.
5. **Attach the new sterile caps to the catheter aseptically**. Use caution if tape is used to secure caps to the catheter. Tape can leave residue on the hubs that can make it difficult to disinfect them later. (NOTE: Your clinic may use end caps that kill bacteria i.e., ClearGuard® HD.)
6. **Ensure that catheter is still clamped**.
7. **Remove gloves and perform hand hygiene.**

TO CHANGE A CATHETER DRESSING

Change the dressing at each treatment and teach the patient to keep it clean and dry.[54] Dressings must also be replaced if they become damp, loose, or soiled.

1. **Perform hand hygiene and put on new, clean gloves**.
2. **Clean the skin around the catheter *twice***, starting at the exit site and working outward in a 10 cm circle. Chlorhexidine requires a scrubbing motion.
3. **Gently swab the top and bottom of the tubing** starting at the exit site and working outwards, to clean the section of the catheter next to the skin.
4. **Let dry, then apply an antimicrobial ointment** that does not react with the catheter plastic.[72]
5. **Apply a dressing aseptically**.[72] The dressing should be sterile gauze if the patient's skin is damp and there is drainage. Gauze dressings on short-term catheters must be replaced every 2 days. If the skin is dry and drainage-free, a sterile, transparent, semipermeable dressing that covers the site can be used. Transparent dressings on short-term catheters should be replaced every 7 days in adults until the insertion site is healed (unless it is loose or soiled). Transparent dressings on tunneled-cuffed catheters should be replaced no more than once per week until the insertion site is healed, unless it is loose or soiled).
6. **Look at intact dressings to see if they are loose or soiled, and palpate them for pain or tenderness**.[72]
7. **If the patient has pain, tenderness, or a fever, the dressing should be removed so the site can be examined**.[72]
8. **The patient can shower if a cover is used to keep the dressing dry**. NOTE: One option to protect an HD catheter is to use a pocket, such as a CathGuard™ in place of gauze or tape (see Figure 41). Catheter ends are tucked into the pocket, which then taped in place on the patient's skin.

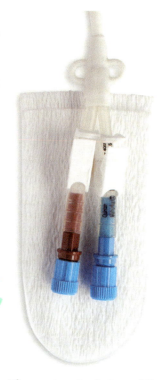

Figure 41: CathGuard™
Photo used with permission from RPC.

Complications of HD Catheters

Infection

Exit site and bloodstream infections are major risks of central venous catheters. Since the catheter is a doorway into the body, infection can go directly into the bloodstream. Catheter infections can cause hospital stays and death for patients. We use aseptic technique to help prevent them.

Catheter Disconnection

"I've seen a death from a catheter that came apart. It is heart wrenching to watch a person take their last breaths while their blood is on the floor. Don't ever cover your access or your face! It just takes a few minutes to bleed to death."

Patient safety is our main concern during HD. A catheter accident can quickly become fatal. Secure the connections and lines, and make sure you can see the catheter or needle site during the treatment. Patients can bleed to death under a blanket, or an air embolus can occur if air is sucked in through a dislodged catheter or tubing. In the event of disconnection, clamp the line clamps and hemostats and call for help. Good catheter care is good patient care.

Catheter Loss

Sometimes a catheter will come out, often when a patient is out of the clinic. Infection may make a catheter more slippery. A catheter may accidentally be pulled or tugged on. Patients may cut a stitch that causes pulling, or the hub of a new catheter may not have had time for tissue to hold it in place. Regardless of the cause, patients need to be taught what to do: **Lie flat (to reduce blood loss), hold pressure on the exit site, and call 911**.

Central Venous Stenosis

Central venous stenosis is a longer-term risk of hemodialysis catheters. How can you tell that this may be a problem? Compare your patient's arms to see if one is larger than the other. Stenosis can cause venous pressures to be high. Recent evidence suggests that venous pressures should be between 100–150 mmHg.[31] Frequent clotting of catheters is another sign of central venous stenosis.

Slow Blood Flow Rate

During an HD treatment with a catheter, watch the blood flow through the dialyzer. Note the arterial and venous pressures on the catheter to reach the prescribed blood flow. Always keep the pre-pump arterial monitor connected and open.

If pressure alarms signal that the blood flow cannot be kept at the prescribed rate:

1. **Look at the patient and the lines** to be sure there is no major bleeding or air entry. Call for help right away if there is.
2. **Next, look for a kink or blockage**. Check again that the catheter is in place.
3. **Move the patient**—lower the head of the chair, have the patient turn his head, cough, etc., to help move the tip of the catheter for better flow. The catheter may be positional.
4. **Flush the catheter with sterile saline** to help further see the condition of the catheter.
5. **"Switch" or reverse the lines** with the permission of the nurse, so blood is pulled through the "venous" limb and returns through the "arterial" limb. Reversing the lines creates recirculation, for less adequate HD. And, it does not fix the problem. Disconnecting lines to switch them is a chance for infection—and you must scrub the hub again.
6. **Ask the nurse to assess the problem**.

If these steps do not bring back the prescribed blood flow, the nurse will alert the nephrologist for further orders.

Improving Vascular Access Outcomes

Continuous Quality Improvement (CQI)

Access is often a challenge to manage. Continuous quality improvement (CQI) can be a powerful tool to help reduce the rate of access problems and reach the best outcomes (see Figure 42).

Collecting data and forming a CQI team are the first steps toward making a plan. Dialysis technicians are vital members of the team. It might be helpful to start a log or database to track access problems at your clinic. The log could include:

- Access type
- Date of placement
- Surgeon
- Type of problem
- Action taken
- Data from the One Minute Check used for access monitoring

Vascular Access

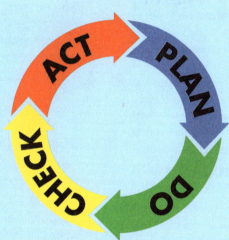

1 Identify Improvement Needs
- Collect data
- Analyze data
- Identify problem statement
- Prioritize activities

2 Analyze the Process
- Select a team
- Review the data
- Study the process/problem
- Identify patterns/trends

3 Identify Root Causes
- Identify probable root causes
- Define/refine the problem

4

ACT — Implement the solution, change or modify facility-wide tests, revise standards and specifications, incorporate revisions into day-to-day practices.

Obtain judgments of improvement achieved (performance, process measurements, outcomes); determine if solution, change, or medication has been successful. **CHECK**

PLAN — Design or redesign policies, procedures, services, or products. Specify objectives or degree of improvement desired.

Deliver care, perform policy or procedure in limited trial run. **DO**

Figure 42: CQI Process

- Clinical observations
- HD dose measures
- Rates of hospitalization, etc.

By charting this information on bar graphs, patterns can be seen. Based on a pattern, your team can make a plan to solve a problem or improve the practice or process. The patterns are only as good as the data. If the wrong data are collected, the patterns will not tell you what is going on.

Your plan should include your goals, steps to take, timetable, and a staff member to take charge of each step. Do the plan on a small scale as a trial run. (For example, try improved methods for handling access sites.) Then collect more data to check the results. Did the plan work? If it did, implement the plan in day-to-day practice and move on to another problem. If the plan did not work, rework it and try again. Recheck past findings at a later date to detect any changes.

HD clinics must report vascular access infections on their billing claim forms to CMS.[75] Any infections should be addressed through your Quality Assessment Performance Improvement (QAPI) plan and your CQI meetings.

Clinical Practice Guidelines

The KDOQI guidelines provide ways to check and preserve a patient's access. You can help protect patients' accesses when you use good technique to put in needles, help patients put the right pressure on needle sites after a treatment, and report problems to a nurse or doctor right away. The HD staff can think of ways to use the guidelines each day. The end result will be better access care for patients.

Three of the *KDOQI Guidelines for Vascular Access* are part of the ESRD Networks' Clinical Performance Measures (CPMs) project. Each year, data are collected on the percent of fistulas in new and ongoing HD patients, the percent of patients with catheters, and the way grafts are monitored for stenosis. These data are now part of the CROWNWeb data collection. Infections are reported in the CDC's National Healthcare Safety Network database, at http://www.cdc.gov/nhsn/datastat/index.html.

Patients whose accesses do not work well will not get good dialysis. They may become uremic and feel ill, tired, and not well enough to work or do other things that matter to them. Patients may lose their HD lifeline, which must then be repaired or replaced—if there is a site left. Access problems use staff time, disrupt schedules, and reduce clinic income while patients are in the hospital, too. For all of these reasons, there are two national efforts to improve access outcomes. Both share ways to assess and preserve blood vessels for fistulas and promote early fistula placement when possible:

- **The NKF Kidney Disease Outcomes Quality Initiative (KDOQI™)** – Clinical Practice Guidelines for Vascular Access.
- **Fistula First Catheter Last (FFCL)**. The FFCL has created tools to help with access planning, monitoring, catheter safety, fistula maturity and graft healing. To see these tools, visit www.esrdncc.org/.

Vascular Access Surgeons: Questions Patients Can Ask

Fistulas and grafts are made by vascular access surgeons, who specialize in working with blood vessels. However, not all vascular surgeons focus on dialysis access. They may help people who have had strokes, fix varicose veins, reattach limbs, etc.

"*Practice makes perfect*," as the saying goes, and this does seem to be true of making fistulas for dialysis. Surgeons who made *at least 25 fistulas* while in training had a 34% lower failure rate than those who did not.[76] However, two studies have found that trainees who made fistulas had outcomes just as good as those of fully trained surgeons.[77,78] The Vascular Access Society of the Americas (VASA) is a membership group for vascular access surgeons. VASA puts out the *Journal of Vascular Access*. The group has an annual meeting, and does research to advance the science of dialysis access.

Patients can ask their nephrologist who s/he would go to or send a family member to for a fistula. And, you can suggest that they ask a vascular surgeon two questions:

1. *How many fistulas did you make when you were in training?*
2. *Are you a VASA member?*

Fistula First, Catheter Last (FFCL): Increasing Use of Fistulas in the U.S.

In 2003, the Centers for Medicare & Medicaid (CMS) started to focus on having more fistulas for HD access. (The 2016 goal was 68% fistulas.) There are also new efforts to improve access monitoring and coordination, and to reduce the number of infections.

The FFCL is funded by CMS and supported by the ESRD Networks. FFCL partners are access experts: nephrologists, surgeons, nurses, primary care doctors, patients, and others. The group works to change practice and boost fistula use in HD patients who can have one. FFCL also aims to reduce the number of HD catheters, access infections, and hospitalizations.[22] The effort is guided by the 13 "Change Concepts" below. Clinics can use these concepts to help increase the rate of fistulas in their own patients:

1. **Routine continuous quality improvement (CQI) review of vascular access**
2. **Timely referral to a nephrologist**
3. **Early referral to a surgeon for "fistula only" evaluation and timely placement**
4. **Surgeon selection based on best outcomes, willingness, and ability to provide access services**
5. **Full range of surgical approaches to fistula evaluation and placement**
6. **Secondary fistula placement in patients with grafts**
7. **Fistula placement in patients with catheters, where indicated**
8. **Fistula cannulation training**
9. **Monitoring and maintenance to ensure adequate access function**
10. **Education for caregivers and patients**
11. **Outcomes feedback to guide practice**
12. **Modify hospital systems to detect CKD and promote AV fistula planning and placement**
13. **Support patient efforts to live the best possible quality of life through self-management**

You can help your clinic with FFCL. Take an active role in your clinic's vascular access CQI team. Learn how to cannulate fistulas and grafts. Help your patients understand the differences between the types of access, and why a fistula or graft is better than a catheter. And, work to improve your skills by learning more.

Conclusion

Vascular access is one of the most important and challenging parts of HD. As a dialysis technician, you have a vital role in caring for your patients' accesses. It is your job to learn how to cannulate fistulas and grafts and to observe access sites for problems. Remember that each patient's vascular access is a lifeline and must be treated with a great degree of respect and care. Proper access care and use, along with patient education, can improve and even extend your patients' lives.

References

1. Konner K. History of vascular access for haemodialysis. *Nephrol Dial Transplant.* 2005;20(12):2629-35
2. US Renal Data System 2016 annual data report: Epidemiology of kidney disease in the United States. National Institutes of Health, National Institute of Diabetes and Digestive and Kidney Diseases. Bethesda, MD. (Vol 2, Table G.13: Inpatient utilization by principal diagnosis of hospitalization: Hemodialysis)
3. Lee Y, Song D, Kim MJ, et al. Upper arm basilic vein transposition for hemodialysis: a single center study for 300 cases. *Vasc Specialist Int.* 2016;32(2):51-6
4. Maliska CM, Jennings W, Mallios A. When arteriovenous fistulas are too deep: options in obese individuals. *J Am Coll Surg.* 2015;221(6):1067-72
5. Lok CE, Sontrop JM, Tomlinson G, et al. Cumulative patency of contemporary fistulas versus grafts (2000-2010). *Clin J Am Soc Nephrol.* 2013;8(5):810-18
6. DaVita. How long can an AV fistula last? Available from: https://www.davita.com/kidney-disease/preparing-for-dialysis/planning-for-a-vascular-access/how-long-can-an-arteriovenous-av-fistula-last?/e/5033. Accessed May 2017
7. Al-Jaishi AA, Oliver MJ, Thomas SM, et al. Patency rates of the arteriovenous fistula for hemodialysis: A systematic review and meta-analysis. *Am J Kidney Dis.* 2014;63(3):464-78
8. McGrogan D, Al Shakarchi J, Khawaja A, et al. Arteriovenous fistula outcomes in the elderly. *J Vasc Surg.* 2015;62(6):1652-7
9. Hicks CW, Canner JK, Arhuidese I, et al. Mortality benefits of different hemodialysis access types are age dependent. *J Vasc Surg.* 2015;61(2):449-56
10. Ottaviani N, Deglise S, Brizzi V, et al. Early cannulation of the Flixene™ arteriovenous graft. *J Vasc Access.* 2016;17 Suppl 1:S75-8
11. O'Grady NP, Alexander M, Burns LA, et al. Healthcare Infection Control Practices Advisory Committee. Guidelines for the prevention of intravascular catheter-related infections. *Am J Infect Control.* 2011;39(4 Suppl 1):S1-34
12. Böhlke M, Uliano G, Barcellos FC. Hemodialysis catheter-related infection: prophylaxis, diagnosis and treatment. *J Vasc Access.* 2015;16(5):347-55
13. Ravani P, Palmer SC, Oliver MJ, et al. Associations between hemodialysis access type and clinical outcomes: A systematic review. *J Am Soc Nephrol.* 2013;24(3):465-73
14. Shingarev R, Barker-Finkel J, Allon M. Association of hemodialysis central venous catheter use with ipsilateral arteriovenous vascular access survival. *Am J Kidney Dis.* 2012;60(6):983-9
15. Balasubramanian S, Gupta S, Nicholls M, et al. Rare complications of a dialysis catheter insertion. *Clin Kidney J.* 2014;7(2):194-6
16. Wong K, Marks BA, Qureshi A, et al. Migration of a central venous catheter in a hemodialysis patient resulted in left atrial perforation and thrombus formation requiring open heart surgery. *A Case Rep.* 2016;7(1):21-3
17. Rivara MB, Soohoo M, Streja E, et al. Association of vascular access type with mortality, hospitalization, and transfer to in-center hemodialysis in patients undergoing home hemodialysis. *Clin J Am Soc Nephrol.* 2016;11(2):298-307
18. Fontsere' N, Mestres G, Yugueros X, et al. Effect of a postoperative exercise program on arteriovenous fistula maturation: A randomized controlled trial. *Hemodial Int.* 2016;20(2):306-14
19. Salimi F, Majd Nassiri G, Moradi M, et al. Assessment of effects of upper extremity exercise with arm tourniquet on maturity of arteriovenous fistula in hemodialysis patients. *J Vasc Access.* 2013;14(3):239-44
20. Xi W, Harwood L, Diamant MJ, et al. Patient attitudes toward the arteriovenous fistula: a qualitative study on vascular access decision making. *Nephrol Dial Transplant.* 2011;26(10):3302-8
21. Wong CS, McNicholas N, Healy D, et al. A systematic review of preoperative duplex ultrasonography and arteriovenous fistula formation. *J Vasc Surg.* 2013;57(4):1129-33
22. Thirteen change concepts for increasing AV fistulas. Available at http://fistulafirst.esrdncc.org/ffcl/change-concepts/. Accessed May 2016
23. Mid-Atlantic renal coalition. *Assessment and monitoring of the newly placed AV fistula for maturation.* Available from: http://fistulafirst.esrdncc.org/wp-content/uploads/2014/06/Final-Assessment-of-the-Newly-Placed-AVF-for-Maturation-04-09-10.pdf. Accessed May 2017
24. Beathard, GA. We refuse to give up on nonmaturing fistulas. *Semin Dial.* 2016;29(4):284-6
25. Jaberi A, Muradali D, Marticorena RM, et al. Arteriovenous fistulas for hemodialysis: application of high-frequency US to assess vein wall morphology for cannulation readiness. *Radiology.* 2011;261(2):616-24
26. Centers for Medicare and Medicaid Services. *Conditions for Coverage for End-Stage Renal Disease Facilities: Final Rule,* 73 *Federal Register* 73 (15 April 2008), p. 20459. Available at www.cms.gov/Regulations-and-Guidance/Legislation/CFCsAndCoPs/downloads/esrdfinalrule0415.pdf. Accessed June 2017
27. Fistula First, Catheter Last. Cannulation site selection and preparation. Available from http://fistulafirst.esrdncc.org/wp-content/uploads/2014/06/cannulation_of_the_AVF_Ch5.pdf. Accessed June 2017
28. Carefusion. ChloraPrep® swabstick applicator; application instructions. Available from http://www.carefusion.com/Documents/in-service-materials/IP_ChloraPrep-Swabstick-Poster_IM_EN.pdf. Accessed June 2017
29. Angelini Pharma. Procedure for use: Antisepsis preparation for graft/AVF cannulation. Available from: http://angelini-us.com/wp-content/uploads/2013/02/Preparation_for_Graft-AVF.pdf. Accessed June 2017
30. National Kidney Foundation. KDOQI clinical practice guidelines and clinical practice recommendations for 2006 updates: Hemodialysis adequacy, peritoneal dialysis adequacy, vascular access. [Guideline 3, Table 2] *Am J Kidney Dis.* 2006;48 Suppl 1:S1-S322
31. Parisotto MT, Schoder VU, Miriunis C, et al. Cannulation technique influences fistula and graft survival. *Kidney Int.* 2014;86(4):790-7
32. Ozmen S, Kadiroglu AK, Ozmen CA, et al. Does the direction of arterial needle in AV fistula cannulation affect dialysis adequacy? *Clin Nephrol.* 2008;70(3):229-32
33. Woodson RD, Shapiro RS. Antegrade vs. retrograde cannulation for percutaneous hemodialysis. *Dial Transplant.* 1974;29-30
34. Nesrallah GE. Pro: Buttonhole cannulation of arteriovenous fistulae. *Nephrol Dial Transplant.* 2016;31(4):520-3
35. Muir CA, Kotwal SS, Hawley CM, et al. Buttonhole cannulation and clinical outcomes in a home hemodialysis cohort and systematic review. *Clin J Am Soc Nephrol.* 2014;9(1):110-9
36. O'Brien FJ, Kok HK, O'Kane C, et al. Arterio-venous fistula buttonhole cannulation technique: a retrospective analysis of infectious complications. *Clin Kidney J.* 2012;5(6):526-9
37. Béchade C, Goovaerts T, Cougnet P, et al. Buttonhole cannulation is not associated with more AVF infections in a low-care satellite dialysis unit: a long-term longitudinal study. *PLoS One.* Nov. 17, 2015. Available from https://doi.org/10.1371/journal.pone.0142256. Accessed June 2017
38. Castro MC, Silva Cde F, Souza JM, et al. Arteriovenous fistula cannulation by buttonhole technique using dull needle. *J Bras Nefrol.* 2010;32(3):281-5
39. Ball LK. Improving arteriovenous fistula cannulation skills. *Nephrol Nurs J.* 2005;32(6):611-8

40. Ball LK. The buttonhole technique for arteriovenous fistula cannulation. *Nephrol Nurs J*. 2006;33(3):299-304
41. Ball LK, Mott S. How do you prevent indented buttonhole sites? *Nephrol Nurs J*. 2010;37(4):427-8, 431
42. Collier S, Kandil H, Yewnetu E, et al. Infection rates following buttonhole cannulation in hemodialysis patients. *Ther Apher Dial*. 2016;20(5):476-82
43. Labriola L, Crott R, Desmet C, et al. Infectious complications following conversion to buttonhole cannulation of native arteriovenous fistulas: a quality improvement report. *Am J Kidney Dis*. 2011;57(3):442-8
44. Marticorena RM, Hunter J, Macleod S, et al. The salvage of aneurysmal fistulae utilizing a modified buttonhole cannulation technique and multiple cannulators. *Hemodial Int*. 2006;10(2):193-200
45. Mott S, Prowant BF. The "touch cannulation" technique for hemodialysis. *Nephrol Nurs J*. 2008;35(1):65-6
46. Wani AL, Ara A, Bhat SA. Blood injury and injection phobia: the neglected one. *Behav Neurol*. 2014;2014:471340. doi: 10.1155/2014/471340
47. Peterson AL, Isler WC 3rd. Applied tension treatment of vasovagal syncope during pregnancy. *Mil Med*. 2004;169(9):751-3
48. Kamata T, Tomita M, Iehara N. Ultrasound-guided cannulation of hemodialysis access. *Renal Replace Ther*. 2016;2:7
49. Kumbar L, Soi V, Adams E, et al. Coronal mode ultrasound guided hemodialysis cannulation: a pilot randomized comparison with standard cannulation technique. *Hemodial Int*. 2017 Jan 9. Doi:10.1111/hdi.12535 [Epub ahead of print]
50. Centers for Medicare and Medicaid Services, HHS. ESRD surveyor training interpretive guidance. Final Version 1.1. October 3, 2008 (V Tag 456) Available at https://www.cms.gov/Medicare/Provider-Enrollment-and-Certification/GuidanceforLawsAndRegulations/Downloads/esrdpgmguidance.pdf Accessed June 2017
51. Çelik G, Özbek O, Yilmaz M, et al. Vapocoolant spray vs lidocaine/prilocaine cream for reducing the pain of venipuncture in hemodialysis patients: a randomized, placebo-controlled crossover study. *Int J Med Sci*. 2011;8(7):623-7
52. Kundu S, Achar S. Principles of office anesthesia: part II. Topical anesthesia. *Am Fam Physician*. 2002;66(1):99-102
53. Brouwer, DJ. Cannulation camp: basic needle cannulation training for dialysis staff. *Dial Transplant*. 2011;40(10):434-9 Available from http://onlinelibrary.wiley.com/doi/10.1002/dat.20622/full. Accessed November 2016
54. National Kidney Foundation (NKF). KDOQI clinical practice recommendations for 2006 Updates: Hemodialysis adequacy, peritoneal dialysis adequacy and vascular access. *Am J Kidney Dis*. 48(suppl 1):S1-S322, 2006
55. Merit Medical. HeRO® graft. Available from: https://www.merit.com/peripheral-intervention/access/renal-therapies-accessories/merit-hero-graft/. Accessed June 2017
56. Rothera C, McCallum C, Huang S, et al. The influence of between-needle cannulation distance on the efficacy of hemodialysis treatments. *Hemodial Int*. 2011;15(4):546-52
57. Brouwer DJ. The road to improvement? Part 2. The care and feeding of the AV fistula. *Nephrol News Issues*. 2003;17(7):48-51
58. Dinwiddie LC (ed.). Flipping or rotating fistula needles: readers' responses. *ANNA J*. 1997;24(5):559-60
59. Brouwer DJ, Peterson P. The arteriovenous graft: how to use it effectively in the dialysis unit. *Nephrol News Issues*. 2002;16(12):41-4, 46, 48-9
60. Ball LK. Fatal vascular access hemorrhage: reducing the odds. *Nephrol Nurs J*. 2013;40(4):297-303
61. Centers for Medicare and Medicaid Services, HHS. ESRD surveyor training interpretive guidance. Final Version 1.1. October 3, 2008 (V Tag 405 and 407) Available at https://www.cms.gov/Medicare/Provider-Enrollment-and-Certification/GuidanceforLawsAndRegulations/Downloads/esrdpgmguidance.pdf Accessed June
62. NHS Purchasing and Supply Agency. Evidence review: Redsense blood loss detection device for venous needle dislodgement monitoring in haemodialysis. March 2009. Available from: http://www.renal.org/docs/default-source/patient-safety-docs/patient-safety-reports/redsense---cep08050-mar-09.pdf?sfvrsn=2 Accessed June 2017
63. RedSense Medical AB. Veteran affairs announces that Redsense alarm will be mandatory on patients by November 1, 2010. PRNewswire. August 25, 2010. Available from http://www.prnewswire.com/news-releases/veteran-affairs-announces-that-redsense-alarm-will-be-mandatory-on-patients-by-november-1-2010-101462114.html. Accessed June 2017
64. Ball LK. Are YOU ready for a vascular access rupture? KidneyViews blog. *Home Dialysis Central*, Medical Education Institute, March 12, 2015. Available from http://www.homedialysis.org/news-and-research/blog/91-are-you-ready-for-a-vascular-access-rupture. Accessed November 2016
65. Achneck HE, Sileshi B, Li M, et al. Surgical aspects and biological considerations of arteriovenous fistula placement. *Semin Dial*. 2010;23(1):25-33
66. Mudoni A, Cornacciari M, Gallieni M, et al. Aneurysms and pseudoaneurysms in dialysis access. *Clin Kidney J*. 2015;8(4):363-7
67. Pandolfe LR Malamis AP, Peirce K. Treatment of hemodialysis graft pseudoaneurysms with stent grafts: institutional experience review of the literature. *Semin Inervent Radiol*. 2009:26(2):89-95
68. Beathard G. Fistula First Catheter Last. *A practitioner's resource guide to hemodialysis arteriovenous fistulas*. Available from https://pdfs.semanticscholar.org/b325/92e5b6489aaf6af4a7d4a3987e23dc0e20fc.pdf. Accessed June 2017
69. Agarwal AK. Central vein stenosis: current concepts. *Adv Chronic Kidney Dis*. 2009;16(5):360-70
70. Schild AF, Perez E, Gillaspie E, et al. Arteriovenous fistulae vs. arteriovenous grafts: a retrospective review of 1,700 consecutive vascular access cases. *J Vasc Access* 2008;9(4):231-5
71. End-Stage Renal Disease Network Coordinating Center. *It only takes a minute to save your lifeline*. Available from http://fistulafirst.esrdncc.org/wp-content/uploads/2015/01/patient-complete-guide.pdf. Accessed June 2017
72. O'Grady NP, Alexander M, Burns LA, et al. Centers for Disease Control. *Guidelines for the prevention of intravascular catheter-related infections, 2011.* Available from https://www.cdc.gov/hai/pdfs/bsi-guidelines-2011.pdf. Accessed June 2017
73. National Center for Emerging and Zoonotic Infectious Diseases, Division of Healthcare Quality Promotion. Centers for Disease Control. *Hemodialysis central venous catheter scrub-the-hub protocol*. Available from https://www.cdc.gov/dialysis/pdfs/collaborative/hemodialysis-central-venous-catheter-sth-protocol.pdf. Accessed June 2017
74. California Pacific Medical Center. *Your dialysis catheter*. Available from http://www.cpmc.org/learning/documents/dialysiscath.pdf. Accessed June 2017
75. Medicare Claims Processing Manual. *Chapter 8 – Outpatient ESRD hospital, independent facility, and physician/supplier claims*. Available from https://www.cms.gov/Regulations-and-Guidance/Guidance/Manuals/downloads/clm104c08.pdf, Accessed June 2017
76. Goodkin DA, Pisoni RL, Locatelli F, et al. Hemodialysis vascular access training and practices are key to improved access outcomes. *Am J Kidney Dis*. 2010 Dec;56(6):1032-42
77. McGrogan DG, Maxwell AP, Inston NG, et al. Preserving arteriovenous fistula outcomes during surgical training. *J Vasc Access*. 2014;15(6):474-80
78. Barnes R, Smith GE, Chetter IC. A prospective observational study to assess the impact of operator seniority on outcomes following arteriovenous fistula formation. *J Vasc Access*. 2015;16(5):372-6

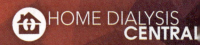

Appendix A:

A How-To Manual: The Art of Teaching Buttonhole Self-Cannulation

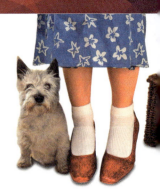

Background

Dialysis needles are large and scary! Fear of needles and pain is a reality for most people on dialysis, especially in the beginning. Some have true phobia, and require special techniques and interventions to self-cannulate. All patients, once they become familiar with dialysis, worry about who will put their needles in (and potentially cause access damage that can lead to a hospital stay, surgery, or loss of their lifeline). Some even avoid travel because they don't want an unknown staff person to cannulate them. All of these fears can reduce quality of life. Patients who cannulate themselves learn to overcome these fears—and this task is not as formidable as it may seem.

Patients who can see and use their hands well enough to self-cannulate are their own best cannulators. Why? Because patients are the only ones who can feel both ends of the needle. They can better control the angle and direction of the needle. They can tell when the tip of the needle is in the vessel. Thus, patients are far less likely to infiltrate themselves than a dialysis staff member or a care partner. A fistula with a consistent cannulator, i.e. a self-cannulator, may work longer and have fewer problems than one with multiple cannulators. There is even some evidence that self-cannulation is more comfortable for the patient, i.e., less painful.[1-2] Surprisingly, there are very few studies in the literature on cannulation technique.

The information in this manual is based on extensive clinical experience and observation. The techniques mentioned in this work have been published in peer-reviewed journals. Can your patients succeed with self-cannulation? The answer is a resounding **YES**! In this **FREE** manual, compiled by the non-profit Medical Education Institute (MEI) for its Home Dialysis Central website (www.homedialysis.org), we will be discussing:

I) **Pre-cannulation Education** – to help patients overcome fear of needles

II) **Tandem-Hand Cannulation** – guided help in learning to cannulate

III) **Touch Cannulation** – a method of holding cannulation tubing, to afford better control

IV) **Buttonhole Technique** – faster and less painful[2] than rope-ladder rotation, but with fewer aneurysms and infiltrations[3]

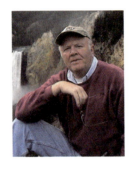

Stuart Mott
Vascular Access Nurse
Columbia, MO

"Because my ultimate aim was to do dialysis at home, I knew I would have to learn to needle myself. But, at first, I could not even watch the nurse needle me! I started by watching her insert needles out of the corner of my eye. Gradually, by an effort of will, I was able to watch the whole process without blinking. I watched her technique very carefully. After doing this for about 6 weeks, I felt ready to take the next step.

I visualized myself asking the nurse to allow me to have a turn myself. Finally I took a deep breath and asked to insert my own needle. It was easier than I thought and the nurse commended me on my excellent technique. These needles were the very fine ones used for local anesthetic. I simply repeated the process, when I felt brave enough, to cannulate with the large dialysis needles."

— Home dialysis patient

I. Pre-cannulation Education: Countdown to Cannulation

Four weeks prior to initiating self cannulation:

Step 1 – Teach the patient:

- How his or her access works, fistula vs. graft
- Importance of the blood flow rate
- Impact of access flow on dialysis adequacy
- Size and type of needles used, including gauge; (17,16,15,14), length (3/5", 1", 1-1/4"); and sharp or blunt
- Presence of any side vessels branching from fistula and why they are important
- How to assess his or her access before each session: Show how you check the pulse and thrill, then have the patient do it; explain how to recognize problems
- Anything else your clinic feels is important

Step 2 – Show the patient how you find the *bruit* with your stethoscope. Describe the sound and what it means. Then, have the patient find the *bruit* with his or her own stethoscope and describe the sound. You can listen to a bruit on this Youtube video: https://www.youtube.com/watch?v=ztt72ik9ouY

Your clinic doesn't use stethoscopes to listen to *bruits*? It should. *KDOQI Vascular Access Guidelines*[4] recommend that patients become familiar with their accesses and check them on a daily basis, including the pulse, thrill, and *bruit*. Training materials such as the *Core Curriculum for the Dialysis Technician*[5] also suggest that the cannulator check the access prior to cannulation, including the *bruit*. It is in your patients' best interests to add this check, and stethoscopes can be very inexpensive.

Three weeks prior to cannulation:

Step 1 – Have the patient assess all aspects of his or her access as you've instructed, making sure that the access is in good condition for cannulation. This must become a ritual.

Step 2 – Discuss proper handwashing (**Fig. 1**) and the need for cleanliness to maintain a trouble-free access. Have the patient show you how to use the proper technique.

Step 3 – Put a glove onto the patient's cannulating hand. (**Fig. 2**) Ask, "What does this feel like to you?" Many will say, "It's like being on TV, you know, like ER." This is a motivational step that can help engage the patient in the process of taking control of his or her care.

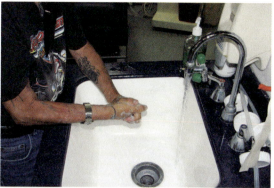

Figure 1

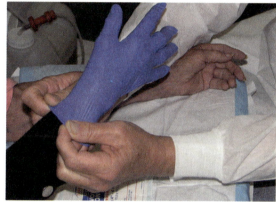

Figure 2

> **WORDS COUNT**
> Avoid using the word "stick," which can stress the patient. Criminals stick up banks and convenience stores; we *cannulate* dialysis accesses!

Appendix A (continued)

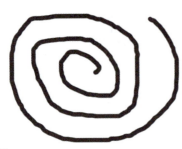

Figure 3

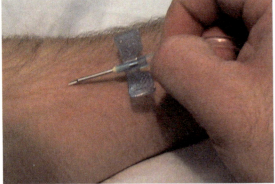

Figure 4 NOTE: Wear gloves to cannulate! This photo omits them only to show the correct finger positions.

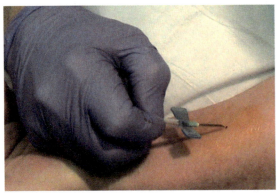

Figure 5

> **NEEDLE LENGTH**
> Consider needle length. Using unnecessarily long needles can frighten patients and increase the risk of infiltration. Most forearm AV fistulas are shallow, so a 3/5-inch long needle will reduce the risk of infiltration and vessel wall damage. An upper arm or leg access will probably require a 1-inch long needle.

Two weeks prior to cannulation:

Step 1 – Have patient assess his or her access.

Step 2 – Have the patient show you how to prepare his or her access for cannulation, following your clinic's Standard Operating Procedure, as you have taught.

Step 3 – Have the patient wash his or her hands and arm.

Step 4 – Follow handwashing with a Betadine® cleanse. Scrub in a spiral (**Fig. 3**) motion, moving outward from the cannulation site. Then, have the patient practice this technique.

One week prior to cannulation:

Have patient demonstrate all of the previous steps.

Step 1 – Following your clinic's policy for needle gauge, explain the types of needles you use and why. (For example, our clinic starts with a 17 gauge needle for one treatment, switches to 16 gauge needles for the next three treatments, then goes to 15 gauge needles.)

Step 2 – Give the patient a blunt needle to practice with at home. During the next week, the patient can wear gloves and touch the needle to the skin at the sites where the Buttonholes will be formed. This practice will help eliminate a lot of the nervousness about the needle and having the needle touch the skin, which can make the process less stressful for the patient when the time comes to cannulate. (**Fig. 4**)

> **Reading glasses**
> Be sure that you and your patients can see the cannulation sites! About 40% of our patients need reading glasses to cannulate. To check vision, place a small black dot on the patient's arm with a Sharpie marker. (**Fig. 5**) Have the patient try to line up the needle tip with the black dot. If they can't do it, they need glasses! A patient who wears bifocals may still need a pair of reading glasses to cannulate with. Local drug and "big box" stores carry reading glasses from 1.5 to 3.0 diopters in the range of $2-5/pair. Keep a few pairs on hand in the clinic for patients—and staff.

II. Tandem-Hand Cannulation

During the precannulation phase, you talked the patient though each step and answered questions. Now, it is time to move on to cannulation itself. NOTE: Wear gloves to cannulate!

Tandem-Hand cannulation,[6] is a hands-on method where you work one-on-one with the patient to insert the needles.

Step 1 – As with all cannulation, manipulation of the needle is the most critical aspect. The first step in using the Tandem-Hand method is learning how to "set" and use the cannulating hand. The hand is anchored by resting it on the patient's arm. This produces a solid base, so that with the fingers "cocked," the needle tip is at the insertion site. Then all you have to do to cannulate is move the thumb and forefinger forward. (**Fig. 6**)

Step 2 – To initiate the self-cannulation process, have the patient place his or her thumb and forefinger directly behind your thumb and forefinger. Have the patient squeeze your fingers—tightly enough to feel your thumb and forefinger moving forward to insert the needle. The patient will feel the needle go through the skin and feel the motion to cannulate at the same time. Follow this practice for several treatments, until the patient is ready to move on to the next step.

When both you and the patient feel comfortable with the process, move on. Talk with the patient. The training time will be different for each patient—and confidence is the key to success. When the patient feels comfortable with and is consistent with the process it is time to move on. (**Fig. 7**)

Step 3 – Now, have the patient trade hand positions. Place your forefinger and thumb directly behind the patient's thumb and forefinger. This lets you have a modicum of control if something should go awry, and provides the patient with a sense of security that eliminates a lot of the stress, hesitation, and jerky movements that could otherwise hinder self-cannulation. (**Fig. 8**)

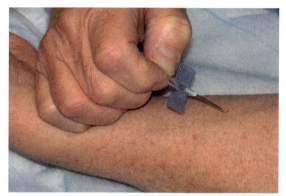

Figure 6 NOTE: Wear gloves to cannulate! This photo omits them only to show the correct finger positions.

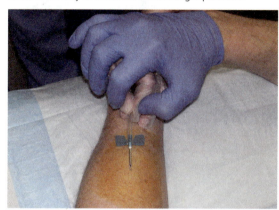

Figure 7

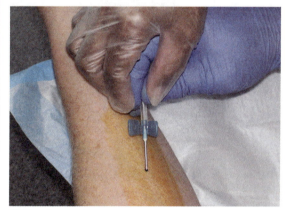

Figure 8

PHOTO DISCLAIMER
Some of the following pictures are shown without gloves so you can better see the position of the thumb and forefinger, which is key to this method. They are not of actual patients, but rather training photos made with a technician.

Appendix A (continued)

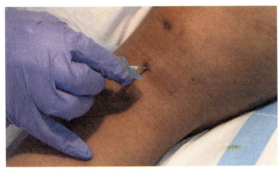

Figure 9

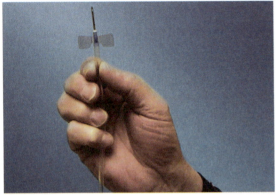

Figure 10

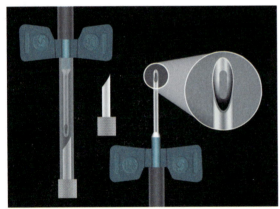

Figure 11

BUTTONHOLE OPTIONS IN EUROPE
Those of you outside the USA have two options that are not available in the USA: a specially designed plastic peg,[8] or a catheter that can be implanted in the needle tract for this purpose.[9]

Step 4 – Continue the Tandem-Hand process until both of you feel comfortable and secure that the patient can cannulate with minimal supervision. Then, remove your hand and allow the patient to self-cannulate alone. Continue to observe closely, offering encouragement, support, and guidance as needed. (**Fig 9**)

Patient can choose not to self-cannulate
If at some point, after sufficient time self-cannulating, the patient prefers to have a staff member cannulate him or her, that option should be available. Try to determine why, though, because it may be something as simple as the need for re-education on some point. Even if a patient chooses not to self-cannulate after this education, he or she will understand the access and cannulation process much better, which will help ease fears—and empower the patient to catch potential staff errors before they can harm the access.

III. Touch Cannulation

Touch cannulation[7] is a method that differs from standard cannulation, in that the cannulator *holds the tubing* [about 1.9 – 2.5 cm (3/4 – 1 inch) behind the needle] *rather than the needle wings*. Holding the tubing allows the cannulator to feel what the tip of the needle is doing. This technique is especially useful for the Buttonhole technique, as it gives the needle tip a little "wiggle room" to find its own way down a Buttonhole tract, preventing damage to the tract. (**Fig. 10**)

IV. The Buttonhole Technique

The Buttonhole technique, or "constant-site" cannulation, was developed by Dr. Zbylut Twardowski[2] and has been in use since 1977 in Europe. With this method, instead of rotating needle sites, needles are placed into the *exact same spot at the exact same angle*. It usually takes 6-8 consecutive treatments to form a tunnel tract. If you have trouble forming a Buttonhole tract, use a sharp needle for another couple of treatments until the tunnel is developed. Once a tract is formed, change to a blunt Buttonhole needle to avoid damaging the tract with the cutting edge of a sharp needle. (**Fig. 11**)

Vascular Access

> **WEAR GLOVES**
> A reminder, anyone who may come in contact with the needle or the patient's skin must wear gloves.

> **BUTTONHOLE TECHNIQUE CAUTION**
> The Buttonhole technique can be used only in an AV fistula—NOT a graft. Fistula walls have muscle fibers that will "snap" shut after the dialysis needle is removed, preventing excess bleeding. Artificial graft walls have no muscle fibers, so "coring" will result: the needle cuts a hole in the graft wall, causing it to leak blood into the surrounding tissue, and creating a risk of exsanguination and death.

It is best if the patient forms his or her own Buttonhole tracts. Why? There are a limited number of positions in which a self-cannulator can comfortably anchor his or her hand to achieve the correct needle angle. It is easier for a patient to duplicate an angle if the site and angle are ones that are best suited to the *patient*—not the staff person. Also, if patients are comfortable only with blunt Buttonhole needles, they may be at a loss if they choose home hemodialysis and later need to start new Buttonholes.

Cannulating Buttonholes

Show the patient how a Buttonhole is like a pierced earring track by sliding a needle into an end-cap. For a shallow forearm AV fistula where you will be using a ³/₅" cannulation needle, use a quarter of a cap, about ¼". For an access requiring a longer needle, such as an upper arm fistula, use the longer needle and an end-cap cut to about ½". (**Fig. 12**)

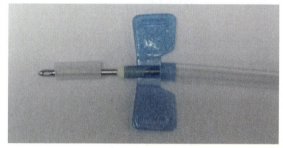
Figure 12

Step 1 – Clean the access site. The fistula must be prepared following established clinic protocol. Remove the scabs covering the tracts from the previous treatment and then wash the Buttonhole sites. (**Fig.13**)

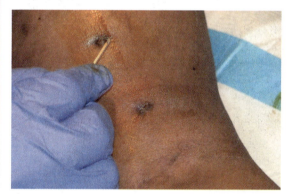
Figure 13

Step 2 – Show the patient how to hold the needle, where to anchor the heel of his or her hand, and how to "cock" his or her fingers in preparation to cannulate. (**Fig. 14**) Demonstrate how you grasp the needle so it's ready to insert: Hold the tubing behind the needle with your thumb and forefinger, then curl all four fingers underneath it. Reiterate hand placement and needle angle. Using a 20° to 25° angle will establish a flap in the vessel wall that will heal well, and reduce the risk of infiltration.

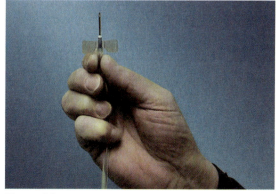
Figure 14

Appendix A (continued)

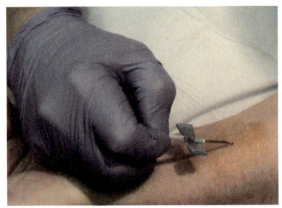

Figure 15

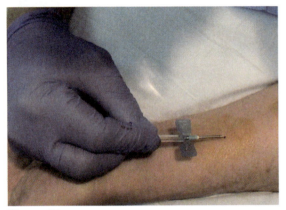

Figure 16

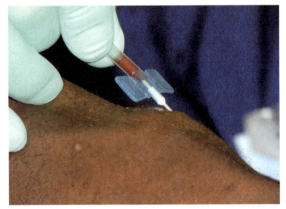

Figure 17

> **SCAB REMOVAL**
> Use of fingernails, toothpicks, and other non-sterile tools has led to Buttonhole tract infections which can result in sepsis.

Step 3 – Have the patient anchor his or her hand in a comfortable position relative to the cannulation site, with fingers cocked, and the needle tip at the buttonhole site. (**Figs. 15 & 16**) Then all he or she needs to do to cannulate is to advance the thumb and finger. Advance the needle to cannulate. If resistance is felt, move your fingers closer to the wings for more stability.

Step 4 – When the patient is ready, have him or her hold the tubing. Following the Tandem-Hand Technique, as outlined above, continue the cannulation process by placing your hand over the patient's hand, so that s/he can guide the needle into the Buttonhole. Watch for the flashback. Then remove your hand so s/he can finish sliding the needle into the access. Avoid sudden, jerky movements. When you take your hand off and the patient finishes, he or she will realize that self-cannulation was a success. This can be an amazing discovery! They may say, "I can do this!" And you can respond, "Yes, you sure can!" (**Fig. 17**)

Conclusion

It is generally accepted that patients who are more involved in their care have better outcomes. They don't rely entirely on their doctors and nurses; they take ownership of their care and control of their lives. They lose their fear of dialysis, of pain, of infiltrations, and of access problems, because they have become empowered and are no longer dependent. You can help! If good education and encouragement are provided, a large number of patients will become self-cannulators, which, in turn, will lighten the staff load. Fewer access problems and hospitalizations translate into money saved, thus lowering the burden of providing dialysis care.

Some of our older population and those with true needle phobia will always want the dialysis staff to cannulate them. This should not, however, relieve them from responsibility for their care. The staff cannulator should start the session with something like "I'll be cannulating you today" and then say, "Please tell me about your access." An empowered patient should be able to provide all the information as outlined above such as thrill, *bruit*, needle angle, deep or shallow, what blood flow was used last session, etc. Offer to answer any questions the patient has. This routine in and of itself is an opportunity to continue the education process, which will help both the cannulator and the patient. With this kind of patient input, cannulation time should be minimal, as the patient will alert the cannulator of any problems that have developed with the access, e.g. areas to avoid, making it easier for the cannulator to be successful on the initial try— which makes everyone happy.

References

1) http://www.esrdncc.org/en/fistula-first-catheter-last/ffcl-for-patients/. Accessed 2/17/17.

2) Twardowski Z, Kubara H. Different sites versus constant sites of needle insertion into arteriovenous fistula for treatment by repeated dialysis. *Dial Transplant* 8:978-80, 1979.

3) Van Loon MM, Goovaerts T, Kessels AGH, van der Sande FM, Tordoir JHM. Buttonhole needling of haemodialysis arteriovenous fisulae results in less complications and interventions compared to the rope-ladder technique. *Nephrol Dial Transplant.* 25:225-230, 2010.

4) *National Kidney Foundation: KDOQI Clinical Practice Guidelines for Hemodialysis Adequacy,* 2000. *Am J Kidney Dis* 37:S7-S64, 2001 (suppl 1)

5) *Core Curriculum for the Dialysis Technician: A Comprehensive Review of Hemodialysis.* Sixth Edition. Module 6: Vascular Access. Developed by Medical Education Institute.

6) Mott S, Moore H. Using 'Tandem hand' technique to facilitate self-cannulation in hemodialysis. *Nephrol Nurs J.* 36(3):313-316, 2009.

7) Mott S, Prowant BF. The "touch cannulation" technique for hemodialysis. *Nephrol Nurs J.* 35(1):65-66, 2008.

8) Toma S, Shinzato T, Fukui H, Nakai S, Miwa M, Takai I, Maeda K. A timesaving method to create a fixed puncture route for the buttonhole technique. *Nephrol Dial Transplant.* 18(10):2118-2121, 2003.

9) Marticorena RM, Hunter J, Cook R, Kashani M, Delacruz J, Petershofer E, Macleod S, Dacouris N, McFarlane PA, Donnelly SM, Goldstein MB. A simple method to create buttonhole cannulation tracks in a busy hemodialysis unit. *Hemodial Int.* Jul;13(3):316-321, 2009.

7 Hemodialysis Procedures and Complications

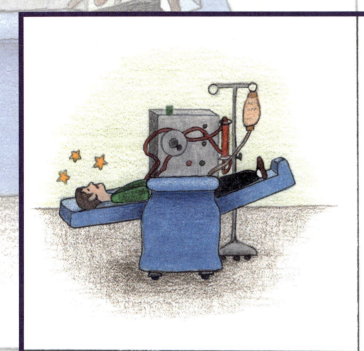
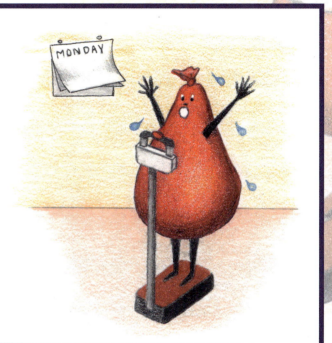
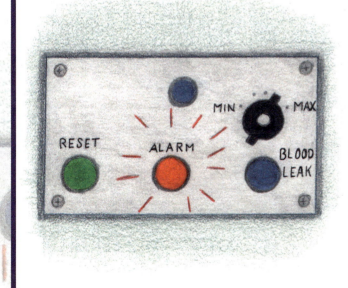
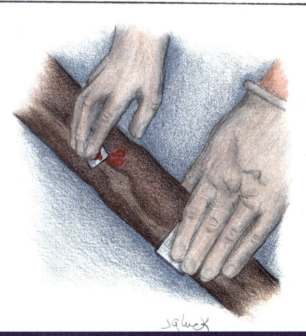

Cover art by Judith Gluck

"This is the first time in nearly 2 years that I have had to have a machine changed out during my run. It was making strange noises and then it just shut off. The girls in this clinic ROCK! My tech was right on top of it and one of the others came over to help her out. I love my clinic."

Objectives

MODULE AUTHORS

Joan Arslanian, MS, MPA, MSN, RN, FNP-BC, CS, CNN, CHN, CPDN

Lynda Ball, MSN, RN, CNN

Silvia German, RN, CNN

Debbie McDillon, MSN, RN, CNN

Heather Paradis, CHT

Eileen Peacock, MSN, RN, CNN, CIC, CPHQ, CLNC

RJ Picciano, BA, CHT, OCDT, CHBT

Tia Sabin, CHT

MODULE REVIEWERS

Rachelle Barclay, RN, CDN

Nancy M. Gallagher, BS, RN, CNN

Melinda Martin-Lester, RN, BA, CNN, CHC

Darlene Rodgers, BSN, RN, CNN, CPHQ

John H. Sadler, MD

Dori Schatell, MS

Vern Taaffe, BS, CBNT, CDWS

Tamyra Warmack, RN

Practice Test Questions at:
www.meiresearch.org/cc6

After you complete this module, you will be able to:

1. Explain your role in preventing the spread of infection in the dialysis clinic.
2. Outline three ways to draw a blood sample.
3. Demonstrate how to draw up and give intravenous medications.
4. Define "body mechanics" and explain how you will use them in patient care.
5. Describe how to set up the hemodialysis machine and extracorporeal circuit.
6. Review the vital signs that are monitored before, during, and after treatments.
7. Explain the procedures done at the beginning, during, and at the end of a routine treatment.
8. List three reasons why it is vital to document patient care.
9. Describe some of the medical and technical complications that can occur during dialysis.
10. Discuss dialysis adequacy and how and why to measure it.

An acronym list can be found in the Glossary.

Introduction

Dialysis is a complex process with many steps. Each step is crucial to keep patients safe and maintain their comfort. You will see that *safety*—for your patients and for you—is a theme in this module and all of the other modules as well. Errors that could harm patients can occur at any step, and you have a major role in being watchful and helping to prevent them. **The more you know and the more vigilant you are, the safer your patients will be, and the safer you will be, too**.

This module covers patient care and treatment tasks you will need to learn to give safe and effective HD treatments, from set-up through clean-up. Your exact tasks will vary with the rules and laws in each state, and with your clinic's policies. Patient assessment is the job of registered nurses, for example. But, you can help when you gather data, note and share your observations and concerns, and give your input into the care plan. You will also learn about procedures and complications that can occur.

Infection Control

"Our staff wash their hands after everything they do, wear protective guards, gloves, and gowns. I can't fault their cleanliness at all. The infection control in our clinic is second to none!"

Infection is the third most common cause of death in HD patients. More than 15% of patient deaths—nearly one in six—are from infections each year; mainly blood infections.[1] Many of these can be prevented—with YOUR help.

Pathogens (bacteria, viruses, fungi) that enter the body can cause infection. The most common ones live on the skin and on *mucous membranes* (e.g., the lining of the nose, mouth, genitals, urinary tract, and bowels). Some are found in the soil, in water, or on clothing. Pathogens can live on *all* surfaces.

Patients who get infections at dialysis often need to be in the hospital, sometimes for weeks. An infection and treatment are painful and costly for the patient and family. It is up to you to give the level of care that you would want for yourself or a loved one.

How Infections Spread

"I know that the staff are supposed to change gloves before each step, but once they do, they sometimes touch things other than my access (i.e., the machine, equipment etc.)."

Germs that are harmless in one place, like the skin or gut, can be lethal in another—like the lungs or bloodstream. Some pathogens are more dangerous than others. And, some are more *communicable* (easy to spread) than others. Healthcare-associated infections (HAIs) are picked up in a hospital or other healthcare setting. Your goal is to prevent them in your clinic.

Infection can occur when pathogens enter your body through:

- **Your mucous membranes** – like a splash in the eye, touching the nose, food poisoning, or a sexually transmitted disease
- **Your lungs** – by breathing in pathogens
- **A break in your skin** – from a scratch, cut, bite, or trauma
- **Your bloodstream** – from a needle or trauma

Whether you will get an infection from a pathogen you are exposed to depends on the type of germ and the strength of your immune system. If you are healthy, your immune system may work quite well. *Patients on HD tend to have weakened immune systems*. So, they are much more vulnerable to infection and they have a harder time fighting one off if they do catch one. In a dialysis clinic, pathogens can be spread by patients, staff, visitors, equipment, water, dialysate, and air (see Table 1).

In most cases, infection is spread by staff who do not wash their hands. The problem of infection in dialysis clinics is getting worse:

- Between 2011 and 2014, the number of clinics cited by CMS surveyors for errors in hand hygiene rose from **31.4%** to **42.4%** (a 35% increase).[2]
- Failure to properly disinfect the dialysis station rose from **29.2%** to **33.6%** (a 15% increase).[2]
- Improper care of HD catheters went up from **9.3%** to **16.9%** (an 83% increase).[2]

Table 1: Infection Transmission in a Dialysis Clinic and How You Can Prevent It

Method of Spread	How it Works	Prevention
Direct Contact *Examples*: Staph skin infection, Mononucleosis	You touch an infected person and get their germs onto your mucous membranes or into a break in your skin.	■ Wear gloves ■ Wash your hands ■ Wear a gown ■ Wear eye protection
Indirect Contact *Example*: Norovirus (a "stomach flu")	You touch a surface, like a machine, with germs on it, then touch your eyes, nose, mouth, or a wound.	■ Wear gloves ■ Wash your hands ■ Clean surfaces
Droplet *Examples*: Common cold, flu, strep throat	Someone with an infection coughs, sneezes, or laughs and spreads germ-filled droplets.	■ Wear a mask ■ Wear eye protection
Fecal-Oral *Examples*: Food poisoning, hepatitis A	Germs in the stool transfer to food or surfaces by unwashed hands or while processing animals for food. You eat the food or touch a surface, then touch your mouth.	■ Wash your hands ■ Wear gloves ■ Clean surfaces
Bloodborne *Examples*: Hepatitis B & C, HIV	Germs from someone's bloodstream get into your blood through a wound, needle stick injury, or exchange of body fluids.	■ Wear gloves ■ Wash hands ■ Use needle precautions
Waterborne *Examples*: Giardia, pyrogenic reactions	Germs in a water supply get into the gut or the bloodstream.	■ Treat dialysis water
Airborne *Examples*: Chicken pox, tuberculosis, measles	A few germs can survive for a long time in a dried out form that can float in the air, like dust. You can breathe these in.	■ Wear a mask ■ Get vaccinated

The care you take can save your patients' lives—or end them. Each time you touch your patients, you could be bringing them an infection that could harm them. Or, you could bring dangerous germs home to *your* family. Be aware of where your hands have been. **Wash your hands and put on clean gloves often, per your clinic's protocol**.

Hemodialysis Infection Control Precautions

"My husband just got out of surgery. The doctor had to remove his leg graft. It had clotted, and has a massive infection."

Centers for Disease Control and Prevention (CDC) rules help prevent infections in HD patients (see Figure 1).[3] The 2008 CMS *Conditions for Coverage* require use of the CDC rules for all dialysis patients.

Hand Hygiene

Washing your hands or using an alcohol-based hand rub is **the single *most* important thing you can do to prevent the spread of infection**. The use of "hand hygiene" protects you *and* your patients. The goal is to remove pathogens that could be transferred to patients, visitors, other staff, or surfaces. Hand hygiene can reduce infection rates, stop an outbreak of disease, and reduce the spread of drug-resistant bacteria.[4]

You may think you know how to wash your hands. After all, you have been doing it since you were a small child. But, we take extra steps in a healthcare setting to stop the spread of infection. Table 2 will tell you when and how to use soap and water vs. alcohol hand gel. NOTE: When you wash your hands as often as you need to, they are likely to become dry and/or chapped. Use hand cream approved by your clinic, after you wash your hands, to prevent dryness and chapping.

Hemodialysis Procedures and Complications

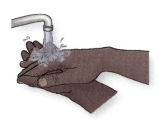
Wash hands before and after removing gloves, or after exposure to body fluids

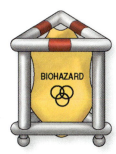
Place infectious waste in color-coded receptacles

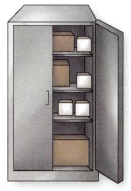
Store properly

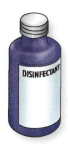
Clean all work surfaces

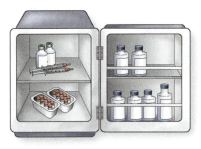
Never mix food and medical supplies in the same refrigerator

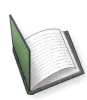
Maintain accurate records

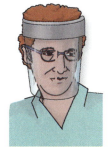
Wear personal protective equipment (PPE)

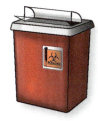
Use sharps box

Figure 1: Components of Dialysis Precautions

When to Wash Your Hands[4]

- When you arrive at the dialysis clinic
- Before you touch a patient (Patients want to see you wash your hands. They are watching!)
- Before and after you insert needle—even though you wear gloves. Gloves are not sterile. They may also have micro holes in them that could let pathogens through, and wearing gloves creates a warm microclimate on your hands that can let more bacteria grow.
- Before you touch any break in the skin—from an HD needle, surgery, a wound, etc.
- Before you put on gloves—NOTE: Take gloves out of box after you wash your hands
- Between tasks and procedures on the same patient to prevent cross contamination of different body sites
- After you touch any type of body fluid or mucous membrane
- After you touch machines, equipment, or computer keyboards
- After you take off your gloves
- When you leave the clinic (whenever you leave the treatment area)—so you do not bring germs home to your loved ones

When and How to Use Aseptic Technique

"It's our lives on the line, and we trust our lives to these professionals."

Germs grow on all surfaces. In the clinic, you will use *aseptic* (free from disease-causing germs) technique to keep objects or areas free from *all* germs long enough to be used for a treatment. Terms that relate to aseptic technique are:

211

Table 2: Hand Hygiene Options

Product	Alcohol Hand Rub[4]	Soap and Water[4,5]
When to Use	When hands are *not* visibly soiled with: ■ Dirt ■ Blood ■ Bodily fluids	■ When you can *see* that your hands are not clean ■ If you touched—or *may* have touched—*C. difficile*, *norovirus*, or *bacillus anthracis* ■ Before you eat ■ After you use the restroom
How to Use	■ Apply gel to the palm of one hand, using the amount called for on the label. ■ Rub your hands together to cover all surfaces of hands and fingers until your hands are dry.	■ Wet your hands with water. ■ Apply the amount of soap the manufacturer suggests. ■ Rub your hands together briskly for *at least 15 seconds*. ■ Cover *all* of your hands and fingers—between fingers and under nails, too. Sing "happy birthday" to yourself *twice*. ■ Hold your hands *up* and rinse with water from your fingers *down* to your wrists. ■ Dry well with a paper towel. ■ Use a paper towel to turn off the faucet (it is dirty). ■ Do not wear artificial nails. Keep nails less than ¼ inch long.

1. **Aseptic** or **Sterile** – *Completely* free of any living microorganisms.
2. **Clean** – Disinfected. Usable for some steps in the treatment, but *not* free of germs (or sterile).
3. **Contaminated** – Dirty. An item that *was* sterile or clean, but then was touched by a non-sterile object. For example, a needle or catheter cap falls onto the patient's lap or the floor. Now it is contaminated and cannot be used, or it could cause an infection.

Learn aseptic technique, understand it, watch closely, and practice it with supervision.

HOW TO USE ASEPTIC TECHNIQUE

■ **Wash your hands before you touch the package of a sterile item**. This will help keep you from getting germs on the item.
■ **Sterile items are sterile *only* if the package is closed and sealed**. Open the package just before you need the item. Once a package is open, airborne dust or droplets can land on it.
■ **Look at sterile packages carefully**. Do not use packages that are wet or may have been torn or punctured. Moisture or tears let pathogens through the wrapper to contaminate the item. A change in the wrapper color could also mean that a package may have been contaminated.

■ **A contaminated object contaminates a sterile one**. For example, when you spike a bag of saline, insert the spike directly into the port. If the tip of the spike touches the outside of the bag or *anything* unsterile—like your gloved hand—the spike is contaminated. Do not use it.
■ **Avoid cross contamination**. Do not handle medicine or clean supplies where used equipment or blood samples are kept.
■ **Before you use a multi-dose medicine vial, scrub the rubber stopper with disinfectant**. Once you open a vial, label it with the date and time and use it up per your clinic's policy (e.g., within 28 days).
■ **All fistula needles, syringe tips, and needles used to give medicines or draw blood must be sterile**. Needles enter the bloodlines or the patient's body. When you start a treatment, do not touch the fistula needle or ends of the bloodlines that are connected to the patient or dialyzer. When you attach a heparin syringe to the heparin line, do not touch the syringe tip or the end of the heparin line. **When in doubt, throw it out.**

Hemodialysis Procedures and Complications

Personal Protective Equipment (PPE)

"My line clotted, so the nurse had to change it. He took the line out, went to the sharps box with the needles, then the trash, and then he wanted to connect my new lines with the same dirty gloves on! I stopped him and said, 'You have to change your gloves.' 'Oh yeah, that's right,' he said."

During a treatment, you can be exposed to blood or body fluids so you need to wear PPE. Wearing this equipment can protect you *and* your patients. For example:

- **You must *wear* gloves when you care for a patient or touch any equipment**. *Wrapping a glove around your finger to silence an alarm is not an appropriate use of protective gear.*
- **You must *change* your gloves often**. Review *How to Use PPE* for some examples.

HOW TO REMOVE GLOVES SAFELY

Gloves that are not used the right way can spread disease. Use these steps to take off your gloves safely so you do not spray droplets of blood or body fluids around the clinic:

- Being careful not to touch your skin, pinch one glove off starting at your wrist and peel it down to your fingertips, inside out. *Never "snap" a glove.*
- Wad up the glove you took off into the palm of your gloved hand.
- With your now ungloved hand, peel the second glove off starting at the *inside* of your wrist. The first glove will now be inside the second glove, which is inside out.
- Throw out the soiled gloves promptly.

Safe Handling of Equipment and Supplies After Treatment

"When I came in, I saw techs washing down the chairs and machines and they would not seat a patient until this was done. They were courteous and professional at all times and there was a certain level of kidding around that relieved the pressure of being there at all."

Your clinic will have policies and procedures for how to handle supplies after treatment. Items used in a treatment may be contaminated with blood or body

---

How to Use PPE[3]

Change your gloves:

- Before you touch any surface—such as a machine, a chart, or a phone
- When they are soiled
- After each patient contact
- Between patients
- After you touch a sharps box or *any object that may be contaminated with blood*
- After you start a treatment

Wear a gown:

- At all times on the treatment floor—before, during, and after patient treatments. Before treatments, you will do tasks where you will handle chemicals. During treatments, blood or body fluids may splash. After treatments, you may touch equipment that is soiled with blood or body fluids.

Wear a face shield and protective eyewear:

- For tasks where droplets of blood or body fluids may spray
- At the start or end of a treatment
- When you troubleshoot a patient's access
- When you inject into the bloodlines or change a transducer protector
- Wear a mask when a catheter is open—your patient should wear a mask too
- For exposure to chemicals, e.g. when setting up the machine

Protect yourself and your coworkers from accidental needle sticks:

- Use needle-free devices and safety needles when you can.
- Never recap a used needle if there is any way to avoid it. If you must recap, use a recapping device or a one-handed method. Learn your clinic's policy and devices, if used.
- Activate the needle/device safety features after use, before you dispose of the needle.
- Do not bend, shear, or break needles.
- Dispose of needles in a sharps box and keep fingers away from the container opening.
- Always point needles away from yourself and be aware of people around you.
- Watch out for sharps that may fall into linen, beds, on the floor, or in waste containers.

213

Module 7

fluids, even if they look clean. So, *all* items—even those placed on top of the machine—must be:[3]
- **Thrown out** if they are disposable
- **Assigned to one patient** so they do not spread germs to another patient
- **Cleaned and disinfected** before they go back to a *clean area* (storage space for sterile and clean items) if they are not disposable

Learn about the "clean" and "dirty" areas in your clinic. There are rules and laws in each county and state for how to identify, handle, package, and transport infectious waste. Your clinic's policies and procedures will be based on these local and state laws. In most cases, you will:
- Throw out needles in sharps boxes. Label these and do not let them get too full.
- Throw out disposable supplies, like gloves, gauze, and gowns in "red" or color-coded garbage bags.
- Place laundry with blood or other pathogens on it in labeled or color-coded, leak-proof bags. (Some clinics *double-bag* all contaminated laundry, putting the materials into two bags.)

Any contaminated gear that is not disposable must be cleaned and disinfected per your clinic's policy. **Keep shared equipment to a minimum**. Learn which products your clinic uses and how to use them the right way.

Bloodborne Diseases

"I just got out of the hospital after a severe staph bloodborne infection. There is not 100% proof that it came from a dialysis needle, but that is what the docs think is most likely."

Three main bloodborne pathogens pose a special risk to HD patients:
- Hepatitis B
- Hepatitis C
- Human immunodeficiency virus (HIV)

CDC Tips to Prevent the Spread of Bloodborne Infection[3]

Personal Hygiene:
- Follow your clinic's hand hygiene policy and teach patients about it. Never eat, drink, smoke, put on makeup or lip balm, or touch your contact lenses in a treatment area.
- If you have a cold or cough—but are not too sick to come in to work—wear a mask all day so you do not spread germs to your patients.
- Patients who come in with coughs or colds should also wear masks.

Avoid Environmental Contamination:
- Never store food or drinks in refrigerators, freezers, shelves, cabinets, or counters where there is blood or other body fluids.
- Wash your hands before you take equipment or supplies off a cart.
- Do not use common carts or common medicine trays in the patient treatment area to prepare or give out medicines.
- Use fresh external venous and arterial pressure transducer protectors for each treatment to keep the machine's pressure monitors free from blood. Change them if they become wet with saline or blood; *do not reuse them*. If the external transducer protector is wet, ask biomed to check the internal one as well.
- Use a dedicated isolation room and machine, and a new dialyzer for patients who test positive for the hepatitis B surface antigen. Bag single-use dialyzers and blood tubing after treatment for safe disposal.
- Promptly clean up any blood.
- After each treatment, clean *all surfaces at the station with an approved disinfectant. These include the chair or bed, counters, and the outside of the machine. Pay special attention to the control panels and other surfaces that are touched a lot and may have blood on them.*
- If the dialyzer and/or blood tubing will be reprocessed, cap the ports and clamp the tubing. Place used dialyzers and tubing in leak-proof bags or tubs to take them from the station to the reprocessing or disposal site.

Hemodialysis Procedures and Complications

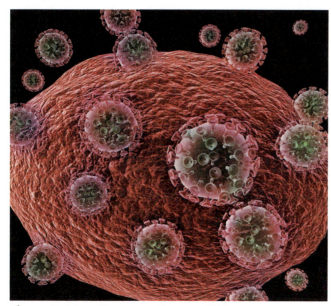

Figure 2: Bloodborne pathogen: HIV

HEPATITIS B (HBV)

Per the CDC, HBV is a highly contagious virus that attacks the liver.[3] Spread through infected blood and body fluids, HBV can cause acute disease or become chronic, where it can lead to liver cancer. The virus is hardy enough to live for 7 days or more on surfaces. Blood spills—even *dried* blood—can be infectious, and must be cleaned with a disinfectant, such as a 1:10 dilution of bleach. HBV outbreaks in HD patients can be prevented. The CDC says they are most often due to:[3]

- A sharp object, like a needle, scalpel, or broken blood tube, breaking the skin
- Broken skin or mucous membranes of the eyes, mouth, or nose coming in contact with blood
- Contaminated surfaces like the machine or chair, or supplies (i.e., clamps)
- Using single-dose drug vials for more than one patient
- Drawing up drugs for injection near areas where blood samples are handled
- Staff who care for HBV-infected and susceptible patients at the same time

Clinics can help avoid the spread of HBV if they:

- Follow the HD infection control precautions with all patients.
- Dialyze HBV-positive patients in a dedicated isolation room. Use a dedicated machine, PPE, instruments, and supplies.
- Do not let staff who care for patients with HBV care for other, susceptible (HBsAg and/or HBsAb negative) patients at the same time.
- Test patients for HBV per the CDC guidelines.
- Do not reuse the dialyzers or bloodlines of HBV-positive patients.
- Vaccinate patients *and staff against HBV.*

HEPATITIS C (HCV)

Like HBV, HCV is a virus that attacks the liver, and infection can be acute—or chronic, and can lead to liver scarring and cancer. HCV is spread by contact with infected blood and the virus can be easily killed with disinfectants and germicides. This virus is not as hardy or as easy to spread as HBV, so patients who have it do *not* need to be in isolation rooms. You can use HD infection control precautions, and dialyzers can be safely reused. The CDC recommends routine testing of dialysis patients for the virus.[3] There is no vaccine to prevent HCV in patients or dialysis staff, but there are medicines to treat this virus.

Outbreaks of HCV in dialysis clinics have been linked to these types of cross-contamination among patients:[3]

- Use of common carts to set up and give out meds
- Sharing of multi-dose drug vials that were on top of machines
- Failure to change or disinfect priming buckets between patients
- Blood spills that were not cleaned up promptly
- Movement of supply carts from one station to the next with both clean supplies and contaminated items. (Examples of these items include small biohazard containers, sharps boxes, and used blood or lab tubes with blood in them.)
- Equipment, machine surfaces, and supplies that were not disinfected between uses

In 2016, the CDC reported that more HD patients had acquired HCV while at dialysis than in the past.[6] It is vital to follow the infection control precautions and use quality improvement steps to find and address gaps. The CDC has tools to help clinics do this.

HUMAN IMMUNODEFICIENCY VIRUS (HIV)

HIV is a bloodborne virus that attacks the immune system and is the cause of acquired immune deficiency syndrome (AIDS). The virus targets T cells, which help fight infection. HIV is spread by blood, semen, vaginal fluids, and breast milk. In the general public, HIV is most often spread through sexual contact and shared IV drug needles.[7]

There have been rare cases of confirmed work-site transmission of HIV to U.S. healthcare staff. Standard HD infection control precautions and safe handling of sharps can help prevent the spread of HIV.[7] You must take HD infection control precautions, but this virus is easy to kill with bleach solution and does not live for a long time on surfaces. So, patients with HIV do not have to be isolated from other patients or use a dedicated machine. Their dialyzers can be safely reused.[3] There are medicines to treat HIV infection, and patients who have this virus need counseling to teach them how to cope and avoid spreading it to others.

Antibiotic-resistant Bacteria

"The graft that was just placed in my arm (my 5th; all have failed, clotted off, or didn't develop) is severely infected. We are trying to overload with antibiotics to hopefully avoid having it removed. Also, I found out I have MRSA."

Viruses are not the only pathogens we need to concern ourselves with. Bacteria are also a threat. While most can be killed with antibiotics, some bacteria in the healthcare setting have become *antibiotic-resistant*. We do not have drugs to treat them, so they can be very dangerous. The bacteria of most concern in a dialysis clinic are covered next.

METHICILLIN-RESISTANT STAPHYLOCOCCUS (STAPH) AUREUS (MRSA)

Staph lives on skin and mucous membranes, and in the respiratory, GI, and urinary tracts. MRSA is a type of staph that can no longer be killed by most antibiotics and can cause severe infections in sites where it does not belong. MRSA is most common in wounds, exit sites, and access sites, and can cause massive flesh wounds, joint damage, pneumonia, and *sepsis* (blood infection) that can be fatal. MRSA most often gets into the bloodstream of HD patients through the vascular access or HD catheter.[3]

Someone may be *colonized* with MRSA—they carry the bacteria but it does not make them sick. Carriers can transmit the bacteria to others, who may become sick.

MRSA causes many infections in the U.S. People with weak immune systems—like HD patients—may be more likely to be infected if they come in contact with MRSA than a healthy person would be. MRSA is very easy to spread. **YOU can spread MRSA on your hands!** MRSA may also be present on equipment and can live for a long time on surfaces.[8]

VANCOMYCIN-RESISTANT ENTEROCOCCUS (VRE)

Enterococcus bacteria live in the intestines and female genital tract. They are harmless to healthy people, but VRE can cause severe infections if it gets into the blood of people with weak immune systems. Data from 23 studies found that about 6% of U.S. dialysis patients (about 1 in 16) carry VRE, and the number may really be higher, since many refused to be tested.[9]

Outbreaks in hospitals have become more common, and have shown that VRE can spread from one patient to another patient through:

- Direct contact
- ***Staff's hands***
- Contaminated equipment or surfaces

Antibiotic-resistant Bacteria Precautions

When we use the CDC's infection control standard precautions, we can help prevent the spread of drug-resistant bacteria. Your clinic may use *extra precautions to treat patients who are at a higher risk to spread disease, such as those who have:*

- An infected skin wound with drainage that seeps out of dressings
- Stool incontinence or diarrhea that cannot be controlled

For these patients, *extra* precautions may mean that you:

- Wear a gown over your clothes. Take off the gown when you are done caring for that patient. If you always wear a gown on the treatment floor, change it before and after that patient.
- Dialyze the patient at a station with as few stations next to it as possible (e.g., at an end or corner of the clinic)
- Use a blood pressure cuff and stethoscope just for that patient

CARBAPENEM-RESISTANT ENTEROBACTERIACEAE (CRE)

CRE are gut bacteria that turn lethal when they get into the bloodstream.[10] They are resistant to all, or nearly all, the antibiotics we have—even our more powerful drugs of last resort. Some CRE germs kill 50% of the patients who get bloodstream infections from them.

Other Infection Concerns

"I'm on PD and have been trying to treat C-diff for nearly 2 months. First round was Vanco for 2 weeks. Still had the diarrhea, so they gave me another drug for 10 days. Was okay for about 2 weeks and then it was back. I'm on my second round of the last drug, and it doesn't seem to be helping. This is starting to affect my social life. I can't do things with my kids and wouldn't even DARE to eat out anywhere...ugh. Help!"

This *Core Curriculum* cannot cover *every* disease that can be found in a dialysis clinic. When patients with weak immune systems and other illnesses come in three times a week, there is a chance for infections—and other problems—to spread from person to person. Here are a few examples of some of the diseases that we do not want to spread.

CLOSTRIDIUM DIFFICILE (C. DIFF)

After a course of antibiotics kills off good gut bacteria, C. diff gut bacteria can grow. The germ inflames the colon, and causes abdominal pain, fever, nausea, loss of appetite, and a large volume of odorous, watery diarrhea.[11] Besides being highly contagious, a C. diff infection can make it a challenge for patients to get to the clinic and stay for their full treatments. The germ can live on surfaces for long periods of time. Hand washing with soap and water and thorough cleaning of all surfaces with bleach can help prevent the spread of C. diff. A blood pressure cuff, etc. should be disposable or used just for the infected patient. Wear a gown over your regular gown when you care for these patients. Patients with C. diff should dialyze at a station as far away from other patients as possible.

TUBERCULOSIS (TB)

Tuberculosis (TB) bacteria attacks the lungs and causes coughing, fever, chills, and night sweats. TB can also attack other parts of the body such as the kidneys, spine, and brain.[12] The disease spreads through tiny airborne droplets that form when someone with *pulmonary* (lung) TB coughs, sneezes, shouts, or sings. Anyone who breathes in the droplets could get TB. Infection is more likely, though, in those with weak immune systems and those who have more contact with someone who has TB.[12]

TB infection can be active or *latent* (inactive). Someone with latent TB will have a positive skin or blood test, but no symptoms of TB, and is not contagious. However, without treatment, the TB may *become* both active and contagious. Active TB can cause a persistent cough, fever, weakness, weight loss, and night sweats. People with TB *must* take all of their medicine. If they do not, a latent infection could become active—and an active one could become drug-resistant.

> ### Precautions to Prevent the Spread of TB[12]
> Clinics can help avoid the spread of TB by taking these steps:
> - Patients should have a TB test when they start at the clinic to see if they have latent TB. If they have ongoing exposure to TB, they should be re-screened once a year.
> - Teach patients who have TB about the latent and active forms.
> - New dialysis staff need to have a TB test. After that, how often you might need re-screening depends on how many patients with TB your clinic sees in a year. If it is less than three patients (low risk), no ongoing screening is required. If your clinic has three or more patients with TB, it is at medium risk, and you will need a TB test once a year.
> - Dialyze patients with infectious TB in an acute care setting or an isolation room with *negative air flow (air is pulled into the room)*.
> - Dialysis staff should wear at least an N95 disposable respirator to care for patients with TB.
> - Ask patients with active TB to wear a surgical mask when they are outside of the isolation room (such as in the waiting room or hallway).

BEDBUGS

Bedbugs are not known to spread disease. However, they are considered to be a pest of public health significance. Bedbug bites can cause allergic reactions and skin infections in some people. If there are bedbugs in your clinic, it may help to use a spray cleaner such as Steri-Fab® after cleaning with bleach. Heat kills all bedbug stages: the eggs, nymphs, and insects. You can give a patient who has bedbugs at home scrubs to wear and use an enviro case to heat his or her clothes for 1.5 hours to kill any bugs or eggs, if your clinic has one. If possible, store the patient's clean clothes until the next treatment and clean the ones s/he wears to the clinic. See Module 2: *The Person with Kidney Failure* to learn more.

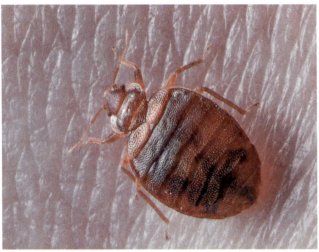

Figure 3: Bedbug - About the Size of an Apple Seed

Giving Medications and Solutions

Each state has rules for what dialysis technicians can do, and which drugs and solutions you can or cannot give. Some states will let you draw up and give heparin and/or normal saline. In other states, you will not be allowed to draw up or give any drug. Learn the rules and laws for *your* state, and the policies and procedures in your clinic. If you live in a state that does let dialysis technicians give some medicines, the next section will help you learn how to give them safely.

Needles

Needles are made of stainless steel and are *never* reused. The slanted part of a needle's tip is called the *bevel*. The diameter of the needle is called the *gauge*. Needles come in different bevel and gauge sizes. **The larger the number, the *smaller* the gauge, so a 17-gauge needle is smaller than a 15-guage**. Needles used for medications are smaller than dialysis needles. *Needles must always be used with aseptic technique*. Throw away used needles in a sharps box.

Syringes

Syringes are made of plastic and are packaged in sterile paper or plastic. They come in different sizes and have three parts (see Figure 4). The top of the syringe is the *tip. A needle connects to a syringe at the tip, so the tip must be sterile at all times.* The outside of the syringe is the *barrel*, which has scales printed on it for measuring the dose. The *plunger* fits into the barrel to push the drug out through the needle.

Safe Use of Syringes and Needles

Wash your hands before you use a syringe and needle. **Use only sterile syringes and needles to avoid contamination**. To prevent accidental needle sticks, do not cut or recap them. Throw out used needles and syringes immediately in a sharps box.

The Occupational Safety and Health Administration (OSHA) Needlestick Safety and Prevention Act requires the use of safety devices like these for sharps in all dialysis clinics:[3]

- Sharps boxes
- Self-sheathing needles
- Needle free systems (see Figure 5)

NOTE: Needles used for Buttonhole cannulation can be used without a device, because they are blunt.

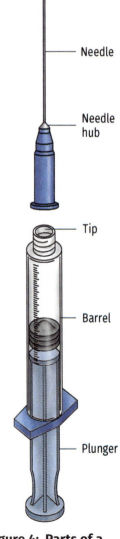

Figure 4: Parts of a Needle and Syringe

Hemodialysis Procedures and Complications

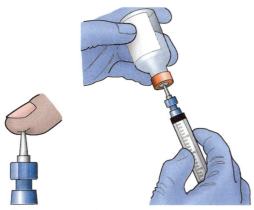

Figure 5: Needleless System

Drawing Up Medicine

CMS rules say clinics must have "clean" areas to prepare, handle, and store medicines. You may not bring multi-dose *vials* (small plastic or glass bottles with sealed rubber caps) from *station to station*—or keep them in your pocket.[13] Learn your clinic's procedure to draw up medicines if this is part of your role. *Never give an unlabeled medicine that you have not drawn into the syringe yourself. Giving the wrong medicine or dose can harm or even kill a patient.*

Vials come in different sizes and may contain one or more doses of a medicine. If your role includes drawing up medicines, you will need to draw up the right amount without contaminating the rest of the vial if the vial holds more than one dose. The standard recommendation from the CDC is that clinics use only single dose vials as much as possible. The rubber caps on vials have a protective metal or plastic cap on top (see Figure 6). The basic steps to drawing up solutions and medicines in a syringe are:

- **Read the drug name and dose on the vial** *before, during, and after* drawing up a solution to be sure you have the right one. Label the syringe with the medicine name, dosage, the date and time, and your initials.
- **Check the expiration date on the vial.** Do not use a vial if the date has passed.
- **Inspect the vial for chips or cracks in the bottle or the cap.** Look at the contents. The liquid should not be discolored and there should be no floating particles. If a vial is damaged or there are issues with the contents, do not use the vial and tell the nurse right away.
- **Remove the protective metal or plastic cap from a new vial.** Then, clean the vial's rubber cap with a disinfectant to wash off any contaminants.
- **Use a single-dose vial only once.** Discard any medicine that is left. *NEVER combine small amounts of leftover medicines from multiple vials into a single vial for use later.*
- **Label each multi-dose vial per your clinic's policy when you open it.**
- **Draw air into the syringe and inject as much air into the vial as solution you want to draw up.** This will keep a vacuum from forming, which would make it hard for you to draw up the solution.
- **After you pull the needle out of the vial, hold the syringe with the needle up.** Tap the syringe a few times to move any air bubbles to the top. Slowly expel any air bubbles out through the needle, and recap the needle safely until you use the syringe.

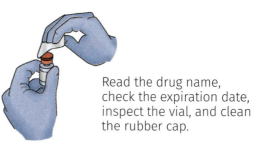

Read the drug name, check the expiration date, inspect the vial, and clean the rubber cap.

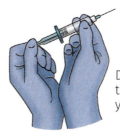

Draw as much air into the syringe as solution you want to draw up.

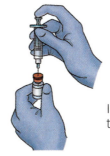

Inject air into the vial to prevent a vacuum.

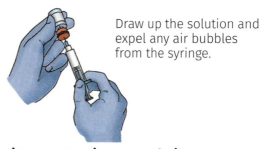

Draw up the solution and expel any air bubbles from the syringe.

Figure 6: Drawing up a Solution

Module 7

Using IV Solutions

Normal saline used during the treatment is given through an *intravenous* (IV; into a vein) bag. You will need to *spike* (open) the bag and let the saline flow through the tubing to *prime* (prepare) it. Spiking the bag and priming the tubing before use pushes all of the air out of the extracorporeal circuit so the air cannot reach the patient's bloodstream.

Spiking an IV bag is done using aseptic technique. The sterile parts of the bag need to remain sterile. Follow your clinic's procedure to connect the IV tubing to the insertion port of the bag (see Figure 7). Here are the steps you may use:

- Place the bag on a flat surface or hang it up on an IV pole.
- Remove the sterile protective cap or tear tab from the port.
- Hold the port firmly in place *without touching it* and insert the spike of the IV tubing into the port. You will have to push hard, and twist the spike back and forth.
- Allow the port and IV spike to touch ONLY each other. If either touches anything else, they are contaminated and you will need to get a new bag, IV set, or both.
- After you spike the bag and attach it to the IV tubing, fill the drip chamber by pinching and releasing. Prime the dialyzer and tubing per your clinic procedure, letting the saline fill the circuit until all of the air is gone. After priming, there must be saline left in the bag. If there is none, change the bag, using the same IV tubing, in case the patient needs more saline during treatment and/or to rinse the patient's blood back at the end of treatment. Consult your clinic's policies and procedures to learn when to change the saline bag, especially if reprocessed dialyzers are used. When a dialyzer is reused, there is a chance that some disinfectant could back up into the saline bag during machine set up and recirculation. Changing the bag keeps any disinfectant from reaching the patient.

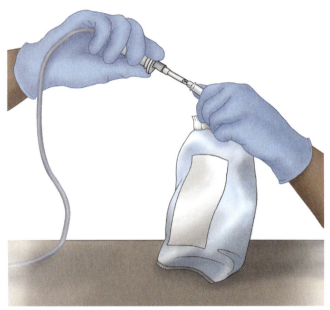

Figure 7: Spiking an IV Bag

Body Mechanics

You will use your muscles and bones on the job to stand, walk, sit, or squat to carry, lift, push, or pull. These tasks can injure your muscles and back. When you use good *body mechanics* (moving your body to prevent injury) you can avoid muscle strain and fatigue (see Figure 8). The three main risk factors for a musculoskeletal injury are:

- Awkward postures
- Repetitive motion
- Forceful exertion

To move well, you need to make friction, leverage, and gravity work for you. Your clinic will show you the basics of good body mechanics. Use what you learn in your day-to-day work.

Lifting and Carrying

There is a right way to lift heavy objects like supply boxes:

- Stand with your feet shoulder-width apart
- Bend from your hips and knees

Hemodialysis Procedures and Complications

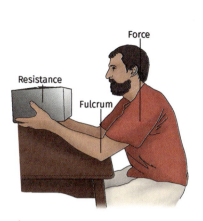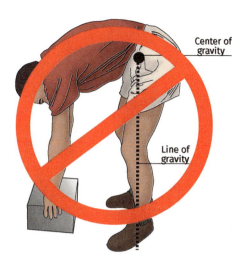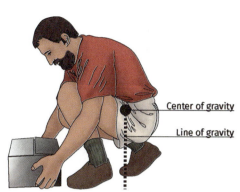

Figure 8: Good Body Mechanics

Never bend at the waist or turn when you lift, push, or pull an object. Pick up the object and hold it close to your body. Bend your knees. Keep your back straight. You want to use your arm and leg muscles—*not* your back. If the object is too heavy for you to lift by yourself, do not try it alone—get help.[14]

Patient Transfers

Many HD patients need help to *transfer* (move from a wheelchair to a treatment chair, chair to bed, etc.). Your clinic will teach you to do a few types of patient transfers. Use the steps you learn to prevent injuries to yourself, other staff, and patients.

Before you move a patient, check his or her general condition. Try not to move a patient who has unusual fatigue, nausea, or an unstable pulse or blood pressure.

An unstable patient may fall. Learn how to reduce the risk of a fall:

- If a patient stands up and is unsteady, help him or her to sit back on the edge of the chair or bed he or she started from.
- If you cannot prevent a fall, try to slowly ease the patient down to the floor, then call for help.

The technique you use for a transfer will vary with how well a patient can stand up and bear weight:

- **Patients who *can* bear their own weight may be able to transfer alone**. A staff member needs to stand by in case the patient needs help. This is especially true after a treatment, when the patient may be dizzy.

- **Patients who *cannot* bear their own weight may need help from more than one staff member**. A lift device is the safest option. Nursing homes minimize manual lifts for safety reasons.[15]

General Tips for Lifting or Moving Patients

- Before lifting or moving, evaluate the patient.
- Get patients to help as much as they can.
- Know your own limits and do not exceed them.
- Get help when you need it.
- Plan ahead and prepare.
- Use chairs, beds, or other surfaces to keep work tasks, equipment, and supplies close and at the right height (i.e., between the waist and shoulders).
- Make sure brakes hold and apply them firmly on beds, gurneys, chairs, etc.
- Use upright, neutral working postures and proper body mechanics.

Patients with Walkers

Patients use walkers for a number of reasons.[16] It can help you to know whether the reason is:

- Poor balance due to dizziness, low blood pressure, inner ear problems, etc.
- Back or leg injuries
- Neuropathy in the feet
- Arthritis
- General weakness or frailty

Module 7

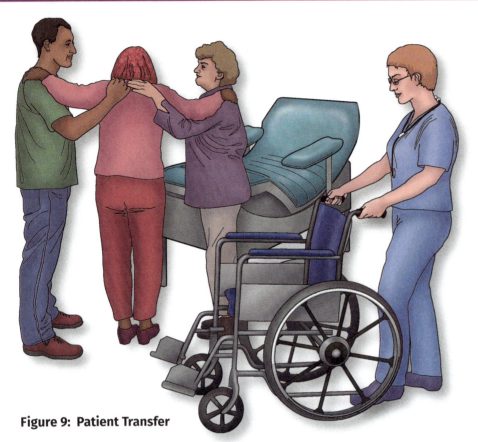

Figure 9: Patient Transfer

- Shortness of breath
- Fear of falling
- Amputation and/or a leg prosthesis
- Trouble walking and carrying something at the same time

You may need to help patients who use walkers to be sure they can balance and will not fall. It may be faster for *you* to put a patient in a wheelchair. But, it is better for the *patient* to use the walker.

Chair-to-Chair Transfers

Some patients can transfer from a wheelchair to the dialysis chair and back after a treatment. Others who use wheelchairs will need help to transfer to the dialysis chair (see Figure 9).

Before you move a patient to or from a wheelchair, lock the dialysis chair and put on the wheelchair brakes. Even with the brakes on, hold the wheelchair in place or put one foot against a wheel during a transfer to keep it from slipping or tipping over.

Stand and Pivot Technique

If a patient can bear enough weight to stand, you may be able to transfer him or her by yourself, using the stand and pivot technique. Use good body mechanics when you do this to prevent back injury:[17]

- Following your clinic's procedure, lock the wheels of the wheelchair.
- Talk the patient through the steps, so s/he can help you as much as possible.
- Put a *gait belt* (heavy canvas belt) around the patient's waist. The belt will help keep the patient stable and help you maintain control during the transfer.
- Help the patient sit on the edge of the chair, with his or her feet flat on the floor and apart.
- Stand in front of the patient and block his or her knees with your legs.
- Have the patient lean forward to help you.
- Help him or her to stand by pulling the belt to bring the patient toward you.
- Slowly pivot to swing the patient's bottom around until you can lower him or her into the other chair.
- Remove the belt.

Using a Slide Board

You can do a chair-to-chair *lateral* (sideways) transfer from the sitting position for someone who cannot bear weight on his or her legs with a *slide board* (smooth board) to reduce friction. When you use a slide board:[18]

- Bring the two sitting surfaces as close together as you can, at a 90° angle.
- Lock the wheelchair (if used).
- Put a gait belt around the patient's waist.
- Scoot the patient's hips to the edge of the bed or chair.

Hemodialysis Procedures and Complications

- Have the patient lean to one side or lift up the patient's leg on the transfer side. Slide the board under the patient's thighs/buttocks at a 45° angle between the sitting surfaces.
- Place the patient's feet on the floor, and put your foot between the patient's feet.
- Put one arm across the patient's body like a seat belt, with your hand on the patient's hip.
- Have the patient lean forward with one hand on the chair he or she is moving *off* of, and the other hand on the board.
- Help the patient scoot over to the new surface and turn. Keep *your* back straight and bend with your knees, so you do not hurt yourself, or sit on a low stool.
- Hold onto the patient until he or she is secure on the new surface. Remove the gait belt and sliding board.
- Have a "spotter" standing by—someone who can help the patient slowly to the floor if he or she slips or the board moves.
- Ask a staff person to hold the dialysis chair to keep it from moving during the transfer.

Portable Lift Devices

Portable lift devices (like Hoyer™ lifts or sling lifts) are used to make lifting safer for you and your patients who cannot bear weight or are very heavy. The weight limit will be in the manual or on the lift itself. Make sure the device will hold the weight of the patient you are moving *before* you try a transfer. Patient transfers with portable lift devices need at least two staff members: one to move the lift and one to pull the patient to the right part of the chair.[19] When you use a portable lift device:

- Make sure the sling is under the patient's body from shoulders to hips.
- Check that the hooks are all in the right slots on the sling holder.
- Raise the patient up just enough to clear the chair.
- Be sure the patient's fingers are clear of any hooks that could pinch.
- Release the patient down into the chair gently.
- Reposition the patient as needed.

During your training, be sure you learn how to operate the lift your clinic uses.

Stretcher-to-Chair Transfers

Some patients, often those from nursing homes, come to dialysis on stretchers:

- If a patient *can* bear some weight, follow your clinic's procedure to place the stretcher in a low position and use the stand and pivot technique.
- If the patient *cannot* bear any weight, use a portable lift device.[17]

Stretcher-to-Bed (Lateral) Transfers

Lateral transfers are used for bed-bound patients. You can use assist devices, like sheets or boards with rollers, to help push and pull a patient from a stretcher to a bed. You will need a few staff members, but these devices avoid the need for a complete lift, so there is less chance of injury.

The surface to which the patient is being moved should be a half-inch or so *lower* than the one s/he is on. Some staff members will push while the others pull the patient onto the new surface.

Documentation

At each HD treatment, we write information that becomes part of a patient's permanent medical record, or chart. *Documentation* or *charting* (writing about the patient's care in the chart) helps the care team track how a patient responds to treatment. **Write so that anyone who reads your notes will know exactly what happened.** You are painting a picture for other staff. Include facts only, NOT your opinions. Proper charting is vital for legal reasons. A patient's record is kept to provide:

- A way for staff taking care of the same patient to share what they know
- A basis to prescribe medical treatment
- A diagnostic tool for the team
- Data for research and quality improvement
- A legal document, admissible in court, as evidence of care the patient did or did not receive. *Legally, if something was not charted, it was not done.*

Each clinic has policies and procedures for how to document patient care. Know your role in documenting in the patient's medical record.

Charting is a record of the care given, the events that occurred, the condition of the patient and response to treatment. It is not the care you intend to give, or the outcome you hope for. NEVER chart any information ahead of time in the patient's medical record.

Electronic Charting

Your clinic probably has electronic medical records. To be sure an electronic chart is not tampered with and to keep confidentiality:

- **Never share your password or computer signature with anyone**. This includes another tech or nurse at your clinic, a temporary worker, or even a doctor.
- Log off if you are not using your terminal, even if you just plan to step away for a moment.
- Follow your clinic's protocol to fix errors. Computer entries are part of the patient's permanent record and cannot be deleted. In most cases, you can X an entry error before you store the entry.
- Stored records have backup files—a vital safety feature. If you accidentally delete part of the permanent record, type an explanation into the file with the date, time, and your initials.
- **Never display patient information**. Do not leave information about a patient on a monitor where others can see it. File printed versions or excerpts of the patient's chart so people who should not have access cannot see them.

Paper Charting: Writing an Entry in the Medical Record

If your clinic uses paper charting or the computers are down, in most cases, entries can be printed or written in script as long as they can be read and are in *ink*. After each entry you make, write your name and title, in the format used by your clinic, for example, "J. Smith. D.T."

What do you do if you make a mistake? You cannot use ditto marks, erase, or use correction fluid; these could lead to legal questions if the chart is used in a court case. Instead, most clinics require you to draw *one* line through the wrong entry. Then, write "error" above the mistake, and write your initials next to it, like this:

Error (A.K.)
Example: Patient dialyzed for 4 hrs. 3.5 hrs.

Never leave lines in a chart partly or fully blank. If the end of a line is not filled in, draw one line through it to keep someone else from charting there after the fact. Record the time on all entries. Read your clinic's policy manual for specific steps. You must be accurate when you chart:

- Be sure the patient's full name is on *each page*, so a page of one patient's chart is not accidentally put in another patient's chart.
- Use **only** abbreviations and initials that are approved by your clinic. Some examples that your clinic may use can be found in Table 3.
- Include the effects and results of all treatments and procedures.
- Include detailed descriptions when you chart about pain, patient complaints, etc. Include what was done for the patient and what the patient's response was to the treatment.
- Symbols can also be confusing and should not be used unless approved by your clinic.

Predialysis Treatment Procedures

Several tasks must be done before a patient's treatment can start. This section will cover:

- The treatment plan
- Setting up the equipment
- Predialysis safety check
- Evaluating the patient

The Treatment Plan

Dialysis is done with a doctor's prescription. Each patient has a treatment plan ordered by a nephrologist. It is vital to know where to find these plans and how to carry them out as ordered. The nephrologist tailors each treatment plan to meet the patient's needs. S/he checks each patient and changes the treatment plan, when needed, by writing new orders.

Hemodialysis Procedures and Complications

Table 3: Abbreviations, Symbols, and Acronyms to Avoid When Charting[20]

Abbreviation to Avoid	Intended to Mean	Misread As	Use This Instead
.5	0.5	5	Use a zero if a number is less than 1
1.0	1	10	Avoid decimal places for whole numbers
x3 D	Days or doses	Opposite – doses or days	Spell out days or doses
cc	Cubic centimeters	"U" or 4	mL
D/C	Discharge	Discontinue (e.g., stop a medicine)	Discharge or Discontinue
HS	Hour of sleep (bedtime)	Half strength	Spell out meaning
IJ	Injection	IV or intrajugular	Spell out meaning
IN	Intranasal	IM or IV	Spell out or write NAS
IU	International unit	IV	Spell out international unit
OD	Once daily	Oculus dexter (left eye)	Spell out meaning
QD	Daily	4 times a day	Daily
QHS	Nightly at bedtime	QHR – every hour	Nightly
QN	Nightly or at bedtime	QH – Every hour	Nightly or at bedtime
Q1D	Once a day	QID (4 times a day)	Daily
QOD	Every other day	QID (4 times a day)	Every other day
µg	Microgram	Mg (milligram)	Mcg or microgram
SC	Subcutaneous	SL (sublingual)	Subcut or subcutaneously
TIW	Three times a week	Three times a day or twice a week	Three times weekly
U	Unit	Zero, 4, or cc	Unit

EQUIPMENT SET-UP

You will set up the equipment before each treatment and check the:

- **Dialysate**
- **Concentrate delivery system**
- **Machine alarms**

Module 4: *Hemodialysis Devices* covers all of the equipment in detail. This section will give you an overview of what you need to do before each treatment.

Mix, Set Up, and Test the Dialysate

As you have learned, dialysate is made up of RO water and two concentrates: acid and bicarbonate. Only a semipermeable membrane keeps the patient's blood apart from the dialysate. The exact make-up of the dialysate is key to your patient's well-being.

Your clinic may buy **acid concentrate** as a *liquid* in single jugs, or in large amounts for a storage tank. It is also sold as a *dry powder* to be mixed in the clinic. **Bicarbonate concentrate** is most often a dry powder. It comes in:

- Single packets to mix one jug
- Large packets to use with a bicarbonate mixer
- Cartridges with dry concentrate that hang on the machine

> **Example: Factors in a Dialysis Prescription**
>
> Dialysis treatment orders are written by the nephrologist and may need to be copied onto the flow sheet. Dialysis treatment orders may include these factors:
>
> - Target weight: **70 kg**
> - Duration: **4 hours (240 minutes)**
> - Frequency: **3 x/week**
> - Dialysate temp: **36.5° C**
> - Dialysate type: **Brand name or Formula**
> - K^+: **2 mEq/L**
> - Ca^{++}: **2.5 mEq/L**
> - Na^+: **138 mEq/L**
> - Dialyzer: **Brand name, high flux, single use**
> - Tubing: **Blood systems**
> - Prescribed Kt/V: **1.4**
> - Max UFR: **< 13 mL/kg/hour**
> - Access type: **AV fistula (Left forearm; Needle gauge – 15 x 1 inch)**
> - Dialysate flow (mL/min): **600**
> - Blood flow (mL/min): **350**
> - Anticoagulant heparin:
>   - 1,000 units pretreatment bolus
>   - 2,000 units hourly
>   - Stop time: 30 minutes prior to the end of treatment

Different manufacturers make the equipment to mix acid and bicarbonate concentrates. Follow your clinic's policies and procedures to mix and test the dialysate concentrates. To learn more about dialysate concentrates, see Module 4: *Hemodialysis Devices*.

The acid and bicarbonate concentrates can be sent to the dialysis machine in one of two ways:
- Through a central delivery system
- By connecting a single jug or "carboy" to each machine.

Your clinic may use central delivery for most patients, *and* jugs for a few. The dialysis machine will mix the concentrates with RO water to make the final dialysate.

Prepare the Dialysis Machine

The steps you will take to get the system ready for your patient will depend on the system your clinic uses, and you may need to:

- Make sure the machine has been internally cleaned and disinfected per clinic policy.
- Rinse out any disinfectant or sterilant that is in the system.
- 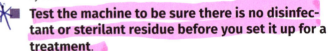 **Test the machine to be sure there is no disinfectant or sterilant residue before you set it up for a treatment**.
- Connect the machine to the acid and bicarbonate concentrates.
- **Check to be sure that the dialysate temperature and conductivity are within limits**.
- If the conductivity is not in the correct range, do a manual check with an independent meter.* Compare the results to the machine readings. Follow your clinic's procedure for how much of a difference in the readings is acceptable, and what to do if the results are outside those limits. *The meter must be verified as accurate using a NIST traceable QC standard solution.
- Check the pH of the final dialysate, as most machines do not display this. Some independent meters will give you the pH. For others, you may need to use test strips. Again, follow your clinic's procedures on how to test and what results are acceptable.
- **Test all of the alarms to be sure they are working**.
- Test the hydraulic pressure on volumetric ultrafiltration machines.
- String the machine with the bloodlines.
- Attach the bloodlines to the dialyzer ports, using aseptic technique.
- Be sure the dialyzer and bloodlines are free of air at the end of the priming and before starting dialysis.

Set Up the Dialyzer and Bloodlines

Giving the patient the prescribed dialyzer and correctly setting up the bloodlines is vital for safety:

1. **Prepare the dialyzer**:
   - For a single-use dialyzer
     - Is it the one the doctor ordered?
     - Check the expiration date.
     - Check to be sure that the protective packaging is intact, the caps are on and there are no cracks or leaks.

Hemodialysis Procedures and Complications

- For a reprocessed dialyzer
  - It has the right patient name label, number of prior uses indicated, and the correct dialyzer for the patient; this information is checked by a second person, preferably the patient
  - There is no evidence of damage or tampering
  - The time since reprocessing is safe per facility policy
  - The ports are capped and not leaking; the fibers are aligned
  - Use a potency test to be sure that the dialyzer **DOES** contain sterilant **BEFORE** you prime it.
  - Use a residual test to be sure that the dialyzer **DOES NOT** contain sterilant **AFTER** you prime it, if the previous results were out of limits.
2. **Document each step in the patient's chart**.

PRIMING AND RECIRCULATION

The inside of the bloodlines are sterile. You must use aseptic technique to take the caps off of the bloodlines so you do not cause an infection. You will learn to **prime** the bloodlines and dialyzer by filling them with normal saline. Priming removes air, glycerin, sterilants, and other residues. Air can be deadly to a patient—and microscopic amounts of air can cause the dialyzer fibers to clot.

Recirculation of the saline keeps the bloodlines ready for use until you are ready to start a treatment. You will start by connecting the venous and arterial bloodlines to form a loop. The prime will flow through the loop (*recirculate*). UF and diffusion help to "dialyze off" any substances that are left. These substances will move from the blood side of the dialyzer to the dialysate side, and then go down the drain. Recirculate the primed dialyzer until treatment begins. This step prevents sterilant rebound from the dialyzer side into the extracorporeal circuit.

NOTE: Your clinic will have a time limit for how long recirculation of the extracorporeal circuit can safely go on. If a circuit exceeds this time limit, follow your clinic's policy. You may need to discard the circuit and start over.

Conduct an Alarm Safety Check

Most dialysis machines do some safety checks for you when you press a button. You need to know *what* the machine is checking. **Do all of the safety checks in Table 4 *before* each treatment—not just at the start of a shift**. Completing this check is key to patient safety. If an alarm is not working and the treatment starts, you could harm the patient.

All alarm checks must pass *before* a machine is used for a treatment. If any alarm checks fail, remove the machine from the patient area for inspection, per your clinic's policy. See Table 5 for safety precautions to take before starting a treatment.

Evaluate the Patient

"I almost died last month of an infection in my blood that wouldn't culture 'til I was in the hospital with a 104° fever. My center was doing twice a month blood cultures that were negative, but when they pulled out my catheter, it WAS infected."

Part of your job will be to look at the patient's condition before a treatment. You will need to compare what you find with data from past treatments. Tell the nurse about any abnormal findings. The nurse will assess each patient to make sure that s/he is well enough to treat in an outpatient setting. The predialysis patient check includes:

- Weight
- *Edema* (Swelling)
- Pulse*
- Blood pressure*
- Respiration rate*
- Temperature*
- Vascular access
- General physical and emotional well-being

* These are the patient's "vital signs." See Table 7 on page 234 to learn more about vital signs.

227

Module 7

Table 4: Predialysis Alarm and Safety Checks

Test these *extracorporeal* alarms	To pass, each alarm must:
■ Air detector ■ Blood leak detector ■ Arterial pressure high/low alarm ■ Venous pressure high/low alarm	■ Stop the blood pump ■ Clamp the venous line ■ Sound an audio alarm ■ Show an alarm message on the screen
Test these *dialysate* alarms ■ Machine conductivity ■ Temperature ■ pH (some machines do not have this) ■ UF check	**To pass, each alarm must:** ■ Go into bypass mode (stop dialysate flow to the dialyzer) ■ Be within limits set by your clinic
Make these *safety* checks ■ Independent conductivity* ■ Independent dialysate pH ■ Absence of disinfectant (after rinsing) ■ Positive germicide test (reprocessed dialyzer) ■ Negative germicide test (reprocessed dialyzer) *NOTE: Some machine manufacturers may not require a conductivity test.	**To pass, each alarm must:** ■ Be within limits set by your clinic and/or the manufacturer

Weigh the Patient

The patient's pretreatment weight is used to decide:
- How much water weight the patient gained since the last treatment
- How much water weight to remove at this treatment

> **Assess Target Weight (TW)**
>
> After a treatment, a patient *at* TW should have:
> - Normal blood pressure for him or her
> - No edema
> - No shortness of breath
>
> After a treatment, a patient *above* TW will still have fluid *on board* (in his or her body) and may have:
> - High blood pressure
> - Edema
> - Shortness of breath
>
> After a treatment, a patient *below* TW may be dehydrated, and may have:
> - Low blood pressure
> - Lightheadedness or dizziness when standing
> - Painful muscle cramps
> - Fatigue that lasts for hours or into the next day

The *target weight* (TW) also known as *dry weight* or *estimated dry weight* is the doctor's best assessment of what a patient's weight would be with no extra water and with a normal blood pressure. The doctor prescribes a TW for each patient. This weight is used to decide how much water to remove during a treatment. In an ideal case, by the end of a treatment the patient will be at or near TW.

FACTORS THAT AFFECT THE TARGET WEIGHT

Weighing the patient accurately is just the *first* step in the vital process of finding out how much water to remove during a treatment. You will need to know:

- How the scale works
- How to balance the scale to make sure it is accurate
- How to position the patient on the scale
  - Have patients who can stand by themselves stand in the middle of the scale.
  - Do not let patients support their weight by holding onto the scale, or a counter, cane, or crutch—the weight will not be accurate. If they cannot stand by themselves, use a wheelchair scale for safety.
  - A patient in a wheelchair must have all four of the wheels on the scale.
  - Weigh the chair without the patient in it and subtract the chair weight from the total weight.
- Your clinic's guidelines on maximum weight gains between treatments

Table 5: Safety Factors in Hemodialysis

I. Know and follow your clinic's policy and procedures to maintain equipment.
II. We use alarms for patient safety. *Do not clear an alarm without checking the patient and the machine to be sure of the cause and correction for the alarm.*

III. Do not solely rely on machine alarms. Understand how the machine should respond to an alarm. For example:
  A. For a conductivity or temperature alarm, dialysate should go to bypass. Check the machine to ensure that it has done so. Know what to do to protect your patient if the machine alarm does not engage. You may need to remove the dialysate hose connectors by hand and take the machine out of service.
  B. If there is an alarm on the blood side (e.g., a high venous pressure), assess the patient and access, and check machine to ensure that the blood pump has stopped and the venous clamp has engaged.

IV. Alarm fatigue – exposure to a large number of alarms can lead to sensory overload and slow, or no response. This can lead to complacency and harm patient safety.[21,22]
  A. Do not override an alarm without finding its cause.
  B. Do not automatically push "reset."

V. Patient concerns
  A. The patient's **vascular access** must be visible at all times during a treatment.[23]
  B. The patient's **face** must be visible at all times.
  C. The **patient** should be visible at all times during the treatment.
  D. Monitor patients' blood pressure per your clinic's policy. This may be at least every 30 minutes, or more often if needed.
  E. Follow your clinic policy about patients eating during treatment. Patients who eat may be at a higher risk of choking or hypotension. If the patient *must* eat, i.e., due to diabetes or treatment schedule, limit the amount of food and avoid high carbohydrate meals.

VI. Staff member concerns
  A. All patient care staff should be certified in CPR per clinic policy. The policy may require an accredited source (e.g., American Heart Association or Red Cross).
  B. All patient care staff must know clinic emergency procedures and their roles in keeping patients safe and protecting themselves.
  C. Always use standard precautions and protect patients from cross contamination.
  D. Use proper patient identifiers before doing patient care or giving medicines. Do not *assume* that you have the correct patient. Assuming patient identity can lead to errors!

VII. Environmental concerns
  A. Clean up any spill immediately.
  B. Minimize clutter to reduce infection control risks for falls.

Table adapted from the *Core Curriculum for Nephrology Nursing*. Module 3 Table 2.1. and used with permission from the American Nephrology Nurses Association.

- When to tell the nurse about abnormal weight changes (too much or too little weight gained)

Many factors besides water gain can affect a patient's weight:

- A hospital stay or illness with loss of appetite, diarrhea, or vomiting can cause weight loss.
- The holidays can cause *real* (muscle or fat) weight gains if patients eat more than usual.
- Patients may lift weights and gain muscle weight.
- Wearing different clothes or shoes can raise *or* lower a patient's weight on the scale.
- Extra items in pockets such as a cell phone or a handful of coins add weight, and so do extra items in a wheelchair, such as a bag or purse.
- *Patients who still make a lot of urine do not need to remove as much water.*

Many patients can tell you if they have gained or lost real weight vs. water weight. Ask your patients to wear similar kinds of clothing and shoes to each treatment, so their weights are more accurate.

Check for Edema

Edema occurs when extra water builds up in the patient's tissues. **Due to gravity, the effects of edema are often seen in the feet or ankles**. Edema may also be seen in the hands, face, abdomen, or back. Asking simple questions like these can help you find problems with edema:

- How do your shoes fit?
- Have you been short of breath?
- Do your rings fit any differently than they normally do?

You can feel for swelling by gently pressing your thumb over the foot, ankle, or shin with slow, steady pressure. If a dent stays in the patient's skin, this is called *pitting edema*, which is more severe. Be sure to learn:

- How your clinic wants you to check patients for edema
- When to tell the nurse about a patient's edema

Take the Patient's Pulse

With each heartbeat, the heart muscle pushes a wave of blood into the arteries. You can feel or hear this pulse wave at several points on the body. You will take a patient's pulse by feeling or listening at a pulse point (see Figure 10) and then you will record the number of beats per minute in the patient's medical record. The rhythm of the pulse can also be recorded. A normal pulse for an adult is between 60 and 100 beats per minute, with a regular rhythm. If the patient's pulse is very fast (*tachycardia*), very slow (*bradycardia*), or irregular (*arrhythmia*), tell the nurse.

Take the Patient's Blood Pressure (BP)

The pulse of each heartbeat causes pressure inside the arteries:

- The highest pressure occurs *during* a heartbeat, when the heart contracts—**systolic**.
- The lowest pressure is *between* beats, when the heart is at rest—**diastolic**.

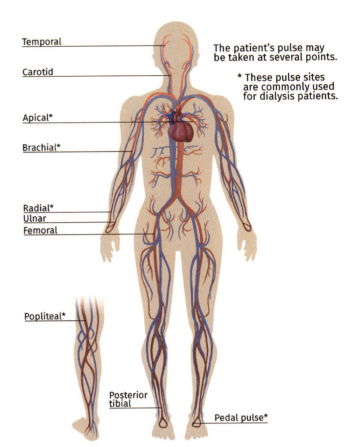

Figure 10: Sites Used for Taking a Pulse

A BP reading records both the high (systolic) and the low number (diastolic). So if a BP reading is 120/70 ("120 over 70"), the systolic pressure is 120 millimeters of mercury (mmHg) and the diastolic pressure is 70 mmHg. You will take BP readings while the patient is seated and standing.

In patients with kidney failure, changes in fluid status are the key reason that BP readings rise or fall. As water weight rises, BP also rises, because more water in the blood raises pressure in the blood vessels. As water weight is removed, the BP drops because the blood volume drops.

To measure blood pressure, you need to put a cuff around the patient's arm (or, in some cases, leg). You will need to learn how to use a cuff properly. **The size and condition of a cuff can change the accuracy of a BP reading**. Inside each blood pressure cuff is a rubber bladder that holds air. The American Heart Association says that cuff bladder length should be 80% of the distance around patient's arm (or leg).[24] The cuff bladder should be at least 40% as wide as the distance between the patient's elbow and shoulder.[24] (See Table

Hemodialysis Procedures and Complications

6 for blood pressure cuff sizes.) Some other tips about blood pressure cuffs include:[25]

- Readings will not be accurate if the cuff Velcro does not stick tightly when the cuff inflates.
- Placing a cuff over thick clothing will cause a lower reading.
- *Too-small* cuffs will read too *high*.
- *Too-large* cuffs will read too *low*.
- BP cuffs that are wrapped too loosely or unevenly will also cause a higher reading.

Table 6: Blood Pressure Cuff Sizes

Distance Around Arm	Blood Pressure Cuff Size
7–9 inches	Small adult cuff
9–13 inches	Standard adult cuff
13–17 inches	Large adult cuff

Look for a horizontal RANGE limits line on the inside of the cuff and a vertical INDEX mark on the outside. To check if the cuff size is right for your patient, place the cuff around the patient's arm or leg and check to see that the INDEX mark is within the RANGE limits (see Figure 11).

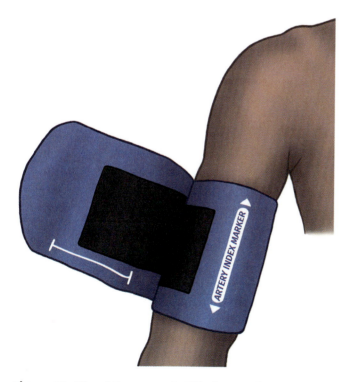

Figure 11: Blood Pressure Cuff Index Marks

Check a BP with the patient's elbow supported at the same level as his or her heart:[26]

- If the BP site (e.g., arm) is *below* heart level, the readings will be too *high*.
- If the BP site is *above* heart level, the readings will be too *low*.

You will most often check a patient's BP on an arm, but may need to check a BP on a leg (see Figure 12) if there is an access in both arms, or a patient has only one arm. Two sites to place the cuff to take a leg BP are:

- Above the knee
- Above the ankle

To keep the patient's leg at heart level, take a leg BP in the *supine* position (with the patient lying flat on his or her back). A leg BP reading tends to be higher than an arm reading. Patients with peripheral artery disease will have lower knee and ankle blood pressures.

HOW TO TAKE AN AUTOMATED BP READING

On the treatment floor of a dialysis clinic, BP readings are most often taken by the dialysis machine. You can leave the cuff on the patient's arm (or leg) and set the machine to take the BP at certain intervals. But, this approach has limits:

- A patient's bradycardia and/or arrhythmia can confuse the system, so take manual BP readings.
- ***Never squeeze the cuff to speed up deflation***: you could damage the internal BP module on the machine.
- Kinked BP lines or loose connections can cause false readings. Check that these are straight and connected before a treatment.

HOW TO TAKE A MANUAL BP READING

You may need to take a manual blood pressure with a stethoscope and a *sphygmomanometer* (blood pressure cuff with a bulb pump). To do this, you will:

1. Place a cuff of the correct sizes on the patient's arm or leg, and position the limb at the patient's heart level. (You can rest the patient's arm on a chairside table.)
2. Put the stethoscope earpieces in your ears.
3. Place the bell of the stethoscope over a pulse point on the patient's arm or leg at the lower edge of the cuff so you can hear the pulse.
4. Twist the valve to hold the air in.

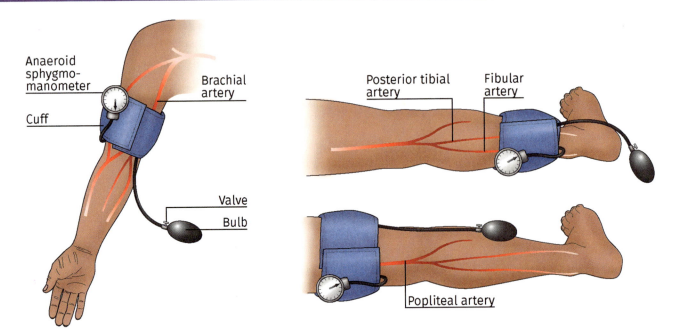

Figure 12: Blood Pressure Sites

5. Inflate the cuff by pumping the bulb until you can no longer hear the pulse.
6. Turn the valve slowly the other way to deflate the cuff.
7. Note at what number on the readout you start to hear the pulse (systolic) and at what number you can no longer hear it (diastolic).
8. Record the reading in the patient's chart.

Count the Respiration Rate

With each breath, oxygen from the air enters the lungs and carbon dioxide leaves them, a gas exchange that affects the health of every cell in the body. The action of breathing in and breathing out is one full breath exchange. Most adults have a regular rate of about 12–16 breaths per minute, but patients may change their patterns if they know you are counting. So, count breaths while you are taking a patient's pulse or checking for edema—and do not tell them that you are doing it.

In dialysis patients, water weight gains may cause water to enter the lungs, which can cause shortness of breath or trouble breathing. Report these symptoms to the nurse. Nurses use the stethoscope to listen to and evaluate breath sounds. They may also use a *pulse oximeter* ("pulse-ox" machine with a sensor probe) to check a patient's blood oxygen level (see Figure 13). The oximeter probe, which looks like a clothespin, is placed on a finger. The machine then shows the oxygen saturation (SaO2). A "pulse-ox" reading of less than 90% is abnormally low. Besides water weight, a low "pulse ox" reading may mean the patient has steal syndrome in a fistula or graft.[27]

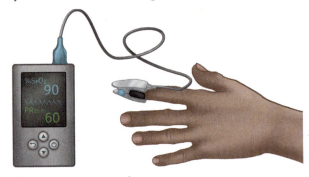

Figure 13: Pulse Oximeter

Take the Patient's Temperature

Different types of thermometers are used to measure a patient's temperature (see Figure 14). No one body temperature is "normal" for all people. HD patients tend to have low temperatures before dialysis, around 96.8° F, and it is normal for their temperature to rise a bit by the end of the treatment.[28]

Note any of these and report them to the nurse:

- **Fever *before* dialysis**. A patient who comes to treatment with a temperature even *slightly* higher than his or her usual may have an infection—even if the reading is just 98 or 99° F.[29] A high temperature before a treatment could be due to:

Hemodialysis Procedures and Complications

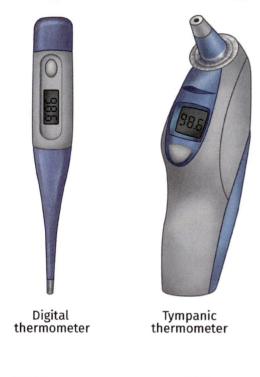
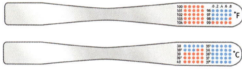

Figure 14: Types of Thermometers

- A cold
- The flu
- A catheter, graft, or fistula infection
- A bladder infection
- A foot infection (common in patients who have diabetes)
- Inflammation, such as *pericarditis* (an inflamed heart sac)

■ **Fever *during* dialysis**. A patient who spikes a fever *during* dialysis may be having a *pyrogenic reaction* (fever response to toxins in the dialysate). This is especially true if more than one patient develops symptoms during a shift.

■ **Fever *after* dialysis**. Pyrogenic reactions can start after dialysis—and so can infections. Ask the patient about any fevers between treatments.

Check the Vascular Access

The vascular access is the patient's lifeline. Before each treatment starts, check the access to be sure it is working. See Module 6: *Vascular Access* to learn how to check the access.

Ask About General Physical and Emotional Health

"This past Saturday after dialysis I had such bad pains in my lower back that I was in tears."

Talk with your patients, ask them questions, and listen to their answers to find out how they are doing before a treatment. **Patients know themselves best**. By talking to and watching them, you can find clues to their general health and emotional well-being. Here are some questions you might ask:

■ *How have you felt since your last treatment?*
■ *Have you had any trips to the emergency room or outpatient procedures?*
■ *Have you felt any chest pain or trouble breathing?*
■ *Have you had any weakness or numbness?*
■ *Are you in any pain today?*
  ➢ You may *see* pain in the patient's facial expression, sweating, or protection of a certain body area.
  ➢ CMS requires that patients get a formal pain rating assessment twice a year.[30] Find out how your clinic does this assessment and your role in it.
■ *Are you having any problems eating or digesting your food?*
■ *Have you been to the doctor or started any new medicines since your last treatment?*
■ *Have you been able to do the things you want to do?*
■ *Have you fallen at home?*
■ *Have you noticed any unusual bleeding?*

You can also learn about patients just by watching them. For example:

■ Did the patient walk into the clinic as well as on other days?
■ Is the patient's speech normal (not slurred)?

Table 7: Vital Signs for Adult Patients on Hemodialysis

Vital Sign/Definition	What You Should Find	Terms
Blood pressure (BP) **Systolic:** Pressure in an artery during a heartbeat. Top number in a BP reading. **Diastolic:** Pressure in an artery when the heart is at rest. Bottom number in a BP reading.	Recommended BP for adults on dialysis:*[31] **Before HD:** < 140/90 or a target set by the patient's doctor. **After HD:** < 130/80 * In children, BP after HD should be 130/80 *or* below the 90th percentile of normal for age, height, and weight.	**Hypertension**—high BP (often with no symptoms) **Hypotension**—low BP **Orthostatic hypotension**—a drop in BP of 15 mmHg or more upon rising from sitting to standing. The patient may feel dizzy and faint.
Pulse The wave of blood in an artery caused by each heartbeat	60–100 beats per minute (with regular rhythm)[32]	**Tachycardia**—fast pulse, > 100 **Bradycardia**—slow pulse, < 60 **Normal sinus rhythm**—normal rate and rhythm **Arrhythmia**—irregular rate and rhythm
Respiration Taking air into and pushing it out of the lungs	12–16 breaths per minute[33]	**Dyspnea**—shortness of breath **Apnea**—no breathing
Temperature The degree of heat in the body of a person	Average is from 96.8–98.6° F or 36–37° C[34] No increases over patient's usual baseline.	**Afebrile**—no fever (up to 37.8° C; 100° F.) **Febrile**—with fever (above 37.8° C; 100° F)

- Does the patient seem confused, agitated, or depressed?
- Is the patient's skin color normal or is it pale or ashen (gray)?

See Module 2 to learn more about patients' health.

Starting a Dialysis Treatment

To start the treatment, you will:
- Verify the patient's dialysis orders
- Calculate how much water to remove
- Cannulate or connect the patient's access
- Draw blood for laboratory testing
- Start the dialysis machine

Calculate How Much Water to Remove

"I don't know how many times I've explained to them that any weight on my body is read by the scale, not just fluid. They laugh in the winter when I take off my thick sweater before weighing, but that's over a kilo right there that they would be trying to suck off of me!"

Ultrafiltration **(UF)—removing water—is one of the three main tasks of dialysis, along with removing wastes and excess electrolytes**. It will be your job to calculate how much water to remove during a treatment—and getting the amount right is vital. A physician decides each patient's target weight. The goal of dialysis is to try to return to target by the end of the treatment. However, if a patient has gained too much water weight between treatments, you may not be able to remove all of the excess in one treatment. Check with the nurse about a safe amount, and talk with the patient about fluid intake between treatments. A safe UF amount depends on the patient's fluid status and how much urine s/he still makes. Some patients may need minimal or no water removal. Others require far more water to be removed. UF is a careful balancing act:

- **Removing *too much* water leads to dehydration, long recovery time, and is linked with a higher risk of death**.[35] When a patient's blood pressure drops, your clinic's policy may be to turn off the UF rate until the BP rises and the patient feels better. While the UF is off, only wastes and electrolytes are removed—not water. Turning off the UF for a time allows the patient's body to "catch up" by giving time for water to shift into the bloodstream, so the BP will rise. NOTE: *Backfiltration* of dialysate into the blood compartment *will NOT occur when the UF is turned down or off.* The usual minimum UF of 300 is solely to reduce nuisance alarms. When the UF must be turned off, *"there is no clinical effect on the machine, hemodialyzer, or the patient."*[36]

- **Not removing *enough* water leaves patients fluid overloaded, harms the heart, and raises the risk of death.**[37]

How do you remove the *right* amount of water safely?

1. **Start with the desired weight loss.** You will need to know:

   - **The target weight**, which is prescribed by the patient's doctor. Changes in the target weight must also be made by the doctor. Discuss patient requests for a change in target weight with the charge nurse.
   - **The patient's pretreatment weight.**
   - **How much (if any) urine the patient makes.** Some patients still make a *lot* of urine, which removes water, but not wastes. Ask them. The patient may be asked to do a 24-hour urine collection to see how much residual kidney function s/he still has. Residual function can also affect the Kt/V (dialysis adequacy). The nurse will provide a toilet "hat," and a collection jug with written instructions.
   - **The maximum UF rate (UFR).** UFRs higher than 10 mL/kg/hour can lead to organ stunning and early death.[38] CMS has set a safety limit of 13 mL/kg/hour, and if a patient gains so much water weight that the UFR would need to exceed this rate, the nurse will need to decide on an intervention and plan of care[39] (see Modules 2 and 3 to learn more about organ stunning).

2. **Add in the patient's fluid intake during dialysis** (see Table 8). In most cases we do not include fluid output during dialysis (e.g., urine, vomit, stool).

   Fluid intake includes:

   - **Saline** in the bloodlines and dialyzer that is infused into the patient at the start of dialysis.
   - **Rinseback** saline used to return the patient's blood back into the body after a treatment.
   - **Ice chips, drinks, and IV medications**, including saline flushes if the patient does not receive heparin during the treatment. A good rule of thumb is to count any fluid in excess of 100 mL.

3. **Enter the total fluid amount (in mL) and the treatment time into the machine.**
4. **The machine will calculate and set an hourly UFR.** Compare the machine UFR with the patient's maximum UFR. Tell the nurse if the machine UFR will exceed that maximum *before* you start a treatment. A patient who has more water to remove than can be done safely during a single treatment may need the doctor to prescribe more time, an extra treatment or two to catch up, or a treatment option that removes more water.

Table 8: Total Water Removal Calculation Example

Target weight	85 kg
Predialysis weight	88.1 kg
Desired weight loss is 3.1 kg (1 kg = 1,000 mL)	3,100 mL
Priming saline	240 mL
Saline rinseback	200 mL
Medications	250 mL
Dietary intake (ice chips, drinks)	120 mL
Total water to remove	**3,910 mL**
3,910 ÷ 4 hours (treatment time) = **977.5 mL/hour** (.977 L/hr)	
The **UFR** would be **977.5 ÷ 88.1 kg** (predialysis weight) = **11.10**, below the 13 mL/kg/hour safety limit.	

NOTE: The Medical Education Institute has developed a free UFR calculator that you or your patients can use, at www.homedialysis.org/ufr-calculator (see Figure 15).

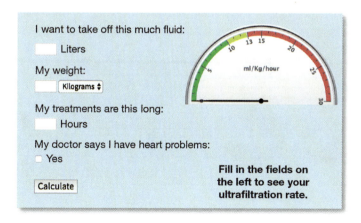

Figure 15: UFR Calculator

Special Concerns for New HD Patients

"My husband still pees, but no matter what his dry weight is, they take 5 kilos off. We have complained about this to his nephrologist, but nothing has been done yet. He has been hospitalized twice because of what they are doing. We are on the waiting list for home hemo."

For many years, U.S. dialysis survival numbers did not include the first 90 days of treatment, when patients were getting used to their new routines. But, as it turns out, those first 90 days are extremely risky. **In fact, the highest risk of death is in the first 2 weeks of HD, and the rate of death in the first 90 days is *twice* what it is later.**[40]

There may be many reasons why the first few weeks and months of dialysis are so dangerous. One of these reasons seems to be **organ stunning**. The highest rate of sudden cardiac death is in the first month of HD, when we are most likely to try to remove too much water and stun the heart (and other organs). And, the highest rate of *stopping* dialysis—which will lead to death—is in the second month of treatment.[41] A study found that between 2004 and 2011, the rate of early withdrawal from dialysis *tripled*. One reason was because patients *"perceive that dialysis has become unduly burdensome."*[42]

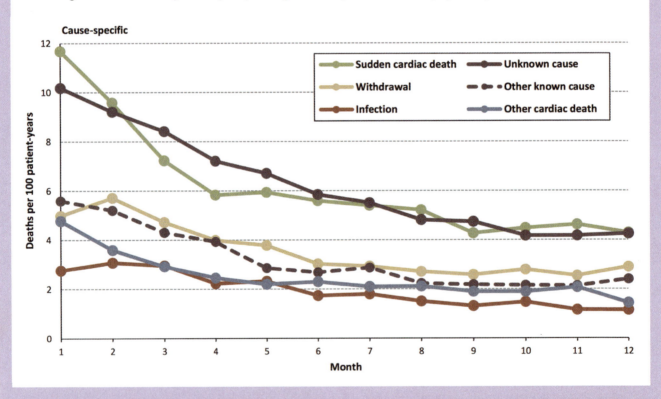

Figure 16: Cause of Death by Month on Dialysis
Graph used with permission from the Peer Kidney Care Initiative, Peer Report: Dialysis Care and Outcomes in the United States, 2016, Chronic Disease Research Group, Minneapolis, MN, 2016.

Be extra gentle with your new patients! Ask them if they make urine, and see if the nurse would like to verify the amount. Do not pull off water that is not there so they cramp and "crash"—*or* leave them fluid overloaded and gasping for breath. Be sure they know about all of the dialysis options and how each one can affect their lives. You can point them to: www.mydialysischoice.org. Your patients are going through a difficult time, and they need the help of the entire care team—and excellent care—to make it through.

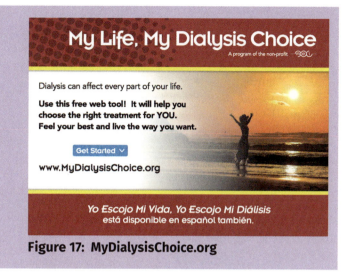

Figure 17: MyDialysisChoice.org

ULTRAFILTRATION PROFILING

The nephrologist can prescribe one of several UF profiles (see Figure 18) designed to reduce symptoms patients may have when water is being removed. The profiles can be set to remove more or less water during each part of the treatment (see Module 4: *Hemodialysis Devices* to learn more). You will input the prescribed profile into the machine.

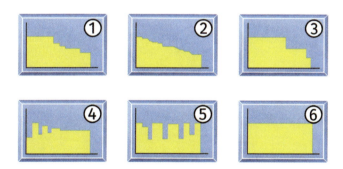

Figure 18: Ultrafiltration Profiles

UFR AND TRANSMEMBRANE PRESSURE

In the past, you would have had to calculate transmembrane pressure (TMP) and input it into the machine to reach the right UF. A dialyzer's KUF and the patient's UF goal were part of this equation.

The KUF is a measure of how water permeable a dialyzer is, and how much fluid can pass through the membrane at a given pressure on the blood side:

- **High efficiency dialyzers have a KUF from 7–15**.
- **High flux dialyzers have a KUF that is greater than 15**.

TMP, as measured by most machines today, is *venous pressure minus dialysate pressure*, in mmHg. TMP can be a positive or a negative number, based on where the machine displays it:

- **Positive** – on the blood side, where pressure should always be higher
- **Negative** – on the dialysate side

Today, you no longer have to manually calculate and control the TMP to reach a patient's UF goal. However, you will need to *check* the TMP, because it may be able to show if there is a problem. For example, there might be pressure changes due to clotting in the dialyzer. You can learn the approximate TMP if you divide the patient's UFR by the dialyzer's KUF. So, a patient with a UFR of 10 and a dialyzer KUF of 18 would have a TMP of about 0.555 (10÷18) (see Module 4 to learn more).

REPLACING FLUID

"So I'm at dialysis & I have about 20 minutes left & this is when the bad stuff always starts happening. They pull too much fluid off. I start getting really hot, my blood pressure drops, I feel like I'm gonna pass out. Ugh, I hate this so much. I want to punch my machine!"

At times, you may need to *give* patients normal saline during a treatment to help them reach their target weight. For example, a patient may come in for a treatment dehydrated and below target weight due

Example of a UF Management Program

Dialysis has always removed water, wastes, and excess electrolytes. But, as you will see in the "adequacy" section on page 264, formulas for dialysis dose do not include ultrafiltration. So, UF was not a strong focus. This has changed in the past few years, since we now know how important it is to remove the right amount of water at a safe UF rate. Yet, changing the practices of busy dialysis clinics is a challenge.

WT in Kg	10 mL	13 mL	15 mL
35	350	455	525
40	400	520	600
45	450	585	675
50	500	650	750
55	550	715	825
60	600	780	900
65	650	845	975
70	700	910	1,050
75	750	975	1,125
80	800	1,040	1,200
85	850	1,105	1,275
90	900	1,170	1,350
95	950	1,235	1,425
100	1,000	1,300	1,500
105	1,050	1,365	1,575
110	1,100	1,430	1,650
115	1,150	1,495	1,725
120	1,200	1,560	1,800
125	1,250	1,625	1,875
130	1,300	1,690	1,950
135	1,350	1,755	2,000 (Max)
140	1,400	1,820	2,000 (Max)
145	1,450	1,885	2,000 (Max)

Figure 19: UF Chart
Image used with permission from RJ Picciano.

The non-profit Centers for Dialysis Care in Ohio has set up an experimental program for the care team to challenge patients' dry weights over a series of treatments.[43] Led by a Fluid Manager, with a nurse "Fluid Champion" in each clinic, they are looking at two ways to monitor patients during HD:

1. A device* that uses a forehead sensor to track pulse rate, strength, rhythm, and changes in oxygen saturation. The device lets staff see on a screen when patients are stressed by the UF rate or amount.

2. A protocol to observe patients and track BP changes during treatment.

When problems are seen by either approach, chair side adjustments are made per a UF chart (see Figure 19).

Green column (UFR is 10 mL/kg/hr): Up to a 200 mL increase in the UF amount is allowed.

Yellow column (UFR is 13 mL/kg/hr): Up to a 100 mL increase in the UF amount is allowed.

Red column (UFR is 15 mL/kg/hr): No increases in UF are allowed. Decreases are allowed.

Interventions for patients with symptoms included:
- Changing the chair to position #2 or #3 (see Figure 20)
- Giving oxygen
- Using a starting dialysate temperature of 35.5° C (which could be reduced to 35° C with a doctor's order)
- Reducing the UF goal
- Reviewing the dialysate calcium and potassium
- Using sequential hemofiltration and dialysis, with a doctor's order
- Measuring BP every 15 minutes

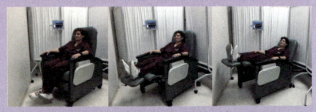

Chair Position #1   Chair Position #2   Chair Position #3

Figure 20: Chair Positions
Images used with permission from RJ Picciano.

The Centers for Dialysis Care continues to track results. They aim to see whether patients can be brought closer to target weight without symptoms, and if the technology helps more than the charts alone.

*CVInsight by Intelomed. Crit-Line® Technology is another option your clinic may use. Learn more in Module 4: Hemodialysis Devices.

to vomiting or diarrhea. Tell the nurse if a patient comes in below target weight. S/he will tell you if saline is needed during the treatment, and, if so, how much. When you calculate the amount of saline that will be needed, you will take into account the saline prime and rinseback as well as dietary intake and IV medicines.

AVOID SODIUM LOADING

Sodium loading means we *add sodium into a patient's blood* instead of removing it (see Table 9). Most standard in-center HD patients who make little or no urine are asked to limit their fluid and sodium intake. But, we can add *far more* sodium than patients can eat into their blood if we use sodium modeling. This can cause high blood pressure, headaches after treatment, and thirst, so patients drink more and come in even more overloaded next time.

For these reasons, the Chief Medical Officers of the largest U.S. dialysis providers agreed that:[44]

1. **A normal level of extracellular fluid should be a main goal of dialysis**.
2. **Fluid should be removed gently; treatments should not routinely be less than 4 hours long**.
3. **Sodium loading should be avoided: dialysate sodium should be 134–138 mEq/L**. Sodium modeling should not be routinely used, and hypertonic saline should be avoided.[45]
4. **Patients should be counseled not to eat too much sodium**.

Cannulate or Connect the Patient's Access

Preserving a patient's access through correct cannulation is one of the most vital tasks you will do. With a fistula or a graft, needles must be placed into the access. Skilled and gentle needle placement helps an access last longer. Good blood flow through the needles helps ensure that a patient will receive a treatment with proper clearances of waste and water from the blood.

Patients whose fistula or graft is not yet ready to use, or who do not have a venous access, must use a hemodialysis catheter. Catheters must be used with great care to prevent infection (see Module 6: *Vascular Access* to learn how to care for and cannulate accesses).

Draw Blood for Laboratory Testing

Dialysis patients have blood drawn to see if their treatments are effective and if any changes need to be made. Refer to your clinic's or lab's procedures for how blood tests must be done. In this section, you will learn the basic steps to draw samples of the patient's blood from the blood tubing port or the needle tubing with a needle and syringe or a vacuum tube.

Table 9: Causes and Prevention of Sodium Loading During HD

Cause	Prevention
Use of dialysate sodium that is higher than the patient's blood sodium. Sodium diffuses into the blood.	**Lower dialysate sodium**, with a doctor's order. Reaching the same sodium level as in the patient's blood reduces sodium transfer.
Use of normal saline (**NS**): Each 1 mL of NS contains 9 mg of sodium. So, 400 mL of NS gives a patient 3,600 mg—nearly twice the common daily diet limit of 2,000 mg.	■ **Give the patient a drink of water** for mild BP drops. ■ **Give 100–200 mL NS** for moderate drops.
Use of hypertonic saline (**HS**): With 2,340 mg of sodium, even one 10 mL vial of HS will give the patient more than his or her daily sodium limit. Some clinics no longer use HS.	**Prevent blood pressure drops**: ■ Use a UFR the patient can tolerate. ■ Run the patient longer.* ■ Offer an extra treatment.*
Use of broth for low blood pressure or cramps. One cup of broth has about 850 mg of sodium—almost half of the daily limit.	
Use of sodium modeling – high dialysate sodium levels at the start of treatment and less later on sodium loads most patients.	**Use UF profiling*** to control water removal rates throughout the treatment.

*With a doctor's order

After you draw the sample, in most cases, you will attach a syringe to the end of the needle tubing. Then, you can flush the line with saline and keep the tubing sterile.

HOW TO DRAW BLOOD FROM AN HD CATHETER

Catheters are "locked" with heparin or saline after each use, to prevent clotting. The first blood from a catheter may be mixed with the locking solution, which could change the results of some blood tests. Follow your clinic's policy to draw blood for tests from a catheter, if this is part of your role. In some states, only nurses can draw blood from a hemodialysis catheter.

HOW TO USE A CENTRIFUGE

A centrifuge (see Figure 21) is a machine that uses centrifugal force to separate red blood cells from blood serum. It may be your job to "spin down" or centrifuge blood samples that require it. A centrifuge may have "holders" with screw-on lids, each of which has blood tube-sized indents to hold several blood tubes. Follow your clinic's procedures to use the centrifuge. **A centrifuge must be balanced at all times**. Only tubes of the same size, filled to the same level, can be across from each other. Start the centrifuge only after you have secured the lid. A centrifuge that is unbalanced will shake and may become unstable. Blood tubes may break, or the centrifuge may even "walk" off of the counter and fall on the floor.

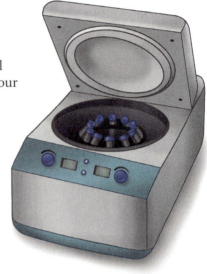

Figure 21: Centrifuge

Tips for Laboratory Testing

- Draw samples from the arterial bloodline injection port or arterial needle tubing.
- Once the samples are drawn, label the test tubes with the correct patient's name.
- You will need to draw most blood samples *before you start a treatment or give saline or heparin*. Some exceptions may include:
  - **Recirculation studies** (a test of how much blood is cleaned during a treatment) are drawn *during dialysis*.
  - **Post-dialysis BUN** (a test of dialysis adequacy) is drawn *after dialysis, using specific timing and technique*.
- **Blood tests can worsen anemia**. Draw the smallest amount of blood your clinic's lab will take for each test. Use pediatric (children's) blood tubes when you can.
- **Use the right tube for the test.** Blood tube tops are color-coded. Some contain chemicals to preserve the blood, clot it, keep it from clotting, etc. If you do not know which tube to use, look in your clinic manual or ask the nurse.
- Always draw blood tubes in the *order your lab requests*. (Chemicals in the tubes may attach to the needle and change results in other tubes if they are drawn in the wrong order.) Gently tip blood tubes back and forth to ensure proper mixing of blood with any additives in the tube. Do not shake blood tubes vigorously; this can damage the blood cells.
- Keep blood tubes upright once you are done mixing the blood with the additives.
- Learn how to process the blood tubes: Some must be refrigerated. Others must sit for 10–20 minutes before spinning in a centrifuge.
- Never place blood sample tubes on warm or hot surfaces (e.g., on top of a dialysis machine).

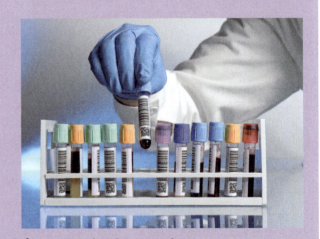

Figure 22: Blood Draw Tubes

If a sample tube breaks:[46]
- Close the centrifuge lid for at least 30 minutes (an hour is better) to let droplets settle, so staff and patients do not breathe them in.
- Use forceps to remove broken tubes so you do not cut yourself.
- Soak the blood tube holders in warm water and your clinic's preferred disinfectant, then rinse and dry.
- Clean all surfaces that become contaminated with blood, per your clinic's protocol.

TESTING BLOOD SUGAR

If your patient has diabetes and shows signs or symptoms of *hypoglycemia* (low blood sugar), tell the nurse. The patient's blood sugar level will need to be tested, most often using a finger stick and a blood sugar meter (see Figure 23). (We do not use blood in the circuit to test blood sugar, because glucometers need to be recalibrated for whole blood testing.) Glucose can be given by mouth (juice, pills, or gel) or IV, as needed. The American Diabetes Association says a patient with low blood sugar may:[47]

- Feel nervous or shaky
- Sweat, have chills, or feel clammy
- Be irritable, angry, sad, or impatient
- Be confused or delirious
- Have a rapid heartbeat
- Feel lightheaded or dizzy
- Be hungry or feel nauseated
- Have blurry vision
- Have tingling or numb lips or tongue
- Report a headache
- Feel weak or fatigued
- Have nightmares or cry out during sleep
- Lack coordination
- Have seizures
- Pass out

Most dialysate has some glucose, which helps keep the patient's blood levels from dropping too low during treatment. The nurse will give you instructions.

Start the Dialysis Machine

Once all of the previous steps are done, you will need to connect the bloodlines to the access. In most cases, the patient will receive the saline prime—but not

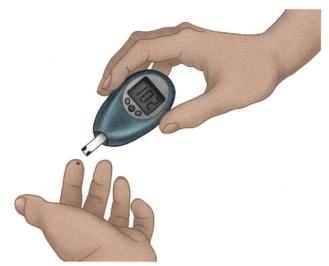

Figure 23: Blood Sugar Meter

always. Follow your clinic's policies and procedures, which may be something like these:

- **If the patient *will* receive the saline prime:**
  ➢ *Drain and discard the prime and fill the lines with fresh saline.*[29] With fresh saline, you will not expose the patient to particles left in the dialyzer from manufacturing. Fresh saline also helps the patient avoid sterilant rebound that could occur after a dialyzer is made or reprocessed.
  ➢ Clamp both arterial and venous lines.
  ➢ Connect the arterial bloodline to the arterial needle.
  ➢ Connect the venous bloodline to the venous needle.
  ➢ Unclamp both lines.
  ➢ Turn on blood pump slowly < 200 mL/min.
  ➢ Take the patient's blood pressure.
  ➢ Slowly raise blood flow to the prescribed rate.

- **If the patient will *not* receive the saline prime:**
  ➢ Stop the blood pump and clamp both lines.
  ➢ Connect the arterial bloodline to the arterial needle and unclamp.
  ➢ Unclamp the venous line placed over the prime waste container.
  ➢ Turn blood pump on slowly < 200 ml/min.[29]
  ➢ Let the extracorporeal circuit fill with blood, while you drain the saline prime into a waste container. Turn off the blood pump and clamp the venous line.
  ➢ **Pay close attention: there is a risk of severe blood loss until you connect the venous line to the access!**

- ➤ Connect the venous bloodline to the venous needle.
- ➤ Turn blood pump on slowly < 200 ml/min.
- ➤ Take the patient's blood pressure.
- After you connect both bloodlines, slowly raise the blood flow to the prescribed rate. Be sure there is no infiltration of the vascular access. The patient should not have pain, swelling, or a *hematoma* (collection of blood) under the skin at the needle site.
- As you do this, make sure there is enough blood flow from the access by watching the arterial and venous pressure monitors:
  - ➤ **The venous pressure should be about half of the blood flow rate**.
  - ➤ **Pre-pump arterial pressure should never exceed -250 mmHg**.
- Set the venous and arterial pressure alarms.
- Once you have started the treatment, document what you have done in the patient's treatment record or flow sheet.
- Before you leave the patient's chair, verify that ALL alarms are set correctly.
- Check that all line connections are secure and that you can see the patient's access.

Monitoring During Dialysis

"I was about 20 minutes from finishing when I started getting cold sweats. Before I could call for help, I was surrounded by two nurses and two techs. I must have passed out, 'cause I was getting oxygen. I'm so appreciative of the staff at my center for their attention and care. I know I'm in very good hands, and I praise the Lord for that!"

After a treatment starts, you will monitor the patient *and* the machine. The purpose of monitoring is to:

- Provide a comfortable and safe treatment for the patient.
- Allow you to note potential problems right away and take appropriate action.
- Detect any unusual machine issue as quickly as you can.

Patient Monitoring

Patient monitoring includes:
- Taking vital signs
- Checking the patient's vascular access
- Keeping an eye on the patient's general condition and response to the treatment
- Giving medicines as ordered
- Monitoring the patient's comfort and safety
- Watching for clotting in the extracorporeal circuit

Taking Vital Signs

You will check the patient's vital signs to ensure a safe and effective treatment. Check blood pressure and pulse every half hour—or more often if a patient has symptoms, is not stable, or as ordered. Compare the results to the predialysis values, per your clinic's policies and procedures.

Teach your patients to recognize and report early signs of low blood pressure (hypotension) so you can take steps before they "crash" and cramp. These may include:

- A racing pulse
- Nausea
- Vomiting
- Light headedness
- Ringing in the ears
- Seeing spots or sparkles
- Sweating
- Restlessness
- Yawning
- Warmth
- Confusion
- Seizure or unresponsiveness (if severe)

Watch the patient's *diastolic* (bottom number) blood pressure. An increase can be a sign of a too-rapid drop in blood volume—and hypotension may follow. Tell the nurse if you find anything unusual.

Hemodialysis Procedures and Complications

Vascular Access

CMS and State Health Departments require that you must be able to see a patient's vascular access at all times during a treatment. **A covered vascular access can be deadly**. Bleeding from bloodlines that come apart or a needle that pulls out could be hidden by a blanket. You might not see the blood in time to prevent fatal blood loss.

You will also check the access (fistula or graft) for:

- Pain or bleeding
- An infiltration or hematoma
- Blood flow that does not reach the prescribed rate
- Arterial and venous pressures that are outside your clinic's limits

Table 10 contains some issues that can be a factor in access bleeding problems and suggested best practices to address them.

Preventing Access Bleeding During Dialysis

"I looked across the aisle and saw a pool of blood under another patient's chair. He was reading and didn't realize anything was wrong."

Access bleeding at dialysis can be fatal for patients. Research suggests that in the U.S.:

- **Each day**, 200 venous needles come out of patients' accesses—and two or more patients have a serious health outcome like a hospital or ICU stay.[48]
- **Each week**, 2–3 patients die due to venous needle dislodgement.[49]
- **Each year**, more than 130 patients bleed to death on dialysis from access or line disconnects.[49]

These numbers are quite likely an *underestimate*. Just five states require dialysis clinics to report unexpected patient deaths.[50] **Monitor each patient at least every 30 minutes**. Walk by and look to ensure that there is no blood on the tape, on the blankets, floor, under chairs, or behind the machines. Check that transducer protectors (if present) are dry, and change them if they become wet.

Teach Your Patients How to React to an Access Rupture

"I had a Band-Aid over my needle scabs, and when I took it off, it felt like warm water was hitting me in the face, and blood sprayed out like a faucet. I ran to the bathroom to get something to stop it and had my brother call 911. I was so scared, I thought I was gonna die. It happened again a month later and they had to re-route the vein."

Most access ruptures occur *away* from dialysis. Teach patients what to do, quiz them once a month, and document that you have done this. Patients need to learn to:[51]

- **Raise their access arm above the level of their hearts to slow the flow of blood**
- **Put their finger in the hole to plug it and apply direct pressure at the bleeding site IMMEDIATELY**. Do *not* apply a tourniquet. Do *not* use towels: they will wick even more blood out of the access.
- **Call 911—*without* letting go of the pressure**. Yell for help if someone is around.
- Not worry about infection or loss of the access, this is an emergency

General Patient Condition

You will learn how patients tolerate a treatment by watching and listening to them. Watch the patient's behavior, appearance, response, and symptoms. **Teach your patients what symptoms to look for (they often do not know until you tell them)**. Ask them to tell you about any symptoms they have. Nervousness, shortness of breath, restlessness or agitation, itching, flushing, fever and chills, sleepiness, and complaints of pain or any discomfort are things that should be noted. Report symptoms or any unusual events to the nurse so the care team can take action early (see Table 12 on pages 248-261).

Giving Medicines

Patients may need some medicines before, during, or after a treatment. The timing depends on whether a medicine will dialyze out, and on your clinic's policies

Module 7

Table 10: Troubleshoot Access Problems[50]

Access Concern	Best Practices to Address the Challenge
Not enough staff to monitor patients' accesses	■ Encourage a ratio of one staff person to four or fewer patients.
Poor preparation of access sites	■ Allow time to carefully inspect the access. ■ Clean and prepare the needle site. ■ Consider shaving the site if hair would keep tape from adhering.
Difficult access sites	■ Match the needle length to the fistula depth.
Poor attention to taping (See Module 6 for step-by-step taping to prevent needle dislodgement.)	■ Ask patients about tape or adhesive allergies. Consider paper or silicone-based adhesive for those with sensitive skin. Test tape before use somewhere *other* than the access. ■ Use a consistent taping technique, per clinic policy and procedure. ■ *Chevrons* (taping around the tubing in a "V" pattern) help fix needles in place to prevent pulling. (Put the chevron tape on *before* the piece that covers the puncture sites. This helps to secure the needles.) ■ Use a long enough piece of tape on both sides of the tubing to be sure the tape will adhere. ■ Clear "window" dressings can cover and fixate the entire access site. ■ Avoid tape tabs—they can catch on objects and dislodge a needle. ■ Consider re-taping or extra taping for patients who sweat a lot.
Poorly securing bloodlines	■ Anchor bloodlines to the *patient*—not to a chair or bed. ■ Put the machine on the same side as the patient's access. ■ Use snap-on clips to keep bloodlines from loosening during HD if your clinic has them, or verify that Luer locks are tightened securely. ■ Loop the bloodlines to allow the patient *some* movement, but not so loosely that they can catch on something.
Obstructed view of the access	■ **Keep every access visible at all times**. ■ Do not obstruct the access with alarms or monitors. ■ Get in the habit of glancing at the floor and chair for blood. ■ Teach patients *why* they must keep their accesses in your view. ■ Offer blankets or suggest warmer clothing if patients are cold.
High access pressure settings to avoid alarms	■ Set the lower limit for the venous pressure alarm as close to the current venous pressure as the machine will allow. ■ **Low venous pressure may not trigger a machine alarm.** A patient can *exsanguinate* (lose a large volume of blood) in minutes. ■ Measure access pressure before each treatment; if it is < 30 mmHg, use an external monitor, such as RedSense®, HEMOdialert™, or an *enuresis* (bedwetting) pad, if available. ■ Have policies and procedures for silencing, changing, or disabling alarms. ■ Set clinic protocols for prompt response to alarms.

and procedures. For example, patients cannot take certain blood pressure pills within a few hours before a treatment. If they did, their blood pressure could drop too low during a treatment.

A nurse may give some medicines, such as IV iron, during a treatment. Others, like some antibiotics, are given near the end of or after a treatment to reduce the chance of the drug dialyzing out.

Patient Comfort and Safety

"I wear hearing aids. Our center got new TVs, so we each have one to look at. I can program mine to have Closed Captions so I can read my programs. I also take a puzzle book to do or play games on my cell phone. And, I take a sign language book so I can learn some signs."

Pay attention to the patient's comfort and diversion during a treatment. Did the patient bring something to do? Is s/he warm enough? Is the chair comfortable, or is an extra cushion needed?

- You can suggest that the patients read, bring coloring books or small handcrafts that can be done without disturbing the needles, listen to radio or podcasts, watch TV or movies, etc.
- Encourage patients to talk to their chair neighbors.
- Take this opportunity to talk with your patients about their needs, education, safety, nutrition, etc.

Anticoagulation

Anticoagulants help prevent clotting, so the patient's blood can flow freely through the extracorporeal circuit. During a treatment, the patient's blood touches foreign surfaces like the bloodlines, dialyzers, and even air in the drip chambers. This contact can cause blood to clot, which could clog the dialyzer and lines. Two common anticoagulants we use are heparin and citrate. Saline flushes may be used for patients who cannot use an anticoagulant.

HEPARIN

The anticoagulant of choice in HD is heparin, because it is easy to give and works quickly. Depending on the patient, heparin is gone from the bloodstream in 30 minutes to 2 hours, so it allows normal blood clotting to resume after a treatment.[52] The patient's doctor prescribes the dose. There are four ways to give heparin (see Table 11); which one is used will depend on the patient's needs and your clinic's procedure.

Learn the signs of heparin or bleeding problems and report any problems to the nurse. Check your patients for signs and symptoms of too much or not enough heparin:

Signs of too much heparin:
- Nosebleeds
- Bleeding in the white part of the eyes
- *Ecchymosis* (bruising)
- Prolonged bleeding from the access after treatment
- Worsening GI, retinal, or menstrual bleeding
- Bloody urine (hematuria)

Signs of not enough heparin:
- Clots in the drip chambers and/or arterial dialyzer header
- Very dark blood in the bloodlines
- Dark blood, shadows or dark streaks in the dialyzer
- Changes in arterial or venous pressures (depends on where clotting has occurred)

Table 11: Four Ways to Give Heparin[52]

Bolus	- Give a bolus loading dose (single amount) 3–5 minutes before a treatment starts. No more heparin is given.
Continuous	- Using a heparin infusion pump, infuse the drug into the arterial bloodline after the blood pump, during the whole treatment (see Figure 24). - You may also use a bolus loading dose before the start of dialysis. - Stop the heparin pump before the end of the treatment, as ordered.
Intermittent (Routine Repeated Bolus)	- Inject a bolus dose of heparin 3–5 minutes before a treatment starts. - You may give more bolus doses of heparin throughout the treatment, as ordered.
"Tight" Heparin A minimal dose may be used for patients who bleed, had a procedure before treatment, or will have a procedure after a treatment or the next day.	- The bolus heparin dose and infusion rate are *just* enough to prevent clotting of the extracorporeal circuit. - Give a bolus dose 3–5 minutes before a treatment starts. - Use the heparin pump to continuously infuse heparin during the treatment, as ordered. - Keep the heparin pump on until the end of the treatment, as ordered.

HEPARIN-FREE DIALYSIS

Heparin-free dialysis can be done for patients who are at a high risk for bleeding (e.g. recent surgery, active bleeding) or are allergic to heparin. Heparin-free dialysis is hard to do well. It requires:

Module 7

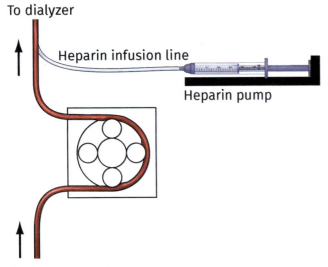

Figure 24: Heparin Pump

- A good arterial blood flow rate of at least 300–400 mL/min.[52] The blood flow rate should keep the arterial pre-pump pressures less than -250 mmHg.
- Normal saline flushes through the dialyzer and lines at regular times (e.g., 100–200 mLs every 30 minutes). These flushes help you to see and prevent clotting, or to see the need to change dialyzer and lines if clotting is seen. NOTE: Saline can also be infused into the atrial line continuously to dilute blood before the dialyzer. If this is done, an IV pump must be used to ensure appropriate pressure in the arterial line.
- A dialyzer with a high UF coefficient, which allows for an increased fluid and solute removal
- A dialysis machine with UF control

NOTE: Add the total fluid amount of all of the saline flushes to the patient's UF goal at the start of dialysis. If this amount is not in the initial calculations, the patient will leave the treatment weighing more than when s/he arrived.

Alternative Acid Concentrates

Certain acid concentrates for dialysate can prevent blood clotting without the use of heparin. Standard acid concentrates use acetic acid. Citrasate® and DRYalysate® use citric acid instead. Computer models can help predict what the patient's calcium level will be.[53]

Machine Monitoring

"I went for treatment yesterday, and came in at my dry weight: 72.5. Treatment went well, but my weight after was 74.7. What's up with that? They said something must be wrong with that machine."

The sensors and detectors on a dialysis machine allow it to:

- Tell you—with audio and visual alarms—if something in the treatment is outside of the *parameters* (limits)
- Check the patient's blood for air bubbles and pressures
- Continually watch how the system's dialysis control functions are working

Technicians monitor dialysis machines by:

- Doing equipment safety tests
- Checking each patient's dialyzer and machine readings
- Quickly responding and correcting alarms when they occur

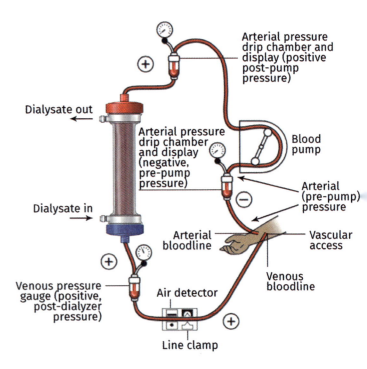

Figure 25: Pressure Monitoring Devices on Arterial and Venous Bloodlines

You will learn what each monitor on the HD machine does and what to do when an alarm sounds. Then, you can act quickly to find the problem. Module 4: *Hemodialysis Devices* covers monitors and alarms in detail. It will be your job to watch the extracorporeal circuit, dialysate circuit, and equipment for problems during treatments (see Figures 25 and 26).

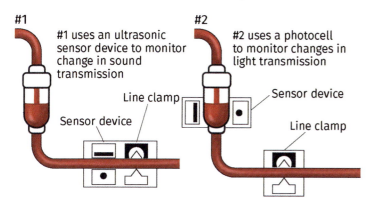

Figure 26: Air Detector

You will need to:
- Look at the dialyzer and bloodlines for air
- Watch for dialyzer blood leaks
- Check for clotting
- Check all of the pressure alarms
- Monitor blood and dialysate flow rates
- Check dialysate temperature and conductivity
- Monitor the amount of fluid removal
- Check the infusion rate, if a heparin pump is used
- Check the tubing connections

These checks help keep patients safe. **Check all systems every half hour or per your clinic's policy**.

Hemodialysis Complications

"I moved and had to switch clinics, and I have been itching like crazy! At first I thought it was my phosphorus, but it's not that high. Plus, I only itch when I'm on the machine. It's so bad I haven't been able to sleep until my treatment is over. I think I may be allergic to the solution."

While HD technology has improved, there is always a risk of complications during a treatment. These can be *clinical* (related to patient care) or *technical* (related to equipment). We will cover both types.

NOTE: Dialysis technician scope of practice laws and rules vary from state to state. In your state, you may or may not be allowed to perform some of the "what to do" steps that you will learn in this section.

Clinical Complications

"Anyone have issues with the dialysis machine driving your blood pressure up instead of down? Mine gets scarily high, 190s/90s. I've been as high as 202 on the first number. I'm afraid I'm going to have a stroke or a heart attack!"

Clinical complications that may occur during a treatment are described in Table 12. Follow your clinic's policies and procedures to prevent or respond to these. Tell the nurse right away if you see a problem so s/he can react.

Module 7

Table 12: Clinical Complications of HD[29,54,55]

AIR EMBOLISM
Air bubbles are carried by the blood stream into a vessel small enough to be blocked by the bubbles.

Causes

- Unarmed or defective air detector, **and**:
  - An empty saline bag
  - Careless IV administration
  - Loose bloodline connections or a leak before the blood pump
  - Separation of an arterial bloodline
- Very cold dialysate that releases a large amount of dissolved air when warmed.
- An uncapped and unclamped catheter, especially when a patient is sitting up.

Signs

- Air or foam in the venous line
- No caps or clamps on catheter

Symptoms

- If the patient is *sitting up*, air may travel to the *brain* and cause:
  - Changes in vision
  - Confusion
  - Slight paralysis of one side of the body
  - Seizure, stroke, coma, or death
- If the patient is *lying down*, air may go to the *heart and lungs*, and cause problems such as:
  - Shortness of breath or coughing
  - *Cyanosis*—blue lips, fingers and toes
  - Irregular heart rhythms (arrhythmias)
  - Chest pain, cardiac arrest, *death*

Prevention

- Secure all blood circuit connections.
- Arm the air detector at all times.
- Look at the venous bloodline from the air detector to the patient *before* you override an air alarm.
- Verify that catheters are clamped if the cap must be removed.
- Remove or clamp empty IV bags or syringes.
- Double clamp the saline line/all stagnant lines.
- Inspect the venous bloodline for air before you connect it to the access.
- Keep the blood pump speed to a rate the access can deliver, so air is not pulled in.

What to Do If This Happens

Your role:
- Clamp the bloodlines and turn off the blood pump to stop the inflow of air.
- Call for help.
- Raise the patient's feet above his/her head. (Trendelenburg position)
- Turn the patient on his or her *left* side so air will rise to the *right* side of the heart.

The nurse will:
- Give oxygen (8 L–10 L).
- Call 911 and the patient's physician.
- Do an EKG if possible.
- Monitor and stabilize vital signs.
- Attach a normal saline line to the arterial cannula or start a new IV for medicines.
- Give saline, if the patient is hypotensive.

ANAPHYLAXIS
Severe allergic reaction

Causes

- Sensitivity to ethylene oxide (ETO), a sterilant (NOTE: Most dialyzers are now sterilized with gamma-radiation and/or steam)
- Taking an ACE inhibitor for blood pressure *and* using AN-69 dialyzer membranes
- Reaction to germicide left in the dialyzer and/or bloodlines
- A medication/blood reaction
- A Type A reaction to a dialyzer membrane

Signs

- A reaction in the first 5–30 minutes of HD
- A reaction 5–10 minutes after a medicine

ANAPHYLAXIS (CONTINUED)

Symptoms

- Trouble breathing (throat may close up)
- Chest tightness
- Tachycardia
- Cardiac arrest
- Hypotension
- Feeling anxious or restless
- Flushing; burning, heat sensation
- Hives and itching
- Tearing up; swelling around the eyes
- Runny nose
- Abdominal cramping
- Numbness and tingling around the mouth
- Low back pain
- Burning and pain at the venous puncture site if disinfectant is infused—usually right away

Prevention

- Avoid drugs patient has a known allergy to.
- Rinse "first use dialyzers" well right before use (per the manufacturer's procedures).
- Rinse dialyzers and bloodlines well during treatment preparation.

What to Do If This Happens

Your role:
- Call for help.
- Stop the suspected treatment (i.e. medicine, the blood pump) to prevent further reaction.

The nurse will:
- Call 911 and the doctor.
- Give oxygen.
- Clamp all lines.
- Stop dialysis and *not* return the blood.
- Monitor vital signs.
- Treat hypotension.
- Give medicines as ordered.

ANGINA
Chest pain due to low oxygen levels in the heart

Causes

- Coronary artery disease (blocked heart arteries)
- Hypotension (makes the heart work harder)
- Anxiety (raises heart rate)
- Anemia
- Cardiac stunning from aggressive UF

Symptoms

- Pain or tightness in chest, arm, or jaw
- Patient may be cold, sweating, and/or have trouble breathing
- Patient may be hypotensive

Prevention

- Monitor BP closely to avoid hypotension.
- Prevent blood loss that could worsen anemia (i.e. clotted dialyzer fibers).
- Treat anemia per the prescription.
- Calculate and set a UF goal of < 13 mL/kg/hr.

What to Do If This Happens

Your role:
- Call for help.
- Slow the blood flow rate and UFR to prevent further fluid loss and heart stress.
- Monitor vital signs.

The nurse will:
- Assess the patient and call the physician.
- Give nitroglycerin, per standing orders.
- Do an EKG if possible.
- Give oxygen if the patient is short of breath.
- Stop dialysis if pain is severe or unresolved.
- Assess dry weight, UFR goal, and UFR.
- Give saline, if patient is hypotensive.

ARRHYTHMIA
Irregular heartbeat

Causes

- Underlying heart disease
- Changes in serum pH or electrolyte levels, especially potassium
- Hypotension
- Heart disease
- Cardiac stunning from aggressive UF

Symptoms

- Irregular pulse (skipped or extra beats)
- Slow or rapid heart rate
- Patient complains of "palpitations"
- Anxiety

Prevention

- Verify dialysate potassium (the doctor may order a higher level if patient is on digitalis).
- Monitor rate *and* rhythm during treatment.
- Monitor blood pressure.
- Monitor the UFR to prevent hypotension.

What to Do If This Happens

Your role:
- Call for help.
- Check vital signs.
- Manually take the patient's pulse.
- If the patient is hypotensive, lower the UFR.

The nurse will:
- Assess the patient.
- Do an EKG if possible.
- Call patient's physician.
- Give medicine(s) as ordered.
- If the patient is hypotensive, give IV fluids.
- Check the dialysate potassium level.
- Discontinue dialysis for severe symptoms.

BLEACH (CHLORINE) OR GERMICIDE EXPOSURE
Bleach in the dialysis water or dialysate causes patient harm

Causes

- Extremely hypertonic solutions

Signs and Symptoms

- Rise or fall in pulse rate
- Cardiac arrest
- Chest pain
- *Cyanosis* (turning blue)
- Hemolysis
- Drop in BP
- Trouble breathing
- Vomiting

Prevention

- Test for bleach or germicide in dialysate and water treatment systems, per clinic policy.
- Test for bleach or germicide in dialysis equipment before the start of treatment, per clinic policy.
- Do not disinfect the dialysate, water systems, or machine while patients are dialyzing.

What to Do If this Happens

Your role:
- Stop the treatment.
- Clamp the venous bloodline so hemolyzed blood does not return to the patient.
- Take blood samples as ordered.
- Take dialysate samples for analysis.
- Save the extracorporeal circuit for analysis.
- Take the dialysis machine off the treatment floor.
- Help identify the source of the bleach.

The nurse will:
- Monitor the patient's oxygen saturation.
- Tell the patient's doctor.
- Monitor the patient's vital signs, breathing, and heart rhythm.
- Help identify the source of the bleach or germicide, and whether it is at the station or is from a central delivery system.

Hemodialysis Procedures and Complications

CARDIAC ARREST
The heart stops beating

Causes

- Extreme hypotension
- Electrolyte imbalance; high potassium
- Arrhythmias
- Heart attack
- Air embolism
- Hemolysis
- Exsanguination (severe blood loss)

Signs

- No apical or carotid pulse
- No breathing
- Loss of consciousness

Symptoms

Men
- Chest, arm, shoulder, or jaw pain/pressure
- Breaking out in a cold sweat
- Indigestion, nausea, vomiting
- Feeling faint, dizzy, or breathless
- Feeling of "impending doom"
- Severe anxiety or confusion

Women
- Pain or pressure from center of chest to arm
- Pain in the upper back, shoulder, throat
- Sweating
- Indigestion, nausea, gas pain, vomiting
- Feeling faint, dizzy, or breathless
- Anxiety
- Sudden severe fatigue or sleep problems

Prevention

- Prevent problems that could cause cardiac arrest, such as shock and rapid potassium shifts.
- Monitor vital signs during treatment.
- Verify that the UF goal is not too high.
- Tell the nurse right away about major vital sign changes and/or patient complaints.
- Check the vascular access and bloodlines to be sure they are securely connected.

What to Do If This Happens

Your role:
- Call for help.
- Stop the treatment, if told to by a nurse. Return the patient's blood.
- Flush the needles or catheter limbs with normal saline to maintain an IV line for fluids and medicines.
- Help with resuscitation as asked.
- Put a backboard under the patient or move the patient to the floor.

The nurse will:
- See if the patient is unresponsive.
- Follow clinic policy for a Do Not Resuscitate (DNR) order if present.
- If the patient has no DNR order or status is unknown, start CPR and use an AED (automatic external defibrillator):
  ➤ Have someone call 911
  ➤ Have someone call the patient's doctor
  ➤ Do CPR until patient responds or paramedics arrive

Module 7

CARDIAC (MYOCARDIAL) "STUNNING"
Drop in blood flow to the heart muscle

Causes

- Aggressive UFR
- Hypotension
- Hypovolemia

Signs

- Symptomatic BP drop
- Muscle cramps
- Chest pain

Prevention

- Lower dialysate temperature.
- Avoid UFRs above 13 mL/kg/hr.
- Use blood volume monitoring if your clinic has this.
- Monitor the patient closely.
- Teach the patient about safe water gains.
- Offer more frequent HD or an extra session for hypervolemia.
- Lengthen treatment time to reduce UFR.
- Reassess target weight.

What to Do If This Happens

Your role:	The nurse will:
■ Monitor blood pressures to prevent significant blood pressure drop. ■ Alert the nurse if you see a high UFR.	■ Know the patient's co-morbidities (i.e., CHF, myocardial fibrosis with LVH) and age. ■ Monitor for high UFRs, and limit them via a doctor's order. ■ Evaluate episodes of hypotension. ■ Give oxygen, as needed. ■ Educate patient on the risks of a high sodium diet that increases fluid intake.

DEATH
The patient passes away at the dialysis clinic

Causes

- Cardiac arrest
- Anaphylactic shock
- Blood loss
- Respiratory failure or stroke

Signs

- Unresponsive
- Not breathing
- No pulse

Prevention

- May or may not be preventable

What to Do If This Happens

Your role:	The nurse will:
■ Do not move the patient. ■ Use screens or curtains for privacy. ■ Do not touch the machine, lines, etc. until you are directed to by a nurse. ■ Gather the patient's belongings, if asked, to give to the family. ■ Do not discuss the patient's outcome with other patients—this would violate HIPAA.	■ Contact the facility medical director. ■ Contact the coroner's office. ■ Call the patient's doctor, family, and a funeral home for transport. ■ Arrange to move the patient's body to await transport.

Hemodialysis Procedures and Complications

DIALYSIS DISEQUILIBRIUM SYNDROME (DDS)
Brain swelling when a rapid drop in BUN level causes water to shift into the brain.
(NOTE: Uncommon these days.)

Causes
- New to dialysis with very high BUN levels
- Skipping several treatments so BUN levels are high

Signs
- During or towards the *end* of treatment:
  - *High* blood pressure (hypertension)
  - Change in level of consciousness
  - Irregular pulse
  - In severe cases: coma and death

Symptoms
- During or towards the *end* of treatment:
  - Nausea and vomiting
  - Blurred vision
  - Headache
  - Tremors/restlessness
  - Behavior changes, seizures

Prevention
- Monitor the patient closely during treatment.
- Tell the nurse right away about vital sign changes or patient complaints.
- When BUN is > 150 mg/dL:
  - Use a smaller (prescribed) dialyzer.
  - Use slower blood and dialysate flows.
  - The nephrologist may prescribe short, slow treatments *daily* for a few days.

What to Do If This Happens

Your role:
- Watch patients for symptoms.
- Tell the nurse if you suspect a problem.
- Stop the treatment, if directed to by a nurse, and return the patient's blood.

The nurse will:
- Assess the patient for disequilibrium or other causes for these symptoms.
- Decrease treatment efficiency:
  - Use a dialyzer with lower clearances.
  - Slow blood and dialysate flow rates.
  - Use a concurrent dialysate flow.
  - Tell the patient's physician.
  - Give medicines as prescribed.
  - Do short, more frequent treatments.
  - Stop treatment if symptoms are severe.

EXSANGUINATION
Life-threatening loss of blood

Causes
- Failure to connect the venous bloodline to the patient when discarding priming saline
- Bloodline separation
- Needle dislodgement
- Fistula or graft rupture
- Dialyzer rupture (blood leak detector fails)

Signs
- Large amount of blood on the patient's clothing, blankets, chair, or the floor
- Pink or red dialysate in the dialyzer compartment and lines, with a blood detector alarm
- Sudden low pre-pump arterial pressure alarm with an air detector alarm

Symptoms
- Blood pressure drops
- Rapid heart rate
- Shortness of breath
- Shock
- Seizures
- Cardiac arrest

EXSANGUINATION
Life-threatening loss of blood (CONTINUED)

Prevention

- Be sure that you always can see the patient's dialysis access and line connections during treatment.
- Tape the needles securely.
- Check all access connections and bloodlines every 30 minutes when you check vital signs.
- Secure looped bloodlines *only* to the patient. Do not make the loops too tight.
- Test all pressure monitors and blood leak detectors before *each* patient.
- Glance at the floors for blood, especially under the chair and behind the machine.

What to Do If This Happens

Your role:
- Call for help immediately.
- Stop the blood pump.
- Clamp both sides of separated bloodlines or a catheter.
- Apply direct pressure to a bleeding site.
- Discard bloodlines and dialyzer and restart treatment, per a doctor's order.
- Secure the dialysis access for possible use to give IV fluids.

The nurse will:
- Monitor vital signs.
- Give oxygen.
- Alert the doctor/nephrologist.
- Give medicine(s) as ordered.
- Call 911.
- Infuse saline or other ordered fluid, if needed, while awaiting EMS.

FEVER AND/OR CHILLS
High temperature, patient shivering

Causes

- Infection (most commonly in a catheter, graft, or fistula, in that order)
- Contaminated reprocessed dialyzer
- Pyrogenic reaction from dialysate water
- Too-hot dialysate
- Too-cold dialysate
- Break in sterile technique

Signs

- **Local infection:** redness, swelling, warmth, or drainage from access or other sites (e.g., feet, wounds)
- **Pyrogenic reaction:** One or more patients with normal temperature(s) develop fever and chills 45–75 minutes after the start of dialysis

Symptoms

- Infection: fever/chills before HD; warmth, swelling, pain, at access or other sites (e.g., feet, skin wounds)
- Shaking (rigors) may lead to a rise in temperature
- Fever, chills develop after HD starts
- Feeling hot (dialysate temperature higher than patient's core body temperature)
- Feeling cold without a fever (cold dialysate)
- Headache
- Nausea and vomiting
- Muscle aches

Prevention

- Practice good hand hygiene and use standard precautions.
- Check the patient's vital signs and tell the nurse right away about major changes.
- Use aseptic technique to set up equipment and place needles.
- Check the patient for *systemic* (whole body) and *local* (one site) infections.
- Check dialysate temperature before treatment.
- Disinfect the dialysis machine and the water treatment system per clinic policy.
- Check reprocessed dialyzers for the proper level of disinfectant and correct dwell time.
- Follow clinic policy for the maximum time saline can be safely recirculated through the extracorporeal circuit before a treatment.

Hemodialysis Procedures and Complications

FEVER AND/OR CHILLS
High temperature, patient shivering (CONTINUED)

What to Do If This Happens

Your role if there is an infection:
- Monitor vital signs including temperature closely and report to nursing staff.

Your role in a suspected pyrogenic reaction:
- Tell the nurse.
- Stop the treatment and follow the nurses' instructions.
- Check vital signs, including temperature.
- Take water and dialysate samples for limulus amoebocyte lysate (LAL) and bacterial testing as directed by the nurse.

If infection is suspected, the nurse will:
- Obtain blood cultures (2 sets) and/or wound culture for drainage, per doctor's order.
- Give medicines as ordered.

If a pyrogenic reaction is suspected, the nurse will:
- Call the doctor.
- Instruct the staff about the care and treatment of the patients who are now on dialysis at the clinic.
- Instruct the staff about the need for water and dialysate samples for culture and LAL and potential isolation of equipment.
- Give medicines as ordered.
- Notify health department if needed.

FIRST-USE SYNDROME
Sensitivity to dialyzer membrane or sterilant gas

Causes
- Reaction to ethylene oxide (ETO), a gas sterilant used in some new, dry dialyzers
- Allergy to the dialyzer membrane or residue from manufacturing. May be more severe in patients on ACE inhibitor blood pressure medicines.

Signs
- Reaction (see symptoms) in the first 5–10 minutes of treatment (20–40 minutes if mild)

Symptoms
- Itching
- Chest and/or back pain
- Shortness of breath
- Hypotension
- Nausea
- General discomfort

Prevention
- Rinse new dialyzers well with normal saline before treatment, per policy.
- Complete reprocessing steps that do not remove the membrane protein coating.

What to Do If This Happens

Your role:
- Tell the nurse if you suspect a reaction.

The nurse will:
- Assess the patient.
- Give oxygen for shortness of breath.
- Stop the treatment, if necessary.
- Give medicines to relieve symptoms and pain, per physician's order.

HEADACHE

Causes
- Hypertension
- Fluid shifts
- Dialysis disequilibrium syndrome (DDS)
- Electrolyte shifts
- Anxiety or tension
- A drop in blood sugar, even in patients who do *not* have diabetes
- Caffeine or alcohol withdrawal, as level drops during dialysis

Signs
- Patient holds head or complains of headache

Symptoms
- Pain in the head or face—can last for hours after a treatment and may be severe enough that patients stop dialysis
- Sensitivity to light and sound

Prevention
- Establish an accurate target weight.
- Calculate desired fluid loss and set the UF goal correctly.
- Encourage the patient to follow fluid and sodium limits and take prescribed blood pressure medicines.
- For DDS, use slower and/or more frequent HD. (A higher dialysate sodium concentrate may help.)
- Check the patient's blood sugar.

What to Do If This Happens

Your role:
- Notify the nurse.

The nurse will:
- Give medicines as ordered.
- Adjust treatment as needed.
- Assess for caffeine withdrawal.

HEPARIN OVERDOSE

Causes
- Error in first heparin bolus dose
- Error in heparin infusion pump setting
- Broken heparin pump delivers too much heparin

Signs
- Bleeding around needle sites at HD
- Needle site bleeding after HD for 20+ minutes
- Wrong amount of heparin left in syringe

Symptoms
- Hemorrhage (excessive bleeding)
- Low BP
- Bruising
- Nosebleeds
- Tarry stools
- *Petechiae* (purple spots where blood has leaked out under the skin)

Prevention
- Draw up the heparin dose correctly.
- Use the prescribed type of heparin.
- Monitor the heparin pump during treatment.

Hemodialysis Procedures and Complications

HEPARIN OVERDOSE (CONTINUED)

What to Do If This Happens

Your role:	The nurse will:
■ Tell the nurse.	■ Take frequent clotting times (if used). ■ Stop the heparin pump, especially near the end of dialysis. ■ If bleeding persists after removing the needles, apply pressure to sites and use a product to stop bleeding quickly. ■ Evaluate the heparin dose for the next treatment. ■ Notify the patient's doctor. ■ Send the patient to a hospital for protamine sulfate, the heparin antagonist, if ordered. ■ Have the patient's access checked for a tear or stenosis.

HYPERTENSION (HTN)
High blood pressure during or after HD treatments

Causes

■ Fluid overload (may be linked to high sodium intake or sodium modeling) ■ Not taking prescribed BP medicine(s)	■ Anxiety ■ Dialysis disequilibrium syndrome (DDS)

Signs

■ Headache ■ Nausea and vomiting	■ Nervousness ■ May have no symptoms (common)

Prevention

■ Encourage the patient to follow fluid and sodium limits and take prescribed BP medicines. ■ Establish an accurate target weight. ■ Calculate fluid loss correctly and set the UF goal accordingly.	■ For DDS, use slower and/or more frequent dialysis. ■ Medicate BP during treatment. ■ Confirm that the patient takes BP medicines correctly (and can afford them).

What to Do If This Happens

Your role:	The nurse will:
■ Monitor vital signs closely. ■ Calculate the UF goal correctly. ■ Encourage patients to follow their fluid and salt limits.	■ Give medicines, as needed if HTN is significant and prolonged. ■ Test the patient's blood sodium levels. ■ Assess whether sodium loading is going on during dialysis. ■ Talk to the doctor to consider a lower dialysate sodium level. ■ Ask the doctor about ambulatory BP monitoring to better see the BP pattern. ■ Talk with the dietitian about sodium in the patient's diet. ■ Consult with MD re: ER evaluation, if BP does not come down before discharge.

HYPOTENSION
Low blood pressure

Causes
- A too-high UF goal
- A too-high UF rate (> 13 mL/kg/hr)
- Taking BP medication before dialysis
- Change from sitting to standing
- Heart disease
- Anemia
- Dehydration (i.e. from vomiting, diarrhea)

Signs
- Gradual or sudden drop in blood pressure
- Sweating or cold, clammy skin
- Patient fans him or herself
- *Pallor* (patient turns white)
- Yawning
- Loss of consciousness

Symptoms
- Dizziness upon standing, feeling faint
- Nausea and vomiting
- *Tachycardia* (rapid heartbeat)
- Feeling warm
- Weakness
- Cramps
- Chest pain
- Headache
- Feeling anxious

Prevention
- Get an accurate weight before treatment.
- Calculate the fluid goal correctly.
- Do not exceed your clinic's UFR goal (i.e., < 13 mL/kg/hr).
- Monitor BP carefully during treatment.
- Teach your patients to recognize early symptoms and report them to staff.
- Ask patients if they are taking their BP medicines as prescribed.
- Encourage patients to follow fluid limits.
- Check patient's BP before and after they stand up to learn which patients have *orthostatic* hypotension (BP drops when they stand).

What to Do If This Happens

Your role:
- Tell the nurse.
- Use a modified Trendelenburg position (elevate legs 30–45 degrees).
- Decrease the UFR.
- Give a saline bolus.
- Keep checking BP until it is restored.

The nurse will:
- Assess the patient.
- Assess patient's need for oxygen.
- Assess patient's UF goal.

HYPOXEMIA
Not enough oxygen in the blood

Causes
- Congestive heart failure (CHF)
- Chronic obstructive pulmonary disease (COPD)
- Wrong dialysate composition
- First-use syndrome
- Non-biocompatible dialyzer membrane
- Anemia < 10 g/dL
- Eating during dialysis
- Warm dialysate (> 36° C)

Signs
- *Cyanosis* (blue lips, nail beds, skin)
- Low blood pressure
- Rise in pulse rate
- Faster respirations or panting
- Oxygen saturation is less than 90%

HYPOXEMIA
Not enough oxygen in the blood (CONTINUED)

Symptoms

- Blurred vision
- Chest pain
- Confusion
- Cramping
- Nausea and vomiting
- Dizziness
- Restlessness
- Shortness of breath

Prevention

- Give oxygen at treatment if Hgb < 10 g/dL.
- Watch for respirations > 24/min.
- Watch for systolic BP < 150 mmHg.
- Watch for a pulse rate < 60 or > 100.
- Watch for oxygen saturation < 90.
- Match bicarbonate dialysate to the patient.
- Use a biocompatible dialyzer membrane.
- The patient maintains an ideal dry weight.
- Use cooler dialysate (< 36° C).
- Discourage eating right before and during dialysis for affected patients.

What to Do If This Happens

Your role:
- Check the dialysate composition.

The nurse will:
- Give the patient oxygen.
- Support the patient's blood pressure.

MUSCLE CRAMPS

Causes

- Stunning from aggressive UF
- A too-high UF goal
- Hypotension
- Changes in blood chemistries, especially sodium, calcium, or potassium*

*NOTE: The response to changes in blood chemistry varies from patient to patient.

Signs

- Patient calls out or cries
- Patient stands or grabs the painful muscle

Symptoms

- Painful muscle cramps (spasms) – most often in the hands and feet or abdomen

Prevention

- Get an accurate weight before treatment.
- Calculate the desired weight loss and set the UF goal correctly.
- Verify the machine setting before you start a treatment.
- Do not exceed the UFR goal per your clinic's policy (i.e., < 13 mL/kg/hr).
- Use the prescribed dialysate.
- Encourage patients to follow their salt and fluid limits.

What to Do If This Happens

Your role:
- Decrease the UFR.
- Apply warm moist compresses to the affected area to relax the muscle.
- Gently massage the area.

The nurse will:
- Give oxygen per physician order.
- Give saline per clinic policy.
- Help patient stretch affected muscles, such as bend the fingers or foot back and forth.
- Verify that the patient's BP supports standing up before letting the patient do so.

Module 7

NAUSEA AND VOMITING	
Causes	
■ Hypotension ■ Food poisoning or GI virus ■ Dialysis disequilibrium syndrome ■ Pyrogenic reaction	■ Allergy to a dialyzer membrane ■ Medication reaction or interaction ■ Other GI problem
Symptoms	
■ Nausea, vomiting ■ Possible low—or high—blood pressure	■ Possible diarrhea and headache
Prevention	
■ Get an accurate weight before treatment. ■ Calculate the fluid goal correctly. ■ Do not exceed your clinic's UFR goal (i.e., < 13 mL/kg/hr).	■ The patient's doctor can prescribe medicine to reduce nausea. ■ Discourage eating at dialysis or suggest minimal intake if the patient must eat.
What to Do If This Happens	
Your role: ■ Give the patient an emesis basin. ■ Offer the patient a cool, wet washcloth and/or water to rinse his/her mouth. ■ Check the patient's vital signs. ■ Decrease the UFR for low blood pressure and give normal saline. ■ If available, offer scrubs if the patient's clothes are soiled.	**The nurse will:** ■ Check with the physician about anti-nausea medicine. ■ Reduce dialysis efficiency if dialysis disequilibrium syndrome is suspected. ■ If the patient has a fever, follow the steps for fever and/or chills.

PRURITUS Itching	
Causes	
■ Uremia ■ Dry skin ■ High serum phosphorus: calcium-phosphate crystals form in the skin	■ Secondary hyperparathyroidism ■ Allergic reaction to a medicine, needle, tape, dialyzer, gloves, bleach used to clean the chair, etc.
Signs	
■ Reddened skin ■ Seeing the patient scratching ■ Crusting on the skin ■ Increased serum phosphorus level	NOTE: Painful purple skin sores that develop suddenly and get worse quickly may be a sign of *calciphylaxis*. This problem requires special treatment.
Symptoms	
■ Severe itching *all* the time—high phosphorus levels are likely	■ Severe itching on dialysis *only*—allergy is likely
Prevention	
■ Keep the skin clean and dry. ■ Dialyze the patient as prescribed. ■ Ask patients if they take their phosphate binders with meals and snacks. ■ Refer to the nurse to suggest skin lotions.	■ Rinse the dialyzer with extra saline or ask the doctor to prescribe a different one. ■ Change the needle and/or tape for access itching. ■ Refer to the nurse for a medicine review.

PRURITUS
Itching (CONTINUED)

What to Do If This Happens

Your role:	The nurse will:
■ Tell the nurse.	■ Assess the patient. ■ Give medicine per physician's order ■ Suggest follow up (e.g. skin care, dietary consult).

SEIZURE

Causes
- Severe hypotension
- Electrolyte imbalance
- Seizure disorder
- Dialysate composition error
- Dialysis disequilibrium syndrome
- Low blood sugar
- Air embolism

Signs
- Change in level of consciousness
- Twitching, jerking of the arms and legs

Symptoms
- Patients with seizure disorders may have a change in vision (an "aura") that alerts them to a pending seizure.
- Patients may feel twitching, panic, or lightheadedness before a seizure.

Prevention
- Avoid rapid drops in BUN during HD.
- Monitor BP changes during HD.
- Give oxygen to patients who have heart or lung disease.
- Adjust the UFR to avoid hypotension and brain "stunning."
- Monitor the patient throughout treatment for signs and symptoms of treatment and equipment complications.
- Make sure the patient is taking anticoagulant medicine if prescribed.

What to Do If This Happens

Your role:	The nurse will:
■ Tell the nurse. ■ Check the patient's vital signs if you can. ■ Put something soft under the patient's head if s/he is on the floor. ■ Protect the access arm from needle dislodgement if you can. ■ Decrease the UFR for low blood pressure and give normal saline. ■ Stop the treatment if the patient is unresponsive, per the nurse.	■ Call the doctor. ■ Check glucose and track blood sugar. ■ Give medicines as ordered. ■ Treat dialysis disequilibrium syndrome. ■ Give oxygen for severe seizures. ■ Track low blood pressure, if present. ■ Insert a plastic airway and turn the patient's head to the side. ■ Call 911 for transport to the hospital.

Technical Complications

"I started with a 1,500 bolus of heparin, 1,500 for the second and third hour, and none in the last hour. In the last 2 weeks I have gone to a 2,200 bolus with 2,200 for 2nd and 3rd hour. Now I'm doing a 3,000 bolus and then 2,200 for the 2nd and 3rd and I'm still clotting the machine!"

Table 13 describes the technical complications that may occur during HD. Follow your clinic's policies and procedures to prevent or react to a complication. Tell the nurse right away if any of these problems occur.

Table 13: Troubleshooting Patient Problems at Dialysis

What You See	Possible Causes	What to Do: ALWAYS alert the nurse, and:
Air or foam in the bloodlines or collapse of the arterial bloodline	■ Empty saline bag ■ Under-filled drip chambers ■ A disconnect in the extracorporeal circuit ■ A needle that comes out of the vascular access while the blood pump is running	■ Check to see if the air detector clamp is on and secure on the venous bloodline below the drip chamber. If not, *clamp the line right away before the air reaches the patient*. ■ Verify that the blood pump has stopped. ■ Aseptically disconnect the patient from the extracorporeal circuit. ■ Remove all air from the extracorporeal circuit before resuming the treatment.
Bright (cherry) red blood in lines	■ *Hemolysis* (red blood cells bursting) ■ Pre-pump negative pressure too high (> -250 mmHg) ■ Kinked bloodline or too much blood pump occlusion ■ Dialysate contains zinc, copper, nitrates, or chlorine/chloramines ■ Too-warm dialysate ■ Germicide left in reprocessed dialyzer	■ Stop the treatment. ■ **Do not return the patient's blood**—it may contain lethal levels of potassium from the burst blood cells. ■ Do not use that machine for another patient. Remove it from the treatment floor and label it. ■ Check all other patients for signs and symptoms, in case hemolysis is caused by a faulty dialysate. ■ Keep and bag all supplies from the affected patient's treatment. Label "do not destroy." ■ Enlist experts to help find the cause.
Dark blood in the lines; clots seen in extracorporeal circuit during rinseback	■ Clotting ■ Not enough anticoagulant ■ Decreased blood flow rate ■ Low arterial drip chamber level ■ Frequent alarms stopped the blood pump ■ Air in the circuit (could be microbubbles in the dialyzer)	■ Give heparin as prescribed. ■ Respond promptly to alarms. ■ Check the patient's access and report any unusual findings (reduced bruit or thrill, cool skin). ■ Ensure that all air is removed from the extracorporeal circuit during priming.
Machine shuts down and alarms	■ Machine is unplugged ■ Machine failure ■ Power outage	■ Know how to free the venous line from the air bubble detector and hand crank to return the patient's blood. ■ If the whole clinic is affected, follow your clinic's policy and procedures.
Blood pooled on the floor or on the patient's clothes	■ Exsanguination ■ Separated bloodlines ■ Ruptured access ■ Dislodged needle	■ Stop the blood pump and clamp both sides of a separated line. ■ Apply pressure to a bleeding site or use a tourniquet if pressure will not stop the bleeding. ■ Do not return the patient's blood if the lines have separated. ■ Tighten all extracorporeal connections. ■ If ordered, give saline and oxygen and call 911.

Post-dialysis Procedures

"One of my dialysis nurses sat and talked me through an anxiety attack on Friday. The fact that she cared enough to sit with me, and help me work through it is amazing. I'm so grateful for each and every one of the staff I cross paths with three times a week!"

At the end of a treatment, you will have another set of steps to do. These include:

- End the dialysis treatment
- Take the patient's vital signs and weight
- Document the treatment
- Clean up the equipment

End the Dialysis Treatment

At the end of each treatment, you will need to follow your clinic's policies and procedures to:

- Draw any post-dialysis blood samples the doctor ordered.
- Turn off the heparin pump, if one was used. The doctor may order this to be done 30 minutes before the end of the treatment.
- Check the patient's blood pressure and pulse.
- Reduce the UFR and blood flow rate.
- Rinse the patient's blood back by infusing normal saline until the fluid in the venous bloodline is pink. At this point, your clinic's policy may direct you to either:
  - Remove the arterial needle from the patient's access and stop the bleeding.
  - Take the patient's vital signs before you remove either of the needles.

Follow your clinic's protocol for the order of these steps:

- Take the patient's sitting and standing blood pressure to check for *orthostatic hypotension* (a drop in arm blood pressure of 15 mmHg or more when the patient stands). If this is present, the patient may need extra saline to stabilize his or her vital signs.
- Remove the arterial needle and stop the bleeding (if you have not yet done so), then remove the venous needle and do the same.

Look at the dialyzer after the blood rinseback to assess the number of clotted fibers and/or clots in the headers (see Figure 27). Report dialyzers that do not clear well to the nurse.

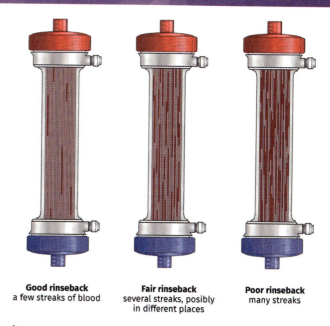

Good rinseback a few streaks of blood
Fair rinseback several streaks, posibly in different places
Poor rinseback many streaks

Figure 27: Good, Fair, and Poor Rinsebacks

Take the Patient's Vital Signs and Weight

"When they take off too much, I get a headache, cramps so bad my bones feel like they will break, dizzy especially when standing, cramping, lose my voice, get a washed out feeling."

After dialysis:

- Check the patient's vascular access (see Module 6) and general condition.
- The patient's BP should be about the same as it was at the start of treatment—or lower. Patients whose BP is very low are at risk of falls—or car accidents if they drive home. Your clinic will tell you what the patient's BP needs to be before s/he can leave. If the patient's BP is too low for safety, your clinic may have you:
  - Let the patient sit for a couple of minutes to let water shift back into the bloodstream.
  - Give the patient a glass of water.
  - If pressure is still low, consider giving normal saline to prevent cardiac stunning (see page 252 for information on cardiac stunning).
- Take a post-dialysis weight and compare it to the target weight and the pre-dialysis weight.
- Tell the nurse about any changes or abnormal findings, like fever and if the patient did not reach their weight loss goal or lost too much weight, before the patient leaves the clinic.

Module 7

Document the Treatment

Remember, if you do not chart it, it was not done. Follow your clinic's policy to document *all* aspects of each patient's treatment.

Clean Up the Equipment

"We have vinyl flooring in our clinic & it gets scuffed up real bad & you can see all the blood stains. Plus, there's trash everywhere on the floor. They have someone every once in a while sweeping it up but they never pick up everything."

REUSED DIALYZERS

If your clinic reuses dialyzers, you will prepare them for reprocessing after a treatment. This may mean that you:

- Circulate leftover saline from the bag and any remaining heparin through the extracorporeal circuit to flush out some of the blood in the dialyzer.
- NOTE: Fill the dialyzer *all the way up* with saline. Air will cause any blood that is left to clot.
- Take the dialyzer and bloodlines off of the HD machine.
- Throw away the bloodlines and disposable equipment as biohazard waste.
- Cap all ports of the dialyzer.
- Per your clinic's policy, bag the dialyzer. This step helps to prevent cross-contamination. Place the bag in the refrigerator to reduce pathogen growth. Or, reprocess the dialyzer immediately.

See Module 5 to learn more about reprocessing dialyzers.

SINGLE-USE DIALYZERS

If your clinic does not reuse the dialyzer, throw it out per your clinic's policy. Remove and disinfect clamps and other non-disposable items, per your clinic's policy, before they are used for other patients.

DISINFECT THE EQUIPMENT

To kill germs, you must disinfect equipment that will be used for another patient. Otherwise, germs could transfer to the next patient who uses it:

- Clean the dialysis chair and outside of the machine well with a disinfectant after each treatment.
- Pay special attention to knobs and other surfaces that may have been touched and contaminated during the treatment.
- Disinfect the internal pathways of the machine regularly with heat and/or chemicals. This must be done at least at the end of each treatment day, but may be done more often. Check your clinic procedures to find out when this should be done. Rinse dialysate out of the machine before disinfecting with heat and/or chemicals. Vinegar or citric acid are most often used for this rinse.

Heat disinfection is a 3-cycle process built into some machines:*

1. During a **warm-up** cycle, water is heated to 85° C–95° C.
2. In a **recirculation** cycle, hot water passes through the hydraulic circuit for 20–60 minutes to disinfect the machine, then the hot water is drained out and cool water flows in.
3. At the **normalization** cycle, the temperature-regulating mechanism goes back to normal.

*NOTE: Some dialysis machines use heated citric acid for disinfection.

Chemical disinfection is a 3-cycle process as well (water fill, circulation, rinse). The machine runs with disinfectant instead of dialysate. The disinfectant mixes with treated water and follows the dialysate path. Then, a rinse cycle washes it out.

Before you start a treatment after disinfection, test the rinse water to prove that no disinfectant is left in the machine, where it could harm or kill patients. Machines must be on a regular disinfection schedule. This includes back-up machines that are not used for treatments, isolation machines, etc. All machines have limits on how long they can sit between disinfection cycles. Most must be disinfected at least every 48 hours, even if they are not used.

Measuring Dialysis Adequacy

"The problem is, they don't up my Kt/V because they feel minimum is good enough. Which, in some cases, it's not. I have adequate clearance but feel lousy most of the time."

"Adequate" treatment means that a patient is getting at least the minimum dose of dialysis that Medicare requires. However, research finds that more hours of dialysis are better for patients. Standard in-center HD survival in the U.S. does not compare well with the rest of the Western world—in large part because treatment times are so short: often less than 4 hours.[56]

Never tell patients that they need less treatment time just because their "adequacy numbers are good." Why not? Because the dose of dialysis is based *only* on blood levels of *urea* (blood urea nitrogen, or BUN). Urea is a small molecule protein waste that is easy and inexpensive to measure—but not very toxic. Unlike any other wastes, urea freely diffuses between all of the fluid spaces in the body. This means that:

1. Removing urea is very easy to do.
2. Not removing enough urea is a clear sign of poor dialysis.
3. Removing a lot of urea does not mean that the treatment is removing other wastes that really *are* toxic—and can cause long-term damage.

Other, "middle molecule" wastes like beta-2 microglobulin (β_2M) are larger and harder to remove during a 4-hour session. These wastes can build up over time to damage nerves, destroy joints, break bones, and harm soft tissues.

In addition, our measures of adequacy do not include ultrafiltration. But, we now know that using a safe UF goal and UF rate at each treatment is vital to how patients feel, and even how long they may live.

Urea Kinetic Modeling (UKM)

"It's my second month using the new dialyzer, and my labs are even better! Clearance 1.6. I've never had it that high. Phosphorus 3.3! Potassium 4.9. I could not be more happy about using that filter!"

UKM can help a doctor prescribe treatment, predict how much treatment time a patient should have, and find out if s/he eats enough protein. A pre- and post-dialysis BUN blood sample are needed, along with pre- and post-dialysis weights.

The UKM formula, Kt/V, is an equation for the amount of dialysis a patient is receiving. The formula estimates the removal of urea (BUN) during dialysis. Because Kt/V includes treatment and patient specific data, it is so complex, that it is calculated by a computer in the lab. Here is what Kt/V stands for:

- **K** = dialyzer urea **clearance of blood** in mL/min. K is affected by the dialyzer type and blood and dialysate flow rates.
- **t** = **time** on dialysis in minutes. T is affected by the minutes of treatment time and number of treatments. It is important that a patient stay for his or her entire treatment and does not skip treatments.
- **V** = **volume** of water (in mL) that a patient's body contains. A person's height, weight, sex, age, and any amputations are included in the estimate of V.

Drawing Pre- and Post-dialysis BUN

"Ask for a full copy of your labs monthly, not just the report card the dietitian gives you. I noticed my hemoglobin dropping, talked to the clinic nurse, and she called the kidney doc. Learn how to read your lab report. Ask until you can. I watch my BUN and creatinine levels, too. When you feel crummy there is a reason."

Predialysis and post-dialysis BUN samples are drawn each month for Kt/V. *Draw the predialysis and post-dialysis BUN samples during the same treatment.*[30]

HOW TO DRAW A PREDIALYSIS BUN SAMPLE

- Do not dilute the sample with saline or heparin.
- Draw the sample just before a treatment begins.
- For patients with **fistulas or grafts**:
  - Take the sample from the arterial needle before you connect the arterial blood tubing.
  - Or, flush the needle and take the sample *just* before a treatment.
- For patients with **HD catheters**, you or the nurse (depending on your state) will:
  - Withdraw any heparin and saline from the arterial port, following your clinic's protocol.
  - Connect a new syringe to the arterial lumen to draw the sample.

HOW TO DRAW A POST-DIALYSIS BUN SAMPLE

The post-dialysis blood sample should be drawn at the end of the ordered treatment (see Table 14), using a **slow-flow method** (100 mL/min for 15 seconds) or a **stop-dialysate-flow method** (for 3 minutes). These measurements should be done at least monthly as the KDOQI guidelines recommend.[57] Please refer to your clinic's policy for how to draw this sample.

Table 14: Options to Obtain the Post-dialysis BUN Sample

A. Slow-Flow Method
1. At the end of the treatment, **turn off the dialysate flow**.
2. Decrease the **UFR** to 50–100 mL/hr, the lowest TMP/UFR setting, or off, according to your clinic policy.
3. Slow the **blood flow rate** to 100 mL/min for 15 seconds (longer if the bloodline volume to the sampling port exceeds 15 mL, or if your clinic policy calls for it). To prevent pump shut-off as the blood flow rate is reduced, you may need to manually reduce the venous pressure limits.
4. Shut off the blood pump or leave it running at 100 mL/min while you draw the sample.
5. After you take the sample, stop the blood pump (if you did not stop it before) and disconnect the patient per your clinic protocol.

B. Stop-Dialysate Flow Method
1. At the end of the treatment, **turn off the dialysate flow** (or put the machine into bypass).
2. Decrease the **UFR** to 50 mL/hr, to the lowest TMP/UFR setting, or off, according to your clinic policy.
3. **Wait 3 minutes**. Do NOT reduce the blood flow rate during this 3-minute time.
4. Draw the blood from the sampling port on the inlet bloodline, the arterial needle tubing, or the arterial port of the venous catheter.
5. After you draw the sample, return the patient's blood in the bloodlines and dialyzer per protocol.

Minimum Delivered and Prescribed Dose of Dialysis

The 2015 KDOQI guidelines say to use UKM as a measure of the minimum delivered and prescribed dose of dialysis. Medicare rules require clinics to report UKM as well. As you have learned, UKM is better, since it includes aspects of the treatment (dialyzer, flow rates, time, etc.) *and* patient factors such as body size.

KDOQI guidelines set standards for the *minimum* delivered and prescribed doses of dialysis. This is a *floor*—not a ceiling. It is the least possible amount of dialysis to keep the patient alive: more is better for patients who want to feel well, do the things that matter to them, and live longer.

KDOQI guidelines recommend a target Kt/V of 1.4 for patients treating three x/week, and a minimum Kt/V of 1.2.

Factors that Affect the Dialysis Treatment

A number of factors can affect the delivered dose or "adequacy" of treatment.

DIALYZER CLEARANCE FACTORS

Dialyzers vary in size, porosity, and surface area. Each can affect how much dialysis a patient receives. Other treatment factors like these can also reduce clearance and the treatment:

- Poor blood flow from the patient's access
- Poor dialyzer function due to not enough heparin or air trapped in the fibers due to rapid priming (clotting of dialyzer fibers)
- Wrong estimates of dialyzer performance
- Wrong blood flow rate settings
- Blood pump calibration errors
- Reduced blood pump speed, due to a patient's low blood pressure or muscle cramps
- Wrong dialysate flow rate settings that do not match the doctor's orders
- *Access recirculation* (cleaned blood coming back through the venous needle is pulled back into the arterial needle—instead of going to the bloodstream)

TIME FACTORS

Factors that affect the patient's treatment time, like these, will also affect adequacy:

- Stopping a treatment early
- Frequent alarms that stop the blood pump (extra-corporeal arterial or venous pressure)
- Frequent alarms that send dialysate to the drain on bypass

Losing just 5 minutes from each treatment over a year adds up to 13 hours—more than three standard HD treatments. Standard HD treatment replaces only a small amount of normal kidney function. **Patients get 0% kidney replacement on non-treatment days, so each minute is needed**. Longer treatment times offer a lower UFR, which is safer for the heart and other organs. Removal of "middle molecule" wastes is better with longer and/or more frequent treatments. When you can (with approval of the charge nurse), add time at the end of the treatment to make up for a slow blood flow rate, blood pump shut-off, or bypass. If a lot of time is lost and the clinic is too busy to add time, a patient may need to come for an extra treatment.

WHAT TO DO IF UKM RESULT IS VERY LOW

Repeat the measure (unless the reason is obvious). Reasons for very low results may include:

- Interrupted treatment(s)
- Too-low blood or dialysate flow
- A problem sampling the pre- and/or post-dialysis blood

If no reason for a sudden drop is apparent, then suspect a problem with needle placement, like accidental needle reversal, or recirculation.

Dialysis Dose and Patient Well-Being

Dialysis should control or reduce the complications of kidney failure. Patient well-being is a way to tell if dialysis is adequate, but a patient who receives poor dialysis may have few symptoms in the short-term. Severe problems may occur in the long-term. He or she is likely to develop nerve damage, joint and bone pain, and die sooner.

In the short term, poor dialysis can cause uremia, which can decrease the patient's appetite. A malnourished patient may lose weight (muscle). He or she may have no appetite, and have low BUN and serum albumin levels. Malnutrition is a risk factor for hospital stays and death.

It is wise to measure adequacy with more than one test. Besides UKM, we look at the patient's nutritional status and sense of well-being. These measures serve as a check for the quality of the treatment. They also help alert you to problems and help the doctor tailor the prescription to meet the patient's needs.

Conclusion

Dialysis is a complex process. You must learn many patient care and technical skills to provide safe and effective patient care. You will work with your teacher to practice the skills you read about in this module. Before you work on your own, you will need to show that you can complete all of these skills correctly. Learning these skills so you can successfully care for patients can help you to be part of improving people's lives each day that you work.

Module 7

References

1. United States Renal Data System. *2016 USRDS Annual Data Report: Epidemiology of Kidney Disease in the United States.* National Institutes of Health, National Institute of Diabetes and Digestive and Kidney Diseases. Bethesda, MD, 2016 (Reference Tables, Volume 2, Table H.12_HD). Available at https://www.usrds.org/reference.aspx. Accessed February 2017
2. Kari J, Messana J, Frank K, et al. The ESRD Core Survey: working together to improve care. Available at http://education.kidney.org/content/esrd-core-survey-working-together-improve-care. Accessed July 2016
3. Centers for Disease Control and Prevention. Recommendations for preventing transmission of infections among chronic hemodialysis patients. *Morbidity and Mortality Weekly Report (MMWR).* 2001;50(RR05). Available at https://www.cdc.gov/mmwr/preview/mmwrhtml/rr5005a1.htm. Accessed January 2017
4. Centers for Disease Control and Prevention. Guideline for hand hygiene in health-care settings. *Morbidity and Mortality Weekly Report (MMWR).* 2002;51(RR16). Available at www.cdc.gov/mmwr/preview/mmwrhtml/rr5116a1.htm. Accessed May 2016
5. United States Department of Labor. Occupational Safety and Health Administration. *Bloodborne pathogens* (1910.1030). Regulations (Standards – 29 CFR). Available at https://www.osha.gov/pls/oshaweb/owadisp.show_document?p_table=standards&p_id=10051. Accessed June 2017
6. Centers for Disease Control and Prevention. *CDC urging dialysis providers and facilities to assess and improve infection control practices to stop Hepatitis C virus transmission in patients undergoing hemodialysis.* Available at http://emergency.cdc.gov/han/han00386.asp. Accessed July 2016
7. Centers for Disease Control and Prevention. *HIV Transmission.* Available from http://www.cdc.gov/hiv/basics/transmission.html. Accessed July 2016
8. Coughenour C, Stevens V, Stetzenbach LD. An evaluation of methicillin-resistant Staphylococcus aureus survival on five environmental surfaces. *Microb Drug Resist.* 2011;17(3):457-61
9. Zacharioudakis IM, Zervou FN, Ziakas PD, et al. Vancomycin-resistant enterococci colonization among dialysis patients: a meta-analysis of prevalence, risk factors, and significance. *Am J Kidney Dis.* 2015;65(1):88-97
10. Centers for Disease Control and Prevention. *Carbapenem-resistant Enterobacteriaceae in healthcare settings.* Available at https://www.cdc.gov/hai/organisms/cre/index.html. Accessed July 2016
11. Centers for Disease Control and Prevention. *Clostridium difficile infection information for patients.* Available at https://www.cdc.gov/hai/organisms/cdiff/cdiff-patient.html. Accessed July 2016
12. Centers for Disease Control and Prevention. *Basic TB facts.* Available at https://www.cdc.gov/tb/topic/basics/default.htm. Accessed July 2016
13. Centers for Medicare & Medicaid Services. *ESRD Core Survey Field Manual*, Version 1.7. Available at https://www.cms.gov/Medicare/Provider-Enrollment-and-Certification/GuidanceforLawsAndRegulations/Downloads/ESRD-Core-Survey-Field-Manual.pdf. Accessed January 2017
14. *Proper body mechanics.* 2011. Available at https://www.drugs.com/cg/proper-body-mechanics.html. Accessed January 2017
15. Collins JW, Nelson A, Sublet V. *Safe lifting and movement of nursing home residents.* Department of Health and Human Services. Centers for Disease Control and Prevention. National Institute for Occupational Safety and Health. NIOSH Publication Number 2006-117. February 2006. Available at www.cdc.gov/niosh/docs/2006-117/pdfs/2006-117.pdf. Accessed January 2017
16. Walker-Facts.com. *Do I need a walker? Physical considerations in choosing a walking device.* Available from http://www.walker-facts.com/Physical-Considerations.asp. Accessed July 2016
17. Shepherd Center. *Pivot transfer.* Available at: http://www.myshepherdconnection.org/sci/transfers/pivot-transfer. Accessed January 2017
18. California Department of Social Services. *Transfer techniques.* Available at http://www.cdss.ca.gov/agedblinddisabled/res/VPTC2/4%20Care%20for%20the%20Caregiver/Transfer_Techniques.pdf. Accessed January 2017
19. U.S. Food and Drug Administration. *Medical devices: patient lifts.* Available at https://www.fda.gov/MedicalDevices/ProductsandMedicalProcedures/GeneralHospitalDevicesandSupplies/ucm308622.htm. Accessed January 2017
20. Institute for Safe Medication Practices. *ISMP's List of error-prone abbreviations, symbols, and dose designations.* Available at https://www.ismp.org/tools/errorproneabbreviations.pdf. Accessed January 2017
21. Cvach M. Monitor alarm fatigue: an integrative review. *Biomed Instrum Technol.* 2012;46(4):268-77
22. Horkan AM. Alarm fatigue and patient safety. *Nephrol Nurs J.* 2014;41(1):83-5
23. Centers for Medicare & Medicaid Services, HHS. ESRD surveyor training interpretive guidance. Final Version 1.1. October 3, 2008 (V Tag 407) Available at https://www.cms.gov/Medicare/Provider-Enrollment-and-Certification/GuidanceforLawsAndRegulations/Downloads/esrdpgmguidance.pdf. Accessed June 2017
24. Pickering TG, Hall JE, Appel LJ, et al. recommendations for blood pressure measurement in humans and experimental animals: part 1: blood pressure measurement in humans: a statement for professionals from the subcommittee of professional and public education of the American Heart Association Council on High Blood Pressure Research. *Circulation.* 2005;111:697-716
25. Canaan A. *How to determine the correct blood pressure cuff size.* October 16, 2015. Available at https://www.livestrong.com/article/167914-how-to-determine-the-correct-blood-pressure-cuff-size/. Accessed January 2017
26. McEvoy M. *5 Errors that are giving you incorrect blood pressure readings.* Updated October 14, 2016. Available at https://www.ems1.com/ems-products/Medical-Monitoring/articles/1882581-5-errors-that-are-giving-you-incorrect-blood-pressure-readings/. Accessed January 2017
27. Spergel LM. *Management of steal syndrome.* Fistula First. Available at http://fistulafirst.esrdncc.org/wp-content/uploads/2014/07/11_Management_of_Steal_Syndrome.pdf. Accessed June 2017
28. Daugirdas JT. Chronic hemodialysis prescription, in Daugirdas JT, Blake PG, & Ing TS, *Handbook of* Dialysis, (5th ed). Philadelphia, Wolters Kluwer Health, 2015
29. Speranza-Reid JE. Hemodialysis: complications of hemodialysis: prevention and management. In Counts CS (ed): *Core Curriculum for Nephrology Nursing* (6th ed). Pitman, NJ, American Nephrology Nurses Association, 2015, pp. 69-166
30. Centers for Medicare & Medicaid Services. *ESRD Quality Incentive Program.* Available at https://www.cms.gov/Medicare/Quality-Initiatives-Patient-Assessment-Instruments/ESRDQIP/index.html . Accessed March 2017
31. National Kidney Foundation. K/DOQI clinical practice guidelines for cardiovascular disease in dialysis patients. *Am J Kidney Dis.* 2005;45(4) Suppl 3:S1-154
32. Laskowski ER. *What's a normal resting heart rate?* Mayo Clinic. August 22, 2015. Available at https://www.mayoclinic.org/healthy-lifestyle/fitness/expert-answers/heart-rate/faq-20057979. Accessed June 2017
33. Potter PA, Perry AG. Principles for nursing practice, in: *Basic Nursing—Essentials for Practice* (5th Ed). St. Louis, MO, Mosby, 2003, pp.176, 195, 203-4, 208, 210, 212

34. Salai PB. Patient management – the dialysis procedure, in Counts CS (ed): *Core Curriculum for Nephrology Nursing* (5th ed). Pitman, NJ, American Nephrology Nurses' Association, 2008, p. 688
35. Jadoul M, Thumma J, Fuller DS, et al. Modifiable practices associated with sudden death among hemodialysis patients in the Dialysis Outcomes and Practice Patterns Study. *Clin J Am Soc Nephrol*. 2012;7(5):765-74
36. Tom Folden, Fresenius Medical Care. Customer letter dated March 15, 2005.
37. Onofriescu M, Siriopol D, Voroneanu L, et al. Overhydration, cardiac function and survival in hemodialysis patients. *PloS One*. 2015;10(8):e0135691
38. Flythe JE, Kimmel SE, Brunelli SM. Rapid fluid removal during dialysis is associated with cardiovascular morbidity and mortality. *Kidney Int*. 2011;79(2):250-7
39. Centers for Medicare & Medicaid Services. *Measures Assessment Tool (MAT)*. Version 2.5. Available at https://www.cms.gov/Medicare/Provider-Enrollment-and-Certification/GuidanceforLawsAndRegulations/Dialysis.html. Accessed December 2016
40. Chan KE, Maddux FW, Tolkoff-Rubin N, et al. Early outcomes among those initiating chronic dialsyis in the United States. *Clin J Am Soc Nephrol*. 2011;6(11):2642-9
41. Peer Kidney Care Initiative. Dialysis care & outcomes in the United States. Peer Report. 2014. Available at http://www.peerkidney.org. Accessed June 2017
42. Charnow, JA. Early dialysis withdrawal on the rise. *Renal Neph News*. Available at http://www.renalandurologynews.com/kidney-week-2015-dialysis/early-dialysis-withdrawal-on-the-rise/article/452060/. Accessed 3/9/2016
43. Picciano RJ. Identifying the value of technology in fluid management. *Nephrol News Issues*. 2016; July:20-21. Available at http://www.nephrology-digital.com/July2016/Default/11/0##&pageSet=11&contentItem=0. Accessed June 2017
44. Weiner DE, Brunelli SM, Hunt A, et al. Improving clinical outcomes among hemodialysis patients: a proposal for a "volume first" approach from the chief medical officers of US dialysis providers. *Am J Kidney Dis*. 2014 Nov;64(5):685-95
45. Agarwal R. How can we prevent intradialytic hypotension? *Current Opinions in Nephrology and Hypertension*. 2012;21:594-599. doi:10.1097/MHN.Ob013e3283588f3c
46. Gleason J. The basics of centrifugation. Clinfield. November 21, 2011. Available at http://clinfield.com/2011/11/basics-of-centrifugation/. Accessed July 2016
47. American Diabetes Association. Hypoglycemia. Available at http://www.diabetes.org/living-with-diabetes/treatment-and-care/blood-glucose-control/hypoglycemia-low-blood.html. Accessed July 2016
48. Hurst J. Venous Needle Dislodgement-A Universal Concern. *European Nephrology*. 2011;5(2):148–51
49. Sandroni, S, Sherockman T, Hays-Leight K. (PUB 354 2008). Catastrophic Hemorrhage from Venous Needle Dislodgement during Hemodialysis: Continued Risk of Avoidable Death and Progress toward a Solution. Presented at ASN/Renal Week, Philadelphia, Nov 2008
50. Morales M, Padilla-Kastenberg G. Venous needle dislodgement in dialysis clinic settings: A compilation of best practices and prevention. *Renal Business Today*. Special Report. February 2013
51. Ball LK. The art of making your fistula or graft last. Home Dialysis Central. Available at http://www.homedialysis.org/life-at-home/articles/art-of-making-your-fistula-or-graft-last. 2013
52. Davenport A, Lai KN, Hertel J, et al. Anticoagulation, in Daugirdas JT, Blake PG, Ing TS (eds): *Handbook of Dialysis* (5th ed). Philadelphia, PA, Lippincott Williams & Wilkins, 2015, p 258
53. Thijssen S, Kossmann RJ, Kruse A, Kotanko P. Clinical evaluation of a model for prediction of end-dialysis systemic ionized calcium concentration in citrate hemodialysis. *Blood Purif*. 2013;35(1-3):133-8
54. Sherman RA, Daugirdas JT, Ing TS. Complication during hemodialysis. Daugirdas JT, Blake PG, & Ing TS, *Handbook of Dialysis*, (5th ed). Philadelphia, Wolters Kluwer Health, 2015
55. Kotanko P, Levin NW. Common clinical problems during hemodialysis, in Nissenson AR, Fine RN (eds): *Dialysis Therapy* (4th ed). Philadelphia, PA, Saunders Elsevier, 2008, p. 415
56. Tentori F, Zhang J, Li Y, Karaboyas A, et al. Longer dialysis session length is associated with better intermediate outcomes and survival among patients on in-center three times per week hemodialysis: results from the Dialysis Outcomes and Practice Patterns Study (DOPPS). *Nephrol Dial Transplant*. 2012;27:4180-88)
57. KDOQI clinical practice guideline for hemodialysis adequacy: 2015 update. *Am J Kidney Dis*. 2015;66(5):884-930.

8 Water Treatment

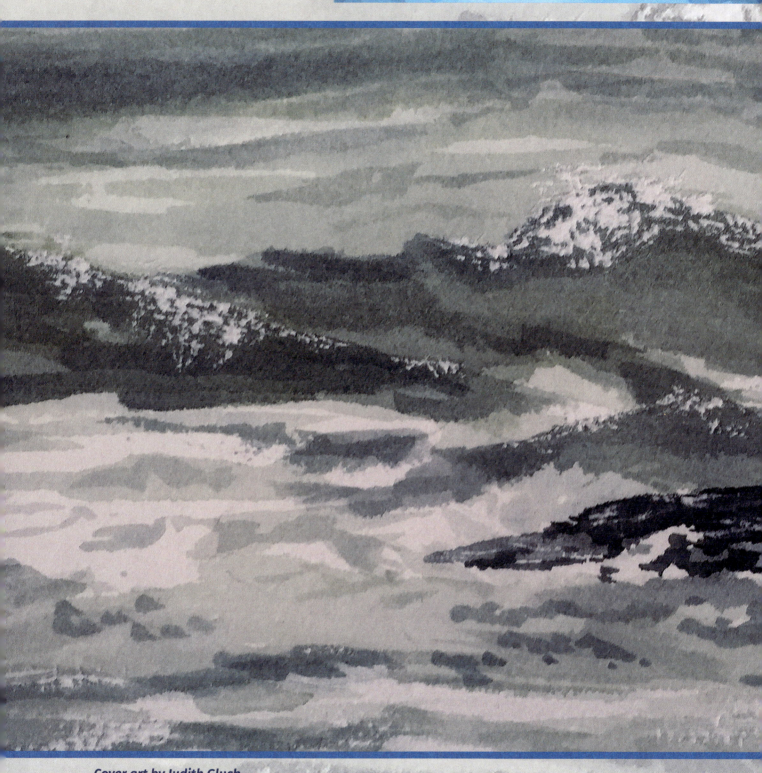

Cover art by Judith Gluck

"Recently, a curious thing happened to me on home hemo—my hemoglobin fell from around 12 to 7, out of the blue. It turned out that I had been having long-term hemolysis (red blood cell destruction). To address the problem, they gave me a larger carbon tank. The theory is that the smaller tank was sometimes overwhelmed by extra chlorine or fluorides added seasonally to our city's water supply."

Objectives

MODULE AUTHORS

Danilo B. Concepcion, CBNT, CCHT-A, FNKF

Scott Hansen

Charles H. Johnson, CHT

Heather Paradis, CHT

Philip Varughese, CHT, CCNT

MODULE REVIEWERS

Debra Barker, RN

Nancy M. Gallagher, BS, RN, CNN

Eric Greenberg, NJ T1&W1 Licensed Operator

Glenda M. Payne, MS RN, CNN

Darlene Rodgers, BSN, RN, CNN, CPHQ

John H. Sadler, MD

Dori Schatell, MS

Vern Taaffe, BS, CBNT, CDWS

Tamyra Warmack, RN

After you complete this module, you will be able to:

1. Explain why we treat water for dialysis.
2. List the parts of a dialysis clinic's water treatment system.
3. Discuss the purpose of water softeners, carbon tanks, reverse osmosis, deionization, and ultraviolet irradiation in water treatment for dialysis.
4. Describe how to test the water treatment system for bacteria.
5. Outline a typical water treatment monitoring schedule.

An acronym list can be found in the Glossary.

Practice Test Questions at:
www.meiresearch.org/cc6

Introduction

In dialysis, we use water to mix concentrates and germicides, flush out and reprocess dialyzers, and rinse out jugs. When we are healthy, we can handle some *contaminants* (harmful substances) in our drinking water. Our digestive tracts and kidneys can help protect us. Hemodialysis (HD) patients do not have those protections. Their blood comes in contact with large volumes of water in dialysate through the dialyzer membrane at each treatment. Using purified water for HD is vital. Contaminated water can cause illness—and death.

To keep patients safe, *all* water for HD is passed through a water treatment system.

This system is made up of a several components; each removes some contaminants until the water is safe to use. This module covers why and how we treat water before it is used for HD. It describes:

- Common contaminants found in water
- The parts of a water treatment system
- How and why we monitor the system

Water Supply

Dialysis water starts out as tap water that has been treated to be safe for drinking. Tap water comes from one of two sources—which can also interact with each other:[1]

1. **Ground water** comes from wells and springs. It is often higher in ions (e.g., iron, calcium, magnesium), but lower in *microbes* (e.g., bacteria, viruses, endotoxins) than surface water.
2. **Surface water** comes from lakes, ponds, rivers, and reservoirs. Surface water may be higher than ground water in pesticides, industrial waste, sewage, and microbes.

Drinking Water Contaminants

We call water the *universal solvent*. It dissolves more substances than any other liquid.[2] As rainwater falls through the air toward earth, it picks up contaminants like carbon dioxide and sulfur dioxide gases. These dissolve in the water to make weak carbonic and sulfuric acids: acid rain. When acid rain flows over limestone and other minerals, the acid dissolves *them*. This process forms calcium carbonate and calcium sulfate—common impurities in tap water (see Figure 1).

Other substances also dissolve in water, such as:

- Sodium chloride (salt)
- Fluoride
- Nitrate salts
- Pesticides

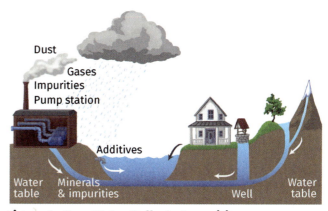

Figure 1: How Water Collects Impurities

All tap water has *some* contaminants. Which ones occur in your water will depend on what is nearby, the season, and the types of industry in the area. Fertilizers and pesticides can show up in water in farm regions, for example. When you are responsible for dialysis water treatment, you will need to be aware of the challenges that affect your local water in the short or long term. For example:

- **Severe storms or floods** can overwhelm water treatment systems and let raw sewage wash into water, as with "Superstorm" Hurricane Sandy in 2012.[3]
- **Pharmaceutical drugs** can be present at low levels in even treated drinking water, because so many medicines are flushed down or excreted into toilets.[4]
- **Hydraulic fracking** pumps a cocktail of chemicals (such as benzene and formaldehyde) into the ground to obtain natural gas from shale. These chemicals can seep into local water.[5]
- **Chemical spills** can contaminate water supplies, such as the coal processing tanks that leaked into a river in West Virginia in 2014, polluting the water for 300,000 people.[6]

Drinking Water Standards

U.S. drinking water is regulated by the Environmental Protection Agency (EPA) to protect us all from harm. All *public* water supplies must at least meet the minimal standards set by the Safe Drinking Water Act, which passed in 1974 to make water safe for the public to drink. States monitor and enforce the law, and your state may also have set more stringent rules than the EPA. A system is "public" if it:[7]

- Has at least 15 service connections
- Serves at least 25 people per day for 60 days of the year

Certain other water systems do not have to meet EPA Safe Drinking Water standards:[8]

- "Small" water systems that serve fewer than 3,000 people (small systems may still need to meet stringent state standards, however)
- Water systems in disadvantaged areas that serve fewer than 500 people
- Private wells that serve fewer than 25 people
- Towns that receive variances for the presence of certain chemicals in the water supply

As you can see in Appendix A: EPA Tap Water Standards, *many* contaminants can make their way into drinking water. We must remove these before the water can be used for HD.

Tap Water Treatment

To help keep us all safe, tap water is tested and treated with several steps that include:[9] (see Figure 2).

- **Coagulation and flocculation**. Dirt and many dissolved particles have a negative charge. So, chemicals like *alum* (an aluminum compound) with a positive charge are added to the water as a first treatment step. These neutralize the charge, then bind (coagulate) with particles to form larger clump, or "floc." Alum is called a *flocculant* for this reason.
- **Sedimentation**. The heavy clumps settle to the bottom of the water.
- **Filtration**. Clear water on top of the sediment is passed through a series of filters, like gravel, sand, and charcoal to remove dissolved particles of varying sizes.
- **Disinfection**. Chlorine or chloramine is added by public systems to kill microbes and parasites. Chloramines are made by mixing chlorine and ammonia. They are used by cities when a long-acting chlorine is needed, for example, when a water distribution system is large. These compounds can also form in nature, when chlorine combines with organic material. In most cases, public systems use monochloramine. Some towns switch back and forth between chlorine and chloramines. Some use other products like chlorine dioxide. You can ask for a "Consumer Confidence Report" (CCR) from your water supplier to learn what is used in your area, and when.[10] The EPA requires each water supplier to put out an annual report by July 1 of each year.
- **Fluoride** is added by public water treatment systems to prevent tooth decay. Levels of fluoride in drinking water may vary from day to day.
- Some cities change the water **pH** (acid/base level) to reduce the amount of metals that might *leach* (dissolve) out of the water system's pipes and into drinking water.[11]

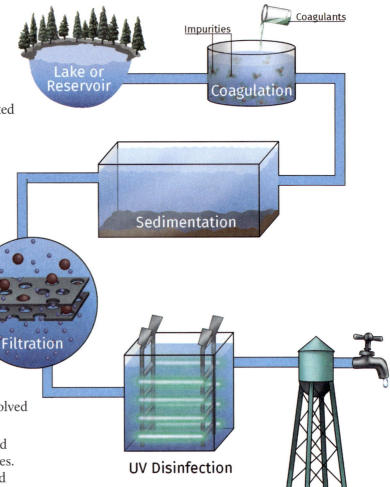

Figure 2: Water Treatment Steps

Dialysis Water

People with healthy kidneys drink about **10–14 liters** of water or other beverages each week. People who do standard in-center HD have their blood exposed to **270–576 liters** of water per week in the dialysate and through a dialyzer membrane (see Figure 3).[12] High-flux HD membranes, which have large pores, allow chemicals or *endotoxins* (toxic bacterial wall fragments) to pass into the blood. Longer and/or more frequent HD can expose patients to even *more* water. Thus, HD water must be *far* cleaner than drinking water, and must meet at least the minimum standards for:

- Bacteria
- Endotoxins
- Metals
- Trace elements
- Salts
- Other substances

AAMI Standards for Dialysis Water

The Association for the Advancement of Medical Instrumentation (AAMI) writes the guidelines for dialysis water. These become *standards* when the American National Standards Institute (ANSI) approves them. Some products that make water safe to drink can harm patients and machines. So, we must test and treat tap water to meet ANSI/AAMI standards for HD. If HD water treatment fails, we can use tap water *only* if the levels of all contaminants still meet the standards.[13]

In the *Conditions for Coverage*, the Centers for Medicare and Medicaid Services (CMS) adopted **ANSI/AAMI RD52:2004** and **RD62:2001** for water treatment.[14] Newer standards, which tend to be more stringent, have since been published by AAMI—but have not been adopted by CMS. These are:

- **ANSI/AAMI/ISO 13959:2014** - *Water for hemodialysis and related therapies*
- **ANSI/AAMI/ISO 23500:2014** - *Guidance for the preparation and management of fluids for hemodialysis and related therapies*
- **ANSI/AAMI/ISO 26722:2014** - *Water treatment equipment for hemodialysis and related therapies*
- **ANSI/AAMI/ISO 11663:2014** – *Quality of dialysis fluid for hemodialysis and related therapies*

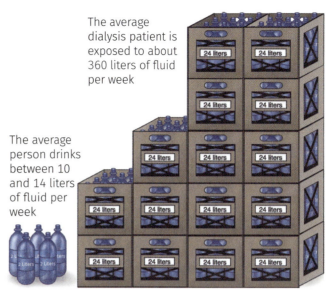

Figure 3: Water Volumes

This module refers to the *Conditions for Coverage* that are in effect now. But, the *Conditions* let clinics choose to adopt newer standards as policy as long as those standards are *more strict*. Many clinics do so as a matter of best practice.[15]

HD uses such a large volume of water that even tiny amounts of contaminants can harm patients. Low-level water contamination can cause chronic inflammation. Some researchers believe that this inflammation may be one of the reasons why U.S. patients tend to die sooner than patients in other countries that have higher water standards.[16] Use of *ultrapure* water—with far fewer microbes—does reduce inflammation.[17] But, controlled studies have not yet been done to prove whether the use of water that is more pure really does help people to live longer.[18]

Home Dialysis and Water Treatment

Water used for home HD must be tested, too, and some patients may have private wells. If well water quality does not meet the standards for HD, the clinic may need to offer a machine that uses bags of dialysate and does not require water treatment.

CHEMICAL CONTAMINANTS

AAMI lists allowable amounts of chemicals in water used for HD (see Table 1).

Table 1: *Chemical* Contaminants: ANSI/AAMI Standards for HD Water[19] vs EPA Standards for Drinking Water[20]

Contaminant	Dialysis Maximum Allowable Level (mg/L)	EPA Drinking Water Standard
Aluminum	0.01	No mandatory standard
Antimony	0.006	0.006
Arsenic, lead, silver	Each 0.005	0.01; 0.015; no mandatory standard
Beryllium	0.0004	0.004
Cadmium	0.001	0.005
Calcium	2.0 (0.1 mEq/L)	No mandatory standard
Chloramines	0.1	4.0
Chlorine (free)	0.5	4.0
Chromium	0.014	0.1
Copper, barium, zinc	Each 0.1	1.3; 2; No mandatory standard
Fluoride	0.2	4.0
Magnesium	4.0 (0.3 mEq/L)	No mandatory standard
Mercury	0.0002	0.002
Nitrates (as N)	2.0	10
Potassium	8 (0.2 mEq/L)	No mandatory standard
Selenium	0.09	0.05
Sodium	70 (3.0 mEq/L)	No mandatory standard
Sulfate	100	No mandatory standard
Thallium	0.002	0.002

BACTERIAL CONTAMINANTS

Some bacteria help us. Others, *pathogens*, cause disease. Bacteria that are harmless on our skin may become pathogens if they enter our blood. There are two types of bacteria:

- *Gram-positive* bacteria turn **purple** when using Gram's stain.
- *Gram-negative* bacteria do not retain any stain.

Both types of bacteria can form **biofilm**—slime that anchors them in place on surfaces like jugs, pipes, tanks, or feed hoses. Biofilm is a *major* problem for water treatment systems. The slime chains, called *glycocalyx*, let nutrients in and keep out disinfectants. With the right pH, food, and a warm temperature, bacteria can multiply quickly and can be very difficult to kill.

An **action level** is the point at which measures must be taken to maintain the AAMI standards. Your clinic must show that it took some type of action—such as disinfection or retesting—to lower the bacterial count if this level is reached. The action level is lower than the maximum allowable level on purpose. The lower level allows time to fix a problem before it becomes more serious. The ANSI/AAMI standards for bacteria in U.S. dialysis water that have been adopted by CMS are:[19, 21]

- In **conventional** dialysate, bacteria must not exceed 200 colony forming units (CFU; number of living bacteria) per mL.
- The ANSI/AAMI *action level* for bacteria in water for **conventional** dialysate is 50 CFU/mL.
- For **ultrapure** dialysate, the maximum allowable level should be less than 0.1 CFU/mL.

If water at your clinic exceeds the action level, the Medical Director will decide what to do.[21]

2014 ANSI/AAMI Standards of Bacteria in Dialysis Water[22]

- < 100 CFU/mL (half of the previous level)
- Action level of ≥ 50 CFU/mL

ENDOTOXINS AS A CONTAMINANT

Endotoxins form part of the cell walls of some Gram-negative bacteria. Some endotoxins are shed while bacteria are alive—and when they die, large amounts are released. Since endotoxins are not alive, we cannot kill them. *Endotoxemia* (endotoxins in the blood) can cause inflammation. One study followed 306 HD patients for up to 42 months. The researchers found that the higher the blood level of endotoxins, the more inflammation patients had.[23] Endotoxins can pass into the patient's blood through an intact dialyzer membrane. If this happens, a *pyrogenic reaction* may occur, and the patient may have:

- Chills and/or fever
- Low blood pressure
- Nausea and vomiting
- Muscle aches

The ANSI/AAMI standard adopted by CMS says that the endotoxin level must be:[19,21]

- **Conventional** dialysate must have a level less than 2 EU/mL (endotoxin units/mL), with an *action level* of 1 EU/mL.
- **Ultrapure** dialysate must have an endotoxin level less than 0.03 EU/mL.

> **2014 ANSI/AAMI Standards of Endotoxins in Dialysis Water[22]**
>
> - < 0.25 EU/mL with an *action* level of ≥ 0.125 EU/mL

Design of a Dialysis Water Treatment System

An HD water treatment system purifies tap water to make it safe for dialysis. Good system design is vital to protect patients. Each dialysis water treatment system is customized to a clinic. All systems will have each of the components in Table 2. Some may *also* have add-ons to make sure the water will meet the ANSI/AAMI standards CMS has adopted—or higher ones.

A team of water treatment experts who know the impact of each part of the system on patients should design the system. They must think about how the local water supply and treatment may change with the seasons. The clinic's medical director must ensure that the system can deliver dialysis quality water and make sure the system stays in good working order.

Table 2: Key Components for All Dialysis Water Treatment Systems[12]

Component	Purpose
Incoming Water (cold and hot)	Basis of dialysis water
Blending Valve	Mixes hot and cold water to reach an RO membrane industry standard temperature, around 77° F
Backflow Prevention Device	Keeps treated dialysis water from backing up into the tap water system
Booster Pump	Keeps water pressure consistent so the RO system has a constant flow
Multimedia Filter(s)	Layers of media ranging in size from gravel to sand trap large particles
Water Softener	Removes minerals that could form scale on the RO membrane
Brine Tank	Contains salt pellets to make brine for the water softener
Primary Carbon Tank	Removes chlorine and chloramines
Secondary Carbon Tank	CMS requires at least two tanks
Cartridge Filter	Placed before the RO to catch carbon fines, resin beads, debris, and other particles that could damage the RO
Reverse Osmosis (RO) Pump	Increases water pressure across the RO membrane; made of high grade steel, inert plastics, or carbon graphite-wetted parts
RO Membrane(s)	Purify water to ANSI/AAMI standards

We use river terms to refer to the location of each part of a water treatment system: upstream and downstream:

- *Raw (tap) water* from outside the clinic is **upstream**.
- Water in the system moves **downstream**.
- An upstream component always comes before a downstream component.

How will you know where the parts of *your* clinic's water treatment system are? Medicare requires each clinic to have a schematic drawing of your system with each part labeled—including which way the water flows in the pipes.[24]

Water treatment systems will have some or all of the parts shown in Figure 4, based on what is in the raw (tap) water. Each system must be tailored to a clinic, so the components may or may not be in the same order as you see in the figure.

Each component of a dialysis water treatment system serves one of three main functions:

1. **Pretreatment** – preparing the water before it reaches the fragile *reverse osmosis* (RO) membrane
2. **Purification** – ensuring that the water is free of chemicals and germs
3. **Distribution** – bringing the product water to the point of use

Pretreatment Components

- A **backflow prevention device** may be first in line, to keep chemicals used for treating dialysis water from backing up into a city water supply.
- A **temperature blending valve** will mix hot and cold water to ensure feed water that is at a safe temperature for the RO.
- A **booster pump** will push water through the system at a safe rate. The pump is downstream from the backflow prevention device and temperature blending valve. Pressure gauges are placed before and after the booster pump.
- A **prefilter** is placed just before the RO to remove *carbon fines* (small pieces of carbon), resin beads, and other debris. Prefilters are low-cost and protect the expensive RO filter, so it is good practice to change them often.
- **Pressure gauges** should be placed before and after a filter to check for clogging.
- **Chemical injection systems** may be used to alter the feed water pH if needed.
- **Sediment filters** remove particles that could damage the RO.
- **Carbon tanks** remove chlorine and chloramines that could harm patients or the RO.
- **A water softener** may be used to remove some minerals from the feed water.

Purification Components

- The **RO system** produces product water by "rejecting" contaminants.
- **Deionization (DI)**—*if used*. A carbon filter must always come before a DI system so cancer-causing nitrosamines cannot reach patients.[25] And, an ultrafilter, or other way to remove microbes, must be used after (downstream) the DI tank to capture microbes.[25]
- **UV light** keeps microbes that might have slipped past the RO from reproducing. A UV light may be placed with pretreatment components, after the carbon tanks, to reduce the levels of microbes going into the RO system.
- **Submicron** and **ultrafilters** back up the UV light and remove microbes that remain. Most often, they are placed just before the distribution piping. These must be downstream from DI tanks, if DI is the last step in water treatment.[25]

Distribution System

- A **distribution pump** will send the water to the stations—or to a **storage tank**.
- Unused water may go to the **drain**.

The number and order of devices can be set up to suit the needs of any clinic. Medicare requires all systems to have at least two carbon tanks in series (water flows through the first tank, then through the second tank).[26] Some other components may be optional, depending on what is in the source water.

Water in the system must always be kept moving. Microbes grow faster in stagnant water. In most clinics, after the last point of use, a **return loop** carries water back through the system. This prevents stagnant spots and lets the clinic use less feed water. Product water made by the water treatment system flows into a **distribution system** to be used for dialysate.

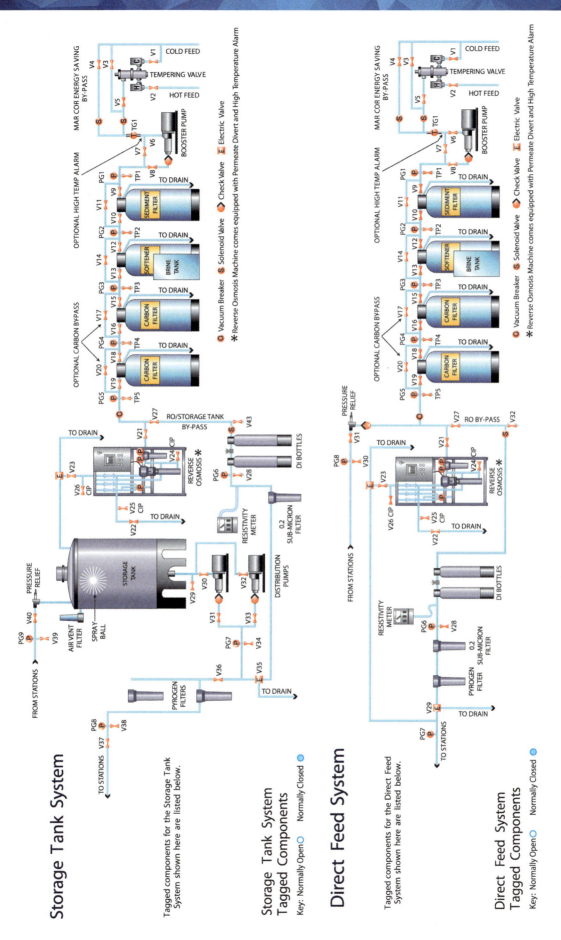

Figure 4: Water Treatment Systems
Images used with permission from Mar Cor Purification.

Parts of a Water Treatment System

Each part of the water treatment system removes different contaminants. The goal is to produce **product water** at the end that is safe for HD (see Figure 4). In this section, we will first describe how reverse osmosis (RO) works, because it is the most vital component. Then, we will explain how other parts of water treatment protect the RO and complete the system.

All device systems used to treat water for HD must be approved by the U.S. Food and Drug Administration (FDA) 510(k). All HD water treatment equipment bought since May 30, 1997 must have FDA 510(k) clearance as well.[27]

Reverse Osmosis (RO)

RO is the heart of a dialysis water treatment system—and is the most costly and delicate part. As part of the purification process, RO is a way to remove solutes from a solution. An RO system has a pressure pump and one or more semipermeable membranes. Pretreatment parts of the water treatment system that you will learn about next help to protect the fragile RO membrane from damage.

HOW RO WORKS

In osmosis, water moves on its own through a membrane to dilute a higher solute level on the other side (see Module 3: *Principles of Dialysis*, to learn more about osmosis). RO uses a hydraulic pressure pump to *push* feed water with high solute levels through a membrane. Water that has passed through the membrane is pure enough to use for HD (see Figure 5). Salts and other contaminants are sent to the drain. A **waste** or **reject** stream of water may be sent to the drain as well—or some systems will send this water back to the start of the loop to be processed again to reduce water waste.[12]

The membrane is the key part of the RO system. It filters out, or *rejects*:
- Metals
- Salts
- Chemicals
- Bacteria
- Endotoxins
- Viruses

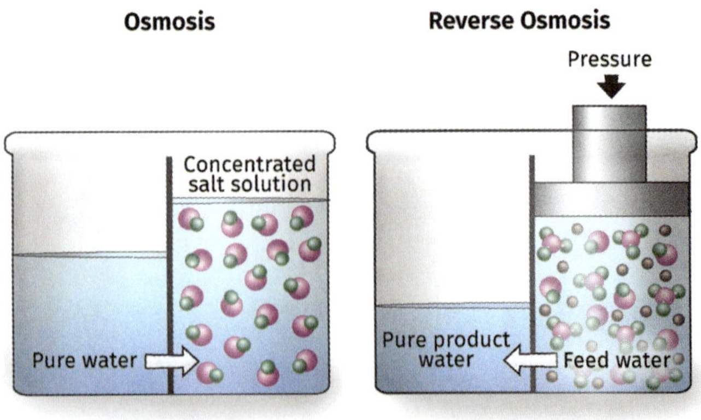

Figure 5: Reverse Osmosis

Green Dialysis and Reuse of RO "Reject" Water

At a flow rate of 500 mL/min, an RO can "reject" 2/3 of the water sent to it.[28] This rejected water is already highly filtered, and most is more than pure enough to meet EPA drinking water standards.[29] What if instead of sending this water to drain, all U.S. clinics reused it? One estimate suggests that we could save enough water to supply a city the size of Salt Lake City, Utah for an *entire year*.[29] We cannot do this yet in the U.S., but perhaps one day it will be possible. Dual-stage systems with break tanks and recovery loops waste less water than other systems.

The most common type of RO membrane is *thin film composite* (TFC), made of polyamide. TFC membranes have a thin, dense membrane over a thick, porous substructure for strength. They are wound in a spiral around a collecting tube (see Figure 6). RO can reject 95–99% of charged ionic particles (e.g., aluminum) and nearly all organic and inorganic substances.[12]

However, TFC RO membranes do have some limits:
- They must be disinfected on a regular schedule.
- They break down when exposed to chlorine and chloramines, so these must be removed before they reach the membrane.[12]
- Use of peracetic acid for disinfection at above a 1% dilution risks damage to the membrane.[12]
- Scale can build up and clog the membrane. Routine cleaning is needed per the manufacturer's instructions to strip off scale build-up.

Water Treatment

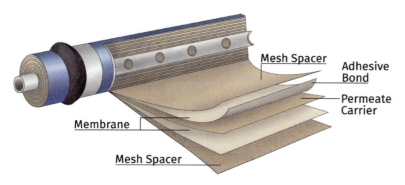

Figure 6: Spiral-wound RO Module

CENTRAL RO SYSTEMS

A central RO system will produce pure water for a small, medium, or large number of dialysis stations. As these systems are in use whenever treatments are done, they do not have a lot of down time when water can stagnate inside. These systems are designed to be easy to use and to disinfect. When present, a backwashing feature, which allows water to flow the reverse of the usual direction, can reduce scale deposits and bacterial growth on the membrane. Some manufacturers offer a dual-stage system with two in-line RO filters. Heat or chemical disinfection may be offered.

PORTABLE RO SYSTEMS

Compact portable RO systems are mainly used for HD in hospitals or at home and usually serve only one station (see Figure 7). They work the same way as central RO systems, but differ in:

- How often they are disinfected
- How often they are used
- ANSI/AAMI standards and CMS rules

Pretreatment parts of a portable water treatment system are similar to those used for central systems. These units may be loaded onto a cart with the portable RO.

The biggest downside of portable RO systems is bacterial growth. These units tend to have a greater chance for stagnant water than central RO systems. Between treatments, bacteria and endotoxins can reach high levels in any water that is left inside. A good maintenance and disinfection plan must be in place to combat this issue. A portable RO system should be run daily to avoid long periods of no water flow. Some manufacturers use one or both of two ways to reduce the risk of bacterial growth in their portable RO systems:

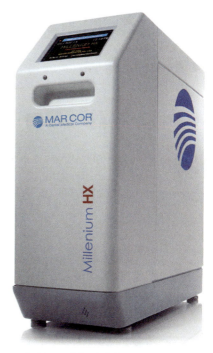

Figure 7: Portable RO System
Image used with permission from Mar Cor Purification.

- Heat and automated disinfection
- An auto-flush feature to avoid stagnant water

PROTECTING THE RO MEMBRANE

The safety of dialysis relies on having an intact RO membrane to filter water so it is pure enough to meet the standards. To protect the membrane, we take a number of steps to ensure that the feed water that reaches it:

- Has particles filtered out that could tear the membrane or cause a build-up of scale
- Is not too hot or too cold

Each of these steps is done by the pretreatment components of the water treatment system, so we will cover them next.

Pretreatment Components

No one pretreatment system will fit every clinic. The clinic's raw (tap) water will dictate the types of pretreatment components that are part of your clinic's water treatment system.

Module 8

Table 3: Benefits and Concerns of Portable RO Systems

	Benefits	Concerns
Portable RO	■ Can trend impending failure of the system ■ Some systems use automated heat disinfection daily or weekly (also true of some central RO systems) ■ A failed system can be easily replaced with a second unit ■ Smaller size makes it possible to move the RO—with the dialysis machine—to the point of use, or to use the RO in the home setting	■ Failure can delay treatment (also true of central RO systems) ■ Bacterial and endotoxin levels must be controlled (also true of central RO systems) ■ May or may not be heat tolerant (also true of central RO systems) ■ Frequent disinfection is required ■ The loaded cart may be unwieldy and heavy

BACKFLOW PREVENTION DEVICE

Plumbing codes require backflow prevention in water treatment systems. Federal or state laws tell us which type of device to use. For dialysis, we must use a **Reduced Pressure Backflow Assembly** (RPBA). With an RPBA in place, contaminants taken out—or chemicals added by the water treatment system—cannot get back into the feed water. A certified backflow assembly tester must check the device each year.[12]

TEMPERATURE BLENDING VALVE

The RO works best when the feed water stays between 77–82° F (25–28° C). The temperature blending valve mixes hot and cold water to keep the water in this range:

- A 1° **F** *drop* leads to a 1.5% drop in product water flow and an *increase* in solute removal.[12]
- A 1° **C** *drop* leads to a 3% drop in product water flow.[12]

Permanent damage to RO membranes may occur if the feed water temperature is above 95° F (35° C). To track the temperature, a gauge (see Figure 4) is placed downstream from the temperature blending valve.

BOOSTER PUMP

All water treatment systems need a certain rate of water flow and pressure to force water through the components. If the flow or pressure is not high or consistent enough, a booster pump can help.[12]

ACID FEED PUMP

An RO membrane works best with water pH range from 5.0 to 8.5.[12] If the feed water pH is above 8.5, carbon filters and RO will not work as well. A chemical injection system called an acid feed pump may be used to lower the pH by injecting a small amount of hydrochloric or sulfuric acid into the feed water. Chemical injection systems have:

- A reservoir to hold the chemicals
- A metering pump to control the level of chemicals added to the water
- A mixing chamber in the feed water line

SEDIMENT FILTERS

All raw (tap) water has particles. Sediment filters and multimedia filters (Figure 8) have either:

- Pores of various sizes to strain out particles, solutes, and other substances
- Layers of different sized media, so each layer can trap smaller particles

As particles build up in the bed, the open channels where water can pass through begin to clog. Resistance then lets less water reach the other water system parts.

CARBON TANKS

If patient's blood is exposed to chlorine, *hemolysis* (destruction of red blood cells) can occur, which can be fatal. Free chlorine may break down some RO membranes, as well. Carbon adsorption systems, or "carbon filters," remove free chlorine, chloramines, and other harmful solutes:

- Free chlorine – we keep levels at or below 0.5 mg/L[19]
- Total chlorine – we keep levels at or below 0.1 mg/L[19]
- Pesticides
- Industrial solvents
- Some trace organic (living or dead) substances

Water Treatment

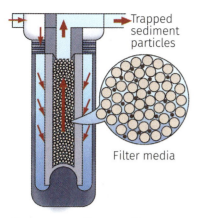

A sediment filter, such as this one, acts as a sieve to trap particles of a certain size. Raw water enters the filter, passes though the filter media (where particles are trapped), and exits the filter.

Figure 8: Sediment Filter

Carbon tanks contain very porous, *granular activated charcoal* (GAC). With its large surface area, GAC adsorbs low molecular weight particles from water, like a magnet attracts iron. **Use only virgin carbon**.[19] Regenerated carbons may have residual contaminants that could harm people on dialysis. GAC:

- May be made of coal, coconut shells, peach pits, wood, or bone.
- Should be acid-washed to remove ash and metals that could leach out.[19]
- Comes in particle or "mesh" sizes. Use a 12 x 40 or smaller mesh size.
- Needs an iodine rating (a measure of carbon adsorption) greater than 900 to remove enough chloramines.[19]

The water treatment system must have at least *two carbon tanks in series* (see Figure 9).[26] The first, or primary tank is called the "worker;" the second or later ones are "polishers." Each tank must have enough carbon to adsorb the chlorine and chloramines in the time the water flows through it. This time span is called *empty bed contact time* (EBCT). EBCT is calculated based on the volume of GAC and the maximum water flow rate. CMS requires *at least 10 minutes* of total EBCT (or 5 minutes per tank) to reduce total chlorine to a level that is safe for dialysis.[30]

WATER SOFTENER

Hard water contains minerals that could build up on the surface of the fragile and costly RO membrane as "scale" and cause damage. A water softener can "soften" water by removing some of the calcium and magnesium (see Figure 10).[12]

> **How to Calculate EBCT**
>
> We use the formula: **EBCT = (7.48 x V) ÷ Q**[19]
>
> - **V** = volume of carbon in cubic feet (cf)
> - **Q** = water flow rate in gallons per minute (gpm)
> - **7.48** is the conversion factor for gallons to cf
>
> For example, if you have a flow rate of 10 gallons per minute and want an EBCT of 10 minutes, your calculation would be:
>
> - **V = (Q x EBCT) ÷ 7.48**
> - **V = (10 x 10) ÷ 7.48 = 13.37**
>
> You would need two tanks totaling at least 13.37 cf.

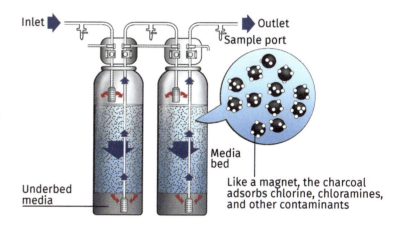

Figure 9: Carbon Tanks

Water softeners work by **ion exchange**, which takes place in a "bed" of tiny round beads of polystyrene resin. The beads are coated with sodium ions, which have a weak bond to the resin. As hard water goes through the softener, the resin attracts the stronger, positively charged ions of calcium and magnesium. Ions of calcium and magnesium are removed (traded) for sodium ions, which then form sodium chloride (salt). The resin gives up sodium ions of equal charge.[12] When the resin has all the calcium and magnesium it can hold, and all of the sodium ions have been used up, the resin bed is *exhausted*. At this point, it must be *regenerated*: a salty "brine" solution is used to saturate the beads with sodium again.

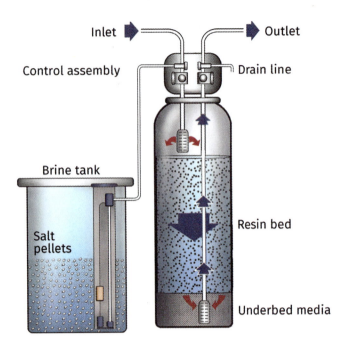

Figure 10: Water Softener

Purification Components

The next group of components removes solutes and particles from feed water and keeps microbes from growing. The RO is the main water purifier. Deionization *may* be part of the system. If so, there are cautions for patient safety. Submicron and ultrafilters remove tiny particles and microbes. Ultraviolet filters keep bacteria in the feed water from multiplying.

ULTRAVIOLET (UV) LIGHT

The UV light uses invisible UV radiation to destroy microbes that pass through the other components. UV changes the DNA of the microbes so they die or cannot multiply.[12]

A low-pressure mercury vapor UV lamp is housed inside a clear quartz sleeve. Feed water flows over the quartz and is exposed to the UV light (see Figure 11). To work, the light must be sized to handle the highest water flow rate your clinic uses.

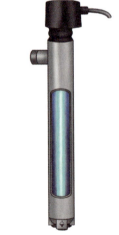

Figure 11: UV Light

We do not rely solely on UV light in dialysis. Because a UV light fades over time, microbes can become resistant to it. You must replace the light source each year or continuously monitor its strength. We also use other means, such as ultrafilters, to remove bacteria.

SUBMICRON AND ULTRAFILTERS

Submicron filters are membrane filters with pore sizes of less than 1 micron that are used to reduce levels of microbes. **Ultrafilter** pore sizes are even smaller, ranging from .05 microns down to .001 microns to catch the smallest microbes (see Figure 13).[19]

Distribution System

Distribution systems carry the product water to the point of use. Pipes to carry dialysis water must be made of a material that can be disinfected and is *"inert,"* so it will not release contaminants into the product water. Pipes may be made from:

- Polyvinyl chloride (PVC)
- Polypropylene (PP)
- Teflon® tubing
- New plastics, such as cross-linked polyethylene (PEX), if chemical or heat disinfection are used. NOTE: Some local or state codes do not permit the use of PEX for dialysis.

Water distribution loops should be as short as possible. It is vital to avoid sharp angles and dead ends where stagnant water could encourage the growth of bacteria. There are two types of distribution systems (see Table 4):

- An **indirect feed system** uses a storage tank.
- A **direct feed system** does not.

INDIRECT FEED SYSTEM

An **indirect feed** system feeds RO water into a storage tank. Product water is pumped through pipes to points of use. Unused product water is sent back to the storage tank by a return loop. There is continuous flow in the loop, even when the RO is *not* running.

Water Storage

The storage tank must have a tight-fitting lid and be vented by a hydrophobic 0.2 micron air filter. The tank should also have a cone- or bowl-shaped bottom. This ensures that the tank will empty all the way, and will be easy to disinfect and rinse. A centrifugal pump made of inert materials is needed to move product water out of the storage tank and through the piping.[31]

Deionization (DI)

DI can make very pure product water by removing solutes using an electrical charge. Clinics may use DI to "polish" the water if RO alone does not result in water that meets AAMI standards.[12] DI has some benefits: it rejects less water than an RO unit, and can reach higher inorganic purity. But, there are some risks to patients with DI, as well.

DI tanks (see Figure 12) have beds of electrically charged resin beads. These beads attract and hold particles with a positive (*cation*) and a negative (*anion*) charge:

- Anions are exchanged for hydroxyl (OH^-) ions.
- Cations are exchanged for hydrogen (H^+) ions.

The OH^- and H^+ ions combine to make pure product water (H_2O).

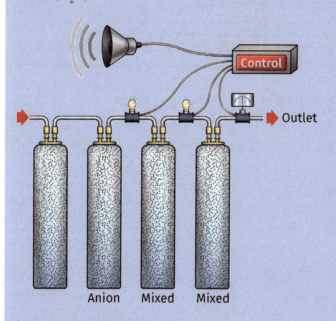

Figure 12: DI Tanks

Types of DI Systems

There are two types of DI systems:

- **Dual bed** DI systems keep anion and cation resin in separate tanks or tanks in a series, where the water goes through both a first and a second tank.
- **Mixed bed** tanks contain both cation and anion resin beads. Mixed bed tanks make higher quality water than dual bed systems.[12]

The most common configuration for DI use is to have two mixed beds.

Risks of DI

Medicare strongly urges that clinics not use *only* DI as the primary way to purify water for dialysis. DI is good at taking out ions we do not want—but it can be very risky for patients:

- **Water from exhausted DI tanks may have high levels of harmful ions**. *DI failure has caused patient deaths*. In one case, 12 patients became severely ill—and three died—when a failed DI let lethal levels of fluoride through.[32]
- **Treated water may become very acidic (low pH) or alkaline (high pH)**. If all of the hydrogen and hydroxyl ions in a DI tank are exhausted, the resin beads will *release* ions they had removed. The level of contaminants released can be much *higher* than the level in the feed water. So, an exhausted DI can serve as a multiplier of contaminants.
- **Use of DI to treat water with chlorine will form cancer-causing nitrosamines**.[12] DI does *not* remove non-charged particles—like bacteria and endotoxins.
- **In fact, the resin bed can support the *growth* of bacteria**.
- **A DI unit can fail catastrophically with no warning**.
- **At a neutral pH, aluminum does not carry a charge—so DI will not remove it**.

DIRECT FEED SYSTEM

A **direct feed** system takes RO water directly to the product water loop for distribution. Unused product water goes back to the RO system or the drain. There is no storage tank, and water flow in the loop occurs *only* while the RO is running.

To calculate the flow rate per second in a direct feed system, install a flow meter at the end of the loop and know the size of piping used. Water flowing at 10 gallons per minute will move much faster through a 1/2-inch pipe than it will through a 1-inch pipe.

Module 8

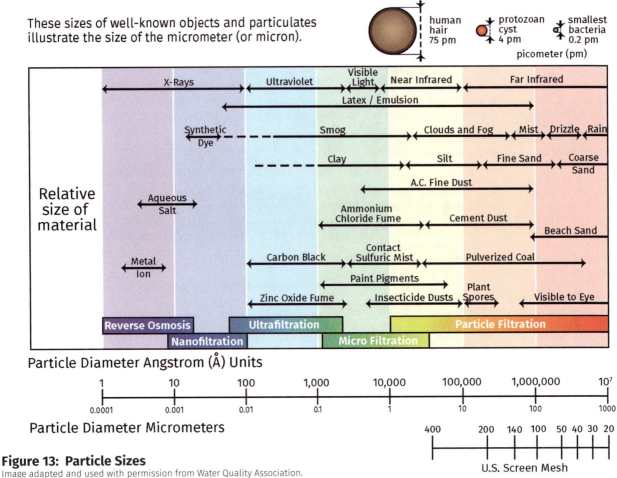

Figure 13: Particle Sizes
Image adapted and used with permission from Water Quality Association.

Table 4: Direct vs. Indirect Feed Distribution Systems

	Benefits	**Concerns**
Direct	■ No added burden for control of bacteria or endotoxins in a storage tank. ■ With continuous use during the treatment day, there is no need to run the system for 15 minutes before each shift or every 4 hours prior to testing for total chlorine.	■ If all of the dialysis stations are not in use, more purified water is wasted. ■ Malfunction will cause immediate loss of water to the point of use. ■ There is no distribution loop flow when the system is off.
Indirect	■ Less water waste, since the RO system is in use only when filling the storage tank. ■ There is constant distribution loop flow.	■ Bacteria can grow if the storage tank is poorly designed or maintained. ■ The system must be in use for 15 minutes before testing for total chlorine. ■ An ultrafilter or other bacterial control device should be used downstream of the storage tank either in the water system or on each dialysis machine.[33]

Monitoring a Water Treatment System

NOTE: In 2014, AAMI released a Technical Information Report. This report, *Water Testing Methodologies*, can help your clinic choose tests to monitor dialysis water.

Water treatment systems are key to dialysis care, but can harm patients if they are not working well. Table 5 lists the tests we use to monitor each system for flow, pressure, temperature, % RO rejection, hardness, total chlorine—and *total dissolved solids* (TDS). TDS is the sum of all of the ions in a solution. We measure TDS through conductivity or resistivity. The result helps to assess the performance of the RO.

Water treatment monitoring is a key part of your clinic's quality improvement program. The *only* way to know if your clinic's system is working is to test each part. If there is a change—such as how your town treats feed water—you may need to test more often or change parts of the system (see Table 6).

All dialysis clinics must keep in close contact with the local water treatment plant. Each clinic should send a letter to the plant at least once a year. The letter will remind the plant that a dialysis clinic is present and needs updates on the status of water treatment. If water treatment changes, too much of a substance is present, water mains are flushed, etc., the plant needs to alert the clinic.

How to Monitor and Maintain Water Treatment System Components

PIPES
Disinfect pipes *at least* monthly to prevent bacterial growth.[34] Make sure the pipes and fittings are compatible with how you disinfect them (see Table 7).

BACKFLOW PREVENTION DEVICE (BPD)
The main problem with BPDs is that they may reduce water flow and pressure. They must be tested once a year by someone who is licensed to test them. If both pre- *and* post-device pressure can be checked, a drop of greater than 30 pounds per square inch (psi) between the two measures may suggest that the filter is blocked and maintenance is needed.[35]

> **Monitoring the Backflow Prevention Device**
> If you can only measure post-pressure, make sure there is enough pressure and flow to operate your system. Watch for pressure change over time to see if the device is plugging up. The correct pressure level will vary with each system. Find the baseline, then check for changes. On average, a large RO will need about 30 psi at 10–12 gallons per minute.

TEMPERATURE BLENDING VALVE
To protect the RO membrane and have a high enough flow of product water, keep feed water at a level suggested by most manufacturers: 77–82° F (25–28° C). If the temperature varies, the amount and quality of the product water will vary as well. Feed water that is too hot can destroy an RO membrane.

> **Monitoring the Temperature Blending Valve**
> Check the temperature blending valve each day by measuring the temperature after the valve. The temperature should be within the set range, and should not change much from day to day—unless the device fails.

SEDIMENT FILTERS
These filters are prone to clogging as they trap particles, which reduces the flow of water. To reduce clogging, the filter may be *backwashed*. If your system requires this, once a day, water is forced backwards through the filter from bottom to top, then flushed to the drain. Backwashing rinses out trapped particles and fluffs up the media layers to help reduce channeling. Some systems will backwash automatically, or you may need to do this by hand.

Water pressure going in and out of the sediment filter is measured with gauges to check for a pressure *change* called Delta (Δ) pressure, or ΔP. As the filter clogs, the pressure reading before the filter rises—so the ΔP increases, while downstream flow declines. The ΔP limit is set by your clinic's policy. If the pressure exceeds this limit, you need to backwash the filter, replace it, or have it serviced.

Module 8

Table 5: Water Treatment Testing[19,22,33,36]

What to Test and Where	Which Test(s) and How Often	Requirement
RO Product Water		
Water coming out of the RO product port	Colony count and limulus amoebocyte lysate (LAL) at least monthly	Recommended
RO Loop Pre		
Water exiting the water storage tank, before UV or ultrafilters	Colony count and LAL at least monthly	Recommended
RO Loop Return		
Water returning from the treatment floor, before returning to the water storage tank or RO system	■ Colony count and LAL monthly ■ AAMI chemical analysis at least once a year	Mandatory Mandatory
Bicarb Mixer		
Water feeding the bicarb mixer (water—not bicarb—sample)	Colony count and LAL at least monthly	Recommended
Acid Mixer (e.g., Granuflo®)		
Water feeding the acid mixer (water—not acid—sample)	Colony count and LAL at least monthly	Recommended
Dialysis Machine Connection Line		
Sample from dialysis connection line to the RO loop	Colony count and LAL at least quarterly for two machine connection lines or any line that shows discoloration	Mandatory
Dialysis Machines Fed by a Central RO System		
Dialysate sample from dialysate sample port as specified by the machine manufacturer	Colony count and LAL on all machines once per year	Recommended or per your clinic policy/state requirement
Tap Water		
Feed water port located prior to all pretreatment devices	Full AAMI chemical analysis, colony count and chloramines, and LAL, prior to installing the system, once a year for chemical contamination, and for seasonal changes or water line repairs	■ Mandatory at install ■ Testing purified water recommended annually to ensure the safety of patients. Persistent high levels of chemicals in the tap water would trigger an analysis to find the source.
Portable RO Machines		
Product water sample	■ Colony count and LAL at least monthly in clinics; at least quarterly at home ■ AAMI chemical analysis at least once a year	■ Mandatory ■ Mandatory
Dialysis Machines Fed by Portable RO Machines		
Dialysate sample from dialysate sample port as specified by the machine manufacturer	Colony count and LAL at least monthly	Mandatory
Total Water Hardness		
Water exiting the water softener tank	Start and end of each treatment day	Recommended
Total Chlorine		
Water exiting carbon tank #1 (before carbon tank #2)	■ Before the first patient shift ■ Every 4 hours for the rest of the day	■ Mandatory ■ Mandatory

Water Treatment

Table 6: Water Monitoring Log Example

	Expected Range	Mon	Tues	Wed	Thu	Fri	Sat
Date							
Gauge Readings							
Press. Gauge #1 (psi) (Pre-Mixed Bed)							
ΔP-Mixed Bed*							
Press. Gauge #2 (psi) (Pre-Softener)							
ΔP-Softener							
Press. Gauge #3 (psi) (Pre-Carb 1)							
ΔP-Carbon Tank #1							
Press. Gauge #4 (psi) (Pre-Carb 2)							
ΔP-Carbon Tank #2							
Softener Timer Check							
Temperature (° F)							
Press. Gauge #5 (psi) (Pre-Filter)							
Press. Gauge #6 (psi) (Post-Filter)							
ΔP-RO Prefilter							
Feed Water TDS							
Product Water TDS							
Percent Rejection							
Feed Flow							
Permeate Flow							
Feed Pressure							
Permeate Pressure							
Water Tests							
Post-Softener Hardness #1							
Post-Softener Hardness #2							
Logged By (initials):							
Chloramines Tests (< 0.1 mg/L)							
Before 1st patient shift							
Before 2nd patient shift							
Before 3rd patient shift							
Audit (initials):							

* The Greek letter delta (Δ) means "change."

Module 8

Table 7: Common Disinfectants Compatible with Piping Material Used in Water Distribution Systems

Material	Bleach	Peracetic acid	Formaldehyde	Hot Water	Ozone
Acrylonitrile butadiene styrene (**ABS**)		✓			
Chlorinated PVC (**CPVC**)	✓	✓	✓		✓
Cross-lined polyethylene (**PEX**)	✓	✓	✓		✓
Glass	✓	✓	✓	✓	✓
Polyethylene (**PE**)	✓	✓	✓		✓
Polypropylene (**PP**)	✓	✓	✓	✓	✓
Polytetrafluoroethylene (**PTFE**)	✓	✓	✓	✓	✓
Polyvinylchloride (**PVC**)	✓	✓	✓		
Polyvinylidene flouride (**PVDF**)	✓	✓	✓	✓	✓
Stainless steel (**SS**)	✓	✓	✓	✓	✓

NOTE: Table 7 is not exhaustive. Verify that your system will not be harmed by the germicide before use. Consider joint and pipe fitting materials and the germicide concentration, as well.

Table adapted with permission from AAMI. Copyright 2004, Association for the Advancement of Medical Instrumentation, ANSI/AAMI RD52:2004 *Dialysate for Hemodialysis*. Table 2.

Monitoring the Sediment Filters

Check all filters periodically by measuring pressure before and after each filter at normal operating flow rates. If the ΔP exceeds your clinic's policy, replace or backwash the filter.[37] If a filter comes with a backwash timer, check the timer setting. **Be sure the filter will backwash only when no one is dialyzing.**

WATER SOFTENER

We regenerate the water softener by flushing the resin bed first with water and then with *brine* (highly concentrated salt water). The resin beads exchange the calcium and magnesium ions, and are again coated with sodium ions. The unwanted positive ions are then rinsed to the drain.

Most clinics have *permanent* water softeners. These have automatic timers and brine tanks that hold salt pellets and water to form brine. They are regenerated on-site every day or every other day. Clinics that are small or have local codes that restrict regeneration may have exchangeable water softeners. A vendor takes these offsite on a set schedule to regenerate them.

Monitoring the Water Softener

You must test the water softener at the end of each day by testing the water hardness after the softener.[38] Test at the start of each day to ensure that the softener is working:

- Hardness should not exceed 1 grain per gallon (gpg), which equals 17 parts per million (ppm). Test strips or the EDTA method may be used to test water hardness.
- The salt tank should be at least half full.[38]
  - If the brine level is too high, a "salt bridge" may occur—salt hardens at the top so the tank *looks* full, even though there is no salt beneath.
  - If the brine level is too low, the concentration of brine may be too weak to regenerate the softener.

Check the regeneration timer setting. Be sure it is set to regenerate when the clinic is closed.

Never let a water softener regenerate during dialysis. If it did, high levels of sodium could enter patients' blood. High sodium levels should trigger the RO system alarm, if an error is made. CMS requires the RO system to interlock with the softener timer so that the RO will not work during regeneration.[39]

Water Treatment

CARBON TANKS

As water flows through carbon tanks, it pushes around the carbon granules inside. Water channels form in the carbon, forcing the water to flow through faster—so it is not cleaned as well. We cannot disinfect *or* regenerate carbon tanks; we can only backwash them and replace them. Backwashing GAC tanks is vital to prevent premature breakthrough of chlorine into the water.

Backwashing "fluffs" the carbon granules to expose new surfaces, remove water channels, and prolong the life of the GAC. However, backwashing does NOT remove substances the carbon has adsorbed. When the GAC in the tank can no longer adsorb enough chlorine, the water leaving the tank will have higher chlorine levels. When this happens, the tank is "exhausted." The first tank is removed, the second tank may be moved into the first spot, and a fresh tank placed in the second spot.[40] New carbon tanks must be rinsed before use.[12]

Monitoring the Carbon Tanks

The water system must be working for at least 15 minutes before you run your first test. If you take a sample when you start up the system, you will be testing water that has been in the tank overnight.[41] This will not give you a true sample of what the carbon tank will produce at normal flow rates. Use test strips that are sensitive enough to ensure that the levels do not exceed the maximum allowed.[41] If the carbon tank comes with a backwash timer, check the timer setting for the correct time. **Be sure it will only backwash when no one is dialyzing.**

RO DEVICE (OPERATING PARAMETERS)

If the RO membrane is not working, water quality or quantity will be reduced. Each RO device has its own baseline levels of pressure and flow to tell you how well it is working. Check pressure in several places including:[42]

- Incoming water (Pressure needs to be enough to maintain flow through the RO device. This is most often 10–12 gpm at 30–40 psi, but will vary with each system.)
- The pump that pushes water through the membrane
- The product water

Water flow is also measured in several places with flow meters:

- **Product flow** tells you how much purified water is getting through the membrane.
- **Waste flow** tells you how much reject water is being flushed down the drain.
- **Direct systems** may measure how much product water is recirculated through the system to blend with the incoming feed water.

Monitoring the RO Device

Check the RO operating parameters each day for flow and pressure. Pressure and flow in an RO system are related. If you reduce the RO pump pressure, product water flow will drop and wastewater flow will increase:

- If the product water flow drops without a change in pump pressure, the RO membrane may be clogging up.
- A change in the pressure reading from baseline, between the pump and rejection pressures, could mean a fouled or torn membrane.

You will need to know the baseline values for all pressures and flows in your system, and check on any deviations. Analyze the trends to watch for even small changes over time.

We also monitor water quality by checking TDS levels in the RO water. This will be discussed in detail later in this module.

RO systems must be disinfected with either heat or chemicals. Some benefits of heat (thermal) disinfection are:

- There are no toxic chemicals to clear from the system.
- Heat disinfection tends to be a more automated process that can be done as needed.

Module 8

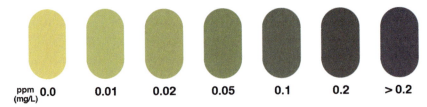

Figure 14: Test Strip
Image used and adapted with permission from RPC.

Some heat disinfection systems allow for a *total system disinfection* that includes the RO, the water loop, *and* the dialysis machines, with little or no staff time required other than for monitoring.

Follow the manufacturer's guidance to disinfect the RO membrane. The RO manufacturer will suggest a type of disinfectant and how often to use it.

UV LIGHT

Over time, the radiant energy of a UV light fades. The quartz sleeve must be cleaned to stay clear so the water is exposed to the light. The lamps must be replaced before they weaken, and at least annually.

Monitoring the UV Light

With older UV light systems, we track hours of use and change the bulb at set times. The light wavelength used must be 254 nanometers and must provide a dose of radiant energy of 30 milliwatt-sec/cm^2.[43]

Newer systems have a UV-intensity meter to check the radiant energy output. If the radiant energy falls below 16 milliwatt-sec/cm^2 (the smallest dose that will kill microbes), a visual alarm will go off to tell you that it is time to replace the bulb.[43]

SUBMICRON AND ULTRAFILTERS

These filters remove microbes from the water:

- Submicron filters reduce the level of bacteria.
- Ultrafilters remove both bacteria and endotoxins.

Over time, these filters can become overgrown with microbes. Routine bacterial and endotoxin testing will reveal issues. The filters must be cleaned, disinfected, or replaced per your clinic's guidelines.

Monitoring Submicron and Ultrafilters

Clean and disinfect these filters on a set schedule or when the ΔP between the inlet and outlet filter gauges exceeds the limit set by your clinic.[44]

WATER STORAGE TANK

Since chlorine is removed during pretreatment, **there is nothing in the product water to prevent the growth of microbes**. The storage tank and pipes are thus perfect spots for bacteria to grow and form biofilm. It may be necessary to *scrub* the inside of the tank to dislodge biofilm. A well designed tank will drain and refill a few times a day, so the water does not stagnate.[45]

Monitoring a Water Storage Tank

We must clean and disinfect the storage tank, distribution piping, and hose to the dialysis machines at least once a month. These steps must also be taken after any invasive repair to the water treatment system. Follow your clinic policies and the manufacturer's guidance.

DI SYSTEMS (OPERATING PARAMETERS)

DI has no moving parts, so monitoring is straightforward. Pure water from a fresh DI tank system has a resistivity of 18.3 megohms-cm.[46] DI must be monitored by resistivity *all the time.* This allows the tanks to be exchanged before exhaustion occurs and contaminants breakthrough into the water. DI tanks used in dialysis must use a **resistivity meter** with an alarm that can be heard and seen in the patient care room(s).[47]

CMS requires in-center DI systems to have an automated way to keep water from an exhausted tank from reaching patients.[47] Water with resistivity of less than 1 megohm-cm is not safe for dialysis. A stop-valve or divert to drain system must be used.

When resistivity of the product water drops below 1 megohm-cm:
- The alarm sounds.
- The product water is sent to the drain or kept from reaching the point of use.

Portable DI tanks are used in a clinic, but regenerated off-site.

Analyze Water Quality

Water must reach the ANSI/AAMI standards your clinic uses. To ensure that the limits set in ANSI/AAMI for the contaminants from Table 1 are met, do a chemical analysis:[19]
- When the RO system is installed
- When RO membranes are replaced
- At least once a year thereafter

RO Water Quality

The RO membrane is the most important part of the RO system.
- **We test RO performance with *percent rejection***, a measure of how well the membrane removes TDS in the water, in parts per million (ppm). Keep the percent rejection of an RO system at a level that will assure AAMI-quality water. **The percent rejection formula is**:[19]

$$\frac{\text{Feed water conductivity minus permeate conductivity}}{\text{Feed water conductivity}} \times 100$$

For example, we will say that input TDS is 100 ppm, and output TDS is 8 ppm. Enter these into the formula:

$$\frac{100 - 8}{100} \times 100$$

The result is $\frac{92}{100} \times 100 = 92$ (percent)

You have a 92% rejection of TDS.

- **We measure RO product water quality with *conductivity***—the level of TDS in the water, in ppm. The conductivity monitor should account for temperature to give a consistent reading.

CMS requires us to take action when the percent rejection is less than 90%. Your state may have even more stringent limits. Set the alarm level at a percent rejection that assures AAMI-quality water. Percent rejection alone does not reflect water quality. *The percent rejection level will depend on your product water analysis.* Clinics with low TDS feed water can have a rejection rate well below 90%—and still produce AAMI quality water in the single digit TDS. AAMI does not say that <90% is *unsafe*, but that it requires an action. The action is to validate that your system delivers safe quality product water. Record the rejection rate at the time of each chemical analysis of your RO product water.

DI Water Quality

Since DI water is more pure than RO water, its conductivity is too low to check accurately. Instead, we monitor DI product water for *resistance* to the flow of electricity. This is the *inverse*, or opposite, of conductivity. **Patients must not be dialyzed with DI water that has resistivity less than 1 megohm-cm, measured at the DI output.**[46] You will need to know how the monitor on your clinic's DI system works, as they vary. Most often, an LED will tell you the water quality.

> **Analyze DI Water Quality**
>
> Monitor water quality continually. CMS requires that resistivity be checked and documented on a log twice each day of use.[46] You must be able to hear and see water treatment alarms in the patient care room(s). Keep the resistivity of DI water greater than 1 megohm-cm.

Module 8

Table 8: Monitoring Guidelines for Water Purification Equipment, Distribution Systems, and Dialysate[8,19]

Component	What to Monitor	Special Interval	Normal Interval	Specification*
Sediment Filter	Pressure drop across the filter	NA	Daily	Pressure drop less than XXXX
Sediment Filter Backwashing Cycle	Backwash cycle timer setting	NA	Daily – start of day	Backwash clock set to XX:XX
Cartridge Filter	Pressure drop across the filter	NA	Daily – end of day	Pressure drop less than XXXX
Water Softener	Product water softness	NA	Daily – end of day	Hardness as calcium carbonate less than 1 grain/gallon, unless otherwise specified by the RO manufacturer
Water Softener Brine Tank	Level in tank of undissolved salt	NA	Daily – end of day	Salt level at XXX
Water Softener Regeneration Cycle	Regeneration cycle timer setting set to the correct time	NA	Daily – start of day	Softener timer set to XX:XX
Carbon Adsorption Beds	Sample of water post primary carbon tank for total chlorine	NA	Before starting each patient shift or every 4 hours	Less than 0.1 mg/L of total chlorine
Chemical Injection System	Level of chemical in the reservoir, injector function, value of the controlling parameter (e.g., pH)	NA	Daily	Chemical level in reservoir is greater than or equal to XXX; controlling parameter is in the range of XX-XX
Reverse Osmosis	Product water conductivity, total dissolved solids (TDS) or resistivity, and calculated rejection rate	NA	Per the manufacturer's recommendations (continuous monitors)	Rejection is greater than or equal to XX%
Reverse Osmosis	Product and reject flow rates, and calculated recovery	NA	Daily (continuous monitors)	Product water flow rate greater than X.X gpm; recovery in the range of XX-XX%
Deionizers	Product water resistivity	NA	Continuous	Resistivity greater than 1 megohm-cm
Ultrafilters	Pressure drop across the filter	NA	Daily	Pressure drop less than XXXX
Water Storage Tanks	Bacterial growth and endotoxisn	Weekly, until a pattern of consistent compliance with limits can be shown	NA	†Bacterial count less than action level of 50 CFU/mL; endotoxin level of less than 0.125 EU/mL[22]
Water Distribution Piping System	Bacterial growth and endotoxins	Weekly, until a pattern of consistent compliance with limits can be shown	Monthly	†Bacterial count less than action level of 50 CFU/mL; endotoxin level of less than 0.125 EU/mL[22]

Water Treatment

Table 8: CONTINUED

Component	What to Monitor	Special Interval	Normal Interval	Specification*
UV Light Sources	Energy output	NA	Monthly	Light output greater than XXX and to safe levels XXX after rinsing
Ozone Generators	Concentration in the water	NA	During and after each disinfection	Ozone concentration greater than XXX
Hot Water Disinfection Systems	Temperature and time of exposure of the system to hot water	NA	During each disinfection and prior to each use	Temperature not less than XX° C; minimum exposure time at temperature is greater than or equal to XX minutes. Safe temperature (XXX) for use.
Dialysate	Bacterial growth and endotoxins	NA	Monthly: rotate so at least two machines are tested each month and each is tested at least once a year	†Bacterial count less than action level of 50 CFU/mL; endotoxin level of less than 0.125 EU/mL[22]
Dialysate	Conductivity and pH	NA	Each treatment	Conductivity within ±5% of the nominal machine value; pH in the range 6.9 – 7.6

* NOTE: It is not possible to state operating ranges for each device in the table, since some values are specific to the system used in your clinic. Where there are Xs in the table, the clinic should define a range based on the manufacturer's instructions or measurements of system performance.

† Bacteria and endotoxin levels from ANSI/AAMI 23500:2014. *Guidance for the preparation and quality management of fluids for hemodialysis and related therapies.*

Table adapted with permission from AAMI. Copyright 2004, Association for the Advancement of Medical Instrumentation, ANSI/AAMI RD52:2004 *Dialysate for hemodialysis*. Table 4

Monitor Water for Bacteria and Endotoxins

Contamination of water by microbes is a health risk for patients. Test your clinic's water for bacteria and endotoxins at least once a month; more often if problems occur. CMS requires us to take water samples using the *worst-case* scenario. For this reason, you will take cultures just before you disinfect the system.[48] Test water that is:

- Used to make reprocessing chemicals
- Used to rinse and clean (reprocess) dialyzers
- From a storage tank, if one is used
- Leaving the RO unit (or deionizer, if used)
- At the start, middle, and end of the distribution loop
- Used to make concentrate solutions
- Used to make dialysate; test at the point it enters the dialysis machine

HOW TO TEST FOR BACTERIA

Even small amounts of disinfectant can keep microbes from growing in a culture. Most clinics now use a transfer device to move the sample to a media tube. If your clinic does *not* use a transfer device:

1. Use alcohol on the outside (only) of the sample ports.
2. Let the sample ports dry fully before you draw the culture sample(s).
3. Run water for one minute and then collect the sample in a sterile cup.
4. Use a pipette to put 0.1 to 0.5 mL of water from the cup onto the culture medium.
5. Process samples for bacteria testing within 1–2 hours or put them in a refrigerator right away and process them within 24 hours.

You will test the samples using one of two techniques:[22,49]

- **Membrane filter technique** (preferred). You aseptically filter a known volume of sample water through a .45 μm membrane filter onto culture medium in an agar plate.
- **Spread plate technique**. You spread at least 0.5 mL of the sample water directly onto the culture medium in an agar plate.

There are two AAMI approved culture methods to test for bacteria:[49]

1. Tryptone glucose extract (TGEA) or Reasoner's 2A with 4% sodium bicarbonate (or equivalent). Do not use blood or chocolate agar. Use an incubation temperature of 17° C to 23° C for 168 hours (7 days).

2. Trypticase soy agar (TSA), a soybean casein digest agar, or standard methods agar and plate count agar (TGYE) incubated at 35° C for 48 hours.

HOW TO TEST FOR ENDOTOXINS

Dialysis water is tested for endotoxins with a limulus amoebocyte lysate (LAL) test.[50]

Most clinics send samples out for testing. There are several methods of LAL testing, all based on the fact that horseshoe crab blood will gel when endotoxins are present.

- The simplest test is a *gel clot test*. When positive, the blood will clot within a certain time at a certain temperature if the sample has endotoxins above the reaction value (or *lambda*). This test is qualitative only, so a positive result means that there are more endotoxins than the threshold level.
- Turbidometric and chromogenic tests are quantitative. They will tell you the level of endotoxins in the sample.

Portable endotoxin meters now are available. These use the turbidometric method and give results in less than 5 minutes. They are very cost-effective for immediate ("stat") testing, where a central lab would charge a higher rate.[51]

DISINFECT THE SYSTEM TO REMOVE BIOFILM

Mature biofilm is almost impossible to remove. In some cases, we must replace all or part of the distribution system to remove biofilm.[35] Good distribution system design and a robust schedule of disinfection can help control biofilm levels. The most common type of water treatment system disinfection is chemical (e.g., bleach). Ozone and heat can also be used in systems made of materials that will not be harmed by these methods. Test and disinfect on a routine schedule—do *not* wait to reach an action level. This approach works better and is less costly than trying to remove biofilm that has formed.

In a 2016 study from Japan, researchers cut out parts of the HD piping system and tested several disinfectants on the biofilm.[52] They used a scanning electron microscope to look at the remaining biofilm. In their results:

- **Sodium hypochlorite** (bleach) did *not* remove biofilm well at room temperature or when heated to 80° C for 2 hours.
- **Acetic acid** worked best when heated, but removed only surface biofilm and not deeper layers.
- **Peracetic acid** worked well at room temperature *and* when heated—and reached deeper layers of the biofilm.

Monitor Water for Chemicals

Conduct a chemical analysis of the water at least once per year. Draw the sample from a sample port right after the RO or DI system. Per CMS, the water treatment system must operate within the AAMI standards at all times. AAMI has set the maximum allowable levels of contaminants that can be in the product water (see Table 1).

TOTAL CHLORINE

Total chlorine is composed of free chlorine and chloramines. Free chlorine and chloramines are strong *oxidants*: they react with oxygen to destroy cell walls. Both may be added to city water to kill bacteria. The carbon tank will remove these chemicals by adsorption. However, we cannot predict when the tank will "exhaust" and lead to breakthrough, so we must test often. Chlorine products used in water treatment include:

- **Chlorine gas** (often used to kill bacteria, fungi, and viruses in drinking water)
- **Chlorine bleach**

The importance of careful testing for chlorine cannot be stressed enough. Patients who are exposed to dialysate with these contaminants will be harmed and could die. The danger we see in dialysis is destruction of red blood cells. Patients in one clinic where chloramine levels climbed in 4 months from < 0.1 mg/mL to 0.27 mg/mL developed anemia.[53] Patients exposed to higher levels of chloramines may have:

- *Methemoglobinemia* - red blood cells that cannot carry oxygen
- *Hemolysis* - red blood cells that burst open
- *Hemolytic anemia* - a shortage of red blood cells due to red blood cell breakdown

We can test for total chlorine in one of three ways:

1. Test strips made to test low level total chlorine
2. N, N-diethyl p-phenylenediamine (DPD) test kit
3. A digital chlorimeter, typically based on the DPD method

Some test strip brands tend to be more accurate, as the results tend to not be affected by other interfering substances that may be in the sample. Test strips also have fewer chances for error. Since we read these tests by looking at colors, the person doing them must pass a color blindness test, or a digital meter must be used:[41, 54]

- The limit for free chlorine is **0.5 mg/L**.
- The limit for total chlorine is **0.1 mg/L**.

There is no direct test for chloramines, so to measure chloramines you must do *two* tests, one for *total* chlorine and one for *free* chlorine. The chloramine level is the difference between the two results. So, if your measured total chlorine is 1.2 ppm and your free chlorine is 0.8 ppm: 1.2 – 0.8 = a chloramine level of 0.4 ppm.

CMS and AAMI permits testing for total chlorine only, *if*:

- The test used is sensitive enough to detect low levels and *if* action is taken for any results greater than 0.1 ppm
- A zero reading for total chlorine means that the amount of chlorine in the water is less than the *sensitivity* (lowest detectable level) of the test

SODIUM AND POTASSIUM

ANSI/AAMI says water used for dialysis should contain **no more than 70 mg/L (3.0 mEq/L)** of sodium and **8 mg/L (0.2 mEq/L)** of potassium.[19] Sodium and potassium are removed by RO or DI.

> **Frequency of Total Chlorine Testing**
> CMS requires that we test for total chlorine:[41]
> - At the start of each treatment day
> - At the start of each patient shift
> - Every 4 hours if your clinic does not have set shifts

CALCIUM AND MAGNESIUM

Hard water contains calcium and magnesium. If too-high levels of these minerals reach patients, the result may be **hard water syndrome**, which can cause:

- Nausea and vomiting
- Muscle weakness
- Severe headaches
- Skin flushing
- High—or low—blood pressure
- Calcium crystals in the soft tissues of the patient's body over time, causing pain, injury, or death

Too much calcium or magnesium can also cause scale to form, which can clog equipment and damage the RO membrane. The ANSI/AAMI standards are **no more than 2 mg/L (0.1 mEq/L)** of calcium and **no more than 4 mg/L (0.3 mEq/L)** of magnesium.[19] Calcium and magnesium are removed by the water softener.

FLUORIDE

Water treatment needs to protect patients from high levels of fluoride. Many dialysis patients are prone to bone disease. Some who have long-term exposure to fluoridated water develop *osteosclerosis* (hardening of bone and/or bone marrow). Other symptoms of too much fluoride may include:

- Nausea and vomiting
- Muscle twitching
- Low blood pressure
- Seizures
- Heart arrhythmias

ANSI/AAMI says there should be **no more than 0.2 mg/L** of fluoride in dialysis water.[19] Fluoride is removed by RO or DI.

NITRATES

Nitrates can be found in harmful amounts in water from some wells, due to bacteria or farm fertilizers. Nitrates can harm patients by keeping red blood cells from using oxygen. This is called *methemoglobinemia*. A patient with this problem will have *cyanosis*—blue skin, lips, gums, and fingernail beds—from the lack of oxygen. They may also have low blood pressure and nausea.

ANSI/AAMI recommends a nitrate limit in dialysis water of **no more than 2.0 mg/L**.[19] Nitrates are removed by RO or DI.

SULFATES

Sulfates (salts or esters of sulfuric acid) in levels greater than 200 mg/L can cause:

- Nausea and vomiting
- Metabolic acidosis (high blood acid levels)

ANSI/AAMI recommends a sulfate limit in water used for dialysis of **no more than 100 mg/L**.[19] Sulfates are removed by RO or DI.

ALUMINUM

Aluminum, a common earth metal, may occur in the local water supply. Or, it may be added as alum to make water clearer by removing algae, sediment, and silt. In healthy people, only small amounts of aluminum are absorbed from the diet, and the kidneys remove the rest.

When the kidneys fail, aluminum can build up in the brain and bones. High aluminum levels are a cause of anemia in dialysis patients. Damage to the nervous system and fatal *encephalopathy* (brain disease) can also occur. Called *dialysis dementia*, this problem can lead to:

- Confusion
- Loss of short-term memory
- Personality changes
- Speech problems
- Muscle spasms
- Hallucinations
- Seizures
- Impaired thinking
- Death

Long-term exposure to high levels of aluminum has also been linked with aluminum-related bone disease (ARBD), which can cause:

- Bone pain
- Muscle weakness
- Fractures

Dialysis water and equipment are key sources of toxic aluminum for patients. Ionized aluminum in water can cross the dialyzer membrane and move into the patient's blood. In 1996, a water pipe into a clinic in the Netherlands was replaced. The new pipe had aluminum in its mortar that leached into the water. Ten patients died of sepsis, convulsions, and coma—with blood aluminum levels more than 25 times normal.[55] Clinics should check the design of all of their water systems, and test patients' blood aluminum levels.

Since aluminum builds up in the bodies of dialysis patients, ANSI/AAMI says levels in dialysis water should be *very* low—**no more than 0.01 mg/L**.[19] Aluminum can be removed by RO or DI. Aluminum levels in local water supplies can vary with the season. And, aluminum is *amphoteric*: it can react as an acid *or* a base, depending on the conditions. Experts suggest that we test for aluminum in dialysis water more than once a year.

COPPER AND ZINC

Water, especially acidic water, can leach copper out of plumbing pipes. The use of galvanized iron in the water treatment or distribution system can cause high zinc levels in the water. In the patient's body, too much **copper** can cause:

- Nausea
- Vomiting
- Headaches
- Chills
- Pancreatitis (painful inflammation of the pancreas)
- Metabolic acidosis
- Liver damage
- Fatal hemolysis

High **zinc** levels can cause:

- Nausea and vomiting
- Fever
- Anemia

ANSI/AAMI says an upper limit for copper and zinc in dialysis water should be **no higher than 0.1 mg/L**.[19] Copper and zinc can be removed by RO or DI.

ARSENIC, BARIUM, CADMIUM, CHROMIUM, LEAD, MERCURY, AND SELENIUM

Table 1 shows the EPA levels for these trace metals in drinking water and the ANSI/AAMI standards for dialysis water. Each of these metals can be removed by RO or DI.

Patient Monitoring

We monitor water quality to protect patients and to protect equipment so it can protect patients. Failure of one or more parts of the water treatment system can cause serious illness—or death. Patient monitoring that would reveal problems with water quality should include:

1. **Routine blood tests** – High levels of toxic substances in patients' blood (e.g., aluminum), or substances that should not be found in the blood, need more study.

2. **Patient symptoms** – At the start of or during treatment, patients may have acute (sudden onset) symptoms. If this occurs, *assume that there is a problem and take immediate action to find the cause.* There could be many causes for some symptoms, like nausea or low blood pressure—and water may be one of them.

If two or more patients have similar symptoms at the same time, suspect a problem with a water treatment system. NOTE: there may be a problem with the delivery system as well, if a central concentrate or dialysate delivery system is being used. Knowing the first and last dialysis station in your clinic's water loop can help you troubleshoot. If two or more patients at the distal (far) end of the loop start to have symptoms, while patients at the start of the loop do *not*, the cause may be something other than the water, e.g., a common medicine vial. Logic would suggest that a central RO cause would lead to a cascading or domino event that would affect patients at the start of the loop first.

If you think there may be a water quality problem, put the dialysis machine in bypass mode, and check the water treatment system right away. In some cases, treatment will be stopped. Table 9 lists some patient symptoms and the water contaminants that may cause them.

Table 9: Symptoms that May be Related to Water Contamination[12]

Sign or Symptom	Possible Water Contaminant-Related Cause
Anemia	Aluminum, chloramines, copper, zinc
Bone Disease	Aluminum, fluoride
Hemolysis	Chloramines, copper, nitrates
Hypotension	Bacteria, endotoxins, nitrates, calcium, magnesium
Metabolic acidosis	Low pH, sulfates, copper
Muscle weakness	Calcium, magnesium
Nausea and vomiting	Bacteria, calcium, copper, endotoxin, low pH, magnesium, nitrates, sulfates, zinc
Neurological deterioration	Aluminum
Fever, chills	Bacteria, endotoxins, copper, zinc
Severe headaches	Copper
Hypertension	Calcium, magnesium, copper, sodium
Liver damage	Copper

Conclusion

A well-designed water treatment system can protect your patients. Knowing why and how we treat the water and the type of system used in your clinic is crucial. You play a vital role in making sure that water is safe for patient use. Each time you check a monitor, record a meter value on a log sheet, or test a part of your clinic's system for microbes, you are helping to ensure safe, quality patient care.

Appendix A: EPA Tap Water Standards

Table A1: EPA Standards for *Inorganic Chemicals* in Tap Water[56]

Contaminant	Maximum Contaminant Level (MCL) in mg/L	Potential Health Effect (from long-term exposure above the MCL)
Antimony	.006	Blood cholesterol rise, blood sugar drop
Arsenic	.01	Skin or circulatory damage, cancer risk
Asbestos fibers	7 million/liter	Risk of benign intestinal polyps
Barium	2	Increase in blood pressure
Beryllium	.004	Intestinal lesions
Cadmium	.005	Kidney damage
Chromium	.1	Allergic dermatitis
Copper	1.3	GI distress in short term. Kidney or liver damage in long term.
Cyanide (free)	.2	Nerve damage or thyroid problems
Fluoride	4.0	Bone disease, mottled teeth in children
Lead	.015	Children: developmental delays Adults: kidney problems, high blood pressure
Mercury (inorganic)	.002	Kidney damage
Nitrate (as Nitrogen)	10	Shortness of breath, blue-baby syndrome in infants under 6 months
Nitrite (Nitrogen)	1	Shortness of breath, blue-baby syndrome in infants under 6 months
Selenium	0.05	Hair or fingernail loss, numbness in fingers or toes, circulatory problems
Thallium	.0002	Hair loss, blood changes, kidney, liver, or intestinal problems

Table A2: EPA Standards for *Organic Chemicals* in Tap Water[57] (NOTE: These are uncommon, unless there is a specific hazard)

Contaminant	MCL (mg/L)	Potential Health Effects (from long-term exposure above the MCL)
Acrylamide	*	Nerve or blood problems, cancer risk
Alachlor	.002	Eye, liver, kidney, spleen problems, anemia, cancer risk
Atrazine	.003	Cardiovascular or reproductive problems
Benzene	.005	Anemia, drop in platelets, cancer risk
Benzo(a)pyrene (PAHs)	.0002	Reproductive problems, cancer risk
Carbofuran	.04	Problems with blood, nerves, reproduction
Carbon tetrachloride	.005	Liver problems, cancer risk
Chlordane	.002	Liver or nerve problems, cancer risk
Chlorobenzene	.1	Liver or kidney problems
2,4-D	.07	Kidney, liver, adrenal gland problems
Dalapon	.2	Minor kidney changes
1,2-Dibromo-3 chloropropane (DBCP)	.0002	Reproductive problems, cancer risk
o-Dichlorobenzene	.6	Liver, kidney, or circulator problems

Table A2: CONTINUED

Contaminant	MCL (mg/L)	Potential Health Effects (from long-term exposure above the MCL)
p-Dichlorobenzene	.075	Anemia, liver, kidney, spleen damage, blood changes
1,2-Dichloroethane	.005	Cancer risk
1,1-Dichloroethylene	.007	Liver problems
cis-1,2-Dichloroethylene	.07	Liver problems
Trans-1,2-Dichloroethylene	.1	Liver problems
Dichloromethane	.005	Liver problems, cancer risk
1,2-Dichloropropane	.005	Cancer risk
Di(2-ethylhexyl) adipate	.4	Weight loss, liver problems, possible reproductive problems
Di(2-etheylhexyl) phthalate	.006	Reproductive problems, liver problems, cancer risk
Dinoseb	.007	Reproductive problems
Dioxin (2,3,7,8-TCDD)	.00000003	Reproductive problems, cancer risk
Diquat	.02	Cataracts
Endothall	.1	Stomach and intestinal problems
Endrin	.002	Liver problems
Epichlorohydrin	**	Cancer risk, stomach problems
Ethylbenzene	.7	Liver or kidney problems
Ethylene dibromide	.00005	Liver, stomach, kidney, reproductive problems, cancer risk
Glyphosate	.7	Kidney, reproductive problems
Heptachlor	.0004	Liver damage, cancer risk
Heptachlor epoxide	.0002	Liver damage, cancer risk
Hexachlorobenzene	.001	Liver, kidney, reproductive problems, cancer risk
Hexachlorocyclopentadiene	.05	Kidney or stomach problems
Lindane	.0002	Liver or kidney problems
Methoxychlor	.04	Reproductive problems
Oxamyl (Vydate)	.2	Slight nervous system effects
Polychlorinated biphenyls (PCBs)	.0005	Problems with skin, thymus gland, immune, nervous, and reproductive systems, cancer risk
Pentachlorophenol	.001	Liver or kidney problems, cancer risk
Picloram	.5	Liver problems
Simazine	.004	Problems with blood
Styrene	.1	Liver, kidney, or circulatory problems
Tetrachloroethylene	.005	Liver problems, cancer risk
Toluene	1	Nervous system, kidney, liver problems
Toxaphene	.003	Kidney, liver, thyroid problems, cancer risk
2,4,5-TP (Silvex)	.05	Liver problems
1,2,4-Trichlorobenzene	.07	Changes in adrenal glands
1,1,1-Trichloroethane	.2	Liver, nervous, or circulatory problems
1,1,2-Trichloroethane	.005	Liver, kidney, or immune system problems

Table A2: CONTINUED

Contaminant	MCL (mg/L)	Potential Health Effects (from long-term exposure above the MCL)
Trichloroethylene	.005	Liver problems, cancer risk
Vinyl chloride	.002	Cancer risk
Xylenes (total)	10	Nervous system damage

* Water systems must certify in writing that acrylamide does not exceed 0.05% dosed at 1 mg/L (or equivalent)
** Water systems must certify in writing that epichlorydrin does not exceed 0.01% dosed at 20 mg/L (or equivalent)

Table A3: EPA Standards for Disinfectants in Tap Water[58]

Contaminant	MCL (mg/L)	Potential Health Effects (from long-term exposure above the MCL)
Chloramines (Cl_2)	4.0	Eye/nose irritation, stomach upset, anemia
Chlorine (Cl_2)	4.0	Eye/nose irritation, stomach upset, anemia
Chlorine dioxide (ClO_2)	.8	Anemia; infants/children: nervous system effects

References

1. Winter TC, Harvey JW, Franke OL, et al. 1998. Ground water and surface water: A single resource. US Geological Survey Circular 1139. Available at https://pubs.usgs.gov/circ/circ1139/pdf/circ1139.pdf. Accessed January 2017
2. US Geological Survey. USGS Water Science School. Water, the universal solvent. Available at http://water.usgs.gov/edu/solvent.html. Accessed July 2016
3. Fisher SC, Phillips PJ, Brownawell BJ, et al. Comparison of wastewater-associated contaminants in the bed sediment of Hempstead Bay, New York, before and after Hurricane Sandy. *Mar Pollut Bull*. 2016;107(2):499-508
4. Furlong ET, Batt AL, Glassmeyer ST, et al. Nationwide reconnaissance of contaminants of emerging concern in source and treated drinking waters of the United States: Pharmaceuticals. *Sci Total Envir*. 2017;579:1629-42
5. Carpenter DO. Hydraulic fracturing for natural gas: impact on health and environment. *Rev Environ Health*. 2016;31(1):47-51
6. Lan J, Hu M, Gao C, et al. Toxicity assessment of 4-Methyl-1-cyclohexamethanol and its metabolites in response to a recent chemical spill in West Virginia, USA. *Envir Sci Technol*. 2015;49(10):6284-93
7. Understanding the Safe Drinking Water Act. United States Environmental Protection Agency. Available at https://www.epa.gov/sites/production/files/2015-04/documents/epa816f04030.pdf. Accessed January 2017
8. Centers for Medicare and Medicaid Services, HHS. ESRD surveyor training interpretive guidance. Final Version 1.1. October 3, 2008 (V Tag 593) Available at https://www.cms.gov/Medicare/Provider-Enrollment-and-Certification/GuidanceforLawsAndRegulations/Downloads/esrdpgmguidance.pdf. Accessed June 2017
9. Centers for Disease Control and Prevention. *Water treatment*. Available at http://www.cdc.gov/healthywater/drinking/public/water_treatment.html. Accessed June 2017
10. Centers for Disease Control and Prevention. *Consumer confidence reports (CCRs): A guide to understanding your CCR*. Available at http://www.cdc.gov/healthywater/drinking/public/understanding_ccr.html. Accessed July 2016
11. United States Environmental Protection Agency. *Secondary drinking water standards: Guidance for nuisance chemicals*. Available at https://www.epa.gov/dwstandardsregulations/secondary-drinking-water-standards-guidance-nuisance-chemicals. Accessed January 2017
12. Layman-Amato R, Curtis J, Payne GM. Water treatment for hemodialysis: An update. *Nephrol Nurs J*. 2013;40(5):383-404, 465
13. Centers for Medicare and Medicaid Services, HHS. ESRD surveyor training interpretive guidance. Final Version 1.1. October 3, 2008 (V Tag 182) Available at https://www.cms.gov/Medicare/Provider-Enrollment-and-Certification/GuidanceforLawsAndRegulations/Downloads/esrdpgmguidance.pdf. Accessed June 2017
14. Centers for Medicare and Medicaid Services. *Conditions for Coverage for End-Stage Renal Disease Facilities: Final Rule*, 73 Federal Register 73 (15 April 2008), p. 20477. Available at www.cms.gov/Regulations-and-Guidance/Legislation/CFCsAndCoPs/downloads/esrdfinalrule0415.pdf. Accessed January 2017
15. Payne GM. *Dialysis Water and Dialysate Recommendations: A User Guide*. Arlington, VA. Association for the Advancement of Medical Instrumentation. 2014
16. Upadhyay A, Jaber BL. We use impure water to make dialysate for hemodialysis. *Semin Dial*. 2016;29(4):297-9
17. Kwan BC, Chow KM, Ma TK, et al. Effect of using ultrapure dialysate for hemodialysis on the level of circulating bacterial fragment in renal failure patients. *Nephron Clin Pract*. 2013;123(3-4):246-53

18. Glorieux G, Neirynck N, Veys N, et al. Dialysis water and fluid purity: more than endotoxin. *Nephrol Dial Transplant* 2012;27(11):4010-21
19. Association for the Advancement of Medical Instrumentation. *Dialysate for hemodialysis* (ANSI/AAMI RD52:2004). Arlington, VA, American National Standard, 2004. Dialysate for Hemodialysis. Approved August 9, 2004, by the American National Standards Institute. Sections: 3.21, 4.1.1, 4.3.2.1, 4.3.2.2, 6.1, 6.2.5, 6.2.7
20. United States Environmental Protection Agency. *National Primary Drinking Water Regulations*. Available at https://www.epa.gov/sites/production/files/2016-06/documents/npwdr_complete_table.pdf. Accessed June 2017
21. Centers for Medicare and Medicaid Services, HHS. ESRD surveyor training interpretive guidance. Final Version 1.1. October 3, 2008 (V Tag 178) Available at https://www.cms.gov/Medicare/Provider-Enrollment-and-Certification/GuidanceforLawsAndRegulations/Downloads/esrdpgmguidance.pdf. Accessed June 2017
22. Association for the Advancement of Medical Instrumentation. ANSI/AAMI 23500:2014 *Guidance for the preparation and quality management of fluids for hemodialysis and related therapies*. Arlington, VA, American National Standard, 2014. Approved August 15, 2014, by the American National Standards Institute, Inc.
23. Feroze U, Kalantar-Zadeh K, Sterling KA, et al. Examining associations of circulating endotoxin with nutritional status, inflammation and mortality in hemodialysis patients. *J Ren Nutr*. 2012;22(3): 317-26
24. Centers for Medicare and Medicaid Services, HHS. ESRD surveyor training interpretive guidance. Final Version 1.1. October 3, 2008 (V Tag 187) Available at https://www.cms.gov/Medicare/Provider-Enrollment-and-Certification/GuidanceforLawsAndRegulations/Downloads/esrdpgmguidance.pdf. Accessed June 2017
25. Centers for Medicare and Medicaid Services, HHS. ESRD surveyor training interpretive guidance. Final Version 1.1. October 3, 2008 (V Tag 204) Available at https://www.cms.gov/Medicare/Provider-Enrollment-and-Certification/GuidanceforLawsAndRegulations/Downloads/esrdpgmguidance.pdf. Accessed June 2017
26. Centers for Medicare and Medicaid Services, HHS. ESRD surveyor training interpretive guidance. Final Version 1.1. October 3, 2008 (V Tag 192) Available at https://www.cms.gov/Medicare/Provider-Enrollment-and-Certification/GuidanceforLawsAndRegulations/Downloads/esrdpgmguidance.pdf. Accessed June 2017
27. United States Department of Health and Human Services. Food and Drug Administration. *Guidance for the content of premarket notifications for water purification components and systems for hemodialysis*. May 30, 1997. Available at http://www.fda.gov/downloads/medicaldevices/deviceregulationandguidance/guidancedocuments/ucm080215.pdf. Accessed January 2017
28. Agar JWM. Personal viewpoint: Hemodialysis—water, power, and waste disposal: rethinking our environmental responsibilities. *Hemodial Int*. 2012;16(1):6-10
29. Agar JWM. Reusing dialysis wastewater: the elephant in the room. *Am J Kidney Dis*. 2008;52(1):10-2
30. Centers for Medicare and Medicaid Services, HHS. ESRD surveyor training interpretive guidance. Final Version 1.1. October 3, 2008 (V Tag 195) Available at https://www.cms.gov/Medicare/Provider-Enrollment-and-Certification/GuidanceforLawsAndRegulations/Downloads/esrdpgmguidance.pdf. Accessed June 2017
31. Centers for Medicare and Medicaid Services, HHS. ESRD surveyor training interpretive guidance. Final Version 1.1. October 3, 2008 (V Tag 211) Available at https://www.cms.gov/Medicare/Provider-Enrollment-and-Certification/GuidanceforLawsAndRegulations/Downloads/esrdpgmguidance.pdf. Accessed June 2017
32. Arnow PM, Bland LA, Garcia-Houchins S, et al. An outbreak of fatal fluoride intoxication in a long-term hemodialysis unit. *Ann Intern Med*. 1994;121(5):339-44
33. Association for the Advancement of Medical Instrumentation. ANSI/AAMI 13959:2014 *Water for hemodialysis and related therapies*. Arlington, VA, American National Standard, 2014. Approved August 15, 2014, by the American National Standards Institute, Inc.
34. Centers for Medicare and Medicaid Services, HHS. ESRD surveyor training interpretive guidance. Final Version 1.1. October 3, 2008 (V Tag 219) Available at https://www.cms.gov/Medicare/Provider-Enrollment-and-Certification/GuidanceforLawsAndRegulations/Downloads/esrdpgmguidance.pdf. Accessed June 2017
35. Kasparek T, Rodriguez OE. What medical directors need to know about dialysis facility water management. *Clin J Am Soc Nephrol*. 2015;10(6):1061-71.Doi:10.2215/CJN.11851214
36. Association for the Advancement of Medical Instrumentation. ANSI/AAMI 26722:2014 *Water treatment equipment for hemodialysis and related therapies*. Arlington, VA, American National Standard, 2014. Approved August 8, 2014, by the American National Standards Institute, Inc.
37. Centers for Medicare and Medicaid Services, HHS. ESRD surveyor training interpretive guidance. Final Version 1.1. October 3, 2008 (V Tag 188) Available at https://www.cms.gov/Medicare/Provider-Enrollment-and-Certification/GuidanceforLawsAndRegulations/Downloads/esrdpgmguidance.pdf. Accessed June 2017
38. Centers for Medicare and Medicaid Services, HHS. ESRD surveyor training interpretive guidance. Final Version 1.1. October 3, 2008 (V Tag 191) Available at https://www.cms.gov/Medicare/Provider-Enrollment-and-Certification/GuidanceforLawsAndRegulations/Downloads/esrdpgmguidance.pdf. Accessed June 2017
39. Centers for Medicare and Medicaid Services, HHS. ESRD surveyor training interpretive guidance. Final Version 1.1. October 3, 2008 (V Tag 190) Available at https://www.cms.gov/Medicare/Provider-Enrollment-and-Certification/GuidanceforLawsAndRegulations/Downloads/esrdpgmguidance.pdf. Accessed June 2017
40. Centers for Medicare and Medicaid Services, HHS. ESRD surveyor training interpretive guidance. Final Version 1.1. October 3, 2008 (V Tag 194) Available at https://www.cms.gov/Medicare/Provider-Enrollment-and-Certification/GuidanceforLawsAndRegulations/Downloads/esrdpgmguidance.pdf. Accessed June 2017
41. Centers for Medicare and Medicaid Services, HHS. ESRD surveyor training interpretive guidance. Final Version 1.1. October 3, 2008 (V Tag 196) Available at https://www.cms.gov/Medicare/Provider-Enrollment-and-Certification/GuidanceforLawsAndRegulations/Downloads/esrdpgmguidance.pdf. Accessed June 2017
42. Centers for Medicare and Medicaid Services, HHS. ESRD surveyor training interpretive guidance. Final Version 1.1. October 3, 2008 (V Tag 200) Available at https://www.cms.gov/Medicare/Provider-Enrollment-and-Certification/GuidanceforLawsAndRegulations/Downloads/esrdpgmguidance.pdf. Accessed June 2017
43. Centers for Medicare and Medicaid Services, HHS. ESRD surveyor training interpretive guidance. Final Version 1.1. October 3, 2008 (V Tag 214) Available at https://www.cms.gov/Medicare/Provider-Enrollment-and-Certification/GuidanceforLawsAndRegulations/Downloads/esrdpgmguidance.pdf. Accessed June 2017

44. Centers for Medicare and Medicaid Services, HHS. ESRD surveyor training interpretive guidance. Final Version 1.1. October 3, 2008 (V Tag 207) Available at https://www.cms.gov/Medicare/Provider-Enrollment-and-Certification/GuidanceforLawsAndRegulations/Downloads/esrdpgmguidance.pdf. Accessed June 2017
45. Centers for Medicare and Medicaid Services, HHS. ESRD surveyor training interpretive guidance. Final Version 1.1. October 3, 2008 (V Tag 209) Available at https://www.cms.gov/Medicare/Provider-Enrollment-and-Certification/GuidanceforLawsAndRegulations/Downloads/esrdpgmguidance.pdf. Accessed June 2017
46. Centers for Medicare and Medicaid Services, HHS. ESRD surveyor training interpretive guidance. Final Version 1.1. October 3, 2008 (V Tag 202) Available at https://www.cms.gov/Medicare/Provider-Enrollment-and-Certification/GuidanceforLawsAndRegulations/Downloads/esrdpgmguidance.pdf. Accessed June 2017
47. Centers for Medicare and Medicaid Services, HHS. ESRD surveyor training interpretive guidance. Final Version 1.1. October 3, 2008 (V Tag 203) Available at https://www.cms.gov/Medicare/Provider-Enrollment-and-Certification/GuidanceforLawsAndRegulations/Downloads/esrdpgmguidance.pdf. Accessed June 2017
48. Centers for Medicare and Medicaid Services, HHS. ESRD surveyor training interpretive guidance. Final Version 1.1. October 3, 2008 (V Tag 254) Available at https://www.cms.gov/Medicare/Provider-Enrollment-and-Certification/GuidanceforLawsAndRegulations/Downloads/esrdpgmguidance.pdf. Accessed June 2017
49. Centers for Medicare and Medicaid Services, HHS. ESRD surveyor training interpretive guidance. Final Version 1.1. October 3, 2008 (V Tag 257) Available at https://www.cms.gov/Medicare/Provider-Enrollment-and-Certification/GuidanceforLawsAndRegulations/Downloads/esrdpgmguidance.pdf. Accessed June 2017
50. Centers for Medicare and Medicaid Services, HHS. ESRD surveyor training interpretive guidance. Final Version 1.1. October 3, 2008 (V Tag 258) Available at https://www.cms.gov/Medicare/Provider-Enrollment-and-Certification/GuidanceforLawsAndRegulations/Downloads/esrdpgmguidance.pdf. Accessed June 2017
51. Williams KL. *Endotoxins Pyrogens, LAL Testing, and Depyrogenation*, (2nd ed). New York, Marcel Dekker, Inc., 2001, pp. 27-56
52. Isakozawa Y, Migita H, Takesawa S. Efficacy of biofilm removal from hemodialysis piping. *Nephrourol Mon.* 2016;8(5):e39332
53. de Oliveira RM, de los Santos CA, Antonello l, et al. Warning: an anemia outbreak due to chloramine exposure in a clean hemodialysis unit—an issue to be revisited. *Ren Fail.* 2009;31(1):81-3
54. Centers for Medicare and Medicaid Services, HHS. ESRD surveyor training interpretive guidance. Final Version 1.1. October 3, 2008 (V Tag 177) Available at https://www.cms.gov/Medicare/Provider-Enrollment-and-Certification/GuidanceforLawsAndRegulations/Downloads/esrdpgmguidance.pdf. Accessed June 2017
55. de Wolff FA, Berend K, van der Voet GB. Subacute fatal aluminum poisoning in dialyzed patients: post-mortem toxicological findings. *Forensic Sci Int.* 2002;128(1-2):41-3
56. United States Environmental Protection Agency. *Ground water and drinking water. National primary drinking water regulations.* (Table of Regulated Drinking Water Contaminants: Inorganic Chemicals.) Available at https://www.epa.gov/ground-water-and-drinking-water/national-primary-drinking-water-regulations#Inorganic. Accessed January 2017
57. United States Environmental Protection Agency. *Ground water and drinking water. National primary drinking water regulations.* (Table of Regulated Drinking Water Contaminants: Organic Chemicals.) Available at https://www.epa.gov/ground-water-and-drinking-water/national-primary-drinking-water-regulations#Organic. Accessed January 2017
58. United States Environmental Protection Agency. *Ground water and drinking water. National primary drinking water regulations.* (Table of Regulated Drinking Water Contaminants: Disinfectants.) Available at https://www.epa.gov/ground-water-and-drinking-water/national-primary-drinking-water-regulations#Disinfectants. Accessed January 2017.

9 Emergency Planning and Response

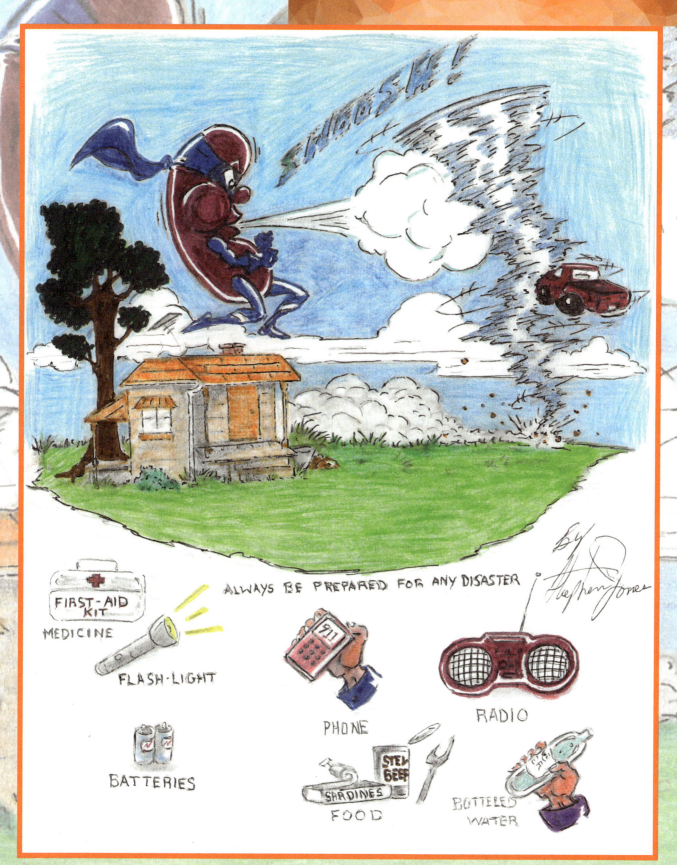

Cover art by Stephen Jones

"A year ago we had a massive chemical leak that contaminated the water for more than 300,000 people in our area. We could not drink it, bathe in it, wash with it, or cook with it. There could be no contact with the skin. The only safe use was to flush. Clearly, the water could not be used for dialysis. Our center closed for a day to clean all the machines and then opened with water from tanker trucks like you see for milk. Our time on the machines was cut to 3 hours to save water, and that went on for 10 days. I think they must have preplanned, because it came together too fast to just be pulled together on the fly. I was impressed!"

Objectives

MODULE AUTHORS

Danilo B. Concepcion, CBNT, CCHT-A, FNKF

Norma Gomez, MBA, MSN, RN

Lisa Hall, MSSW, LICSW

Heather Paradis, CHT

Dori Schatell, MS

MODULE REVIEWERS

Nancy M. Gallagher, BS, RN, CNN

Robert P. Loeper, MBA, PMP

Darlene Rodgers, BSN, RN, CNN, CPHQ

John H. Sadler, MD

Vern Taaffe, BS, CBNT, CDWS

Tamyra Warmack, RN

After you complete this module, you will be able to:

1. Describe the regulations and oversight of dialysis emergencies.
2. Compare the major types of emergencies and threat levels.
3. Outline the steps in emergency preparedness.
4. List at least three topics to include in patient education about emergencies.
5. Summarize a plan for emergency response.

An acronym list can be found in the Glossary.

Practice Test Questions at:
www.meiresearch.org/cc6

Introduction

"In middle Tennessee this week, 18 people died due to the ice storms. Six people were in car crashes, and one lady was trapped and couldn't get to her dialysis. Two elderly people literally froze to death after falling outside and not being able to get up. The other nine died due to cold related incidents. And we're in for another round of ice this weekend and after it warms up, we are in for major flooding."

If you watch the news, it seems as if nearly every day some part of the U.S. is having some type of emergency—an event that requires help or relief, often due to something unexpected. Safe dialysis treatments require a care team, power, water, equipment, and an intact building, at the very least. Any of these can be interrupted by a local or regional emergency. These events may be rare—but since dialysis is a life-saving treatment, it is vital to be prepared.

Emergencies largely fall into two main groups:
- **Natural disasters** – such as earthquakes or mudslides; snow, ice, or rain storms; tornados, hurricanes, floods (see Figure 1).
- **Man-made disasters** – such as a fire, a burst dam, an act of terrorism or workplace violence, an outbreak of disease, an airplane crash, biological warfare.

Emergencies are challenging in dialysis because:
- **We cannot predict them**. We may know that a dangerous storm is heading our way. But, we do not know what *sort* of damage it will inflict—perhaps none and perhaps total destruction. Some events like bombings, a car driving into a clinic wall, or earthquakes cannot be predicted at all.
- **They are disruptive**. If roads are closed or trees are down, staff members may not be able to get to the clinic even if it is untouched by the disaster (see Figure 2). Power outages can render perfectly good equipment useless unless a clinic has back-up generators. If the power is on—but the clinic is flooded—it is not safe to try to do dialysis.
- **You *and* your patients may need to be self-sufficient**. In a large-scale disaster that shuts off roads, power, and communication, it could take days—or longer—for help to arrive. Meanwhile, you or your patients may be trapped at home or at the clinic and will still need food, shelter, etc. Your patients will still need dialysis, too. For a few days, they can limit their diet and fluid intake, but patients who need dialysis and cannot get it risk hospital stays and death.

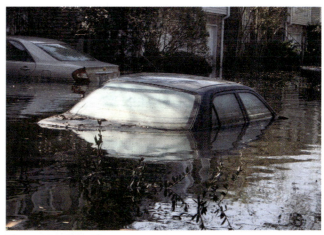

Figure 2: Flooding

There are excellent manuals about how to prepare for dialysis emergencies, and we will refer you to those in the Resources section (Appendix A) at the end of this module. Our effort here is not to duplicate them. But, they are largely written for administrators and those who will direct planning efforts on behalf of dialysis clinics. In this module, we focus on what *your* role may be in an emergency of any kind.

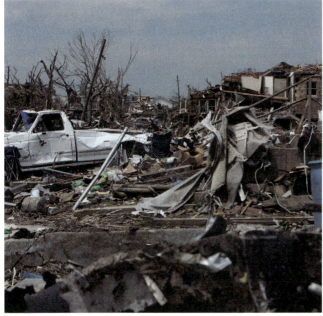

Figure 1: Natural Disasters

Regulations and Oversight of Dialysis Emergencies

Emergencies tend to be complex, and can disrupt a number of functions. Everything from power to transportation to water to communication may be affected. To perform dialysis, the setting and equipment must be safe for patients. It is no surprise, then, that a number of agencies have laws and rules about how to plan for and handle emergencies.

Conditions for Coverage

In 2016, CMS set new rules for disaster planning and response for all dialysis clinics. In short, clinics must:[1]

- Write a disaster plan for all potential emergencies in their region. The plan must take into account both medical and non-medical, and natural and man-made disasters.
- Evaluate and train staff at least once a year on emergency procedures. The training must include use of emergency equipment. Patient care staff must also keep up their CPR certification.
- Include how they will cooperate with other state and local efforts.
- Track the location of patients and staff during an emergency.
- Consider safe evacuation and a means to shelter in place.
- Maintain documentation and confidential medical records.
- Have all necessary equipment on hand.
- Develop a communication plan with contact information.
- Train patients at least once a year on what to do, where to go, and whom to contact during an emergency. Clinics must also teach patients how to disconnect from the dialysis machine.
- Contact the local disaster management agency at least once a year. Clinics must work with the local Health Care Coalition to coordinate planning and drills.
- Show that patient care staff have CPR certification.
- Conduct both large scale and smaller scale disaster drills at least once a year (unless there has been an actual disaster).

The Joint Commission (TJC)

TJC checks to make sure that the healthcare settings they inspect offer safe, effective, high-quality care. In dialysis, the TJC visits only hospital-based clinics. CMS state surveyors inspect outpatient clinics. Both TJC and CMS require dialysis clinics to make a plan to prepare for emergencies, and to practice their plans twice a year. You may be asked to take part in TJC community based drills or to help make sure that your dialysis clinic is ready.

Local and State Rules

Review the local and state rules for emergency preparedness (e.g., state board of nursing). You will need to know *your* state's rules—and they may go beyond what CMS requires. For instance, the state of Oregon requires:

- Two emergency preparedness drills per year
- Hazard vulnerability analysis
- Enough supplies on hand for staff and patients to shelter in place for 2 days
- Posting a detailed evacuation plan for patients to view
- Notifying the state if there is an evacuation

Kidney Community Emergency Response (KCER) Program

KCER, formed in 2006, helps ESRD Networks, kidney groups, and others prepare for response to and recovery from disasters that could harm kidney patients.

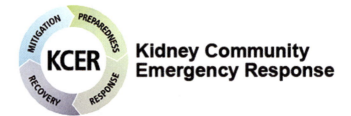

Figure 3: KCER Logo

Emergency Planning and Response

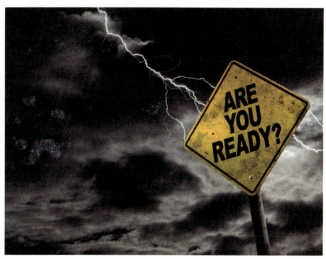

Figure 4: Are you Ready?

KCER is a program under contract with CMS. Health Services Advisory Group (HSAG) currently holds the KCER contract.

KCER partners represent the kidney community:
- Patient and professional groups
- Nurses
- Technicians
- Dietitians
- Social workers
- Nephrologists
- Dialysis providers
- Transplant centers
- Hospitals
- Suppliers
- ESRD Networks
- State emergency and State Survey Agency representatives
- Federal agencies, including the FDA, CDC, NIH, and CMS

KCER in Action

A slow moving weather system brought 10–20 inches of rain to south central and southeastern Louisiana on August 11, 2016, an area with 76 dialysis clinics and about 3,685 patients. This led to:
- Major flooding affecting more than 10,000 homes and businesses
- 70 closed roads due to high water, including 3 major highways
- Mass evacuations: 46 shelters had more than 10,000 occupants
- No power to 41,000 customers
- An overloaded 911 system, so many calls could not get through

KCER hosted daily status calls with LDOs, ESRD Networks, CMS, Health Departments, health care staff, and kidney patient and professional groups from August 15 – August 24, 2016. These calls addressed:
- Tracking dialysis clinic closures and patients
- Shelter triage for dialysis patients
- Pharmacy issues
- Boil water advisories
- Care for dialysis patients in nursing homes that were impacted
- Patient and staff evacuations from flooded homes
- Coordinating transportation with the National Guard
- Coast Guard rescues of patients from their homes
- Sending PD supplies to shelters
- Support for dialysis staff (day care, transportation, gasoline)
- Bringing in nurses and technicians from outside the region to help with patient care
- Timely Survey and Certification inspection of dialysis clinics
- Media alerts for dialysis patients

KCER was able to work swiftly with ESRD stakeholders and state and federal agencies. First, the members identified and prioritized what needed to be done. Then, they implemented action plans and tracked progress until the disaster was over.

Types of Emergencies

"I have been through a few hurricanes in south Florida as well as snow/ice storms on the East coast. The entire staff and patients go in as soon as a storm warning was issued. Each patient is dialyzed for 2 hours. We are given a list of supplies to have on hand in case of no power. After the hurricane was over, we got calls on how and where to go if our regular center was not up and running, but most clinics now have generators if you can get to the clinic."

Not everyone can expect the same type of emergency, and knowing what types of events tend to occur in your area will help you to make some preparations in advance. You need to know whether to anticipate hurricanes or earthquakes, blizzards or tornadoes. Do you have a nuclear power plant nearby, or is there a chemical manufacturing site, or a military base in the neighborhood? All of these known "risks" will give you clues to what might go wrong in an emergency. In addition, local emergencies can happen anywhere. What if there was a fire in the building next door, or a power outage? What if a car drove through the front door of your clinic? (This has happened more than once!) Would you know what to do?

Your dialysis clinic will have an emergency plan that follows all of the guidance set out by the federal and local governments. This plan will have detailed instructions for you to follow. As you go through orientation in your clinic, you will learn about:

- The plan itself
- Risks in your local area, region, and state
- Resources for your patients—and for you, in case you and your family are affected by an emergency
- Tasks you will need to do for each type of emergency and how to complete them
- How to help your patients to be prepared and what you can do to help other staff members

Pay attention to all of these instructions...many lives may depend on it!

Prepare for Emergencies

"A motor in one of the mixing machines in the water room caught on fire. I was asleep when a tech started shaking me. The alarm was loud! She said, 'We have a fire. I need to do an emergency take-off.' She clamped the two lines, put caps on the tubes hanging from my arm and said "go, go, go!" I grabbed my coat and headed for the parking lot. A lady was sitting in the lobby in a wheelchair, so I pushed her outside and gave her my coat. It was amazing to see my dialysis family helping each other. A big burly guy had his arm around a little old lady, keeping her warm and safe while he guided her outside. The nurses brought out a crash cart and evacuation cart. We were able to go back into the lobby while the firefighters did their job. About an hour later we were put back on the machines. Everybody was late getting out of there but the staff did a tremendous job! Whew!"

Learning your clinic's plan and your role in it will help you to help your patients and coworkers in an emergency. Expect to take part in training and disaster drills to be sure the team and patients are ready to respond. You may be asked to do tasks like removing all trash from the clinic floor. If your clinic is planning to close due to a storm or event, you may also be asked to secure all medical waste containers in the medical waste room.

Anticipate, Plan, Train

The Emergency Preparedness plan for your clinic will need to be easy to understand. Your clinic will share versions of the plan with all staff and patients in forms that will work best for each of you. Your clinic plan must fit into your *community's* plan. So, your clinic will need to work with local hospitals and emergency operations centers (EOCs). The plan should address the types of natural disasters that may occur in your area as well as man-made emergencies.

Know Your Part in the Communication Plan

Your clinic will set up a telephone "call tree," so staff can share the tasks of calling all of the other staff and patients (see Figure 5). Be sure you know your role in the call tree. During an emergency, your clinic will need to stay in constant communication with your ESRD Network. KCER has resources to help both patients and clinics.

Emergency Planning and Response

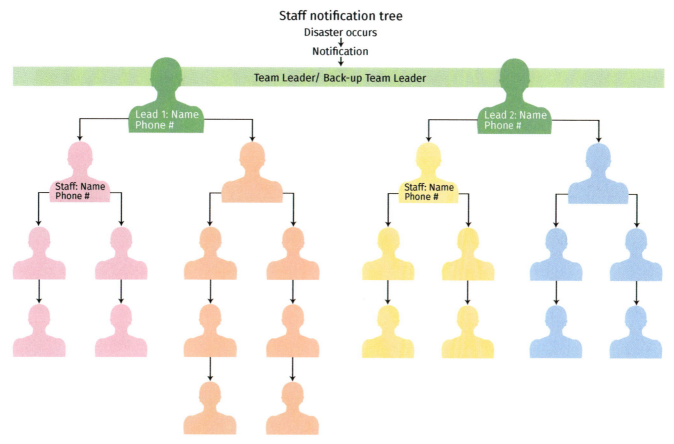

Figure 5: Example of a Call Tree

Many types of emergency can disrupt communications. Your clinic will have to look at its needs in advance and decide who (by title, not name) will be in charge of communications. Your clinic's plan may include options for reaching staff and patients, such as:

- **Set up call fowarding** on the clinic phone if it is closed for emergencies
- **Cell phones** - if cell towers are down, these will not work
- **Satellite phones**
- **Analog phones** - these may work when power is out, but phone companies may no longer support them. Know where your analog phones are kept, and where the wall jacks are located. An analog phone can use a fax machine wall jack.
- **Text messaging** - these *may* go through even if cell service is spotty
- **Walkie-talkies**
- **Toll-free numbers**
- **Notes on the clinic door**
- **Newspaper ads**
- **Public service announcements on radio and television**

Plan for Clinic-level Events

Every clinic staff member must learn the clinic's emergency plan. Your clinic will need to talk with the local EOC and Red Cross about local shelters before any event occurs. Setting up timely transport to your clinic or back-up clinic will be vital as well. In addition:

- A clinic's basic plan should work for any type of disaster. Ensure that your local power and water company knows that your dialysis clinic exists and will be dialyzing patients up to and possibly through the emergency. Make sure that they understand what dialysis is and have updated contact information for the clinic administrator.
- The plan should include a way to keep up-to-date contact information on hand for staff, patients, doctors, local hospitals, vendors, and patient transport.
- Patients who are vulnerable year-round may have the most trouble coping with change in an emergency. Your clinic plan should include social worker guidance for these patients.

311

Module 9

Throughout the year, staff and patients need to learn how to prepare for emergencies. Some parts of the country have seasonal events such as hurricanes or floods, but an event can occur at any time. Your clinic should assess its plan once a year. Using Quality Improvement (QI) techniques will help you identify parts of the plan that need to be updated (see page 319).

WHO IS IN CHARGE

Your clinic will choose someone to be in charge in the event of a disaster. This role may be called *Emergency Manager* (EM) or *Incident Commander* (IC). S/he must assess the impact of an event on patients, staff, and the building before, during, and after the event. Your clinic will need to be sure that these items (see Figure 6) are easy to find quickly:

- A clinic floor plan with gas, power, water lines, and shut-offs
- Water treatment and dialysis schematics
- How to make water treatment safe after a disaster that requires drinking water to be boiled
- Plywood or plastic to cover broken windows
- Emergency food, water, and blankets if your clinic must have them on hand to shelter patients and staff on-site
- A generator, if present, fuel, safe fuel handling and storage guidance, and monitoring (Federal rules do not require a generator, but your state may)
- Emergency standing orders in each patient's chart, in case treatments must be changed.*

* Electronic health record systems may not work if the power goes out. Staff must be trained on the use and storage of paper charts in case they are needed.

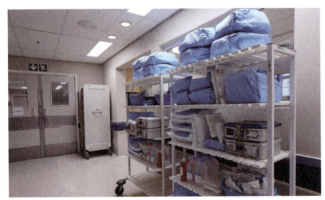

Figure 6: Emergency Supplies

EVACUATION DRILLS

An emergency that occurs in your clinic may mean that you will need to evacuate. Routine drills will reinforce the steps for patients and staff. The EM or IC will ensure the patient and staff evacuation is done safely and efficiently. If staff will need to work extra shifts in a disaster, the administration should make sure they have enough time off to take care of their homes and loved ones before the event.

BACK-UP CLINIC

Each dialysis clinic must have a "back-up" clinic for patients in case they must close. Choosing just one back-up clinic has two main challenges:

- A nearby clinic may be easy to reach—but could be affected by the same event that closes your clinic.
- A far away clinic can cause transportation issues.

It is a good idea for your clinic to arrange for multiple back-up clinics—both near and further away.

If your clinic cannot safely do dialysis, the EM or IC will need to ensure that patients and staff can reach the back-up clinic for treatment. Contact patients about an emergency as soon as you can, and be sure they know where to go if your clinic must close:

- A notice taped on the inside of the clinic door can give the name, address and phone number of the back-up clinic. Use brightly colored paper to post your sign.
- A staff member may be assigned to go to the clinic and help arrange patient transport.

Staff members going to back-up clinics may need further training if the equipment and water system is not what they are used to. No staff member should use equipment without training. Staff members may need to set up childcare and transportation to work extra shifts. Plans should be in place to address issues like these.

Even when clinics can stay open, there may be issues:

- Some parts of the country may not include dialysis patients on their emergency and special needs lists. Your social worker should be able to register dialysis patients for the special needs shelter if there is one.
- Special needs shelters may not be able to safely care for dialysis patients.

- Law enforcement officials may enforce a curfew and not allow staff into certain areas (see Figure 7). Your administrator should register all staff with the EOC. This will allow you to enter an evacuation zone or be allowed in as soon as the evacuation is lifted.
- Red Cross volunteers and local police may need education about the need for dialysis to ensure that patients can reach the clinic.

NOTE: Sending patients to local hospitals is not a plan. Hospitals will be in use for critical medical emergencies.

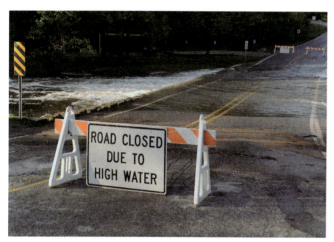

Figure 7: Roadblock

Dialysis During Hurricane Andrew

During Hurricane Andrew, patients were sent to clinics more than an hour away since the storm zone was so large. Buses and vans picked up patients in the morning at the clinic parking lot and brought them back in the late afternoon. Communicating with the back-up clinic was vital to ensure that patients had food and water on the long trips to and from the clinics.

EMERGENCY DISCONNECTION

You may need to evacuate patients from the clinic when staying in the treatment room is unsafe. Patients who just ended a treatment or have not yet started one can be sent out right away, per their triage level. Patients who are on dialysis during an emergency will need to stop. Those who can disconnect themselves without staff help and can walk should be the first to evacuate.

When a room full of patients must come off of the machines urgently, it helps when they can disconnect themselves. Some of your patients may be able to do this IF you teach them how. They will need to prove to you that they understand what to do—and what could go wrong. Cutting the access line without clamps, for example, can cause severe blood loss and death. You will also need to know if your patients' hands are strong and dexterous enough to use a clamp or a scissors. You can check to see if this ability changes over time by letting the patient show you how when you disconnect at the end of a routine treatment.

There are two main emergency disconnect techniques. Both are effective and quick, and each has pros and cons:

1. **Clamp and Cut**. You or the patient clamp the lines and then cut the lines between the *access clamp* and the *bloodline clamp*, which can be done with one hand. But:
   - There is a risk of cutting the access line.
   - A scissors must be available *and* disinfected. A scissors that is kept on the machine must be disinfected after each patient's treatment and replaced. One option is to keep scissors in plastic bags at a clean space, perhaps in a bin or a duffle bag. During an emergency, assign a staff person to bring the bags to each station. In this way, the supplies will stay clean and it is easy to maintain inventory control.

2. **Uncouple a Luer-connection**. No scissors is needed, and the access line cannot be cut by accident. However, this process takes two hands. Some otherwise able patients might not be able to do this, depending on their access.

Plan for Area or Regional Events

If an event affects a large area, some patients may not be able to receive dialysis for 3 days or longer.

- **If they must take shelter in place**, they will need to start the "3-day Emergency Diet" (see Appendix B).
- **If they can reach a back-up clinic**, they can receive care there.

- **If they must evacuate**, they may not be able to go to your clinic's planned back-up clinics. They may be able to stay in special needs shelters or reach other clinics. Special needs shelters may have arrangements with a nearby dialysis clinic. However, this may not be the clinic of choice. It is always best for patients to bring their dialysis prescription, medicines, and medicine list with them.

Your clinic may *receive* patients from a disaster zone. These patients may not have their medical records, so your clinic will need to have procedures in place to accept and treat them.

Even if your area is not prone to floods, protect documents—damage to your clinic's roof or windows from any cause could allow rain in. Keep paper records at least 24" off the floor in plastic tubs (see Figure 8), and be sure to include:

- Patient medical records
- Reuse data
- Progress or communications logs
- Manual treatment flow sheets for at least three treatments
- Medication labels for the next three treatments
- Patient treatment information
- Rounding reports
- Home patient treatment records
- Vendor information

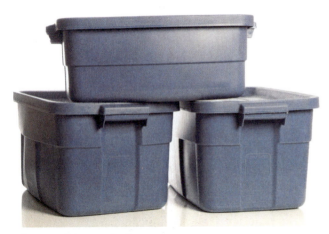

Figure 8: Records Storage

If your clinic uses electronic records, ensure proper shut down of the system in an emergency. Store back-up records off-site in a safe place, or in the cloud.

The biomed department should raise all machines off the floor, if possible, to prevent damage to electrical parts if water is present. Machines are often double bagged, from the top down and from the bottom up. Secure water systems to prevent damage from flooding and overflowing drains.

Patient Education for Emergencies

"I'm into my 4th day without treatment due to the blizzard...been carefully monitoring my fluids/food and I feel okay...but I'm looking forward to treatment in about 14 hours."

People on dialysis are highly vulnerable when a disaster strikes. If they are trapped in their homes (and do not do home dialysis), they may not be able to get to the clinic to do their treatments. In a major emergency, it could take a week—or more—for help to arrive. So, patients need to prepare ahead of time and have what they need on hand where they can find it.

You can help your patients to think about how to be ready for the unexpected. Patients should:

- **Take part in clinic disaster drills**. These are a good way to practice.
- **Review clinic's disaster information**. Each patient needs to know how to contact the clinic if there is no power or phone service.
- **Learn how your clinic will reach them in an emergency**. Outreach may include TV announcements, text messages, signs on the clinic door, etc.
- **Be prepared for the kinds of emergencies that happen in the area**. Each part of the country has different risks, and the same ones that can affect your dialysis clinic can also have an impact on patients in their homes.
- **Collect vital papers in one spot and keep them dry**. Identification, insurance forms, medicine lists, phone numbers for loved ones and the clinic and their doctors will all be important. Patients should have a copy of their dialysis orders and flow sheets and medicine prescriptions in case they need to go to a back-up or other clinic. A zip-top plastic bag can help to keep these papers together and dry.

Emergency Planning and Response

- **Tell you their evacuation plans**. Find out where your patients plan to go and how to contact them. CMS requires all dialysis clinics to account for all patients and staff during and after a disaster.
- **Keep a 2-week supply of medicines at all times**. If a patient has to leave home, it could take time to replace vital medicines.
- **Keep a 2-week supply of home dialysis supplies if they dialyze at home**. Patients who do peritoneal dialysis or home hemodialysis will need supplies, and may want to buy a generator.
- **Talk to their families about disaster planning**. Dialysis affects the whole family, and families need to know what to do and how to support a patient who cannot get to treatment.
- **Gather supplies for the 3-day emergency diet and ask questions if they need to**. Patients need to have clean water on hand and keep a supply of the foods on the list. Some patients even buy freeze dried food or military "meals ready to eat" (MREs) to have on hand.
- **Learn about safety**. Will patients be able to wash their hands if the water is shut off? Can they stay warm safely if it is cold outside, or keep cool in a heat wave? Do they know what to do if power lines are down around them or floodwaters are rising? Do they know the safest route to evacuate, if this is necessary, or where the local shelter is that can handle people with medical needs? If not, you and the other staff members can help them find out.

NOTE: Always carry identification yourself! If a curfew is put in place because of an event, you and your patients will need proof of identity to get into and out of the affected area.

Responding to Emergencies

"I live in New York and this morning we had an ice storm and the roads were slippery. My put-on time is 6:30 am and I arrived at the center at 6:15, but did not get put on until after 7:00 am because some of the staff had trouble getting to work. Next, being short staffed, someone forgot to prime the water pump and all the machines failed!"

Set Up a Command Center

When there is an emergency, someone will need to be in charge. That person is often referred to as the "incident commander." You will need to know who is in charge and pay close attention to the instructions that you receive from that person. S/he is relying on you to do your job as part of the emergency preparedness team.

Triage

Any event that causes patients to miss treatments should include a *triage* system to sort people by how ill or injured they are. A triage nurse will assess patients and decide when and where to schedule treatments. S/he will also assess the patients for any psychosocial issues and work with the social worker to obtain services as needed. The social worker will work with the patients on transportation for scheduled treatments. If the patient is triaged to a back-up clinic, contact information for the clinic will be given to the family.

Assess Damage to the Building and Equipment

If a clinic is damaged, a structural engineer must declare it to be safe for use before treatments can resume. The lease and insurance plan will determine who must make repairs. The biomedical technician must inspect the machines and water treatment system to be sure they are safe for use. Dialysis machines can be damaged by smoke, fire, water, etc. Water cultures may be needed if there is flooding.

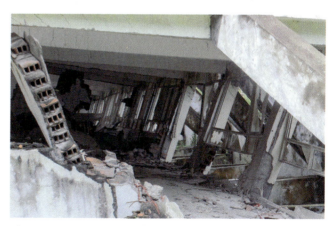

Figure 9: Damaged Building

Maintain Staffing

The greatest asset to any dialysis clinic is the staff. Any catastrophic event will produce issues and problems. During a crisis, all staff should be briefed at least daily and when things change, so you all have the information you need to provide safe patient care. Taking rest breaks—even if they must be short—and eating healthy foods can help keep you going. Keeping a sense of humor, stretching, and taking slow deep breaths may reduce stress at least a little. Be sure that all those affected by the disaster know where to find the local care and comfort centers.

Patient schedules, times, and days, may need to be changed. If there has been damage to the clinic, some stations may be closed. A physician's order is needed for any changes to patient prescriptions.

CMS suggests that during an emergency, your clinic may wish to:[1]

- Provide food and water for staff, as restaurants and grocery stores may be closed
- Have an Employee Assistance Program counselor available to address mental health issues
- Identify and resolve issues between staff. Managers should provide guidance and timely problem solving
- Remind staff to use their own family disaster plans to deal with child or elder care and pets
- Develop a shift rotation that best suits the disaster and the staff on hand
- Help with staff transportation, when possible
- Consider the need for housing, if staff come from other clinics or local staff homes are damaged by the disaster
- Offer incentives to encourage staff members to come to work during a disaster

Administrative issues may arise, such as delays in payroll, patient billing, and vendor payments. If banks are not open, other ways to provide you with your paycheck may be needed.

Recovering from an Emergency

"We had a tornado warning today while at dialysis. I was asleep and my tech was rinsing back my blood and trying to wake me up. I said, 'I'm done?' She's like, 'No, there's a tornado warning and we have to get you guys to a safe place, do you understand what I'm saying? At first I thought I was dreaming, but nope all real. The team did an amazing job getting everyone to safety. I don't even know if I received my full treatment, but I'm just glad everyone is safe."

Plan for Patient Care

The key focus of any recovery plan is to care for patients and staff first. The goal is to resume treatments as soon as it is possible and safe to do so. The severity of a disaster will then dictate the extent of the recovery. Recovery can be as simple as cleaning—or as complex as a full repair, renovation, or replacement of a clinic.

ARRANGE TO DIALYZE PATIENTS

If your clinic is the one providing back-up care, treatments may need to change to fit in more patients. In this case, the Medical Director's emergency prescription orders will be used. If your clinic is closed, patients will need to use a back-up clinic. You may be asked to help the back-up clinic with its patient care or equipment needs. If so:

- Keep records of the time you spend, for pay purposes.
- If another clinic borrows supplies from yours, track those as well.

CHECK TRANSPORTATION

Roads may be closed in an emergency, or patients may not have working cars. CMS says that patients are responsible for their own transportation.[1] And, dialysis staff should *not* transport patients in their private vehicles.[1] Firefighters and ambulances may not be able to transport patients for routine dialysis. Instead, your clinic's plan should include private transport options such as:

- Buses
- Taxis
- Light rail
- Non-emergency medical transport
- Volunteers
- Church groups
- Community agencies

You may be asked to contact patients and/or these companies to help ensure that patients can receive their treatments.

Emergency Planning and Response

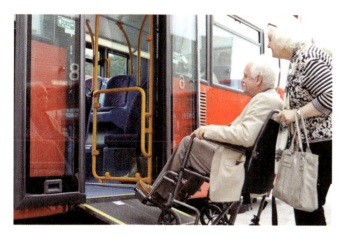

Figure 10: Bus Transportation

FIND MISSING PATIENTS AND STAFF

After any emergency your clinic will need to know if everyone is safe. Staff and patients can be displaced, and may need to be tracked down. If patients evacuate, finding them again may involve the Network and other sources. Notices in local papers may be used to tell patients how to reach your clinic. From your Emergency Preparedness plan, you will know to check:

- The gathering place outside of your clinic if you had to evacuate
- The central call-in phone number for messages from patients and staff
- The back-up clinics (one close by and one far away)
- The local ESRD Network and KCER to see if anyone called in

Physical Plant Safety

Once patients are taken care of, you can then focus on physical plant issues such as:

- Assessing and repairing clinic damage
- Assuring water quality, from the tap source to the product water

BUILDING ASSESSMENT

Enter a damaged building only after it is deemed to be safe. Always use the buddy system, and never enter a building alone. First walk around the building and check for down trees, power lines, sink holes, etc. Emergency responders should be able to help determine the safety of a structure. The clinic emergency team may include staff and/or outside professionals. They should have the knowledge and skills to assess the electrical, structural, plumbing, and information systems of your clinic. Key tasks include:[1]

- Quickly assess the systems and estimate the time it will take to address any damage.
- Identify clinic assets (such as costly equipment) and take steps to protect them, such as moving them to a safer location.
- Report the assessment to the medical director and the charge nurse.
- Work with local government agencies to reopen the clinic, if businesses in the disaster zone were asked to close.
- Work with the management team to identify losses and file insurance claims.
- Notify the medical director of all actions taken.

Finding a Missing Patient

Mr. Smith, a 65 year old male living alone, had informed the staff during pre-hurricane training that he was not evacuating and could be reached at his home after the event. Staff tried for 5 days after the hurricane to contact Mr. Smith—with no answer. His medical record noted no family.

Concerned, the staff asked local law enforcement for help, but the officers were overwhelmed with looting and did not have time to investigate. The staff continued to try to find someone who knew what happened to Mr. Smith; one staff member even drove through the neighborhood asking neighbors, and still no one knew where he was. A missing persons notice was placed in the newspaper.

About 2 weeks after the hurricane, Mr. Smith called the clinic. He said he was fine and had just seen his name in the paper. He had decided to leave after all to visit a friend in a city about 150 miles away, and would be home in a week. The staff were happy to hear from him, but told him how worried they were and emphasized how important it is for him to let them know his plans.

317

WATER QUALITY ASSESSMENT

The clinic water supply could be altered by a disaster. Both the amount of water and its quality could be affected (see Module 8 to learn more about water treatment). **If the building did *not* flood**, the power is on, and water is flowing—even if there is a "boil water alert"—the CDC suggests that you:[2]

- Flush all pretreatment equipment to drain for at least 30 minutes to remove stagnant water.
- Test levels of free chlorine and chloramine in the building's source water. (Expect it to be higher than normal.)
- Test chlorine and chloramine after the primary carbon tank. Verify that the water is < 0.5 ppm free chlorine, or < 0.1 ppm chloramine (or < 0.1 ppm total chlorine).
- If chlorine or chloramines after the primary carbon tank are ≥ 0.5 ppm or ≥ 0.1 ppm, respectively, promptly change the primary carbon tank. For systems with a secondary carbon tank, test the levels after the secondary tank.
- If chlorine and chloramine are below these levels (0.5 ppm or 0.1 ppm), turn on the reverse osmosis (RO) machine.
- Flush the distribution system (to drain if possible).
- Disinfect the RO and the distribution system and rinse. Test for residual disinfectant levels to ensure proper rinsing.
- Replace all cartridge filters.
- Compare the product water quality to your past data.* A large change could mean that the RO membranes are damaged, or the quality of the feed water is much worse. If the total dissolved solids (TDS) are more than 20% higher than the past readings, you may want to use the deionization (DI) tanks to polish the product water. Follow the DI with an ultrafilter to reduce the risk of bacterial growth.
- Increase the frequency of monitoring:
  ➤ Check chlorine/chloramine hourly.
  ➤ Verify hourly that product water quality is acceptable.
  ➤ Monitor water cultures and endotoxin at least weekly. If possible, test for endotoxin on-site daily.
- Draw water cultures and endotoxin tests as soon as possible. If you can test for endotoxin on-site, do this before treating patients. Report the results to the medical director.
- Expect more particles in the water. Monitor the pressure drop across pretreatment components. Backflush as needed.
- Plan to re-bed the carbon tanks as soon as possible.
- Send a sample of product water for an AAMI analysis as soon as is practical.
- Clean the RO membranes as soon as is practical.

*If the product water TDS is high and the % rejection is in line with past data, the RO membranes are most likely good. (The tap and feed water may have a higher than usual level of contaminants.) DI polishing will help cope with the extra burden in the feed water. If the product water TDS is high and the % rejection is *lower* than in the past, the RO membranes are probably bad and should be replaced promptly. DI polishing may or may not be needed once the RO membranes are replaced.

DIALYSIS MACHINE ASSESSMENT

To ensure that the machines are safe to use:

- Rinse the dialysis machines and chemically disinfect them. When you use chemical disinfection, test for residual levels to ensure proper rinsing.
- Bring up the conductivity and "self-test" the machines to verify proper working condition. If a machine fails the "self-test," perform needed repairs prior to using that machine.

NOTE: If your clinic *did* flood, the clean-up of water treatment and machines is far more complex and will take more time. Please see the CDC guidelines for recovery of a flooded building at https://www.cdc.gov/disasters/floods/.

Emotional Recovery After a Disaster

It can take time to recover from the shock of a disaster, especially if it causes loss or change. Healthcare staff can help meet patient needs and support their coping after a disaster causes stress. Patients whose stress goes on long after the event is over may need to see a licensed mental health professional who can assess for post-traumatic stress disorder (PTSD; see below) and help the patient return to normal.

Emergency Planning and Response

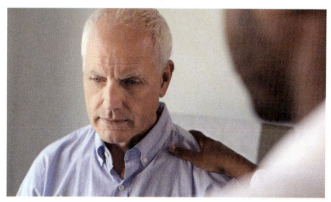

Figure 11: Person in Shock

DISASTER-RELATED STRESS

Everyone who sees or lives through a disaster is affected in some way. And, everyone has different ways of coping. Profound sadness, grief, anger, and concern for the safety of loved ones are normal. Many seek counseling for disaster-related stress, particularly if it lasts a long time or disrupts day-to-day functioning. Some signs of disaster-related stress are listed in Table 1, and some ways to ease the stress are listed in Table 2.

Table 1: Signs of Disaster-related Stress

Trouble sharing your thoughts with others	Tunnel vision or muffled hearing
Sleep problems	Cold or flu-like symptoms
Trouble keeping balance in life	Disorientation or confusion
Feeling easily frustrated	Not wanting to leave home
More use of drugs or alcohol	Depression, sadness
Shorter than usual attention span	Feeling hopeless
Headaches or stomach upset	Mood swings or bouts of crying
Overwhelming guilt and self-doubt	Fears of crowds, strangers, or being alone

Post-traumatic stress disorder (PTSD) is a long-term stress response that can be triggered by a disaster or a health crisis.[3] A study done after Hurricane Katrina found that nearly one in four hemodialysis patients had symptoms consistent with PTSD.[4] And, a study done after an outbreak of severe acute respiratory syndrome (a flu-like disease that can be lethal and has no cure) found that 58% of patients—and more than 40% of healthcare staff—had PTSD. Fears of disease, worries about family, anxiety about the unknown, and guilt were factors. Some doctors (16%) refused to even treat these patients.[5]

Quality Improvement (QI)

After an event is over, you will want to review what went right and what did not. An After Action Review (AAR) is an important QI task for future emergency preparedness. An AAR should be done about 2 weeks after the event. Your Administrator will want to identify gaps in your Clinic Emergency Plan by asking each person on the team two questions:

1. *What did I need that I didn't get?*
2. *What would I have done differently?*

Your administrator should document the AAR discussion and present the results at the next QAPI meeting. The Clinic Emergency Plan can then be updated and improved. Even if you do not have a disaster, your clinic must assess its plan at least once a year and update it to be sure that you are ready for anything (see Table 3).

Table 2: Ways to Ease Disaster-related Stress

Set small goals to tackle big problems	Do not make any big life changes
Breathe deeply each day, as often as possible	Consult a counselor if needed
Talk to people who care about you	Allow yourself time to recover
Keep a journal	Get outdoors – take a walk, enjoy nature
Avoid drugs or alcohol	Try to be patient when dealing with others
Keep your routines as normal as possible	Help others through their problems
Spend time by yourself	Watch your diet – avoid caffeine and sugar
Don't watch disaster-related news	Use humor: watch a funny show or tell jokes

Table 3: Sample Disaster QI Plan

Action/Issue	Lead	Start Date	Timeline	Finish Date and Initials	Comments
Review emergency disconnect plan with all patients	Charge Nurse for each shift	1/10/17	Quarterly	3/1/16 GH 6/1/16 MT 9/1/16 LM	▪ Quarterly review, copies of plan for each patient ▪ Missed nocturnal shift Q2
Update emergency contact info for staff and patients	Secretary	1/10/17	Quarterly	3/2/16 CC 6/10/16 CC 9/15/16 CC	▪ Missed doctors Q1 Plan in place to contact doctors' offices quarterly
Identify shelter locations	Social worker	5/1/17	Annually	5/4/17 HJ	▪ Added shelter addresses/local Red Cross contacts to Emergency manual
Transportation needs for all patients – include home patients	Social worker and Secretary	5/1/17	Annually	5/1/17 HJ	▪ All in-center patients have phone numbers & where they will be in a hurricane. ▪ Two home patients missing contact info. Working with primary nurse

Conclusion

We cannot always prevent a disaster. But when we plan ahead and are ready, we can help reduce the danger to our patients and ourselves. Good handling of an emergency gives your patients confidence in your knowledge and ability to provide safe dialysis care.

Appendix A: Resources

Dialysis Disaster Preparedness

- ESRD Network Cordinating Center. www.esrdncc.org
- KCER Coalition. (866) 901-3773. www.kcercoalition.com
- National Kidney Foundation Emergency Resources. www.kidney.org/help
- Centers for Medicare & Medicaid Services (CMS). (2008). *Disaster Preparedness: A Guide for Chronic Dialysis Facilities*, Second Edition. Publication number HHSM-500-2010-NW007C. Retrieved from http://www.therenalnetwork.org/home/resources/Disaster_Preparedness_-_A_Guide_for_Chronic_Dialysis_Facilities_-_Second_Edition.pdf

Contact Information for the National Forum of ESRD Networks

- PO Box 203 Birchwood, WI 54817. Phone: (715) 354-3735 Fax: 1-888-571-2065. http://esrdnetworks.org

Water Treatment Resources

- Northwest Renal Network document *Monitoring Your Dialysis Water Treatment System* https://www.nwrn.org/files/WaterManual.pdf
- Association for the Advancement of Medical Instrumentation, *Recommended Practices for Dialysis Water Treatment Systems (RD 52 and RD 62* http://www.aami.org
- *Guidelines for Dialysis Care Providers on Boil Water Advisories* https://www.cdc.gov/dialysis/guidelines/water-use.html

Medical Device Resources

- *Medical Devices that Have Been Exposed to Heat and Humidity* https://www.fda.gov/MedicalDevices/Safety/EmergencySituations/ucm056086.htm
- *Medical Devices Requiring Refrigeration* https://www.fda.gov/MedicalDevices/Safety/EmergencySituations/ucm056075.htm

Flood Clean-up Resources

- Fact Sheet: *Flood Cleanup - Avoiding Indoor Air Quality Problems* https://www.epa.gov/sites/production/files/2015-09/documents/floods.pdf
- *Tips about Medical Devices and Hurricane Disasters* https://www.fda.gov/MedicalDevices/Safety/EmergencySituations/ucm055987.htm

Post Trauma Resources

- Department of Homeland Security – http://www.ready.gov/coping-with-disaster
- Centers for Disease Control – https://emergency.cdc.gov/coping/index.asp

Appendix B:
3-Day Emergency Diet Plan for Dialysis Patients

How to change your diet when you cannot get dialysis

The tips and meal plans in this list do not replace dialysis. But, if you can't get treatment, they will work for up to 5 days. This diet is *much* stricter than what you may be used to, but it is only for a short time. If you can, keep these foods on hand so you are ready if there is an emergency.

Talk with your dietitian about YOUR diet.

Floods. Landslides. Blizzards. Earthquakes. Disasters like these seem to be happening more and more these days. And, when they do, you need a plan to stay safe if you can't get dialysis. Using a meal plan like this one can help you keep your blood levels in a safe range.

Here are some helpful tips for emergencies:
- Limit meat to just 3 to 4 ounces each day. (A serving about the size of the palm of your hand.) This is about half the meat you normally eat.
- Avoid all high-potassium fruits and vegetables.
- Lower your fluids to 1 to 2 eight ounce cups a day.
- Choose low-salt foods.
- If the power is out, eat foods from your refrigerator on the first day.
- Open the refrigerator or freezer as little as you can, to keep food cold.
- Freezer foods can be safe to eat *while they have ice crystals in the center*. This may be for up to 3 to 4 days.
- Once you open a refrigerated or frozen food, eat it within 4 hours or throw it out if you can no longer keep it cold. You don't want to get food poisoning.

Emergency Diet:
Meat and other protein (3 to 4 servings each day)
- 1 egg
- 1 ounce fresh meat, fish, tofu, poultry
- ¼ cup frozen or canned meat, fish or poultry. (Use unsalted, or rinse off salt with clean water.)
- ½ can Ensure® Plus, Boost Plus®, Nepro®
- 2 tablespoons unsalted peanut butter
- 1 ounce or 1 slice cheese
- ¼ cup cottage cheese
- 1 cup macaroni and cheese dinner

Fats and oils (6 or more servings each day)
- 1 teaspoon butter, margarine, mayonnaise, or vegetable oil

Bread, starch and cereals (6 to 10 servings each day)
- 1 slice white bread
- 4 slices Melba toast
- 5 crackers with unsalted tops
- Cereals: 1 cup Puffed Wheat, Puffed Rice, Shredded Wheat, or Cream of Rice
- ½ English muffin or bagel
- 2 graham crackers
- 1 cup unsalted cooked rice, noodles or pasta
- 6 shortbread cookies or vanilla wafers

Fruits (4 choices only each day)
- 15 grapes
- ½ cup applesauce
- ½ cup blueberries, blackberries, strawberries, or raspberries
- 1 small apple
- ½ cup pears, plums, pineapple, or cherries

Vegetables (1 choice only each day)
- ½ cup green beans, peas, or corn
- ½ cup carrots
- ½ cup summer squash
- ½ cup zucchini
- ½ cup beets

Beverages (1 to 2 choices each day)
- 1 cup water, coffee, or tea
- 1 cup soda pop (not cola)
- ½ cup evaporated milk
- 2 ½ tablespoons powdered milk mixed with water
- ½ can (4 ounces) Ensure Plus®, Boost Plus®, or Nepro®
- ½ cup Hi-C®, Kool-Aid, Tang, or Crystal Light
- ½ cup juice (cranberry, apple, or grape)
- ½ cup soy, almond, or rice milk
- ½ cup non-dairy creamer
- ½ cup half and half

Other (Use these if you want to)
- Vinegar, spices and herbs, horseradish, lemon, lime, Tabasco, mayo packets

Other – If you do not have diabetes
- Hard candy, jelly beans, cream mints, jam, marshmallows, maple syrup, chewing gum, gumdrops, honey, jelly, sugar

Tips if you do have diabetes:
- Don't eat highly concentrated sweets. Use more fats and oils for extra calories.
- Plain cookies, doughnuts, or cake are okay when you eat them with meals.
- Use unsweetened canned fruit or juices, sugar-free Kool-Aid, or diet soda pop.
- Avoid beer, wine, and hard liquor.
- Be ready in case your blood sugar drops. Have sugar, honey, juice, glucose paste, or gel cake frosting on hand.

EMERGENCY SAMPLE MENU:
You can rotate these options for up to 5 days. **Limit your total fluid intake to 1 to 2 cups a day. One 8-ounce bottle of water should last a whole day.**

Nutritional Information (average per day):
Calories: 2,000; Protein: 50 g; Carbohydrates: 250 mg; Sodium: 1,500 mg; Potassium: 800 mg

Sample 1
Breakfast
- ½ cup canned fruit, drained
- 1 cup cereal
- ½ cup boxed milk

Lunch
- Peanut butter and jelly crackers
  - 20 crackers with unsalted tops
  - 4 tablespoons unsalted peanut butter
  - 4 tablespoons jam
- ½ cup fruit, drained

Snack
- 6 vanilla wafers
- ½ cup fruit, drained

Supper
- Tuna dip and chips
  - ½ cup low sodium canned tuna
  - 2 packets mayonnaise
  - 20 unsalted tortilla chips
- ½ cup applesauce

Snack
- 2 graham crackers
- 1 tablespoon unsalted peanut butter

Sample 2
Breakfast
- ½ cup canned fruit, drained
- 1 protein bar
- 4-6 ounces canned or boxed juice

Lunch
- Chicken and crackers
  - 20 crackers with unsalted tops
  - ½ cup canned chicken
  - 2 packets mayonnaise
- ½ cup canned fruit, drained

Snack
- 6 vanilla wafers
- ½ cup canned fruit, drained

Supper
- Peanut butter and jelly crackers
  - 20 crackers with unsalted tops
  - 4 tablespoons unsalted peanut butter
  - 4 tablespoons jam
- ½ cup canned fruit, drained

Snack
- 2 graham crackers
- 1 tablespoon unsalted peanut butter

Module 9

MAKE AN EMERGENCY FOOD KIT:

A food kit will help you to fix meals even if you can't use your kitchen. Store your kit in a clean, dry place such as a duffle bag or plastic bin with a label and date. Look over your kit once a year. Use up the food in it and add a fresh supply. Pack the foods from the menus *and* the other emergency items below:

- Emergency diet list and menus
- Gallon jugs of distilled water
- A sharp knife
- Matches in a waterproof container
- Three plastic mixing bowls with lids
- Forks, knives, spoons, and paper plates
- A manual can opener
- A flashlight and extra batteries
- Candy (gumdrops, jellybeans)
- A roll of aluminum foil for leftovers
- Measuring cups
- A radio with a new battery and extra batteries
- A refrigerator thermometer

NOTE: Keep a week's worth of your medicines in a clean, dry place you can reach. Add some phosphate binders. Do you have diabetes? If so, include those medicines, too.

Emergency Diet Shopping List

- 6 (8 ounce) boxes of soy, almond, or rice milk
- 6 (4 to 6 ounce) cans or boxes of apple or cranberry juice
- 1 box of Puffed Wheat, Puffed Rice, or Shredded Wheat
- 3 Zone Perfect® or Luna® Protein bars
- 1 box crackers with unsalted tops
- 1 large bag unsalted tortilla chips
- 6 (4 ounce) cans low-sodium tuna or chicken
- 1 jar unsalted peanut butter
- 1 jar jam or jelly
- 1 box graham crackers
- 1 box vanilla wafers
- 12 (4 ounce) cans of pears, peaches, cherries, applesauce, or pineapple
- 6 (8 ounce) bottles of water
- 12 single serve mayonnaise packets
- Small box plastic spoons
- Small box plastic forks
- Small box plastic knives
- Paper plates
- Pack of 8 ounce plastic cups
- Can opener
- Napkins or roll of paper towels
- Hand sanitizer
- Box of disinfecting wipes

Disclaimer

The work upon which this food list is based was performed under Contract Number HHSM-500-2016-00016C, funded by the Centers for Medicare Medicaid Services, an agency of the U.S. Department of Health and Human Services. The content of this list does not necessarily reflect the policies or positions of the Department of Health and Human Services, nor does mention of trade names, commercial products, or organizations imply endorsement by the U.S. government. The authors assume full responsibility for the accuracy and completeness of the ideas presented.

References

1. Centers for Medicare & Medicaid Services. 42 CFR Parts 403, 416, 418 et al. Medicare and Medicaid Programs; Emergency Preparedness Requirements for Medicare and Medicaid Participating Providers and Suppliers; Final Rule. *Federal Register* 81(180) Friday, Sept. 16, 2016
2. Centers for Disease Control and Prevention. *Technical considerations when bringing hemodialysis facility's water systems back online after a disaster.* Available at: https://www.cdc.gov/disasters/watersystems.html. Accessed February 2017
3. American Psychiatric Association. *American Psychiatric Association: Diagnostic and statistical manual of mental disorders, (5th ed).* Arlington, VA, 2013
4. Hyre AD, Cohen AJ, Kutner N, et al. Prevalence and predictors of posttraumatic disorder among hemodialysis patients following Hurricane Katrina. *Am J Kidney Dis.* 2007;50(4): 585-593
5. Maunder R The experience of the 2003 SARS outbreak as a traumatic stress among frontline health-care workers in Toronto: lessons learned. *Philos Trans R Soc Lond B Biol Sci.* 2004;359(1447):1117–25

Glossary and Index

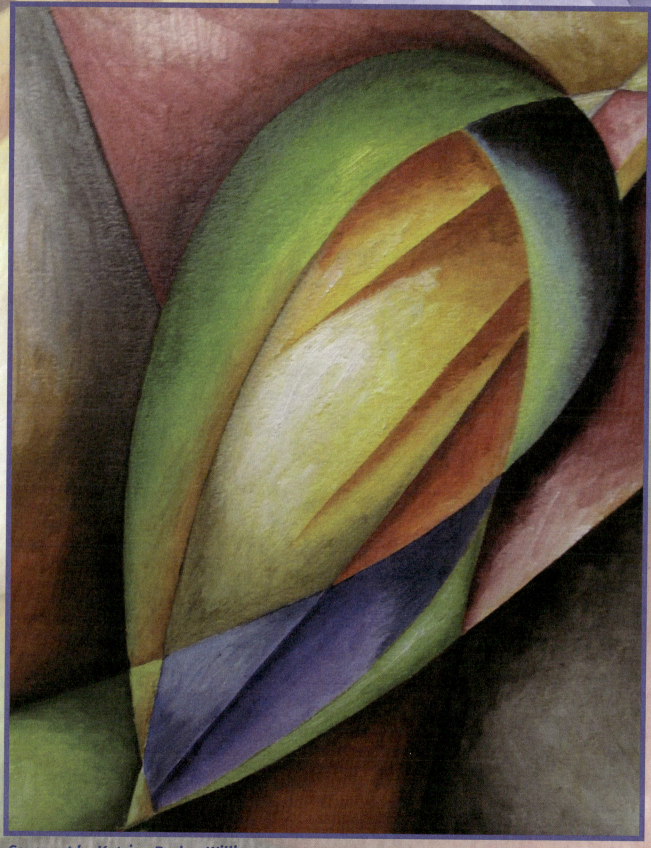

Cover art by Katrina Parker Williams

Glossary

Acronyms

Acronym	What it stands for	Meaning
AAKP	American Association of Kidney Patients	Voluntary organization of and for kidney patients. Free membership for patients.
AAMI	Association for the Advancement of Medical Instrumentation	Organization that sets standards for dialysis equipment, fluids, and water
ACT	Activated clotting time	A test for blood clotting
AHA	American Heart Association	Voluntary organization
AIDS	Acquired immune deficiency syndrome	A disease that attacks the immune system itself
AKF	American Kidney Fund	Voluntary organization
AKI	Acute kidney injury	Sudden episode of kidney failure
ALS	Amyotrophic lateral sclerosis	Neurologic disease; "Lou Gehrig's disease"
ANNA	American Nephrology Nurses' Association	Voluntary nursing organization
ANSI	American National Standards Institute	Oversees guidelines and standards in different businesses to protect people and the environment
APD	Automated peritoneal dialysis	PD with cycler exchanges
ARBD	Aluminum-related bone disease	Bone disease caused by aluminum exposure
ARBSI	Access-related bloodstream infection	Bloodstream infection from a vascular access
AV Fistula	Arteriovenous fistula	Artery + vein vascular access
AV Graft	Arteriovenous graft	Artery + man-made vessel + vein access
$\beta_2 M$	Beta-2 microglobulin	Protein that causes amyloidosis
BONENT	Board of Nephrology Examiners, Nursing and Technology	Group that offers the CHT exam
BP	Blood pressure	A vital sign
BSI	Bloodstream infection	Infection in the bloodstream; one cause can be from a central venous catheter
BUN	Blood urea nitrogen	Measure of protein
C	Centigrade	Metric temperature measure
Ca^{++}	Calcium	An electrolyte
CAPD	Continuous ambulatory peritoneal dialysis	PD with manual exchanges
CBC	Complete blood count	Common blood test
CBNT	Certified in Biomedical Nephrology Technology	Dialysis technician certification
CCHT	Certified Clinical Hemodialysis Technician	Dialysis technician certification
CCHT-A	Certified Clinical Dialysis Technicians – Advanced	Advanced dialysis technician certification
CCNT	Certified in Clinical Nephrology Technology	Dialysis technician certification
CCPD	Continuous cycling peritoneal dialysis	PD with cycler exchanges
CDC	Centers for Disease Control and Prevention	U.S. government agency that protects health and responds to disease threats
CDWS	Certified Dialysis Water Specialist	Dialysis water specialist certification
CFU	Colony-forming units	Measure of bacteria in water

Glossary

CFU/mL	Colony-forming units per milliliter	Measure of bacteria in water
$CH_3CO_2^-$	Acetate	Forms when acetic acid reacts with bicarbonate
$C_6H_5O_7^{3-}$	Citrate	Synonym for citric acid
$C_6H_{12}O_6$	Glucose	Blood sugar
CHF	Congestive heart failure	A condition in which the heart pumps weakly
CHT	Certified Hemodialysis Technician	Dialysis technician certification
CKD	Chronic kidney disease	Slow process of nephron loss
Cl^-	Chloride	An electrolyte
cm	Centimeters	Metric measure of length
CMS	Centers for Medicare & Medicaid Services	U.S. Medicare and Medicaid oversight agency
C-NET	Center for Nursing Education and Testing	Agency that surveys dialysis nurses and technicians about their job tasks
CNNT	Council of Nephrology Nurses and Technicians	NKF professional council that dialysis technicians can join
CO_2	Carbon dioxide	A gas
COPD	Chronic obstructive pulmonary disease	A lung disease that makes breathing difficult
CPR	Cardiopulmonary resuscitation	Chest compressions done if the heart stops
CQI	Continuous quality improvement	Process to improve healthcare quality
CROWN-Web	Consolidated Renal Operations in a Web-enabled Network	Computer system to collect dialysis data from all United States clinics
CRRT	Continuous renal replacement therapy	24-hour/day dialysis done in intensive care units
CUA	Calcific uremic arteriolopathy (or calciphylaxis)	Syndrome of calcification of the blood vessels, blood clots, and skin necrosis
Da	Dalton	Molecular weight measure
DAT	Damage assessment team	A group your clinic puts together to assess the clinic and equipment after a disaster
DDS	Dialysis disequilibrium syndrome	Brain swelling that can occur when water moves into the brain tissues through osmosis due to too-rapid waste removal
ΔP	Delta pressure	Change in pressure level
DFC	Dialysis Facility Compare	Website built by Medicare to help dialysis patients and families assess dialysis care quality
DI	Deionization	Process to remove ions from dialysis water
DOPPS	Dialysis Outcomes and Practice Patterns Study	International study of dialysis patients
DPC	Dialysis Patient Citizens	Non-profit organization made up of dialysis and pre-dialysis patients and their families
DRA	Dialysis-related amyloidosis	Chronic progressive condition caused by the build-up in the body of a protein called $\beta_2 M$
DRI	Dietary references intake	Recommended daily amount
EBCT	Empty bed contact time	How long feed water must touch GAC in a carbon tank
ECD	Expanded criteria donor	Deceased donor kidney from an older person or one with an illness
EDW	Estimated dry weight	Patient's weight with no extra water in the blood

Glossary

eGFR	Estimated glomerular filtration rate	An approximation of percent kidney function
EGHP	Employer group health plan	Health plan through work
EM	Emergency manager	Designated disaster leader for a dialysis clinic
EMLA	Eutectic mixture of local anesthetics	Numbing cream
EOC	Emergency operations centers	Central command center for local emergencies
EPA	Environmental Protection Agency	U.S. agency that protects air and water
EPO	Erythropoietin (hormone)	Tells bone marrow to make red blood cells
ePTFE	Expanded polytetrafluoroethylene	Graft material
EPTS	Estimated post-transplant survival	An estimate of how long a kidney recipient may live after the transplant
ESA	Erythropoiesis-stimulating agent	Synthetic version of a hormone made by kidneys. Helps patients grow their own red blood cells
ESRD	End-stage renal disease	Kidney failure requiring dialysis or a transplant
EU	Endotoxin units	Measure of endotoxin in water
F	Fahrenheit	U.S. temperature measure
GED	General Educational Development	A substitute for a high school diploma
GFR	Glomerular filtration rate	Measure of kidney function
GI	Gastrointestinal	Pertaining to the gut
GPG	Grains per gallon	Measure of water hardness
GPM	Gallons per minute	Rate of water flow
H^+	Hydrogen	A chemical element
H_2O	Water	Two hydrogen plus one oxygen molecules
HAI	Healthcare-associated infections	Infections patients get at dialysis or a hospital
HBcAb	Hepatitis B core antibody	Tests exposure to hepatitis
HBsAB	Hepatitis B surface antibody	Tests immunity to hepatitis
HBsAg	Hepatitis B surface antigen	Tests infection with hepatitis
HBV	Hepatitis B	A virus that attacks the liver
HBV	High biological value (protein)	Animal protein
HCO_3^-	Bicarbonate	A buffer
HCV	Hepatitis C virus	A hepatitis virus that attacks the liver
HD	Hemodialysis	Use of a filter to remove water/wastes from blood
HDF	Hemodiafiltration	A form of dialysis that injects sterile replacement fluid into patients' blood to remove more water
HDU	Home Dialyzors United	Non-profit home dialysis patient organization
HeRO	Hemodialysis reliable outflow	Central vein graft plus implanted catheter option
Hgb	Hemoglobin	Red blood cell pigment
HHD	Home hemodialysis	HD done by the patient and/or a partner at home
HIPAA	Health Insurance Portability and Accountability Act	Law that protects privacy of patient information
HIS	Health information systems	Computer charting systems
HIV	Human immunodeficiency virus	The virus that causes AIDS
HPTH	Hyperparathyroidism	Disease where too much PTH is made

Glossary

HIPAA	Health Insurance Portability and Accountability Act	Law that protects privacy of patient information
HIS	Health information systems	Computer charting systems
HIV	Human immunodeficiency virus	The virus that causes AIDS
HPTH	Hyperparathyroidism	Disease where too much PTH is made
IC	Incident commander	Designated disaster leader for a dialysis clinic
ICH CAHPS	In-center Hemodialysis (ICH) Consumer Assessment of Healthcare Providers & Systems (CAHPS) survey	Survey given twice/year to in-center HD patients to measure satisfaction with dialysis care
ICU	Intensive care unit	A constant-observation unit of a hospital used for the most critically ill patients
IDH	Intradialytic hypotension	Drop in systolic blood pressure of ≥ 20 mmHg or a drop in mean arterial pressure of 10 mmHg
IDPN	Intradialytic parenteral nutrition	Tube feeding during dialysis
IJ	Internal jugular	Best vein for a central venous catheter
IV	Intravenous	Into a vein or veins
IVC	Inferior vena cava	Large vein that brings lower body blood to the heart
JAS	Juxta-anastomotic stenosis	Narrowing of an access vein
K	Clearance	Removal of a substance across a membrane
K^+	Potassium	An electrolyte
KCER	Kidney Community Emergency Response	A coalition of groups that come together for disaster planning and response
KDIGO	Kidney Disease: Improving Global Outcomes	Global clinical practice guidelines
KDOQI	National Kidney Foundation Kidney Disease Outcomes Quality Initiative	U.S. clinical practice guidelines
KDPI	Kidney donor profile index	Estimate of the chance of failure of a deceased donor kidney transplant, including donor factors
kg	Kilogram	Metric measure: 2.2 pounds
KoA	Mass transfer coefficient	How well a solute will pass through a membrane
KP	Kidney pancreas transplant	Dual transplant for a patient with diabetes
Kt/V	Clearance multiplied by time divided by volume	Measure of dialysis dose based on urea clearance
KUF	Coefficient of ultrafiltration	How much water will pass through a membrane in 1 hour at a given pressure
L.M.X.	Lidocaine cream	A numbing cream used for dialysis needles
LAL	Limulus amoebocyte lysate	A test for endotoxin in dialysis water
LBV	Low biological value (protein)	Plant-based protein
LDO	Large dialysis organization	Company with many clinics; the two largest dialysis companies are DaVita and Fresenius.
LED	Light-emitting diode	Tiny, long-lasting light bulb

Glossary

mg	Milligrams	A unit of measurement
mg/dL	Milligrams per deciliter	A unit of measurement
mg/L	Milligrams per liter	A unit of measurement
Mg++	Magnesium	An electrolyte
MHZ	Megahertz	Measure of sound frequency
mL	Milliliters	Metric measure of volume
mL/kg	Milliliters per kilogram	1,000 mL of fluid = 1 kg of mass weight
mL/min	Milliliters per minute	A unit of measurement
mmHg	Millimeters of mercury	Measure of pressure
mmol/L	Millimoles per liter	Measure of flow rate
µmol/L	Micromoles per liter	A unit of measurement
MOA	Memorandum of agreement	An arrangement between two clinics to provide emergency back-up care for each other's patients
MRB	Medical Review Board	Clinician group that advises an ESRD Network
MRE	Meals ready to eat	U.S. field rations for troops, sometimes used as emergency food in disasters
MRSA	Methicillin-resistant Staphylococcus aureus	An antibiotic resistant bacteria
Na+	Sodium	An electrolyte
NANT	National Association of Nephrology Technicians/ Technologists	Voluntary dialysis technician/technologist organization
NCC	National Coordinating Council	Group that oversees the ESRD Networks
NIH	National Institutes of Health	U.S. agency that supports medical research
NIOSH	National Institute for Occupational Safety and Health	U.S. agency that studies workplace safety
NKF	National Kidney Foundation	Voluntary health organization for kidney disease
NNCC	Nephrology Nursing Certification Commission	Group that offers the CCHT exam
NNCO	National Nephrology Credentialing Organization	Group that offers the CCNT, CBNT, and CDWS exams
NSAIDs	Non-steroidal anti-inflammatories	Medications that relieve or reduce pain and can increase the risk of kidney failure
OH-	Hydroxyl ions	Oxygen plus hydrogen
OSHA	Occupational Safety and Health Administration	U.S. agency that protects workers
P	Phosphorus	An electrolyte
P.A.S.S.	Pull the pin, Aim nozzle at base of flames, Squeeze handle, Spray from side to side	Memory device to help recall the steps to use a fire extinguisher
P4P	Pay for performance	Incentive payment program to improve care
PAN	Polyacrylonitrile	Dialyzer membrane material
PD	Peritoneal dialysis	Removing water and wastes from the blood using the lining of the abdomen (peritoneum)
PDCA	Plan, Do, Check, Act	Some of the steps in CQI
PEL	Permissible exposure limit	Highest safe exposure level to a toxic chemical

PES	Polyethersulfone	A dialyzer membrane material
PEX	Cross-linked polyethylene	A plastic used for water pipes
pH	Acid-base measurement	A measure of the hydrogen ion concentration in a liquid with values from 0 (acid) to 14 (base) with the middle (pH 7) being neutral.
PHI	Personal health information	Information protected by the HIPAA law
PICC	Peripherally inserted central catheter	Tube placed in an arm that reaches a central vein
PKD	Polycystic kidney disease	Genetic disease that causes kidney cysts to form
PMMA	Polymethylmethacryate	Dialyzer membrane material
PPE	Personal protective equipment	Masks, gown, and gloves to protect from germs and chemicals
PPM	Parts per million	Measure of a chemical in air or a fluid
PPS	Prospective payment system	Bundled payment
PSf	Polysulfone	Dialyzer membrane material
PSI	Pounds per square inch	Measure of pressure
PTFE	Polytetrafluoroethylene	A plastic used for water pipe
PTH	Parathyroid hormone	Tells the bones to release calcium
PTSD	Post-traumatic stress disorder	A long-term stress response to a traumatic event
PVC	Polyvinyl chloride	A plastic used for water pipes
QA	Quality assurance	Process for writing and testing policies
QAPI	Quality Assessment and Performance Improvement	CQI required by CMS
Qb	Blood flow rate	Rate of blood during dialysis
QC	Quality control	Process to meet standards
Qd	Dialysate flow rate	Rate of dialysate during dialysis
QI	Quality improvement	A process to assess and improve an outcome
QIP	Quality Incentive Program	Pay for performance
R.A.C.E.	**R**escue, **A**ctivate the alarm, **C**ontain the fire (if small), or **E**vacuate	Steps to take in a fire
RD	Renal dietitian	Staff person who helps patients plan meals
RIJ	Right internal jugular	Preferred central venous catheter site
RLS	Restless legs syndrome	A "creepy crawly" feeling and compulsive need to move the legs that can disrupt sleep
RO	Reverse osmosis	A water purification step
RPA	Renal Physicians Association	Voluntary organization
RSN	Renal Support Network	Voluntary organization
SaO_2	Oxygen saturation	Level of oxygen in the blood
SC	Sieving coefficient	Percent of the total volume of a solute (in solution) that can potentially be removed from a solution by convection (solute drag), i.e. how much a membrane will allow to pass through
SDS	Safety data sheet	Information about chemicals
SLE	Systemic lupus erythematosus	A disease that can cause kidney damage
STEL	Short-term exposure limit	Chemical exposure per 15 minutes

Glossary

TB	Tuberculosis	A bacterial lung disease
TCV	Total cell volume	Volume a dialyzer will hold
TDS	Total dissolved solids	All organic and inorganic substances in water
TFC	Thin film composite	Common RO membrane material
THM	Trihalomethanes	Cancer causing substances
TJC	The Joint Commission	Organization that sets standards for hospitals and clinics
TMP	Transmembrane pressure	Pressure difference across the dialyzer membrane
TPN	Total parenteral nutrition	Tube feeding that provides most or all nutrition
TSA	Tryptic soy agar	Medium to grow cultures from water samples
TSAT	Transferrin saturation	Measure of iron storage
TW	Target weight	Patient's weight with no extra water in the blood; sometimes called estimated dry weight (EDW)
TWA	Time-weighted average	Chemical exposure per 8 hour shift
UF	Ultrafiltration	Removal of water in dialysis
UFR	Ultrafiltration rate	Rate of water removal
Unit/kg	Units per kilogram of body weight	Measure of drug dose
UNOS	United Network for Organ Sharing	Keeps the U.S. transplant list
URR	Urea reduction ratio	Amount of urea removed during a dialysis treatment
USRDS	United States Renal Data System	National data system to collect, analyze, and distribute information on chronic kidney disease
UV	Ultraviolet	Invisible spectrum of light
VRE	Vancomycin-resistant Enterococcus	An antibiotic resistant bacteria

Glossary

Abscess (AB-sess)
An infection under the skin that may look like a blister or pimple filled with fluid or pus. If needles are placed into or near an abscess, infection of an access or other tissues may occur.

Access
See: Vascular Access

Acid (ASS-id)
A substance with a pH below 7.0 that can donate a hydrogen ion (H⁺). In the human body, acids form when protein and other foods are broken down by digestion. To help balance pH levels in the body, dialysate has an acid concentrate and a bicarbonate concentrate. *See also:* Buffer, Dialysate.

Acquired Immunodeficiency Syndrome; AIDS
AIDS is the most severe phase of HIV infection. AIDS damages the immune system, so people who have it are prone to other "opportunistic" infections that healthy immune systems can fight off. *See:* Human Immunodeficiency Virus.

Adequacy
See: Hemodialysis Adequacy, Peritoneal Dialysis Adequacy.

Adsorb (Ad-SORB)
Attract and hold. The dialyzer membrane adsorbs blood proteins to the walls of the hollow fibers during a treatment. This can make reused dialyzers more biocompatible than new ones—if bleach is not used to remove the blood protein coating.

Advance Directives (Ad-VANCE Dir-EC-tives)
A way for a patient to outline his or her wishes for healthcare treatment in case s/he can no longer share them. A living will is one type of advance directive and states the patient's wishes. A durable power of attorney for healthcare decisions is another. This form names someone who knows the patient's wishes to make decisions for him or her. Patients should give their families and all healthcare providers a copy of the advance directive to keep on hand. Advance directives can be changed at any time, and a new copy shared with family and healthcare providers.

Air Detector (Air De-TEC-tor)
A device that checks blood in the venous line of the extracorporeal circuit for air. Air in a patient's bloodstream can stop the blood flow or heartbeat, causing death. If the detector finds air, an alarm will sound, the blood pump will stop, and the venous bloodline will clamp to keep air from reaching the patient.

Air Embolism (Air EM-bo-liz-um)
Air bubbles enter the bloodstream and flow into a vessel small enough to be blocked by the air. The air in the vessel acts like a blood clot, stopping blood flow. Dialysis machines have an air detector on the venous bloodline to help prevent this problem, which can be fatal.

Albumin (AL-bu-min)
A blood protein. Low serum albumin levels may mean a patient is under-nourished. Malnutrition is common in dialysis patients and raises their risk of death. Low albumin can also be a sign of inflammation, which is common in dialysis patients and can also increase the risk of death.

Alkaline
See: Base.

Alum (AL-um)
An aluminum compound often added to city water supplies to remove sediment and make the water clearer. Aluminum can build up in the bodies and brains of dialysis patients. Aluminum in dialysis water must be kept at low levels with water treatment. *See also:* Encephalopathy, Flocculant.

Aluminum-Related Bone Disease; ARBD
(Uh-LU-min-um Re-LAY-ted bone dis-EASE)
A health problem caused by long-term exposure to aluminum. Aluminum builds up in the tissues at the point where new bone forms and can be seen on X-ray. Symptoms can include deep bone pain, muscle weakness, and fractures. Sources of aluminum include water, medications, and cookware. Phosphate binders with aluminum are also a source, but are rarely used today.

Glossary

Amyloidosis (Am-ih-loyd-OH-sis)
A disease process that occurs when a protein called beta-2-microglobulin ($\beta_2 M$) builds up in soft tissues, bones, and joints. The deposits can cause joint and/or bone pain. High-flux membranes and/or nocturnal hemodialysis remove more $\beta_2 M$, which may help prevent or treat this problem.

Anaphylaxis (Anna-phil-AX-is)
A fast, severe immune response to an allergen that can be fatal. Hives, itching, or wheezing may occur. Blood pressure may drop, and heart rhythm changes can lead to cardiac arrest. Spasms of the breathing passages may cut off air, and the lips, tongue, and throat may swell. Immediate treatment is essential.

Anastomosis (Uh-NAS-tuh-mo-sis)
A surgical connection between two blood vessels. Dialysis needles should not be placed too near the anastomosis in a fistula or graft.

Anemia (Uh-NEE-me-uh)
A shortage of red blood cells, which bring oxygen to all of the body's tissues. Symptoms of anemia include severe fatigue, trouble with mental focus, feeling cold all the time, and many other problems. The problem is common in kidney failure, as damaged kidneys make less erythropoietin. Many patients are also iron deficient. Hemodialysis patients lose blood (with red blood cells and iron) through tests and their treatments as well.

Anesthetic (An-ess-THET-ic)
A drug that numbs part or all of the body to reduce pain. Local anesthetics can be injected into a spot, such as the skin around a puncture site, before needle placement. Or, sprays, gels or creams can be put on the skin in advance to prevent pain at a needle site. General anesthetics cause unconsciousness so surgery can be done.

Aneurysm (An-your-IS-um)
Ballooning or bulging of a weak spot in a blood vessel. Severe bleeding can occur if an aneurysm ruptures, so great care must be taken with a patient who has one. Aneurysms can occur if needles are placed too often into the same small area of a fistula. *See also:* Area Cannulation.

Angioplasty (An-gee-oh-PLASS-tee)
A procedure to open a narrow blood vessel that is used for vascular access repair. A small balloon is threaded through the vessel into the access and gently inflated to push the walls of the vessel open. *See also:* Stenosis.

Antegrade (ANN-tuh-grade)
Forward-moving. In dialysis, a needle can be placed antegrade: in the direction of blood flow toward the heart. Venous needles are always placed antegrade. Arterial needles may be placed antegrade or retrograde, though there is some evidence that antegrade is better.

Anticoagulant (Ann-tie-co-AG-u-lant)
An anti-clotting drug. Anticoagulants, such as heparin, help to keep a free flow of blood in the extracorporeal circuit for hemodialysis.

Antiseptics (Ant-uh-SEP-ticks)
Antiseptics slow or stop the growth of bacteria and viruses. They are used to kill microbes to prevent infection.

Apical Pulse (AY-pick-ul pulse)
A pulse felt on the chest wall over the heart.

Apnea (AP-nee-uh)
A period when breathing stops, typically during sleep.

Area Cannulation (Air-ee-uh Can-you-LAY-shun)
Placement of needles in the same small area of a fistula or graft at each treatment, which can cause a weak spot. The weak spot can bulge out and become an aneurysm (in a fistula) or pseudoaneurysm (in a graft). Area cannulation is poor practice. Use needle site rotation (sometimes called the rope ladder technique) or Buttonhole technique on fistulas. Use only needle site rotation on grafts.

Arrhythmia (Ay-RITH-me-uh)
An irregular heartbeat that may be felt as an extra pulse or heard over the heart.

Arterial Pressure (Ar-TEER-ee-al PRESH-ur)
Pressure measured in the extracorporeal circuit from the arterial needle to the dialyzer. *Pre-pump* arterial pressure is measured from the patient's access to the blood pump. *Post-pump* arterial pressure is measured after the blood pump, but before the dialyzer.

Glossary

Arterialize (Ar-TEER-ee-ul-eyes)
The process of enlarging a vein by connecting it to an artery. Strong arterial blood flow causes the vein to dilate (widen), thicken, and become more muscular, like an artery.

Arteriovenous Fistula
(Ar-TEER-ee-oh-vee-nus FIS-chu-la)
A link between an artery and a vein under the skin of an arm or leg to provide access to the blood. The force of blood from the artery makes the vein larger and thicker. After a fistula matures, it can be punctured with dialysis needles and will allow the blood flow rates needed for dialysis. (*Plural*: Fistulae.)

Artery (AR-ter-ee)
A blood vessel that carries blood away from the heart at high pressure. Arteries bring oxygenated blood to each part of the body.

Ascites (Uh-SITE-eez)
A build-up of fluid in the abdomen. May be caused by liver damage, heart failure, malnutrition, or infection. Ultrafiltration and drainage may be used to remove it.

Asepsis (Ay-SEP-sis)
The absence of pathogens.

Aseptic (Ay-SEP-tick)
Sterile or germ-free.

Aseptic Technique (Ay-SEP-tick teck-NEEK)
A series of steps used to keep a germ-free environment. Hand hygiene is done before touching items in sterile packages. Sterile objects can only touch other sterile objects. The patient's skin is cleaned with disinfectant before placing a needle. Catheter ports are disinfected before connecting lines. Any sterile supplies in wet, damaged, or torn packages are discarded, not used. Peritoneal dialysis exchanges must be done using aseptic technique to prevent infection.

Auscultate (OS-kul-tate)
To listen with a stethoscope. Auscultation is used to help diagnose access problems like stenosis or thrombosis that can change the normal sound of the bruit. *See also:* Bruit.

Automated Peritoneal Dialysis; APD
See: Continuous Cycling Peritoneal Dialysis (CCPD).

Backfiltration (Back-fill-TRAY-shun)
Dialysate crosses the dialyzer membrane into the patient's blood. This problem can be due to a change in the pressure or concentration gradient between the dialysate and blood. If it occurs, endotoxin in the water can cause fever and infection. Backfiltration may be more likely with high-flux membranes, which have larger pores.

Backwashing (BACK-wash-ing)
Forcing water backwards through a filter. This process can be used to remove particles from clogged sediment filters in a water treatment system.

Bacteremia
See: Sepsis.

Bacteria (Back-TEER-ee-uh)
Microscopic, one-celled organisms that can cause disease. Bacteria are classified as Gram-positive or Gram-negative by the color they turn on a test called a Gram's stain. *See also:* Endotoxin.

Base (Bayce)
Chemicals that can accept a hydrogen ion (H+). A substance with a pH of greater than 7.0 is a base, or alkaline. In the body, bicarbonate is a base. *See also:* Buffer, pH.

Beta-2-Microglobulin
See: Amyloidosis.

Bicarbonate (By-CAR-bo-nate)
A buffer that helps neutralize acids that form when the body breaks down protein and other foods—and is then reabsorbed by the kidneys. Dialysis patients may have low bicarbonate levels because their kidneys do not reabsorb it well. Bicarbonate is added to dialysate to help restore blood levels, but it supports bacterial growth, and needs two concentrates (acid and bicarbonate) to keep scale from forming that could harm equipment. *See also:* Buffer.

Binders
See: Phosphate Binders.

Biocompatible (By-oh-com-PAT-ih-bull)
Like the human body. A biocompatible membrane is less likely to cause patient symptoms or trigger immune responses caused by a foreign "invader."

Glossary

Blood Leak (Blud Leek)
The dialyzer membrane tears, letting blood into the dialysate. Severe blood leaks can cause major blood loss. Any blood leak will expose patients directly to the dialysate.

Blood Leak Detector (Blud Leek De-TECK-ter)
An alarm system on the hemodialysis delivery system. It checks used dialysate for blood. The detector shines a beam of light through the dialysate and into a photocell. A break in the light beam caused by blood cells triggers an alarm that stops the blood pump and clamps the venous line. This prevents further blood loss and contamination of the patient's blood with dialysate. *See also:* Hemodialysis Delivery System.

Bloodlines
See: Blood tubing.

Blood Pump (Blud Pump)
Part of the hemodialysis delivery system. It pushes the patient's blood through the extracorporeal circuit at a fixed rate of speed. During a treatment, the blood tubing is threaded between the pump head and rollers. The rollers move blood through the circuit and back to the patient. *See also:* Pump Occlusion.

Blood Pump Segment (Blud Pump SEG-ment)
A durable, larger-diameter section of the arterial blood tubing that is threaded through the roller mechanism of the blood pump. *See also:* Pump Occlusion.

Blood Tubing (Blud TOO-bing)
Part of the extracorporeal circuit that carries blood from the arterial needle to the dialyzer and back to the patient through the venous needle. An arterial segment of the blood tubing is often color-coded red. A venous segment is often color-coded blue. Parts of the blood tubing include patient and dialyzer connectors, a drip chamber or bubble trap, a blood pump segment, and heparin and saline infusion lines.

Blood Urea Nitrogen; BUN (Blud You-REE-uh NY-tro-jen)
Urea, a waste that forms when the body breaks down proteins, is measured as BUN. Failed kidneys cannot remove urea, which builds up in the blood. Easy and low-cost to measure, BUN is used as a stand-in for other wastes that are harder or more costly to measure. BUN levels are the basis of tests to assess the dose of dialysis. *See also:* Hemodialysis Adequacy, Urea Kinetic Modeling, Uremia.

Bolus (BOW-lus)
A single, large amount of something. In dialysis, heparin can be given by bolus. The full prescribed dose is given all at once.

Bone Disease
See: Renal Osteodystrophy, Secondary Hyperparathyroidism.

Brachial Pulse (BRAY-key-ul Pulse)
The pulse felt in the crease of the elbow at the brachial artery.

Brachiocephalic Fistula (Bray-key-oh-suh-FAL-ic FIS-chu-la)
The most common type of AV fistula of the upper arm. It is created by surgically joining the brachial artery to the cephalic vein.

Brine (Brine)
A concentrated saline solution. In dialysis water treatment, brine is used to flush the resin bed of a water softener. This recharges the softener with sodium chloride ions. These ions are then exchanged with calcium and magnesium to soften the water.

Bruit (BREW-ee)
A buzzing or swooshing sound caused by the high-pressure flow of blood through a fistula or graft. The bruit can be heard through a stethoscope at the anastomosis, and for some length along the access. A high-pitched bruit may mean stenosis of the access.

Bubble Trap
See: Drip Chamber.

Buffer (BUFF-er)

A substance that keeps the pH of a solution at a constant level, even when an acid or base is added. Bicarbonate is the buffer used in dialysis to maintain the pH of dialysate.

See also: Acid, Base, Bicarbonate.

Buttonhole Technique (Button-hole teck-NEEK)

Dialysis needles are placed in a fistula (not a graft) into the same holes at the same angle. Over 3–4 weeks, this creates pierced earring-like tracts that guide the needles to the right spots. The patient or same staff person should place the needles. Once tracts are formed, blunt needles are used to avoid cutting new tracts. Buttonhole cannulation is quick to do, less likely to infiltrate, and may cause less pain for the patient. There is a higher risk of infection, however. *See also:* Needle Site Rotation.

Bypass (BY-pass)

A safety feature that shunts dialysate to the drain. Bypass keeps unsafe dialysate from reaching the patient and causing harm. *See also:* Hemodialysis Delivery System.

Calcium (KAL-see-um)

An element that exists as a cation (positively-charged ion). In the body, calcium is an electrolyte needed for nerves and muscles and to form normal bone. It is partly bound to protein in the blood. Too much or too little calcium in dialysate can cause health problems or death for patients. Blood levels of calcium are checked once a month. In a dialysis feed water supply, calcium can combine with other substances to form scale that can clog equipment. *See also:* Electrolyte, Hypercalcemia, Hypocalcemia.

Cannula

See: Shunt.

Cannulate (KAN-you-late)

To put dialysis needles into a fistula or graft. *See also:* Buttonhole Technique, Needle Site Rotation.

Capillaries (KAP-ih-lair-eez)

Tiny blood vessels, where oxygenated blood crosses from arteries into veins. Capillaries are smaller than a human hair; blood cells must line up single file to pass through. Unlike arteries and veins, capillary walls are semipermeable. The walls let oxygen, nutrients, and waste products pass through. In the kidneys, each glomerulus is a ball of capillaries that filters out wastes from the blood.

Carbon Tank (KAR-bon tank)

Water treatment devices that contain granular, activated carbon to adsorb low molecular weight particles from water. Carbon tanks are mainly used to remove chlorine, chloramines, pesticides, solvents, and some trace organic substances from water used for dialysis.

Cardiac Arrest (Kar-dee-ack Uh-REST)

The heart stops beating, which can be a deadly side effect of some dialysis problems. Too-warm dialysate, wrong dialysate concentration, hemolysis, severe blood loss, or air in the bloodstream are risk factors. Hyperkalemia can also cause cardiac arrest.

Cardiac Output (Kar-dee-ack OUT-put)

The amount of blood passing through the heart in a given period of time. Having an AV fistula or graft causes a 10% increase in cardiac output. This causes a 10% increase in the size of the heart. Patients who cannot tolerate this increase in cardiac output cannot have AV fistulae or grafts.

Catabolism (Kuh-TAB-oh-liz-um)

A chemical process that that breaks down protein, forming wastes. These wastes (e.g., urea) are removed by healthy kidneys.

Catheter (KATH-uh-ter)

A plastic tube. In hemodialysis, a catheter can be placed in a large, central vein for short-term or longer-term access. In peritoneal dialysis, a catheter is placed in the abdomen or chest. It is used to infuse fresh dialysate into the peritoneum and drain out used dialysate. *See also:* Presternal Catheter.

Glossary

Cellulose (SELL-you-lowss)
A fiber that forms the cell walls of plants. Cellulose acetate was used as the first dialyzer membrane by Dr. Willem Kolff in 1942. It was also the first substance used to make reverse osmosis membranes for water treatment. Cellulose dissolved in a solution with copper salts and ammonium can be spun into sheets or hollow fibers. Unmodified cellulose dialyzer membranes were the most likely to cause first-use syndrome, because they are not biocompatible. *See also:* First-Use Syndrome.

Central Venous Stenosis
(SEN-tral VEE-nus Steh-NO-sis)
Narrowing of a central vein that can harm vessels in the arm on the same side, so a patient cannot have a fistula or graft. If central venous stenosis is present, the patient may have large, distended veins in the neck or chest. Or, one arm may be swollen so it is much larger than the other.

Chloramine (KLOR-uh-meen)
A mix of chlorine and ammonia. Ammonia may be added to city water to boost the germ-killing power of chlorine. Chloramine is an oxidant that destroys microbes by breaking down their cell walls. Chloramines in dialysis water can cause a deadly health problem called hemolysis (rupture of red blood cells). Carbon tanks are used to remove chloramines from water used for dialysis.

Chloride (Klo-ride)
An electrolyte in dialysate and in the human body. Chloride combines with other elements. It forms sodium chloride, potassium chloride, magnesium chloride, and calcium chloride.

Chlorine (Klo-reen)
This element is a greenish yellow gas that can harm the lungs if it is inhaled. Chlorine is blended with other substances to disinfect surfaces. It may be added to city water to destroy microbes. Carbon tanks in the dialysis water treatment system remove chlorine and chloramines.

Chronic Kidney Disease; CKD
(Krah-nick Kid-nee Diz-eez)
A long, slow loss of nephrons—and thus kidney function. CKD can take many years to progress. It is divided into stages based on the estimated glomerular filtration rate (eGFR). Stage 1 CKD is mild kidney dysfunction. Stage 5 CKD is the most severe form. *See also:* End-stage Renal Disease.

Clearance; K (KLEER-ance)
The amount of blood (in mL) that is completely cleared of a solute in one minute of dialysis at a given blood and dialysate flow rate. Dialyzer clearance affects how much treatment a patient receives. Dialyzer makers test their products with fluids other than blood (in vitro). Thus, clearance of a solute during treatment (in vivo) can vary from the maker's stated clearance. *See also:* Hemodialysis Adequacy.

Coefficient of Ultrafiltration; KUF
(Ko-ee-FISH-ent of ul-tra-fill-TRAY-shun)
How much water a dialyzer will remove from a patient's blood per hour at a given pressure. Also called ultrafiltration factor (UFF) or UF rate (UFR). KUF is stated in milliliters (mL) per hour (hr) of water removed for each millimeter (mm) of mercury (Hg) of transmembrane pressure (TMP): mL/hr/mmHg TMP. The higher the KUF, the more water per mL of pressure will be removed. High-flux and high-efficiency membranes have a higher KUF than conventional ones. A KUF above 8 requires a volumetric control hemodialysis system. These systems precisely control how much water is removed.

Concentrate (KON-sen-trait)
In dialysis, one of two salt solutions (acid and bicarbonate) that are mixed together to form dialysate.

Concentration (Kon-sen-TRAY-shun)
The level of solute dissolved in a measure of fluid. A highly-concentrated solution has more solutes. A less-concentrated (more dilute) solution has less solutes. One task of healthy kidneys is to control the concentration of urine so the right amounts of water and other substances stay in the body. In dialysis, the concentration of each of substance in dialysate must be right for a treatment to be safe and effective.

Concentration Gradient
See: Gradient.

Conditions for Coverage
(Kon-di-shuns for COV-er-ij)

CMS rules that dialysis clinics must follow to receive Medicare and Medicaid payment. In 2008, the *Conditions* were updated for the first time in 32 years. CMS surveyors inspect clinics to ensure that they follow the rules.

Conductive Solute Transfer
See: Diffusion.

Conductivity (Kon-duck-TIV-it-ee)
How well a fluid will transfer an electrical charge; a measure of ions in a solution. A conductivity meter measures the electrolyte level of dialysate to be sure it is within safe limits. *See also:* Electrolyte.

Conductivity Monitor
(Kon-duck-TIV-it-ee MON-it-er)

A device on the dialysis machine that checks the conductivity of dialysate to be sure it is correct. If the level is wrong, an alarm goes off and the machine goes into bypass mode so dialysate is sent to the drain. Conductivity must also be tested with a separate meter.

Congestive Heart Failure; CHF
(Kon-ges-tiv HART Fail-yer)

The heart cannot pump out enough of the blood it receives. Excess blood backs up into the lungs. Fluid overload from too much fluid intake or not enough fluid removal at dialysis may lead to CHF in dialysis patients.

Constant-Site Cannulation
See: Buttonhole Technique.

Contamination (Kon-tam-in-AY-shun)
Something is impure, due to the presence of dirt, blood, or microbes.

Continuous Ambulatory Peritoneal Dialysis; CAPD
(Kon-TIN-you-us Am-boy-la-tor-ee Pair-it-oh-NE-ul Die-AL-uh-sis)

Peritoneal dialysis with manual exchanges done four or five times each day. Exchanges can be done at home or work while the patient goes about his or her day. Each takes about 30 minutes, and gravity is used to drain the PD solution into and out of the peritoneum. CAPD is continuous, so large amounts of wastes do not build up between treatments. This means the diet and fluids tend to be less restricted for CAPD than for standard in-center hemodialysis. Because the patient can dialyze on his or her own schedule, this treatment is work-friendly. *See also:* Exchange, Peritoneal Dialysis.

Continuous Cycling Peritoneal Dialysis (CCPD)
(Kon-TIN-you-us SY-kling Pair-it-oh-NEE-ul Die-AL-uh-sis)

CCPD, or automated peritoneal dialysis (APD), is PD using a cycler machine to do exchanges at night while the patient sleeps. Because the patient's days are free, this treatment is work-friendly. Some patients use a cycler at night and may do one CAPD exchange at mid-day. *See also:* Exchange, Peritoneal Dialysis.

Continuous Quality Improvement (CQI)
(Kon-TIN-you-us Kwal-it-ee im-PROOV-ment)

A way to improve care by choosing an area that needs to be improved, analyzing the process of care, finding root causes of problems, making and using a plan of change, and checking how well it worked.

Continuous Renal Replacement Therapy (CRRT)
(Kon-TIN-you-us Ree-nul re-PLACE-ment Ther-uh-pee)

A slow, ongoing form of dialysis that uses the patient's heart or a blood pump to move blood through an extracorporeal circuit. CRRT is most often done to gently remove extra fluid and some wastes in patients in intensive care who are too ill or unstable for standard hemodialysis. A cartridge with a semipermeable membrane (like a dialyzer) is used.

Convection
See: Solvent Drag.

Countercurrent Flow (Cown-ter-kur-ent FLOW)
Blood flows one way inside a dialyzer, while dialysate flows the other way. This cross flow allows for efficient dialysis because the blood is in constant contact with fresh dialysate.

Glossary

Creatinine (Kree-AT-ih-neen)
A waste product of muscle use that healthy kidneys remove from the blood. Larger people with more muscle tend to have higher creatinine levels. Higher-than-normal creatinine levels may be a sign of kidney disease.

Creatinine Clearance
(Kree-AT-ih-neen KLEER-ance)
A urine test that measures how well the kidneys remove creatinine from the blood in a given time. As kidney disease worsens, creatinine clearance will fall to 10% or less of normal.

Crenation (Kreh-NAY-shun)
Shriveling of blood cells that can occur with exposure to hypertonic dialysate that is more concentrated than the blood. The blood will look dark red. Crenation can be fatal.

CROWNWeb (Krown Web)
Consolidated Renal Operations in a Web-enabled Network. A computer program clinics use to send their required data in real time to CMS.

Cuffed Tunneled Catheters
(Kufft TUN-uld CATH-uh-ters)
These catheters are placed into a large, central blood vessel through a tunnel formed under the skin. Inside the tunnel, tissue grows into an attached cuff. The cuff makes the catheter more stable and is a physical barrier against bacteria.

Cyanosis (Sy-uh-NO-sis)
Bluish skin, lips, gums, and fingernail beds due to lack of oxygen. May occur when dialysate is made from water with high levels of nitrates. Heart or lung disease can also cause cyanosis.

Daily Home Hemodialysis
See: Short Daily Home Hemodialysis.

Dehydration (Dee-hi-DRAY-shun)
The body does not have enough water, due to diarrhea, vomiting, heavy sweating—or removing too much water at dialysis. A dehydrated patient may have low blood pressure, sunken eyes, brain fog, poor skin tone, and be listless. See also: Hypotension.

Deionization (DI) Tank (Dee-ion-iz-AY-shun Tank)
A tank that uses beds of resin beads to remove unwanted ions from water. The unwanted ions are exchanged for hydrogen (H^+) and hydroxide (OH^-) ions to form pure water (H_2O). Optional part of a dialysis water treatment system, depending on the raw, or feed, water. DI does not remove microbes and should only be used temporarily for in-center dialysis.

Delivery System
See: Hemodialysis Delivery System.

Diabetes (die-uh-BEE-tiss)
There are two main types of diabetes, both of which can harm the kidneys. In type 1, the immune system attacks and kills the pancreas beta cells that make insulin. In type 2, the pancreas does not make enough insulin, or the body cannot use what it does make. About 10% of diabetes in the U.S. is type 1, and about 90% is type 2. Type 2 diabetes may be prevented or controlled with diet, exercise, and medication.

Diabetic Nephropathy
(Die-uh-bet-ic Nef-ROP-a-thy)
Kidney disease caused by diabetes. Type 2 diabetes, a shortage of or resistance to insulin, is the number one cause of kidney failure in the U.S. In type 1 diabetes, the immune system destroys the pancreas cells that make insulin. Diabetes is a disease of the blood vessels. It causes heart disease and nerve damage, and is the leading cause of blindness and limb loss in the U.S.

Dialysate (Die-AL-uh-sate)
A precise mixture of treated water and chemicals used in dialysis to form a concentration gradient to remove wastes from the blood. Sodium, calcium, magnesium, chloride, potassium, glucose, and bicarbonate are most often included, at levels close to those of normal blood. Dialysate must be mixed properly or patients can be harmed. See also: Gradient.

Dialysate Delivery System
See: Hemodialysis Delivery System.

Dialysis (Die-AL-uh-sis)

A treatment that is done to remove wastes and excess water from the blood of people whose kidneys have failed. Dialysis may be done using a dialyzer (hemodialysis). Or, the patient's own peritoneum (peritoneal dialysis) may be used as a filter. *See also:* Hemodialysis, Peritoneal Dialysis.

Dialysis Adequacy

See: Hemodialysis Adequacy, Peritoneal Dialysis Adequacy.

Dialysis Dementia

See: Encephalopathy.

Dialysis Disequilibrium Syndrome (Die-AL-uh-sis Diss-ee-kwal-IB-ree-um sin-drum)

Rapid or drastic changes in the patient's extracellular water that affect the brain. Urea transfers more slowly from the brain tissue to the blood, so water can be drawn into the brain and cause swelling. This syndrome occurs most often in acute renal failure or when BUN levels are very high. *See also:* Blood Urea Nitrogen.

Dialyzer (DIE-uh-lie-zer)

A semipermeable membrane in a plastic cylinder that is used as an artificial kidney. Dialyzers are used in hemodialysis to filter wastes and water out of the blood of patients with kidney failure. Ports on the cylinder let blood and dialysate flow in and out. The membrane keeps blood and dialysate apart, but allows an exchange of water and some solutes to occur. *See also:* Hollow Fiber Dialyzer, Semipermeable Membrane.

Dialyzer Reprocessing

See: Reprocessing.

Diastolic (Die-uh-STALL-ic)

The pressure of blood against the arteries when the heart rate is at rest (between beats). It is the bottom number of a blood pressure reading. *See also:* Systolic.

Diffusion (Diff-YOU-shun)

A chemistry principle. Dissolved particles will cross a semipermeable membrane from a higher solute level to a lower one. The process goes on until both sides of the membrane have the same solute level. In dialysis, diffusion removes wastes from the blood. Dialysate has no wastes, so wastes in the blood diffuse across the membrane into the dialysate. The rate of diffusion depends on the concentration gradient, temperature, and size of the wastes and the membrane pores. Diffusion is also called *conductive solute transfer*.

Disinfectant (Diss-in-FECK-tent)

A chemical or process (i.e., heat) that destroys or slows the growth of harmful microbes. To work, disinfectants need time. They must stay moist and in contact with a surface. Some common equipment disinfectants are heat, bleach, formaldehyde, glutaraldehyde, Renalin®, citric acid, and Amuchina®. Disinfectants are also used to clean water treatment ports before taking a water sample and to wipe off surfaces in the clinic.

Distal (DISS-tul)

Far. In anatomy, distal is far from the center of the body. Hands and feet are distal extremities.

Diuretic (Die-your-ET-ick)

A drug that causes someone to make more urine. Some diuretics can cause hypokalemia because they cause a loss of potassium in the urine. Diuretics are first line treatment for high blood pressure. They may be used for kidney patients before they start dialysis. Once the kidneys stop making urine, diuretics no longer work. *See also:* Hypokalemia.

Documentation (Dock-you-men-TAY-shun)

Information about a patient's care entered in the permanent medical record or chart. It is vital to track the patient's progress, to provide a way to follow up on each patient's response to treatment, and to ensure continuity of care. A patient's chart is legal evidence of the care he or she received. A task that is not charted is considered not to have been done.

Drip Chamber (Drip Chaym-burr)

A device that checks arterial or venous pressure in the extracorporeal circuit. A bubble trap in the drip chamber collects any air that enters the blood tubing.

Glossary

Dry Ultrafiltration
See: Isolated Ultrafiltration.

Dry Weight
See: Target Weight.

Dwell Time (Dwell Time)
A waiting period. A disinfectant must dwell in a dialyzer for a time for reprocessing. In a hemodialysis delivery system, it must dwell in the fluid pathways long enough to kill microbes. In peritoneal dialysis, dwell time is how long dialysate must stay in the patient's abdomen before it is drained.

Dyspnea (DISP-nee-uh)
Trouble breathing; shortness of breath. This can be a symptom of fluid overload, anemia, or heart or lung disease. Dyspnea can occur at dialysis due to problems such as an air embolism.

Ecchymosis (Eck-ih-MO-sis)
A bruise or bleeding under the skin. In dialysis patients, an ecchymosis can be a sign that too much heparin has been given. Or, it can mean that not enough pressure was placed on the needle sites after the needles were removed.

Edema (Eh-DEE-muh)
Water retention with swelling in body tissues. Edema occurs due to fluid overload or other health problems, such as congestive heart failure. Swelling may be seen in the patient's eyelids, ankles, feet, hands, abdomen, or lower back area. "Pitting" edema is present when a finger pushed against the skin in a swollen spot, such as an ankle or calf, leaves a dent. Report this to the nurse if you see it. *See also:* Target Weight, Pulmonary Edema.

Electrolyte (Ee-LECK-tro-light)
A compound that breaks apart into ions when dissolved in water. Electrolytes send electrical signals along the nerves to the muscles, including the heart. Healthy kidneys keep electrolytes in balance. Sodium, potassium, magnesium, chloride, and calcium are electrolytes. Each is added to dialysate in precise amounts.

Embolus
See: Air Embolism.

Empty Bed Contact Time; EBCT (Emp-tee Bed CON-tact Time)
The amount of time feed water must stay in contact with the charcoal bed in a carbon tank during water treatment to remove chlorine and chloramines.

Encephalopathy (En-sef-a-LOP-a-thy)
A change in brain function that can be fatal. Patients may seem confused or may lose short-term memory. You may see a change in personality or speech. Muscle spasms, hallucinations, and seizures can occur. Chronic exposure to high levels of aluminum can cause the problem. Aluminum can come from water, some antacids, and cookware.

Endocrine Function (END-oh-crin Funk-shun)
Making hormones—one of the tasks of healthy kidneys. Kidneys make hormones that control blood pressure and tell the bone marrow to make red blood cells. They also convert Vitamin D into an active form the body can use to absorb calcium.

Endotoxin (End-oh-TOX-in)
A toxic part of the cell walls (lipopolysaccharide) of some bacteria, which can be shed while they are alive or when they die. Since endotoxin is not alive, it cannot be killed. Endotoxin can cause pyrogenic reactions. In water treatment and reprocessing, we reduce the bacteria count of the water or remove it with an ultrafilter. *See also:* Pyrogenic Reaction.

End-Stage Renal Disease; ESRD (End-Stage REEN-ul Dis-eez)
A legal term for complete, permanent loss of kidney function. This occurs during the last stage (stage 5) of chronic kidney disease, when dialysis or a transplant is needed for the patient to live. Patients have ESRD when their glomerular filtration rate has dropped to less than 15. *See also:* Chronic Kidney Disease, Estimated Glomerular Filtration Rate.

Equilibrium (Ee-kwa-LIB-ree-um)
A state of balance. Diffusion and osmosis both go on until equilibrium has been reached and the levels of solutes or fluid are equal on both sides of a semipermeable membrane.

Glossary

Erythropoietin; EPO (Uh-rith-ro-PO-uh-tin)
A hormone made by healthy kidneys that tell the bone marrow to make red blood cells. As the kidneys fail, they make less erythropoietin, which can lead to anemia.

ESRD Networks (Ee-ess-ar-dee Net-works)
Entities that were formed by the U.S. Congress in 1978 to oversee dialysis clinics and make sure patients receive high-quality care. Networks collect data, take steps to improve quality, and promote rehabilitation. They handle patient grievances and give resources to ESRD staff and patients. There are 18 regional ESRD Networks in the U.S.

Estimated Glomerular Filtration Rate; eGFR (Ess-ti-may-ted glom-AIR-you-lar Fill-TRAYshun Rate)
The volume of blood filtered by the glomeruli each minute, in mL/min. Chronic kidney disease is divided into stages based on the eGFR. *See also:* End-Stage Renal Disease.

Ethylene Oxide; ETO (Eth-uh-leen OX-ide)
A gas used by some manufacturers to sterilize new dialyzers. Patients who are sensitive to ETO may have first-use syndrome if a new dialyzer is not rinsed well.

Exchange (Ex-CHANGE)
A peritoneal dialysis process of draining used dialysate and replacing it with fresh after a dwell time. Exchanges may be done by hand or with a cycler machine.

Excretory Function (EX-cra-tor-ee Func-shun)
To excrete means to eliminate from the body. The excretory function of healthy kidneys is to remove wastes and excess water as urine.

Exsanguination (Ex-sang-win-AY-shun)
A severe loss of blood that can be fatal. At dialysis, this can occur if a needle is dislodged, a bloodline separates, an access ruptures, or there is a crack in a dialyzer casing. All of these problems can be prevented.

Extracellular (Ex-tra-SELL-you-lar)
Outside the cells. About 1/3 of water in the body is extracellular: between the cells and in the blood vessels. Water must move into the blood vessels for dialysis to remove it. The sodium in dialysate helps draw water into the blood vessels so it can be removed.

Extracorporeal (Ex-tra-cor-POR-ee-ul)
Outside the body. Hemodialysis is an extracorporeal therapy; it takes place outside the body.

Extracorporeal Circuit (Ex-tra-cor-POR-ee-ul sir-kit)
The arterial bloodline, dialyzer, venous bloodline, and extracorporeal circuit monitors. The circuit is an extension of the patient's blood vessels outside of the body. It brings blood from the access to the dialyzer and then back to the patient. *See also:* Blood Tubing, Dialyzer.

Extracorporeal Circuit Monitors (Ex-tra-cor-POR-ee-ul sir-kit Mon-it-ers)
The blood flow monitor, arterial or venous pressure monitors (measured at drip chambers), air detector, and blood leak detector. Each will shut off the blood pump and clamp the venous bloodline if pressure is too high, there is air in the venous bloodline, or there is blood in the used dialysate. *See also:* Air Detector, Arterial Pressure, Blood Leak Detector, Venous Pressure.

Extraskeletal Calcification (Ex-tra-skel-uh-tal Kal-si-fi-CAY-shun)
Calcium phosphate crystals form in blood vessels or soft tissues; though rare, it can cause gangrene, loss of limb, and death. Patients with high blood (serum) levels of calcium and phosphorus are at a higher risk. If you see mottled, painful, purplish skin (often in the same place on both sides of the body), tell the nurse or nephrologist right away.

Feed Water (FEED Wah-ter)
"Raw" tap water before it passes through a dialysis water treatment system.

Femoral Catheter (FEM-oh-rul CATH-uh-ter)
A short-term vascular access placed in the femoral vein in the groin. This vein is easy to reach and leaves blood vessels in the upper body for a fistula or graft. But, the groin is quite prone to infection. It is most often used for critically ill or bedridden patients.

Ferritin (FAIR-uh-tin)
An iron storage protein that is measured with a blood test. Ferritin stores are needed as a building block for red blood cells. Patients may need iron supplements.

Glossary

Fiber Bundle Volume; FBV (Fie-ber Bun-dul VOL-youm)
Also called total cell volume (TCV), FBV is a measure of the volume of fluid the hollow fibers in a dialyzer can hold. FBV is checked before a dialyzer is used and again after each reprocessing. Reprocessing a dialyzer can reduce its FBV.

Fibrin Sheath (Fie-brin Sheeth)
A cluster of blood clotting fibers that builds up on the outside of a catheter lumen. The fibers can form a cap that blocks the end of a catheter and reduces blood flow.

Fibrosis (Fie-BRO-sis)
Overgrowth of scar tissue. Fibrosis can develop in a fistula due to needle punctures for dialysis. Scar tissue can narrow the lumen of the vessel and reduce blood flow.

Filters (Fil-ters)
Devices that pass particles, solutes, and other substances through holes of various sizes.

First-Use Syndrome (First-use SIN-drum)
A reaction to a new dialyzer. Shortly after a treatment starts, patients may feel nervous, itchy, or have chest pain, back pain, or palpitations (skipped or missed heartbeats). First-use syndrome may be due to ethylene oxide gas or manufacturing residues. Preprocessing a dialyzer may help remove some of these.

Fistula
See: Arteriovenous Fistula.

Flocculant (FLOCK-you-lent)
A chemical added to drinking water to remove solid particles and make the water clearer. Alum is one substance that may be used as a flocculant.

Flow (Flo)
A stream. Blood flow to each organ in the body is based on the amount and pressure of blood delivered by the heart, and the resistance the blood meets in the blood vessels. Blood flow in the extracorporeal circuit is based on the blood pump setting, resistance in the extracorporeal circuit, and the access.

Flow Rate (Flo Rayt)
The amount of fluid that flows through the tubing in a given period of time.

Flow Velocity (Flo Vel-OSS-uh-tee)
The speed at which the fluid moves through a given length of tubing.

Fluid Compartments (Flew-id Com-PART-ments)
Three spaces in the body where water is found. Most body water is inside the cells (intracellular). The rest is mainly between cells (interstitial) and in the bloodstream (intravascular). Only about 7% of body water is in the blood, but this is the only water we can reach for dialysis.

Flush
See: Priming.

Formaldehyde (For-MAL-duh-hide)
A poisonous, clear, strong-smelling gas. In liquid form (37% gas in water), it is aqueous formaldehyde, or Formalin®. Formalin is a germicide used to disinfect dialysate delivery systems or reprocess dialyzers. The liquid form is volatile. It changes into a vapor that can penetrate and disinfect even small spaces. Formaldehyde is a known cancer-causing agent. Dialysis clinics must follow OSHA safety rules to keep patients and staff safe.

Free Chlorine (Free KLOR-een)
Chlorine that is not chemically bound to other substances. See also: Chloramine.

Glomerular Filtration Rate (GFR)
See: Estimated Glomerular Filtration Rate.

Glomerulonephritis (Gluh-MEER-you-lo-nef-RYE-tis)
An inflammation that damages the glomeruli. It can be slow and progressive or rapid in onset. It may occur as an immune response to a strep infection. Hypertension often occurs with it.

Glomerulosclerosis (Gluh-MEER-you-lo-skler-OH-sis)
Hardening of the glomeruli due to a disease process.

Glomerulus (Gluh-MEER-you-lus)
A tangled ball of capillaries in each nephron, held together by a membrane called a Bowman's capsule. Water and small solutes are forced through slits in each glomerulus by the pressure of the beating heart to form glomerular filtrate. (*Plural*: Glomeruli.)

Gradient (GRAY-dee-ent)
A difference. A concentration gradient is a difference in the level of solutes between two fluids kept apart by a semipermeable membrane. In dialysis, the fluids are blood and dialysate.

Graft (Graft)
To join one thing surgically to another. In hemodialysis, a graft is a piece of man-made vessel that is used to create a vascular access. One end of the graft is connected to the patient's artery, the other to the vein. A transplanted kidney is also called a graft.

Gram-Negative (Gram-Neg-uh-tiv)
An electrically charged biofilm (slime) that lets bacteria in water cling to surfaces. Biofilm protects the bacteria from disinfectants, and is very hard to remove. It can form on jugs or hoses, or on water treatment components. Achromobacter is one type of Gram-negative bacteria that can form biofilm in dialysis water.

Gram-Positive (Gram-Pos-uh-tiv)
Bacteria that turn purple with a Gram's stain. Staphylococci are Gram-positive bacteria that live on the skin and cause most access infections.

Green Dialysis (Green Die-AL-uh-sis)
An approach to dialysis that aims to reduce the environmental impact of the treatment. Green dialysis may reuse RO reject water, recycle plastic waste, and/or use solar or wind power.

Hand Hygiene (Hand HI-jeen)
Washing hands with soap or using an alcohol-based hand sanitizer. Hand hygiene is a key approach to reduce infection.

Heat Disinfection (Heet Diss-in-FECK-shun)
Heat can be used instead of chemicals to disinfect some types of dialyzers and equipment. The use of heat prevents patient and staff exposure to chemicals. Cellulose dialyzer membranes degrade in heat and cannot be disinfected in this way.

Hemastix® (HEE-ma-stix)
A reagent test strip that reacts to blood. When the blood leak detector shows that there is blood in the used dialysate—but the blood can't be seen—a Hemastix strip is used to check the extent of the leak.

Hematocrit; Hct (Hee-MAT-oh-crit)
A measure of red cells in the blood, stated as a percentage of red blood cells per total blood volume. Routine checks of Hct levels were used to assess anemia in the past, but have been replaced with hemoglobin, which is less affected by changes in blood volume.

Hematoma (Hee-ma-TOE-ma)
A painful, hard, black and blue mass of blood under the skin caused when blood leaks out of a vessel into the tissues. Hematomas can form when dialysis needles are placed, infiltrated, or taken out. A hematoma can compress the access and make a clot more likely. *See also:* Infiltration.

Hemoconcentration (Hee-mo-kon-sen-TRAY-shun)
Dehydration of the blood. This can occur in the extracorporeal circuit if ultrafiltration goes on after the blood pump is turned off. Recirculation can also lead to this problem. Hemoconcentration can lead to blood clotting, which can harm the patient's access.

Hemodialysis; HD (Hee-mo-die-AL-uh-sis)
A treatment that removes excess water and wastes from the blood by passing it through a dialyzer. Blood goes to the dialyzer and back to the patient's body through tubing connected to needles placed in a vascular access or a central venous catheter. Water and wastes pass through a semipermeable dialyzer membrane and into the dialysate. Alarms and monitors help ensure a safe treatment. Patients can learn to do their HD treatments at home or can receive them in a clinic.

Hemodialysis Adequacy (Hee-mo-die-AL-uh-sis ADD-uh-kwa-see)
The least amount of treatment patients need to live, measured with urea kinetic modeling (Kt/V). KDOQI guidelines say the delivered Kt/V must be at least 1.2 (with a prescribed Kt/V of 1.4). *See also:* Urea Kinetic Modeling.

Glossary

Hemodialysis Delivery System
(Hee-mo-die-AL-uh-sis Dee-LIV-er-ee Sys-tem)

A machine that delivers hemodialysis. It has a blood pump, dialysate delivery system, and safety monitors. The blood pump moves blood from the patient's access through the dialyzer and back to the patient. The machine makes dialysate by mixing treated water with two types of concentrate. Safety alarms check flow, temperature, conductivity, pressure, leaks, and, often, the patient's blood pressure.

HeRO; Hemodialysis Reliable Outflow (HEE-row)

A type of graft that can be used for patients with central venous stenosis or blockages. A 6 mm ePTFE graft has an arterial anastomosis on one side. On the other side, it has a 5 mm silicone outflow into a central vein, with the tip placed in the right atrium of the heart. The HeRO is completely under the skin. It has continuous flow from the graft into the out flow component. It is FDA-approved as a graft, and needles are placed in it just like any other graft.

Hemoglobin; Hgb (HEE-mo-globe-in)

The red, oxygen-carrying pigment of red blood cells. Routinely checking Hgb levels lets the care team follow the patient's response to anemia treatment and alerts them to any chronic blood loss. *See also:* Anemia.

Hemolysis (Hee-MOLL-uh-sis)

Red blood cell rupture; a life-threatening problem that needs urgent care from a doctor. Hemolysis may be due to dialysate that is too hot, too dilute, the wrong conductivity, or contains bleach, formaldehyde, chloramines, copper, or nitrates. Some drugs or diseases, and transfusions with the wrong blood type can cause it. Damage to the blood cells from kinked blood tubing can also rupture red blood cells.

Hemolytic Anemia (Hee-mo-LIT-ic Uh-NEEM-ee-uh)

A shortage of red blood cells due to hemolysis.

Hemothorax (Hee-mo-THOR-ax)

A collection of blood in the chest that keeps the lungs from fully expanding, so it is hard to breathe. The problem can occur if a blood vessel is punctured when a central venous catheter is placed.

Heparin (HEP-uh-rin)

A drug used to help blood flow through the extracorporeal circuit. It can be given as a bolus (one dose), intermittently (on and off), or continuously, with a pump.

Heparin Infusion Line
(HEP-uh-rin in-FEW-shun Line)

A small tube that extends from the blood tubing so heparin can be given during dialysis. The line is most often found on the arterial blood tubing segment just before the dialyzer.

Heparin Infusion Pump
(HEP-uh-rin in-FEW-shun Pump)

A pump with a syringe holder, piston, and electric motor used to give heparin. The pump is connected to a heparin infusion line, which is part of the extracorporeal blood tubing. Most dialysis machines have a heparin delivery system. Stand-alone heparin pumps are still used in some settings.

Hepatitis (Hep-uh-TIE-tis)

Inflammation of the liver that can be caused by one of three viruses (A, B, or C). Hepatitis B and C are spread through contact with infected blood or other body fluids, and are a concern for dialysis patients and staff. Hepatitis can cause liver damage or death. Vaccination against the hepatitis B virus should be offered to all staff and patients. Infection control is used to prevent the spread of hepatitis and other diseases.

High-Efficiency Dialysis
(Hi-ee-fish-en-see Die-AL-uh-sis)

Use of dialyzers that can remove more small solutes (e.g., urea) than conventional ones. Larger-gauge needles and blood flow rates from 300–500 mL/min are most often used. The U.S. government requires ultrafiltration control when a dialyzer with a KUF above 8 is used. *See also:* Coefficient of Ultrafiltration.

High-Flux Dialysis (Hi-flux Die-AL-uh-sis)

Use of a dialyzer with a KUF value higher than 8. Ultrafiltration control must be used. High-flux dialyzers can remove more fluid and large wastes, such as beta-2-microglobulin.

High-Output Cardiac Failure (Hi-out-put KAR-dee-ack Fail-your)

The patient's heart cannot work hard enough to pump out the extra blood sent to it by an AV fistula or graft. *See also:* Cardiac Output.

HIPAA; Health Insurance Portability and Accountability Act (HIP-uh)

A U.S. law that in part requires that patients' personal health information be kept confidential.

Hollow Fiber Dialyzer (Holl-oh Fie-burr DIE-uh-lie-zer)

A dialyzer made with thousands of tiny hollow fibers as the membrane, held in place at each end by a plastic potting "clay." The fibers and potting clay are encased in a clear plastic cylinder. During dialysis, blood flows through the hollow tubes, while dialysate flows around them. This type of dialyzer allows for well-controlled and predictable diffusion and ultrafiltration. It is the only type of dialyzer on the market in the U.S.

Homeostasis (Home-ee-oh-STAY-sis)

A constant internal balance in the body. Healthy kidneys help maintain fluid balance, acid/base balance, hormone balance, and electrolyte balance. All of these are key aspects of homeostasis.

Hormones (HOR-moans)

Chemical messages made in one organ or gland that act on another part of the body. Kidneys make hormones that affect red blood cell levels and let the gut absorb calcium.

HIV; Human Immunodeficiency Virus (Aitch-eye-vee)

A virus that attacks the immune system and destroys the white blood cells that fight disease (T-lymphocytes). HIV is spread through blood, semen, vaginal and peritoneal fluids, and breast milk. Over time, people with HIV can develop acquired immunodeficiency syndrome (AIDS). Damage to the immune system from AIDS leaves the body open to infections and cancers that rarely occur in healthy people. There are treatments, but it is best to prevent the spread of HIV with infection control. *See also:* Infection Control, Opportunistic Illness.

Hydraulic Pressure (Hi-draw-lick PRESH-ur)

Water pressure, which can occur in nature (such as by gravity) or be applied (such as with a pump). It affects the amount of water that is removed from the patient during dialysis.

Hydrophilic (Hi-dro-PHIL-ick)

Attracts water.

Hydrophobic (Hi-dro-PHO-bick)

Repels water.

Hyper- (Hi-per)

Beyond, above, more, or too much. For example, hyperactivity is an above-normal activity level.

Hypercalcemia (Hi-per-kal-SEE-me-uh)

Too much calcium in the blood. Symptoms may include weak muscles, fatigue, constipation, loss of appetite, abdominal cramps, nausea, vomiting, and coma. *See also:* Electrolyte, Extraskeletal Calcification.

Hyperglycemia (Hi-per-gly-SEE-me-uh)

High blood sugar levels. Thirst may be a symptom of hyperglycemia in a patient who has diabetes.

Hyperkalemia (Hi-per-ka-LEE-me-uh)

Too much potassium (an electrolyte) in the blood. Patients who have this may have weak muscles, heart rhythm changes, cardiac arrest, or may die. Hyperkalemia can occur if a patient eats too many high-potassium foods, or if dialysate with too much potassium is used. Bleeding, hemolysis, surgery, or fever can also cause this problem because as tissue breaks down potassium is released from cells into the bloodstream. *See also:* Electrolyte.

Hypermagnesemia (Hi-per-mag-nuh-SEE-me-uh)

Too much magnesium (an electrolyte) in the blood. Magnesium is needed for muscle and nerve function. Patients with hypermagnesemia may feel sleepy or have nerve problems, low blood pressure, and slower breathing. In severe cases, cardiac arrest may occur. *See also:* Electrolyte.

Glossary

Hypernatremia (Hi-per-na-TREE-me-uh)
Too much sodium (an electrolyte) in the blood. Excess sodium in the blood causes water to move out of the cells—including red blood cells. It can cause headaches, high blood pressure, confusion, trouble walking and talking, and crenation. *See also:* Electrolyte.

Hyperphosphatemia (Hi-per-fos-fa-TEE-me-uh)
Too much phosphorus in the blood. May occur in patients who eat a lot of protein or dairy foods and do not take enough phosphate binders. Hyperphosphatemia can cause severe itching in the short term and bone damage in the long term. When it occurs with hypercalcemia, it can cause fractures, bone pain, and sharp calcium phosphate crystals in the soft tissues. *See also:* Extraskeletal Calcification.

Hyperplasia (Hi-per-PLAY-ja)
Overgrowth of cells. Clotting in the middle of a vascular access graft is often caused by clumps of platelets that build up where there is hyperplasia.

Hypersensitivity (Hi-per-sens-ih-TIV-it-ee)
Strong immune response to a foreign substance. Can cause inflammation. In dialysis, these occur most often with cellulose dialyzers. *See also:* Anaphylaxis.

Hypertension; HTN (Hi-per-TEN-shun)
High blood pressure. HTN can be a cause or result of kidney failure and is the second most common cause of kidney disease in the U.S. It can raise the risk of a stroke and damage the kidneys, heart, blood vessels, eyes, and other organs. Patients on standard in-center hemodialysis often take more than one blood pressure drug.

Hypertonic (Hi-per-TON-ick)
A solution with a higher concentration than another solution. Use of hypertonic saline (more concentrated than the blood) can draw more water into the blood if a patient feels dizzy or faint. Since its use leaves excess sodium in the blood, this practice has fallen out of favor.

Hypo- (Hi-po)
Below, beneath, or too little. For example, a hypodermic needle is a needle that is inserted beneath the skin.

Hypocalcemia (hi-po-kal-SEE-me-uh)
Not enough calcium (an electrolyte) in the blood. Hypocalcemia can cause tetany—spasms and twitching of the muscles—or seizures. Low blood calcium can occur in kidney disease due to the loss of calcitriol production by the failing kidneys. Calcitriol lets the body absorb calcium from the diet.

Hypoglycemia (Hi-po-gly-SEE-me-uh)
Low blood sugar levels. In a patient with diabetes, this can cause hunger, nervousness, shaking, weakness, sweating, dizziness, sleepiness, confusion, or trouble speaking. The treatment is a fast-acting carbohydrate, like juice.

Hypokalemia (Hi-po-ka-LEE-me-uh)
Below-normal levels of potassium (an electrolyte) in the blood. This is rare in dialysis patients. It can occur if there is too little potassium in the diet or in the dialysate. Hypokalemia can also be caused by a loss of potassium due to vomiting, diarrhea, use of potassium exchange resins, and use of diuretics that increase the loss of potassium in the urine (if the patient makes urine).

Hyponatremia (Hi-po-na-TREE-me-uh)
Below-normal levels of sodium (an electrolyte) in the blood. Without enough sodium, water moves out of the extracellular space and into the cells. This can cause low blood pressure and hemolysis. Symptoms can include muscle cramping, restlessness, anxiety, access pain, headaches, and nausea.

Hypophosphatemia (Hi-po-fos-fa-TEE-me-uh)
Below-normal levels of phosphorus in the blood that can cause changes in heart rhythm or muscle weakness. This is rare in dialysis patients, as phosphorus is found in most foods. It may occur if a patient has a poor diet and takes too many phosphate binders, or in patients who do nocturnal hemodialysis. Low levels of phosphorus can suggest malnutrition.

Glossary

Hypotension (Hi-po-TEN-shun)
Low blood pressure. In dialysis patients, this occurs most often when too much fluid is removed during a treatment or patients take too many blood pressure drugs. Symptoms include severe muscle cramps; headaches; feeling warm, restless, dizzy, faint, or nauseated; or having visual changes. The Trendelenburg position (raising the feet higher than the heart) and giving fluids (i.e., normal saline) help return blood pressure to normal.

Hypotonic (Hi-po-TON-ick)
One solution has a lower concentration than another. Use of hypotonic dialysate (more dilute than the blood) can lead to hemolysis (bursting of red blood cells).

Infection (In-FECK-shun)
Invasion of the body by a pathogen.

Infection Control (In-FECK-shun con-trol)
Steps to prevent the spread of infection. The steps include hand hygiene, aseptic technique, cleaning, disinfecting, and wearing protective gear.

Infiltration (In-fill-TRAY-shun)
Leakage of a substance into body tissues. In dialysis patients, infiltration of blood into the tissues around the access can occur if the needle punctures the back of the vessel wall. To prevent infiltration, place needles with great care.

Inflammation (In-fla-MAY-shun)
Tissue swelling in response to injury, infection, or surgery.

Instill (In-STILL)
To place into or cause to enter. Heparin is instilled into each lumen of a central venous catheter. This practice helps to stop clotting in a catheter between treatments. Dialysate is instilled into the peritoneum for peritoneal dialysis.

Interdialytic (In-ter-die-uh-LIT-ick)
Between dialysis treatments.

Intermittent (In-ter-MITT-ent)
Periodically or not continuously. Heparin can be given intermittently during dialysis.

Internal Jugular; IJ (In-ter-nal JUG-you-lar)
Central venous catheters may be placed in the IJ vein in the neck. This site is less likely to cause central venous stenosis than placement in the subclavian vein.

Interstitial Space (In-ter-STISH-al Space)
The space between the cells or organ tissues.

Intima (In-TEE-ma)
The smooth lining on the inside of blood vessels. The intima is covered with a thin, fragile layer of cells that lets blood flow through the vessel easily. In a fistula or graft, hyperplasia of the intima cells at the anastomosis can cause stenosis, which makes blood clots more likely.

Intracellular (In-tra-SELL-you-lar)
Within the cells. Two-thirds of fluid in the body is inside the cells. Sodium causes fluid to move across cell membranes between the intracellular and extracellular spaces.

Intradermal (In-tra-DER-mal)
Within the skin. Local anesthetics may be injected intradermally.

Intradialytic Hypotension; IDH (In-tra-die-uh-LIT-ick Hi-po-TEN-shun)
A drop in blood pressure that occurs during a dialysis treatment and can lead to organ stunning.

Intramuscular (In-tra-MUS-kew-lar)
Within a muscle. Vaccines may be injected intramuscularly.

Intravascular (In-tra-VAS-kew-lar)
Within blood vessels. Central venous catheters are intravsascular.

Intravenous; IV (In-tra-VEE-nus)
Within a vein. Many medicines are given intravenously.

In Vitro (In VEE-tro)
A Latin phrase that means in an artificial setting. Dialyzer clearance is measured *in vitro* by the manufacturer, using non-blood fluids, like saline. Real dialyzer clearance may vary from the *in vitro* clearance.

Glossary

In Vivo (In VEE-vo)
A Latin phrase that means in the living body of a plant or animal. Tests done on a dialyzer while a patient is being treated are *in vivo*.

Ion (EYE-on)
An electrically-charged particle. Ions can carry a positive charge (cation) or a negative charge (anion).

Ion Exchange (EYE-on ex-CHANGE)
Trading unwanted ions for hydrogen and hydroxyl ions to create pure water. Occurs inside a deionizer for water treatment.

Iron Deficiency (I-urn De-FISH-en-see)
A lack of iron in the body to make red blood cells. Without iron, the bone marrow can't make red blood cells, even if erythropoietin is present. Low levels of iron can cause a form of anemia.

Ischemia (Is-KEE-me-uh)
A lack of oxygen in the tissues due to reduced blood flow. It can be painful. Ischemia of the heart can cause angina pain. Steal syndrome (ischemia of the hand) may cause hand pain; a cold, clammy feeling; and, in extreme cases, painful, non-healing skin ulcers.

Isolated Ultrafiltration; IU (Eye-so-lay-ted Ul-tra-fil-TRAY-shun)
A way to remove water, but not solutes. IU does not use dialysate. It can be done before, after, or without dialysis. The main plus of IU is that patients may tolerate it better than standard dialysis. May be called dry ultrafiltration, sequential ultrafiltration, or pure ultrafiltration.

Isotonic (Eye-so-TON-ick)
One solution with the same osmotic concentration as another. Normal saline is isotonic; it has the same level of sodium as blood.

Kidney Transplant (Kid-nee Trans-plant)
Replacing the failed kidneys with a healthy kidney from a donor. It is possible to receive a living donor kidney from a relative, spouse, friend, or unrelated person. Deceased donor kidneys come from people who have had died. Blood type and other tissue factors are used to "match" a recipient after a medical work-up has been done.

Kt/V
See: Urea Kinetic Modeling.

KUF
See: Coefficient of Ultrafiltration.

Leach (Leech)
Water passes through a substance and dissolves part of it. In water treatment, copper, lead, or galvanized steel should not be used after the blending valve because water can leach copper or zinc from the pipes.

Leak Testing
See: Pressure Testing.

Loading Dose (Lo-ding dose)
A dose of medicine that creates a certain blood level in the body. A loading dose of heparin may be given after both needles are in place, but before a treatment begins. This lets the heparin flow through the patient's bloodstream.

Local Infection (Lo-kul In-FECK-shun)
An infection only in one area—such as in a fistula or graft and the tissues around it.

Lumen (LOO-men)
The inside diameter of a blood vessel or a tube, such as a catheter or needle. In stenosis, the lumen of the vascular access becomes narrower, which limits blood flow.

Lyse (Lize)
To dissolve. One option for treating a blood clot in a vascular access is to use a drug that will lyse the clot.

Magnesium (Mag-NEE-zee-um)
A metallic mineral found in the body as an electrolyte in the intracellular fluid. A small trace of magnesium in body fluids is vital to the nervous system.

Malnutrition (Mal-new-TRISH-un)
A lack of proper nutrition. Many people on dialysis do not get enough protein, which is a risk factor for death. Protein levels are checked with a blood test for serum albumin. This level should be 4.0 g/dL or higher.

Membrane Compliance (Mem-brane Com-PLY-ans)
A measure of how much a membrane will change shape or volume due to pressure.

Membrane Filters (Mem-Brane FIL-ters)
Water treatment cartridges that contain thin membranes with pores of a certain size. Membrane filters remove small particles and some solutes.

Metabolic Acidosis
(Met-uh-BOL-ick Ass-ih-DOSE-iss)
A condition that occurs when the acid/base balance of body fluid and tissues shifts toward acid. This problem is common in dialysis patients. Their kidneys no longer reabsorb as much bicarbonate—a buffer that keeps blood pH stable.

Metabolism (Met-AB-oh-lis-um)
The sum of chemical processes that occurs when some substances are broken down and others are formed.

Microalbuminuria (My-cro-al-byu-min-UR-ee-uh)
Small amounts of albumin (protein) in the urine. Albumin is a large molecule that does not pass through the cell walls of healthy glomeruli. So, microalbuminuria can be an early sign of chronic kidney disease. Blood pressure drugs in the ACE inhibitor or ARB class can slow the rate of kidney disease in some people with microalbuminuria.

Microbe (MY-crobe)
A microscopic living organism, such as bacteria, virus, fungus, or algae.

Microns (My-crons)
A unit of measure for filter pores. Filters with high micron sizes trap larger particles and let smaller ones flow through. A submicron filter may be needed to capture very small particles.

Microorganism (My-cro-ORG-un-is-um)
A microscopic living organism, such as, bacteria, virus, fungus, or algae.

Mineral Bone Disorder (MBD)
See: Renal Osteodystrophy.

Modality (Mo-DAL-uh-tee)
A type of treatment, such as hemodialysis, peritoneal dialysis, or transplant.

Molecular Weight (Mo-leck-you-lar Wait)
A measure of molecule size in Daltons (Da). The sum of the atomic weights of all elements in a molecule of a substance is its molecular weight. Larger molecules (like $\beta_2 M$) have higher molecular weights.

Molecular Weight Cutoff
(Mo-leck-you-lar Wait Cut-off)
The largest solute size that can pass through a given semipermeable membrane.

Molecule (MOL-uh-kyule)
The smallest complete unit of a substance that has that substance's identity.

Morbidity (Mor-BID-ih-tee)
Illness that may be measured as days in the hospital. It is used as one measure of patient outcomes.

Mortality (Mor-TAL-ih-tee)
Death. Mortality is used as a measure of patient outcomes.

Myalgia (My-AL-ja)
Muscle pain.

Myocardial Infarction; MI
(My-oh-car-dee-ul In-FARK-shun)
Blockage of a heart artery that can lead to death or death of part of the heart muscle. The patient may feel severe or crushing chest pain—a "heart attack." *See also:* Arrhythmia.

Myocardial Stunning
See: Organ Stunning.

Nasogastric Tube; NG (Nay-zo-GAS-rick Toob)
A tube that is inserted through the nose into the stomach. Patients who are malnourished may need to be fed through an NG tube.

Glossary

Needle Site Rotation (Nee-dul Sight Ro-TAY-shun)
A needle placement technique that can be used with fistulae and grafts, also called the "Rope Ladder technique." Its aim is to prevent damage that can occur when needles are placed using "area cannulation." Needles are always placed at least 1.5 inches away from the anastomosis and away from the sites used at the last treatment. At each treatment, needle placement then moves up and down the full length of the access. See also: Buttonhole Technique.

Negative Pressure (Neg-uh-tiv PRESH-ur)
Pressure that is less than 0 mmHg. Negative pressure plus positive pressure equals transmembrane pressure (TMP).

Neointimal Hyperplasia (Nee-oh-IN-ti-mul Hi-per-PLAY-ja)
Overgrowth of cells that occurs when smooth muscle cells at the venous anastomosis grow many extra layers of cells. These cells fill up the graft lumen, which means less blood can flow through the graft. See also: Intima.

Nephrologist (Nef-RAH-lo-jist)
A licensed doctor who specializes in kidney diseases.

Nephrology (Nef-RAH-lo-gee)
The study of kidneys.

Nephron (NEF-ron)
A tiny blood purification filter in the kidney, made up of a glomerulus and a tubule. Nephrons filter wastes from the body and keep electrolyte and fluid balance. Each kidney may have about a million nephrons.

Neuropathy
See: Peripheral Neuropathy.

Nocturnal Home Hemodialysis; NHHD (Nock-TER-nal Home He-mo-die-AL-uh-sis)
Hemodialysis done for 8 hours at night, while the patient sleeps at home, 3 to 6 nights per week. Most home hemodialysis programs require the patient to have a partner (who can sleep during the treatments). Both must successfully complete a few weeks of training. Dialysis needles and bloodlines are carefully taped to avoid line separation. Alarms may be used to detect blood. Longer NHHD treatments mean patients have fewer fluid and diet limits. Most need few or no blood pressure drugs. Since days are free, NHHD is work-friendly. Studies show that survival with this treatment is about the same as with deceased donor transplant.

Nocturnal In-Center Hemodialysis (Nock-TER-nal IN-sen-ter He-mo-die-AL-uh-sis)
In-center treatments done for 8 hours at night while the patient sleeps at the clinic. They are done by the clinic staff three nights per week, often from about 8 pm to about 4 am. The longer treatments allow for fewer fluid and diet limits. Most patients need few or no blood pressure drugs. Since the patient's days are free, this option is work-friendly. Studies find fewer hospital stays and better survival with this treatment than with standard in-center hemodialysis.

Normal Saline (Nor-mul SAY-leen)
A sterile salt water solution with 0.9% sodium chloride. This level is equal to the concentration of sodium chloride found in the blood. In hemodialysis, normal saline is used to prime and prepare the extracorporeal circuit. It may also be used for fluid replacement during the treatment.

Nosocomial (Nose-oh-COMB-ee-ul)
Hospital-acquired. The term is used for infections or illnesses patients get during the course of their medical treatment.

Opportunistic Illness (Opp-er-tune-IS-tick Ill-ness)
An illness that tends to occur only when a patient's immune system is impaired. Patients with AIDS, for example, are prone to these illnesses because their immune systems are weakened.

Organ Stunning (OR-gan STUN-ing)
Damage to the heart, brain, gut, and remaining kidney function due to lack of oxygen. This can occur when dialysis removes too much water from the blood, or removes it too quickly for a patient's body to adjust. The patient may have severe muscle cramps, a drop in blood pressure, headaches, nausea, vomiting, and/or chest pain. It may take hours or into the next day to feel well again. Organ stunning is a risk factor for sudden cardiac death—a leading cause of death on dialysis.

Orthostatic Hypotension (OR-tho-STAT-ick Hi-po-TEN-shun)
A drop in blood pressure of 15 mmHg or more that occurs when a person rises from sitting to standing.

Osmolality (Oz-mo-LAL-i-tee)
The total solute concentration of a solution.

Osmosis (Oz-MO-sis)
Movement of water across a semipermeable membrane from a lower solute concentration to a higher one. The movement goes on until the water level is the same on both sides. Osmosis alone is too slow to remove enough water for hemodialysis. So, water movement is aided by using a pump.

Osmotic Gradient (Oz-MOTT-ick GRAY-dee-ent)
A difference in the concentration of solutes on each side of a semipermeable membrane.

Osmotic Pressure (Oz-MOTT-ick PRESH-ur)
A gradient created by using dialysate that has substances—like glucose—that cause fluid to move out of the blood and into the dialysate.

Palpate (PAL-pate)
To examine by touching. Palpating the thrill over a vascular access is one way to know if the access is working (patent).

Palpitations (Pal-puh-TAY-shuns)
Occasional, strong heartbeats. They can be a symptom of cardiac arrhythmia.

Parathyroid Hormone; PTH (Pair-uh-THY-roid Hor-moan)
A hormone produced by the four parathyroid glands in the neck. PTH is released into the bloodstream in large amounts when calcium levels are low or phosphorus levels are high. Too much PTH can cause bone disease.

Patent (PAY-tent)
Open or not blocked. Before each dialysis treatment, patency of the patient's access is checked by listening for the bruit and feeling for the thrill.

Pathogen (PATH-oh-jen)
An agent (such as bacteria) that causes disease in humans.

Patient Outcomes (Pay-shent OUT-comes)
The results of care. Morbidity and mortality are common measures of outcomes. Others, such as the patient's self-rated physical and mental health, are important as well.

Percutaneous (Per-kyu-TAY-ne-us)
Through the skin.

Pericardial Effusion (Pair-ih-car-dee-ul Eff-YOU-shun)
A build-up of fluid in the pericardium, or sac around the heart. In severe cases, this can lead to cardiac tamponade, a life-threatening problem that occurs when fluid pressure makes it hard or even impossible for the heart to beat.

Pericarditis (Pair-ih-car-DIE-tis)
Inflammation of the pericardium, the sac around the heart. Patients with this may have a low-grade fever, low blood pressure, and pain in the center of the chest that may be relieved by sitting up and taking deep breaths. Patients who are uremic or poorly dialyzed may be prone to pericarditis.

Peripheral (Per-IF-er-ul)
Away from the center of the body. For example, peripheral vascular disease affects the limbs, not the core, of the body.

Glossary

Peripheral Neuropathy
(Per-IF-er-ul Noo-ROP-uh-thy)

Nerve damage in the hands and feet that can cause numbness, tingling, burning, pain, and weakness. Diabetes is a common cause. In dialysis patients, neuropathy may be caused by uremic toxins that are not well removed by standard in-center hemodialysis. It can also be caused by vascular access problems, that lead to poor dialysis. Getting more dialysis may help.

Peripheral Vascular Resistance
(Per-IF-er-ul VAS-kyu-lar Re-ZIS-tens)

A measure of how well blood can flow through the blood vessels. A drop in resistance (the blood vessels relax) will lower blood pressure if the heart can't make up for it. A rise in resistance (the blood vessels narrow) will raise blood pressure.

Peritoneal Dialysis; PD
(Pair-it-oh-NEE-ul Die-AL-uh-sis)

Use of the peritoneum as a semipermeable membrane to clean the blood. A surgeon places a catheter in the patient's abdomen or chest wall. The patient is taught to use the catheter to fill the belly with sterile dialysate. Wastes and excess water move from the blood and into the dialysate by diffusion and osmosis during a "dwell" time of a few hours. *See also:* Continuous Ambulatory Peritoneal Dialysis, Continuous Cycling Peritoneal Dialysis, Dwell Time, Peritoneum, Presternal Catheter.

Peritoneal Dialysis Adequacy
(Pair-it-oh-NEE-ul Die-AL-uh-sis AD-uh-kwa-see)

A measure of the treatment dose of peritoneal dialysis. The intent is to ensure that PD patients receive at least the minimum amount of treatment they need to live. The KDOQI guidelines set standards for adequacy and give tips for attaining them.

Peritoneum (Pair-it-oh-NEE-um)

A smooth, thin layer of blood-vessel-rich tissue that covers the inside of the abdominal walls. The peritoneum forms a closed sac. Thus, it can be used as a semipermeable membrane and container for dialysate.

Peritonitis (Pair-it-oh-NIGH-tiss)

An infection of the peritoneum that can occur when aseptic technique is not used for a PD exchange. Peritonitis may cause scarring of the membrane that can make further PD impossible.

Permeable (PER-me-uh-bull)

Allowing substances to pass through. Cell membranes in the body are freely permeable to water, letting it pass in and out. Dialyzer membranes are semipermeable. They let some substances through, but keep others out.

pH (Pee-aitch)

The hydrogen ion concentration of a solution. A solution with a pH above 7 is alkaline, or a base. A solution with a pH below 7 is an acid. A solution with a pH of 7.0 is neutral. Normal body pH ranges between 7.35 and 7.45—slightly alkaline. The pH of dialysate must be kept in a certain range. Bicarbonate-buffered dialysate should have a pH of 7.2 to prevent bacterial growth and scale that could harm equipment. AAMI recommends that water with a pH between 5.0 and 8.5 be used to mix dialysate.

Phosphate Binders (FOS-fate BIND-ers)

Drugs taken with each meal and snack that bind with phosphorous in food and keep it from being absorbed in the gut. The bound phosphorus is then removed in the stool. Patients should take more binders with larger meals and fewer binders with smaller meals or snacks.

Phosphorus (FOS-fer-us)

A non-metallic element. Found in dairy products, meat, poultry, fish, nuts, chocolate, and colas, it is hard to avoid. Too much phosphorus in the blood can cause itching and bone disease. Phosphorus blood levels are checked once a month. Most patients who do standard in-center hemodialysis need phosphate binders. More dialysis removes more phosphorus. Those who do nocturnal home hemodialysis may be able to eat more higher phosphorus foods or may need phosphate supplements instead of binders. *See also:* Secondary Hyperparathyroidism.

Plasma Refill Rate (PLAZ-ma RE-fill Rate)

The rate at which water removed from a patient's blood is replaced by water from in and between the cells. Removing water too quickly can cause blood pressure drops and organ stunning.

Plasticizer (PLAST-uh-size-er)

A chemical that makes plastic flexible. Priming the dialyzer and blood tubing before use with saline helps remove plasticizers that could harm patients.

Platelets (PLATE-lets)
Blood cells that promote clotting by clumping together when "activated" by signals sent by injured cells.

Pneumothorax (Noo-mo-THOR-ax)
Air in the chest that keeps the lungs from expanding. This can occur if a central venous catheter punctures a blood vessel and passes into the space between the lungs and chest wall.

Polycystic Kidney Disease; PKD
(PAH-lee-sis-tick KID-nee Dis-EEZ)
A genetic disease that causes large, fluid-filled cysts to grow in the kidneys, liver, and sometimes the brain. The cysts can become so large and numerous that they crowd out normal kidney tissue. This can cause kidney failure.

Pores (Porz)
Holes. In a semipermeable membrane, pores allow solutes of a certain size range to pass through, but trap larger ones. Dialyzer fibers contain pores, and so do the capillary blood vessels of the peritoneum. Membrane filters and reverse osmosis units also have pores.

Positional (Po-ZISH-uh-nal)
Affected by the patient's body position. When hemodialysis catheters are positional, blood flow can change when the patient moves. If the patient coughs or moves again, blood flow may improve if the catheter moves away from the blood vessel wall.

Positive Pressure (Poz-uh-tiv PRESH-ur)
Pressure greater than 0 mmHg. In dialysis, positive pressure is created when the blood pump pushes blood through the dialyzer. In the dialyzer, positive pressure helps to push fluid through the membrane pores. Positive pressure plus negative pressure equals transmembrane pressure (TMP).

Post- (Post)
After. A post-test is taken after a lesson.

Post-dialysis Pressure
See: Venous Pressure.

Post-Pump (Arterial) Pressure
See: Predialyzer Pressure.

Potassium (Po-TASS-ee-um)
A metallic element and electrolyte. Levels of potassium that are too high or too low can cause illness or death. See also: Hyperkalemia, Hypokalemia.

Pre- (Pree)
Before. A pre-test is taken before a lesson.

Precipitate
See: Scale.

Predialyzer Pressure
(Pre-DIE-uh-lie-zer PRESH-ur)
Positive pressure after the blood pump and before the dialyzer. It is also called post-pump pressure or post-pump arterial pressure.

Preprocessing (Pre-PROSS-ess-ing)
Putting a new dialyzer through all of the reprocessing steps before it is used for the first time. This helps remove substances used in manufacturing that might cause allergies.

Pre-Pump Arterial Pressure
(Pre-Pump Ar-TEER-ee-ul PRESH-ur)
Pressure measured between the patient's arterial needle and the blood pump. It represents the negative pressure created by the blood pump. Arterial pressure monitoring guards against too much suction on the vascular access.

Pressure (PRESH-ur)
Force applied by something that comes in contact with an object. In the body, blood pressure is the force from the heart and resistance in the blood vessels. In hemodialysis, pressure is the flow from the blood pump and resistance in the dialyzer and extracorporeal circuit.

Pressure Gradient
See: Transmembrane Pressure.

Pressure Testing (PRESH-ur Tes-ting)
Pressure or leak testing, ensures that a dialyzer membrane is intact and no blood loss will occur during reprocessing or the next use. Part of the reuse process.

Glossary

Presternal Catheter (Pre-STERN-ul CATH-uh-ter)
A catheter used in peritoneal dialysis that is placed in the patient's chest wall with the tip in the abdomen. The chest wall is thinner and less prone to infection than the abdomen. Presternal catheters can be a good choice for patients who are obese, have ostomies, are very active, or prefer tub baths. Certain parts of the U.S. use these catheters more than others.

Priming (PRIME-ing)
Flushing the bloodlines and dialyzer before a treatment. The process removes air, disinfectants, and some plasticizers. Normal saline is used to prime the bloodlines and blood compartment. Dialysate is used to prime the dialysate compartment.

Product Water (PRAH-duct Wa-ter)
Water that has been forced through a reverse osmosis membrane.

Proportioning System (Pro-POR-shun-ing sys-tem)
A system that will mix concentrate with treated water to make dialysate and send it to the dialyzer. There are two types: fixed-ratio and servo-controlled. Both use dual conductivity meters to check the mixed dialysate and support the system. Having two meters provides a backup in case one meter fails. *See also:* Hemodialysis Delivery System.

Proteinuria (Pro-tee-NUR-ee-uh)
Protein in the urine. When the kidneys are damaged, protein can leak through the glomeruli into the renal tubules, and then into the urine. *See also:* Microalbuminuria.

Proximal (PROX-uh-mal)
Near. In anatomy, proximal is near the center of the body (e.g., the shoulder is proximal to the hand).

Pruritus (Proo-RY-tiss)
Itching. This may occur in patients due to dry skin or a build-up of calcium phosphate crystals in the skin. Good dialysis, managing calcium and phosphorus, limiting hot water showers or bathtub soaks (which dry out skin), and use of some lotions or creams can help reduce pruritus.

Pseudoaneurysm (Soo-doh-AN-your-ism)
A false aneurysm: a bulging pocket of blood most often around a graft. It can occur if a graft has been damaged by repeated punctures in the same small area. A graft with a pseudoaneurysm may need to be repaired or replaced; rupture is a medical emergency.

Pulmonary Edema (Pul-mo-nair-ee Eh-DEE-ma)
Fluid build-up in the lungs. Fluid overload or failure to remove enough water during dialysis can cause pulmonary edema or make it worse. *See also:* Congestive Heart Failure.

Pump Occlusion (Pump Oh-KLU-shun)
The space between the blood pump rollers and the pump housing. The rollers should compress the blood tubing segment against the pump housing enough to close the lumen all the way. Overocclusion leads to high pressure that may crack the tubing. The pump segment could rupture. But, if occlusion is not complete, blood can flow backwards with each pump stroke.

Purpura (PER-pure-uh)
Bleeding under the skin. May be a symptom of too much heparin or a platelet problem.

Pyrogen (PIE-row-jen)
A fever-producing substance, such as endotoxin.

Pyrogenic Reaction (PIE-row-jen-ick Ree-ACK-shun)
A fever caused by pyrogens. Patients may have chills, shaking, fever, low blood pressure, vomiting, and muscle pain. A problem with water treatment or a reprocessed dialyzer that has endotoxin in it can cause this problem.

Radial Pulse (RAY-dee-ul Puls)
The pulse felt on the thumb side of the wrist.

Radiocephalic Fistula (RAY-dee-oh-sef-AL-ick FIS-chu-la)
Connects the radial artery and cephalic vein in the forearm; the most common type of AV fistula.

Reagent (Re-AY-jent)
A substance that reacts when a certain chemical is present. Reagent strips are used to be sure that all chemical residues are gone from a reprocessed dialyzer or the dialysis delivery system. They are also used to test for blood in dialysate.

Recirculation (Re-sirk-you-LAY-shun)
Dialyzed blood mixes with undialyzed blood in the patient's access. Blood going to the dialyzer is diluted with blood that just left the dialyzer. This can occur if there is retrograde flow through the access between the needles. Recirculation of more than 15% leads to poor dialysis.

Rejection (Re-JECK-shun)
The immune system of a transplant patient attacks the new organ, which is foreign to the body. A patient's blood and tissue type are matched to an organ to reduce this risk. Drugs that suppress the immune system are also used to help prevent rejection.

Reject Water (REE-ject Wa-ter)
The waste or reject stream that is sent to the drain, along with any solutes removed by reverse osmosis.

Renal Osteodystrophy (RE-nal Oss-tee-oh-DIS-tro-fee)
Bone disease caused by too-high or too-low levels of parathyroid hormone. See also: Secondary Hyperparathyroidism.

Renin-Angiotensin System (Ren-in An-gee-oh-TEN-sin Sys-tem)
A feedback loop in the body that helps control blood pressure. Renin is an enzyme made by healthy kidneys during stress. Renin combines with another substance to form angiotensin, a hormone that tightens the blood vessels to raise blood pressure.

Reprocessing (Re-PROSS-ess-ing)
Cleaning and disinfecting a dialyzer to be used again by the same patient. Reprocessing dialyzers saves money and helps keep some plastic out of the landfill. The hazardous chemicals used in reprocessing must be handled with care by staff. Rules are in place to protect patients and staff when reprocessed dialyzers are used.

Resistance (Re-ZISS-tense)
A force created by any factor that partly obstructs flow. In dialysis, there is resistance against the flow of blood in the blood vessels or in the extracorporeal circuit. Flow and resistance influence pressure.

Resistivity (Re-ziss-TIV-ih-tee)
A measure of the forces that oppose the flow of electricity through a fluid. See also: Conductivity.

Retrograde (RET-row-grade)
Against the direction of blood flow. In a fistula or graft, retrograde flow is backward, toward the anastomosis. The arterial needle may be placed either retrograde or antegrade in the access. One study suggests that antegrade may be a better choice.

Reuse
Using the patient's reprocessed dialyzer for his or her next dialysis treatment. See: Reprocessing.

Reverse Osmosis; RO (Re-VERS Oz-MO-sis)
A membrane separation process to take solutes out of water. An RO unit is a cartridge that holds a water pressure pump and a semipermeable membrane. The membrane can remove 95% to 99% or more of bacteria, endotoxin, viruses, salts, particles, and dissolved organics. RO is used to treat water for hemodialysis or reprocessing. RO membranes are costly and fragile. To avoid damage, filters are used to remove particles in feed water before the RO membrane.

Rinseback (Rins-back)
Using saline to flush the patient's blood back into the body after dialysis to minimize blood loss.

Roller Pump (Roll-er Pump)
The most common type of blood pump. A motor turns the roller head, pushing blood through the extracorporeal circuit. See also: Pump Occlusion.

Rope Ladder Technique
See: Needle Site Rotation.

Saline Infusion Line (Say-leen In-FU-jun Line)
A line that allows saline to be given to the patient during dialysis. It is connected to the arterial blood tubing segment just before the blood pump so saline can be pulled into the circuit.

Glossary

Scale (Skayl)
Solid particles that settle out of a solution (e.g., water, dialysate) and can clog pipes or harm parts of the water treatment system. Hard water, which has more minerals and salts, can form scale.

Secondary Hyperparathyroidism
(Sec-on-dare-ee Hi-per-pair-uh-THY-roid-ism)

Release of too much parathyroid hormone (PTH) that can lead to bone disease. With too much PTH in the blood, calcium is pulled out of the bones, making them weak. The condition is treated with phosphate binders and calcitriol to reduce PTH, calcium, and phosphorus levels.

Seizure (SEE-zur)
Involuntary muscle spasm and loss of consciousness. Some patients may have seizure disorders. Or, seizures can be a side effect of too-high blood pressure, wrong dialysate, or chemical exposure.

Semipermeable Membrane
(Sem-eye-per-me-uh-bull MEM-brain)

A membrane with microscopic pores that let some substances (such as water) pass through freely, but hold others (such as red blood cells) back. The membrane's pore size affects dialysis efficiency.

Sepsis (SEP-siss)
A life-threatening infection from bacteria that enter the bloodstream. Also called septicemia or bacteremia.

Serum (See-rum)
Blood plasma without the clotting factors. The clear liquid that can be separated from blood after it clots. Many blood tests are run on serum, such as tests for calcium and phosphorus.

Short Daily Home Hemodialysis
(Short DAY-lee Home He-mo-di-AL-uh-sis)

Two and a half to four-hour treatments done at home 5–7 days per week. The patient must complete a few weeks of training. The more frequent treatments mean that patients have fewer fluid and diet limits. Most need few blood pressure drugs. Because the treatments are done on the patient's own schedule, short daily home hemodialysis is work-friendly. Studies show that survival with this treatment is about the same as with deceased donor transplant. While most people who use this option have a partner, the U.S. FDA removed the partner requirement in 2017 for daytime treatments. Patients who do not have partners but can learn and do the treatments themselves now have this option.

Shunt (Shunt)
A tube inserted into the body to move fluid from one place to another. A shunt was the first permanent vascular access used for dialysis in 1960 by Drs. Scribner and Quinton. A Teflon® tube was used to connect a length of Silastic® tubing to a patient's artery and vein. This created a vascular access that could be used for multiple treatments. For the first time, patients with chronic kidney failure could receive dialysis. Since the shunt was outside the skin, it easily became infected or clotted, and is no longer used in the U.S.

Sieving Coefficient; SC (SIV-ing co-ee-FISH-ent)
The amount of solute removed from a solution by convection (solvent drag).

Sodium (SO-dee-um)
An element and an electrolyte. It causes fluid to move across the cell membranes between the intracellular and extracellular spaces. Sodium is present in dialysate, and the amount must be correct. Too little can cause hemolysis; too much can cause crenation.

Sodium Modeling (So-dee-um MOD-el-ing)
Changing the level of sodium in the dialysate during the treatment to remove more water. A doctor's prescription is needed. Most often, the patient starts treatment at a high sodium level, which is then slowly reduced. If the ultrafiltration rate is higher than about 400 mL/hour (the "capillary refill rate"), blood pressure will drop in most patients. Most clinics no longer use sodium modeling, as it *adds* sodium to the blood. Higher blood sodium levels make patients thirsty so they drink more and gain more water weight between treatments.

Solute (SOLL-yute)
A particle dissolved in fluid. Many of the wastes that need to be removed from the blood of kidney patients (such as urea) are solutes. Solute size is measured by molecular weight. Different membranes are more or less efficient at removing solutes of a certain size.

Solution (Sol-OO-shun)
A combination of a solvent (fluid) and a solute.

Solvent (SOL-vent)
A fluid in which substances are dissolved, e.g., water.

Solvent Drag (Sol-vent DRAG)
Molecules of a dissolved substance are dragged along in a solvent that passes through a semipermeable membrane. Solvent drag is also called convection, or convective solute transfer.

Spore (Spor)
The reproductive form of bacteria, fungi, and algae. They are very resistant to heat. Bleach can kill many types of spores. *See also:* Bacteria, Disinfectant, Heat Disinfection.

Standard In-Center Hemodialysis (Stan-dard in-cent-er he-mo-die-AL-uh-sis)
Treatments done in a hospital or clinic three times a week. Clinic staff do the treatments, though some patients may take their own vital signs, place their own needles, and monitor their own treatments. Leading doctors now say that standard treatments should always be at least 4 hours long. They replace only 12–15% of normal kidney function, which is the same level as stage 5 chronic kidney disease. Patients who do these treatments are 50% more likely to die from sudden heart failure on the day after the 2-day no treatment weekend.

Standard Home Hemodialysis (Stan-dard Home he-mo-die-AL-uh-sis)
Dialysis treatments done three days a week or every other day by the patient and a partner at home. The patient and partner are trained for a few weeks. Since the patient can dialyze on his or her schedule, this treatment is work-friendly.

Standing Orders (Stan-ding OR-ders)
Orders that stay the same. They are written by the doctor to meet patients' common treatment needs. The orders should include all aspects of patient care (i.e., blood flow rate, dialysate flow rate, dialyzer, and dialysate composition).

Steal Syndrome (STEEL sin-drum)
A problem that occurs when a fistula or graft "steals" too much blood away from the distal part of the limb (hand or foot). When the access is in use, some of the patient's blood bypasses the hand or foot and goes through the extracorporeal circuit instead. The loss of blood flow (ischemia) can harm tissue. Signs of steal syndrome include coldness, poor function, and even gangrene if it is not treated promptly.

Stenosis (Sten-OH-sis)
Narrowing of a blood vessel. Stenosis slows the flow of blood and causes turbulence inside the vessel. This sets the stage for more serious problems, such as thrombosis.

Stent (Stent)
A small, expanding metal mesh tube held open by rings that can be placed in a blood vessel to help keep the lumen open. A stent may be used to help keep a fistula or graft patent. *See also:* Patent.

Glossary

Sterilant (STAIR-uh-lent)
A germ-killing solution. Sterilants are used in reprocessing dialyzers.

Sterile (STAIR-ul)
Free of all living organisms (bacteria, viruses, microorganisms).

Sterile Technique
See: Aseptic Technique.

Sterilization (STAIR-ul-iz-ay-shun)
A way to destroy bacteria with chemicals or heat.

Subclavian Catheter (Sub-CLAY-vee-an Cath-uh-ter)
A catheter placed in the subclavian vein. The internal jugular vein is preferred, because it is less likely to cause central venous stenosis.

Subcutaneous (Sub-kyu-TAIN-ee-us)
Under the skin. Some medications, such as Lidocaine®, a local anesthetic, are injected subcutaneously.

Surface Area (SIR-fiss ar-ee-uh)
The amount of membrane in direct contact with blood and dialysate. A larger surface area (in hemodialysis or peritoneal dialysis) allows more diffusion. Large surface area dialyzers tend to have more urea clearance. See also: Diffusion.

Systemic (Sis-TEM-ic)
Affecting the entire body. For example, sepsis is a systemic infection.

Systolic (Sis-TOL-ic)
The pressure inside the arteries during a heartbeat. It is the top number of a blood pressure reading. See also: Diastolic.

Target Weight (TAR-get Weight)
Also called "dry weight," this is a patient's weight without excess fluid. When dry weight is reached, there are no signs of fluid overload or dehydration. Breathing is normal, with no signs of fluid in the lungs. And, blood pressure is normal for the patient (not too high or too low). "Target weight" is the goal weight for a given dialysis treatment and is most often determined by the dry weight.

Temperature Alarm (TEM-per-a-cher A-larm)
An indicator that the dialysate temperature is too high or too low. Dialysate that is too hot can cause hemolysis. Too-cool dialysate can cause patient discomfort and reduce the efficiency of the treatment.

Temporary Catheters (TEM-po-ra-ree Cath-uh-ters)
A central venous catheter used for short-term vascular access, for example, when a fistula has not matured. Temporary catheters may be stitched, or sutured, in place.

Thrill (Thrill)
The vibration of blood flowing through the patient's fistula or graft. It can be felt by touching a patient's access.

Thrombectomy (Throm-BECK-to-mee)
Surgery or drug treatment (i.e., with a clot-dissolving drug) to remove a thrombus, or blood clot.

Thrombolysis (Throm-BALL-uh-sis)
The process of injecting a drug to dissolve a thrombus. Surgery may be needed after thrombolysis.

Thrombosis (Throm-BO-sis)
Formation of a thrombus, or blood clot is the most common cause of access failure. Early thrombosis in a graft or fistula is most often caused by surgical problems with the anastomosis. Or, it can be caused by twisting of the vessel or graft.

Thrombus (THROM-bus)
A clot formed in a blood vessel or a blood passage. A clot may occur when platelets are activated by contact with damaged blood vessel walls, dialyzer materials, or from turbulence inside a blood vessel.

Total Cell Volume (TCV)
See: Fiber Bundle Volume.

Total Parenteral Nutrition; TPN (To-tal Pa-RENT-er-al Nu-TRISH-un)
A form of intravenous feeding. It provides nutrients to patients who can't eat or absorb food through their gastrointestinal tracts. Interdialytic parenteral nutrition (IDPN) is TPN given only during dialysis.

Transducer Protectors (Trans-DEW-sir Pro-TEC-tors)

Small plastic caps with filters inside. They keep blood or fluid from getting into the pressure monitors on the dialysis machine. The transducer protectors are connected to the arterial and/or venous pressure monitors. The monitoring lines are connected to the transducer protectors.

Transmembrane Pressure; TMP (Trans-Mem-brane PRESH-ur)

Blood side pressure plus dialysate side pressure across the dialyzer membrane. To keep dialysate from moving into the bloodstream, pressure on the blood side must be equal to or more than that of the dialysate side.

Trendelenburg Position (Tren-DELL-en-burg Pos-ISH-un)

Putting the patient's head at a 45° incline, with his or her legs up. This helps relieve low blood pressure by bringing more blood to the brain. Patients who may have an air embolism should be placed in Trendelenburg position on their left side.

Ultrafilter (UL-tra-fil-ter)

A membrane filter that removes very small particles. It is the most effective water treatment component for removing endotoxin.

Ultrafiltration; UF (Ul-tra-fil-TRAY-shun)

Filtration caused by a pressure gradient between two sides of a filter. The rate of UF depends on the transmembrane pressure and aspects of the dialyzer.

Ultrafiltration Rate; UFR (Ul-tra-fil-TRAY-shun Rate)

The rate at which fluid moves from the blood into the dialysate through the membrane. This rate depends on transmembrane pressure and aspects of the membrane. UFR is calculated by dividing the amount of fluid to be removed by the minutes of treatment. In UF control or volumetric machines, dialysate in flow and out flow are kept in exact balance with special pumps. *See also:* Transmembrane Pressure.

Ultraviolet Light; UV (Ul-tra-VI-oh-let light)

A form of invisible radiation. UV light can destroy microbes by changing their DNA so they cannot grow. Some microbes are more sensitive to UV light than others. UV light is generated by a mercury vapor lamp housed inside a quartz sleeve that emits light at a specific wavelength. Feed water flows over the quartz and is exposed to the UV light.

Urea Kinetic Modeling; UKM (You-REE-uh Kin-et-ic MOD-ul-ing)

A formula used to assess if a patient's dialysis is adequate, based on change in the level of urea in the blood. The results of UKM are described as Kt/V. K is the dialyzer urea clearance in mL/min, t is treatment time in minutes, and V is the volume of blood in the body. *See also:* Hemodialysis Adequacy.

Uremia (You-REE-me-uh)

A build-up of wastes in the blood that occurs in the last stage of kidney failure or in patients who do not get enough dialysis. Patients with uremia may have yellow-gray skin, edema, high blood pressure, flu-like symptoms, trouble breathing, fatigue, weakness, and mental changes. If a patient on dialysis has these symptoms, more dialysis is needed.

Vascular Access (Vas-kyu-lar AX-ess)

A way to gain repeated entry to the patient's bloodstream for hemodialysis. A vascular access must permit high-enough blood flow rates to ensure effective dialysis. There are three types of access. A fistula is a surgical connection between a patient's artery and a vein and is the preferred type of access. A graft connects an artery and vein with a piece of man-made vein. A catheter is a plastic tube placed into a central vein and is the least preferred access, because of the high risk of infection. The vascular access is the patient's lifeline. Great care must be taken to protect it through good cannulation and either needle site rotation or use of the Buttonhole technique.

Vasoconstrict (Vay-zo-con-STRICT)

To tighten the blood vessels.

Vasoconstrictor (Va-zo-con-STRICT-or)

A drug that causes the blood vessels to constrict.

Vein (Vane)

A blood vessel that carries blood back to the heart.

Glossary

Venipuncture (VEEN-ih-punk-shure)

Inserting a needle into a blood vessel. Skilled and gentle venipuncture prolongs access life, enhances comfort, and helps ensure that the patient will get a good treatment. It is vital to rotate sites or use the Buttonhole technique to avoid aneurysms or pseudo-aneurysms. *See also:* Buttonhole Technique, Needle Site Rotation.

Venous Pressure (VEE-nis PRESH-ur)

The measurement of the extra-corporeal blood circuit pressure after the dialyzer and before the blood goes back into the patient's body. It may also be called post-dialyzer pressure.

Venous Pressure High/Low Alarm (VEE-nis PRESH-ur Hi-Lo A-larm)

An alarm that monitors pressure from the monitoring site to the patient's venous puncture site.

Virus (VIE-rus)

A microorganism that must obtain energy and food from other living cells. Many diseases, such as the common cold, measles, polio, and HIV, are caused by viruses. Though tiny, viruses are too large to cross an intact dialyzer membrane. If the membrane is damaged, viruses in the water could enter the patient's blood. Viruses can be killed by a number of chemicals.

Volumetric (Vol-you-MET-rick)

Volume-measuring. Most dialysate delivery systems use fluid-balancing systems. These compare the volume of dialysate going into and out of the dialyzer. These systems make it possible to precisely remove the prescribed amount of fluid.

Water Softener (Wa-ter-SOF-en-er)

A device to reduce the levels of calcium and magnesium that form scale. Water softeners work by ion exchange. Ions of calcium and magnesium are removed from the water by a bed of electrically charged resin beads. They are traded for sodium ions, which form sodium chloride.

Index

A

AAKP (American Association of Kidney Patients), 73
AAMI (Association for the Advancement of Medical Instrumentation), 10, 112, 275–277, 297–299
abscesses, 159, 185, 333
access. *See* vascular access
acetic acid/acetate, 111, 296
acid concentrate, 112, 225–226, 246
acid-base balance, 24. *See also* pH
acids, 333. *See also* pH
acronyms, 326–332
    to avoid when charting, 225
    active listening, 64–65
    acute kidney failure, 24–25
    adequacy
        definition of, 265, 333, 345
        dialyzer clearance factors, 266
        HD, 121
        measuring, 264–267
        patient well-being and, 267
        PD, 354
        time factors, 267
adsorption, 86, 333
advance directives, 333
AIDS (acquired immune deficiency syndrome), 215–216, 333
air detectors, 128–129, 247, 333
air embolisms, 333
AKF (American Kidney Fund), 73
alarms. *See* monitors and alarms
albumin, 25, 38, 333, 351
alcohol hand rub, 212
alkalis (bases), 24, 83–84, 285, 335
allergic reactions, 104, 248–249
alum, 333
aluminum-related bone disease (ARBD), 298, 333
amyloidosis, 34–35, 47, 334
anaphylaxis, 248–249, 334
anastomosis, 151, 152, 156, 157, 334
anemia, 30–31, 334. *See also* bleeding problems; iron deficiency
anesthetics, 334
aneurysms, 179, 334
angina, 249
angioplasty, 181, 334
angiotensin, 24, 357
ANSI/AAMI standards, 138, 140–141, 275–277, 293, 297–299
antegrade placement, 163, 175, 334
anticoagulation, 245–246. *See also* thrombosis
    definition of, 334
antiseptics, 334
anxiety, 63
APD (automated PD), 44–45, 335
apical pulse, 334
apnea, 36, 334
ARBD (aluminum-related bone disease), 298, 333
area cannulation, 172, 179, 334
arm elevation test, 158
arrhythmia, 250, 334. *See also* myocardial infarction
arsenic, 299, 300
arterial pressure, 168–169, 334
arterializing, 152, 335
arteries, 22, 335
arterioles, 23
arteriovenous fistulas, definition of, 335. *See also* fistulas
arteriovenous grafts. *See* grafts
artificial kidneys. *See* dialyzers (artificial kidneys)
ascites, 335
aseptic technique, 211–212, 220, 335
attitude of patients, 66
auscultation, 335. *See also* thrill, bruit, and pulse
automated PD (APD), 44–45, 335
AV grafts. *See* grafts
AVF (arteriovenous fistulas). *See* fistulas

B

B. Braun Adimea, 110
back-eye needles, 162
backfiltration, 107, 234, 335
backflow prevention device, 287
back-up clinics, 312–313, 316
backwashing, 281, 287, 290–291, 335
bacteremia. *See* sepsis
bacteria, 335. *See also* infection
    ANSI/AAMI standards, 276
    antibiotic-resistant, 216–217
    biofilm, 276, 296
    blood cultures, 38
    endotoxins, 277, 296
    Gram-negative, 276, 345
    testing for, 295–296
barium, 299, 300
bases (alkalis), 24, 83–84, 285, 335
Baxter (Gambro) Diascan, 110
bedbugs, 70, 217–218
belief, 68
beta-2 microglobulin (β_2M), 265, 298
bevel, 218
bibag Online dry bicarbonate concentrate, 115
bicarbonate, 111, 335
bicarbonate concentrate, 24, 112, 115, 225–226
BiCart cartridge, 115
binders, phosphate. *See* phosphate binders
biocompatibility, 86, 94, 104–105, 136, 335
biofilm, 276, 296
biologic grafts, 173
"black blood syndrome," 178
bleach, 250, 296
bleeding problems, 36–37, 128, 177, 178. *See also* exsanguination
    dialysis technicians' role in, 37
    first aid for access ruptures, 177
blood, 88, 111
blood clots. *See* thrombosis
blood flow, 104, 192
    countercurrent flow, 339
blood leak detectors, 122, 336
    monitors and alarms, 116–117, 177
blood leaks, definition of, 336
blood loss. *See* bleeding problems
blood oxygen level, 232
blood pressure. *See also* arterial pressure; hypertension (high blood pressure); hypotension (low blood pressure)
    automated readings, 122, 231
        cuff sizes, 231
        kidney functions, 24
        manual readings, 231–232
        monitoring, 242
        risk of drop in, 93
        sites, 232
        taking, 230–232
blood pumps, 124–125, 336. *See also* pump occlusion
blood tests, 38–39, 122, 239–241. *See also* BUN (blood urea nitrogen)
blood components, 37
blood sample tubes, 240
    centrifuging samples, 249–240
    drawing blood, 239–241
    water quality and, 299
blood transfusions, to treat anemia, 31
blood tubing. *See* bloodlines
blood vessels, 22–23, 156. *See also* fistulas; grafts
blood volume monitoring, 129
bloodborne diseases, 214–216
blood–brain barrier, 92
bloodlines (blood tubing), 226–227, 246, 336
    definition of, 189
    troubleshooting problems, 244, 262
body, human, fluid compartments in, 87
body image, 62, 156
body mechanics, 220–223
body temperature, 116. *See also* fever
    taking patients' temperature, 232–233
body weight. *See* target (dry) weight; water weight; weight measurement
bolus, definition of, 336
bone disorders, 33–34, 298, 333, 357, 358
BONENT (Board of Nephrology Examiners Nursing and Technology), 15
bowel control, 70
Bowman's capsule, 23
brachial pulse, 336
brachiobasilic fistulas, 155–156
brachiocephalic fistulas, 155–156, 336
brain stunning, 32
brain swelling, 92, 253
brine, definition of, 336
bruising. *See* ecchymosis
bruit. *See* thrill, bruit, and pulse
bubble traps. *See* drip chambers
buffers, 337. *See also* pH
buildings, during emergencies, 315, 317
BUN (blood urea nitrogen)

Index

blood tests, 38
    definition of, 336
    drawing BUN samples, 265–266
    reasons for measuring, 265
    slow-flow method, 266
    stop-dialysate flow method, 266
butterfly tape technique, 167–168
buttonhole technique, 162, 165–168, 198–205
    aneurysms and, 179
    definition of, 337
    How-To Manual, 198–205
bypass, definition of, 337
bypass mode, 111, 115–117, 228–229, 266–267

C

cadmium, 299, 300
calcification, extraskeletal, 343
calciphylaxis (calcific uremic arteriolopathy), 29
calcitriol (active vitamin D), 24
calcium, 29, 57–58, 111, 297, 337
    blood tests, 38, 39
"call trees," 310–311
calorie intake, 52–53
cannulas. See shunts
cannulation, 152, 239. See also needles; self-cannulation
    area cannulation, 172, 179, a
    avoiding needle stick injuries, 165
    definition of, 337
    for fistulas, 157, 158, 161–168
    for grafts, 174–175
    patient input, 204–205
    practicing, 164
    re-touching a needle site, 160
    site problems, 160
    three-point cannulation, 166
    touch cannulation, 167, 202
CAPD (continuous ambulatory PD), 44, 339
capillaries, 22, 337
carbon tanks, 278, 282–283, 291, 318
    definition of, 337
cardiac arrest, 251, 337
cardiac output, 184
    definition of, 337
cardiac "stunning," 252
carpal tunnel syndrome, 34
carrying and lifting, 220–221
catabolism, 337
catheters, 153–154, 187–191
    care of, 189
    catheter loss, 192
    central venous stenosis, 192
    changing dressings, 191
    checking before treatment, 189
    chevron, 168, 244
    cleaning before use, 189–191
    complications, 191–192
    connection, 189–190
    cuffed, tunneled catheters, 153–154, 340
        definition of, 189, 337
        disconnection, 190–191, 192
        drawing blood from, 240
    exit sites, 189
    femoral, 153, 188–189
    FFCL (Fistula First Catheter Last), 186, 194, 195
    infection, 191
    line reversals, 190
    locking solution, 240
    lumens (catheter chambers), 187, 350
    non-tunneled catheters, 154
    patient teaching, 190
    placement, 187
    pros and cons, 154
    slow blood flow rate, 192
    starting HD with, 189–191
    veins used for, 188–189
CathGuard, 191
CBNT (Certified in Biomedical Nephrology Technology) Exams, 15
CCHT (Certified Clinical Hemodialysis Technician) Exam, 14
CCHT-A (Certified Clinical Hemodialysis Technician - Advanced) Exam, 15
CCNT (Certified in Clinical Nephrology Technology), 15
CCPD (continuous cycling PD), 44–45, 339
CCRT, 339
CDC (Centers for Disease Control and Prevention), 10, 210
    resources, 74, 194, 214
CDWS (Certified Dialysis Water Specialists) Exam, 16
cellulose, definition of, 338
cellulose membranes, 104–105
Centers for Dialysis Care, UF management program, 238
central venous stenosis, 180, 192, 338
centrifuges, 249–240
certification, for dialysis technicians, 14–16
chair-to-chair transfers, 222
charting, 223–224
    abbreviations, symbols, and acronyms to avoid, 225
    correcting errors, 224
chemical contaminants, 275–276, 297–299
chemical disinfection, 264
chest pain (angina), 249
chills, 254–255
chloramines, 297, 338
chlorides, 111–112, 338
chlorine, 250, 282, 292, 296–297, 318
    definition of, 338
    testing for, 296–297
chromium, 299, 300
chronic kidney disease, definition of, 338. See also kidney disease
CHT (Certified Hemodialysis Technician) Exam, 15
citric acid/citrate, 111
concentrate, 246
germicide, 142, 143
CKD. See kidney disease
"clean" areas, 214, 219
cleaning equipment, 264
clearance, 107–109, 110, 183, 266, 338
clinical complications, 247–260
clinics
    budgeting, 8
    "dirty" areas in, 214
    effect of PPS on, 8
clinics, during emergencies, 311–313, 315–316
Clostridium Difficile (C. Diff), 217
clots. See thrombosis
CMS (Centers for Medicare & Medicaid Services). See also Medicare
    on "clean" areas, 219
    Conditions for Coverage, 7, 210, 275–277, 308, 316, 339
    emergency diet plan and, 324
    FFCL (Fistula First Catheter Last), 186, 194, 195
    QIP (Quality Incentive Program), 8, 10
    on UF rate, 32
CNNT (Council of Nephrology Nurses and Technicians), 14
coagulation. See anticoagulation; thrombosis
coefficient of ultrafiltration (KUF), 338
collateral circulation, 178
collecting tubules, 23
communicable diseases, 209. See also bloodborne diseases; pathogens
communication, 64–65. See also confidentiality; patient education
    emergency plan, 310–311
complement activation, 106
computers, electronic charting, 224
concentrates, 24, 112, 115, 225–226, 246
    definition of, 338
concentration, measures of, 83
concentration gradient. See gradient, definition of
Conditions for Coverage. See CMS
conductive solute transfer. See diffusion
conductivity, 111, 115, 339
confidentiality, 14, 64, 71–72
congestive heart failure (CHF), 156, 339
constant-site cannulation. See buttonhole technique
contamination, 300–302. See also bacteria; green dialysis; water
    bacterial, 276, 296
    chemical, 273, 275–276, 297–299
    definition of, 212, 339
    environmental, 214
    equipment after treatment, 214
continence, 70
continuous cycling PD, 44–45
continuous renal replacement therapy (CRRT), 339
convection, 85, 94, 98
clearance, 108
copper, 298–299
countercurrent flow, 104, 339
courtesy, 12–13
CPR, 71–72
CQI (continuous quality improvement), 11–12, 192-193, 339

Index

cramps, 259
CRE (Carbapenem-Resistant Enterobacteriaceae), 217
creatinine, 25, 38, 340
crenation, 340
Crit-Line Technology, 129
CROWNWeb, 340
CROWNWeb data collection, 194
cuffed, tunneled catheters, 153–154, 340
CVInsight, 129
cyanosis, 298, 340
cysts, kidney, 27

D

daily home HD, 47–48
daily self-care treatment. See PD
dalton, definition of, 91
deaths, 25, 252. See also exsanguination; survival rates
    air in bloodstream, 128
    allergic reactions, 104
    cause of by month on dialysis, 236
    clinical complications, 252
    coping with, 71–72
dialysate mistakes, 111
dialysis water quality, 273, 285, 297–299
    electrolyte levels and, 28, 57–58
    emergency planning and, 307, 313
    first-year mortality rates, 236
    foregoing dialysis, 48
    infection, 185, 191, 209
    "killer gap," 46
    malnutrition, 267
    new patients, 51, 54, 236
    water removal calculations and, 234–235
dehydration, 118, 234–235, 340
deionization (DI) systems, 283, 285, 292–293, 340
    resistivity meters, 292–293
    water quality analysis, 293
delivery systems, 112–114, 346
depression, 4, 42, 59–60, 63
devices. See equipment and supplies
diabetes, 26–27
diabetic nephropathy, 340
dialysate, 111–112. See also concentrates; electrolyte balance; water
    analysis devices, 122
    conductivity, 111
    countercurrent flow, 104, 339
    definition of, 340
    delivery, 113–114, 346
    dialysate circuit, 113
    in HD, 88–89
    mixing and testing, 112, 113, 225–226
    monitoring guidelines, 295
    in PD, 97
    pressure, 95
    substances in, 111
    temperature of, 90
dialysis, 3–6, 41–48. See also HD (hemodialysis); kidney disease; PD (peritoneal dialysis); quality
    before and after Medicare, 7
    challenges in, 70–72
    definition of, 341
    doctor's prescription, 224, 226
    guidelines for care, 9–10
    helping patients cope, 59–63
    normal kidney function compared to, 41
    as partial kidney replacement, 4–6
    post-dialysis procedures, 263–264
    predialysis procedures, 224–227
    principles of, 80–98
    special challenges, 70–72
dialysis adequacy. See adequacy
dialysis clinics. See clinics
dialysis dementia. See encephalopathy
dialysis disequilibrium syndrome (DDS), 92, 253, 341
dialysis emergencies. See emergency planning and response
dialysis environment, 2–16. See also quality
    overview of kidney failure and dialysis, 3–6
    payment for dialysis and transplant, 6–8
Dialysis Patient Citizens (DPC), 73
dialysis technicians
    in care team, 50
    certification, 14–16
    groups for, 14
    helping patients cope, 59–63
    online technician discussions, 14
    professionalism, 12–14
    role in patient nutrition, 53, 55
    roles in condition management, 29–37
dialysis water. See water
dialysis-related amyloidosis (DRA), 34–35, 47, 334
dialyzer membranes. See also clearance
    biocompatibility, 104
    Mass Transfer Coefficient, 109
    materials, 104–105
    patient reactions to, 105–106
    pores, 88–89, 107
    surface area, 106
dialyzer reprocessing, 134–147
    automated versus manual, 139
    definition of, 357
    dialyzer efficiency and, 138
    disinfection, 141, 142
    documentation for, 145–146
    germicide removal, 137–138, 144–145
    handling hazardous materials, 142–143
    history of, 135–136
    inspecting, 144, 145
    labeling, 138, 139–140
    medical risks of, 137
    post-dialysis procedures, 264
    pre-cleaning, 140–141
    preparation, 139–140, 144–145, 264
    preprocessing, 140
    QA & QC, 145–147
    reasons for reuse, 136
    reuse statistics, 136
    rinsebacks, 140, 263, 357
    rules for, 138–139
    safety of reuse, 136–138
    storage, 144
    systems diagram, 138
dialyzers (artificial kidneys), 103–110. See also clearance; dialyzer reprocessing; hollow fiber dialyzers
    definition of, 341
    diffusion and, 89–90
    filters, 45
    labeling, 139–140
    post-dialysis procedures, 264
    preparing for first use, 139–140
    priming and recirculation, 227
    rejecting, 142
    setting up dialyzer and bloodlines, 226–227
    testing performance, 141
diarrhea, 53, 58, 106, 216, 217, 229, 239
diastolic blood pressure, 230, 242, 341
diet. See food and drink
dietitians, 50–51, 322
diffusion (conductive solute transfer), 84–85, 88–89, 97, 108, 341
"dirty" areas in clinic, 214
disasters. See emergency planning and response
disinfectants, 141–142, 264, 290, 296, 302, 341
disposal of waste. See waste disposal
distal (far) convoluted tubule, 23
distal, definition of, 341
diuretics, 341
do not resuscitate (DNR) orders, 71–72
doctor's prescription, 224, 226
documentation, 145–146, 223–224, 264
    acronyms to avoid, 225
    definition of, 341
DOPPS (Dialysis Outcomes and Practice Patterns Study), 10, 72
DOQI (Dialysis Outcomes Quality Initiative), 9
drink. See food and drink
drinking water. See water
drip chambers, 123, 245, 341
dry cannulation, 164
dry ultrafiltration. See isolated ultrafiltration
dry weight. See target (dry) weight
dwell time, 5, 136, 342
dyspnea, 342

E

ecchymosis, 245, 342
edema (swelling), 55, 230, 342. See also water weight
    pulmonary, 51, 356
education. See patient education
efferent arteriole, 23
EGHP (employer group health plans), 7
electrolyte balance, 24, 27–29, 57–58
electrolyte definition of, 342
electronic charting, 224

Index

ELISIO dialzyer, 106
embolisms, 333
emergency disconnection, 313–314
emergency food kits, 324
Emergency Manager (EM), 312, 315
    emergency planning and response, 306–324
    buildings, 315, 317, 318
    clinic-level events, 311–313
    CMS Conditions for Coverage, 308
    disaster-related stress, 318–320
emergency menu and diet plan, 322–324
Emergency Preparedness plan, 310
emotional recovery after a disaster, 318–320
    local and state rules, 308
    objectives, 306
    organizations, 321
    patient education, 314–315
    quality improvement (QI), 319–320
    recovering from emergencies, 316–319
    regulations and oversight, 308–309
    resources, 321
    types of emergencies, 310
EMLA (lidocaine-based cream), 170
emotional health, asking about, 233–234
empathy, 60–61
employment, of patients, 68–69
empty bed contact time (EBCT), 283, 342
encephalopathy (dialysis dementia), 298, 342
endocrine functions, 24, 342, 347
endotoxins, 117, 277, 296, 342
end-stage renal disease. *See* ESRD
environmental contamination. *See* contamination; green dialysis
EPA (Environmental Protection Agency)
    drinking water standard, 273–274, 276, 300–302
equilibrium, 342
equipment and supplies. *See also* disinfectants; sterile items
    damage to, 315
    emergency resources, 317–318, 321
    post-dialysis handling of, 213–214, 264
    pre-dialysis set-up, 225–229
equivalent, definition of, 91
erythropoietin (EPO), 24, 30, 343
ESAs (erythrocyte stimulating agents), 31
ESRD (end-stage renal disease), 25
    definition of, 342
ESRD Networks, 9
    contact information for National Forum, 321
    CPMs project, 194
    definition of, 343
    dialysis experience before and after, 7
    KCER work with, 308–309
    Quality Improvement Initiative, 10
    resources, 74
    support for FFCL, 195
ESRD Program, 9. *See also* Medicare

estimated dry weight. *See* target (dry) weight
ethyl chloride "skin freezing" spray, 169, 171
ethylene oxide, 343
evacuations, 310, 312, 314, 317
evaluating the patient. *See* patient evaluation
exchange, definition of, 343
excretory functions, 23, 343
exercise, 69
exsanguination, 128, 177–179, 187, 192, 203, 243, 253–254. *See also* bleeding problems; deaths
    buttonhole technique and, 203
    definition of, 343
extracellular, definition of, 343
extracorporeal circuit, 122–129
    blood pumps, 124–125
    blood tubing, 122–123
    definition of, 343
    heparin pumps, 125–126
    safety monitors, 126–129, 343
    transducer protectors, 123–124
    venous line clamps, 126
extraskeletal calcification, 343
eyewear, protective, 213

F

face shields, 213
false aneurysms, 179–180
family members, in care team, 49–50
FDA (Food and Drug Administration), 10
feed water, 278, 280–282, 284–285, 287, 293, 318, 343. *See also* water
femoral catheters, 153, 188–189, 343
ferritin, 38, 343
fertility, 62–63
fever, 232–233, 254–255
FFCL (Fistula First Catheter Last), 186, 194, 195
fiber bundle volume, definition of, 344
fibers. *See* dialyzer membranes
fibrin sheaths, 98, 135, 156, 182, 344
fibrosis, 31, 171, 344
filters, 344
filtration, 87. *See also* ultrafiltration
financial concerns, 7, 61
first aid for access ruptures, 177
first-use syndrome, 255, 344
fistulas, 151–152. *See also* buttonhole technique; vascular access
    access planning, 154–155
    arm elevation test, 158
    arteriovenous, 151–152
    assessing maturity, 157–158
    assessing patency, 157
    body image and resistance to, 156
    brachiobasilic, 155–156
    brachiocephalic, 155–156, 336
    common sites for, 155–156
    complications of, 175–186
    creating, 155–156
    definition of, 335
    FFCL resource, 186, 194, 195
    high output cardiac failure and, 156

infection, 159
    monitoring and protecting, 171, 172, 187
    needle placement, 159, 161–168
    new fistula cannulation, 158
    primary fistula failure, 152
    pros and cons, 152
    radiocephalic, 155, 356
    removed fistula, 185
    requirements for, 156
    starting HD with a mature fistula, 158–169
    stenosis in, 180–181
    vascular surgeons, selecting, 194
    vessel mapping and fistula surgery, 156–157
fistulograms, 181
fitness, 69
flocculants, 274, 344
flood clean-up resources, 321. *See also* emergency planning and response
flow, definition of, 344
flow rate, 116, 120–121, 183–184, 192, 344
flow velocity, 344
fluid compartments, 87, 344
fluid dynamics, 86–87, 94–95
fluid intake, 53–54, 235
fluid replacement, 237, 239
fluoride, testing for, 297
flushing (priming), 356
flux, 107
food and drink. *See also* dietitians
    3-day emergency diet plan, 322–324
    emergency food kit, 324
    measurement conversions, 56
    for people on standard in-center HD, 52–59
    potassium levels and, 28–29
formaldehyde, 142, 143, 344
free chlorine, 282, 296–297, 318, 344
Fresenius Medical Care, 110, 183
full blood count, 38
fungi. *See* pathogens

G

gauge of needles, 218
germicides
    contact time, 142
    dialyzer reprocessing, 137–138, 142, 145
    exposure to, 250
    hazardous material handling, 142–143
    OSHA environmental exposure limits, 143
    potency test strip or ampule, 144
    removal of, 144–145
germs. *See* pathogens
glomerular diseases, 27, 344
glomerular filtrate, 23, 25
glomerular filtration rate (GFR), 25
    estimated (eGFR), 343
glomerulonephritis, 27
glomerulosclerosis, 27, 344
glomerulus/glomeruli, 23, 345

Index

glossary, 333–362
gloves, 203, 209–210, 213
    removing safely, 213
glucose, 38, 111
glutaraldehyde, 142, 143
government resources, 74
gowns, 213
gradient, definition of, 345
grafts, 152–153
    buttonhole technique not used for, 203
    cannulation sites, 175
    common graft sites, 153
    complications of, 175–186
    'coring' of artificial walls, 203
    definition of, 345
    direction of blood flow, 174
    inserting needles, 174–175
    monitoring and protecting, 175, 187
    needle insertion, 175
    pros and cons, 152–153
    starting HD with, 173–175
    stenosis in, 181
gram atomic weight, definition of, 91
gram molecular weight, definition of, 91
Gram-negative bacteria, 276, 345
Gram-positive bacteria, 276, 345
green dialysis, 130, 280, 345
ground water, 273

H

hand hygiene, 159, 209–212, 345
hard water syndrome, 297
hazardous material handling, 142–143
HBV (hepatitis B), 38–39, 137, 215
HCV (hepatitis C), 39, 215
HD (hemodialysis), 4–5, 45–49, 87–96, 208–267. *See also* adequacy; cannulation; dialysis; needle placement; nocturnal home HD; nocturnal in-center HD; short daily home HD; standard home HD; standard in-center HD; ultrafiltration; vascular access
    bleeding during and after, 177
    clinical complications, 247–260
    definition of, 345
    drawing blood, 239–241
    new patients, 46, 236–237
    post-dialysis procedures, 240, 263–264
    predialysis procedures, 224–227
    safety factors, 229
    schedules, 5
    scientific principles, 87–96
    starting treatment, 234–241
    starting with a catheter, 189–191
    starting with a graft, 173–175
    starting with a mature fistula, 158–169
    technical complications, 261–262
    technician's role, 5
HD care team, 49–51, 155
    questions for, 67
HD catheters. *See* catheters
HD machines, 102–130. *See also* bleeding problems; monitors and alarms
    adequacy monitoring, 121
    advanced options, 121–122
    assessment after emergencies, 318
    dialysate delivery, 113–114, 346
    dialysate mixing, 113
    disinfection schedule, 264
    extracorporeal circuit, 122–129
    health information systems, 122
    monitoring, 288
    post-pump pressure, 95
    preparing, 226
    pre-pump pressure, 95
    saline prime, 241
    single pass machines, 113
    starting, 241–242
    ultrafiltration control, 117–121
headache, 256
headers, cleaning and disinfecting, 141
health information systems (HIS), 122
health insurance, 7–8. *See also* Medicare
    employer group health plans (EGHP), 7
healthcare-associated infections (HAIs), 209
heart attack. *See* cardiac arrest; myocardial infarction
heart disease, kidney failure and, 32
heartbeat, irregular. *See* arrhythmia
heat disinfection, 142, 264, 291–292, 345
Hemastix, 345
hematocrit (Hct), 129, 345
hematomas, 176, 345
hemoconcentration, 345
hemodiafiltration (HDF), 95–96
hemodialysis. *See* HD (hemodialysis)
hemodialysis delivery systems. *See* HD machines
hemoglobin (Hgb), 30, 38, 346
hemolysis, 28, 90, 116, 124, 168, 282, 297, 346
hemolytic anemia, 297, 346
hemorrhage. *See* bleeding problems; exsanguination
hemothorax, 187, 346
heparin, 245–246, 346
    overdose, 256–257
heparin infusion lines, 123, 125, 346
heparin pumps, 125–126
    definition of, 346
heparin-free dialysis, 245–246
hepatitis, 38–39, 137, 215
    definition of, 346
HeRO® grafts, 173, 346
high blood pressure. *See* hypertension
high-efficiency dialysis, 107, 237, 346
high-flux dialysis, 106–107, 237, 346
high-output cardiac failure, 156, 347
HIPAA (Health Insurance Portability and Accountability Act), 14, 64, 71–72
    definition of, 347
HIV (human immunodeficiency virus), 215–216, 347
hollow fiber dialyzers, 103–104. *See also* dialyzers
    definition of, 347
    parts of, 141, 344
    reuse and, 135–136
home dialysis. *See* nocturnal home HD; short daily home HD; standard home HD
Home Dialysis Central, 72
Home Dialyzors United, 73
homeostasis, 23, 347
hope, 67
hormones, 24, 342, 347
Hoyer lifts, 223
HSAG (Health Services Advisory Group), 309
hubs, 166, 189
human body. *See* body.
hurricanes. *See* emergency planning and response
hydraulic pressure, 86, 347
hydrophilic, definition of, 347
hydrophobic, definition of, 347
hygiene, 70, 214. *See also* hand hygiene
hyper-, definition of, 347
hypercalcemia/hypocalcemia, 29, 347, 348
hyperglycemia/hypoglycemia, 347, 348
hyperkalemia/hypokalemia, 28, 347, 348
hypermagnesemia, 347
hypernatremia/hyponatremia, 28, 348
hyperphosphatemia/hypophosphatemia, 29, 348
hyperplasia, 172, 181, 348, 352
hypersensitivity, 348. *See also* anaphylaxis
hypertension (high blood pressure), 26–27, 257, 348
hypertonic, definition of, 348
hypervolemia (fluid overloaded), 118
hypo-, definition of, 348
hypoglycemia (low blood sugar), 241
hypotension (low blood pressure), 93, 242, 258, 349
    orthostatic, 263
hypotonic, definition of, 349
hypovolemia (dehydration), 118, 234–235, 340
hypoxemia, 258–259

I

identification, 314
immune systems, infection and, 209
immunosuppressant drugs, 40
in vitro, definition of, 349
in vivo, definition of, 350
in-center HD. *See* standard in-center HD
Incident Commander, 312, 315
incontinence, 70
infection. *See also* sepsis
    aseptic technique, 211–212, 220
    catheters, 191
    definition of, 349
    fistulas and grafts, 159, 185
infection control, 185, 209–218
    sepsis (blood infection), 25, 137, 185
    transmission, 209–210

Index

infection control, definition of, 349
infiltration, 175–176, 349
inflammation, contaminated water and, 275, 277
inflammation, definition of, 349
inflow stenosis, 180
injections. See needles
instill, definition of, 349
insurance. See health insurance; Medicare
interdialytic, definition of, 349
intermittent, definition of, 349
internal jugular vein, 153, 188, 349
interstitial space, 349
intima, 349
intracellular, definition of, 349
intradermal, definition of, 349
intradermal lidocaine, 169–171
intradialytic hypotension, 32, 349
intramuscular, definition of, 349
intravascular, definition of, 349
intravenous solutions, 220, 339, 349
ion exchange, 350
ions (charged particles), 24, 350. See also electrolyte balance
    water treatment systems, 283, 285
iron deficiency, 31, 38–39, 350
irregular heartbeat. See arrhythmia
ischemia, 32, 350
isolated ultrafiltration, 350
isotonic, definition of, 350
itching. See pruritus (itching)
IV solutions, 220, 339, 349

J

JAS (juxta-anastomotic stenosis), 180
jobs, keeping, 68–69
Journal of Vascular Access, 194

K

kayexalate, 57
KCER (Kidney Community Emergency Response Coalition), 308–309
KDIGO (Kidney Disease: Improving Global Outcomes), 10
KDOQI (Kidney Disease Outcomes Quality Initiative), 9–10, 189, 193–194, 266
kidney disease, 4. See also treatment options
    acute kidney failure, 24–25
    causes of CKD, 25–27
    chronic, 24–27
    complications of, 28
    dialysis as partial kidney replacement, 4–6
    heart disease and, 32
    overview, 3–6
    person with. See person with kidney failure
    PKD (polycystic kidney disease), 27, 74
    problems caused by, 27–37
    risk of ESRD, 25
    routine medical exams, 25
    slowing the loss of kidney function, 25
    stages of, 25
    symptoms of, 30
    types of, 24–25
kidney doctors. See nephrologists
kidney functions, 3–4, 23–24
Kidney School, 72–73
kidney structure, 22–23
    cross section of kidney, 22
    location of the kidneys, 22
kidney stunning, 32
kidney transplants. See transplants
Kiil dialyzer, 135
"killer gap," 46
KoA (mass transfer coefficient), 109
KUF (coefficient of ultrafiltration), 338

L

lab tests. See blood tests
LAL (limulus amoebocyte lysate) test, 296
lateral transfers, 222–223
leach, definition of, 350
lead, 299, 300
leak testing. See monitors and alarms
left ventricular hypertrophy (LVH), 31–32
lidocaine, 169–171
life changes, empathy and, 60–61
Life Options program, 73
lift devices, portable, 223
lifting and carrying, 220–221
LIJ (left internal jugular) vein, 188
limb, definitions, 189
lipectomy, 152
listening, active, 64–65
loading dose, 350
lobes, 22
local and state rules, for emergencies, 308
local anesthetics, 169–171
local infection, 350
loop of Henle, 23
low blood pressure. See hypotension
Luer-connections, uncoupling, 313
lumens (catheter chambers), 187, 350
lyse, definition of, 350

M

magnesium, 39, 111, 297, 350
malnutrition, 51, 52–53, 350
masks, 189
mass transfer coefficient (KoA), 109
measurement conversions, 56
Measures Assessment Tool (MAT), 10
Medicaid health plan, 6
medical devices. See equipment and supplies
medical management without dialysis, 48–49
medical records, 224, 314
Medical Review Board (MRB), 10
medical waste, 130, 136
Medicare, 6, 7–8. See also CMS; ESRD Program; health insurance
    composite rates, 7
    government resources, 74
    number of blood transfusions under, 31
    PPS (Prospective Payment System), 7–8
    QIP (Quality Incentive Program), 8
    right to be active in own care, 170
    waiting period, 7
medications and solutions, giving, 218–220
    monitoring during dialysis, 243–244
    using IV solutions, 220
    medicine vials, 219
Medigap health plan, 6
medulla, 22
MEI (Medical Education Institute), 43, 72–73, 198–205, 235
membrane filters, 107, 296, 351
membrane compliance, 351
    submicron filters, 284, 292
membranes, dialyzer. See dialyzer membranes
mercury, 299, 300
metabolic acidosis, 24, 351
metabolism, 351
methemoglobinemia, 298
Methicillin-Resistant Staphylococcus Aureus (MRSA), 216
metric system, temperature conversions, 99
microalbuminuria, 351
microbes. See microorganisms
microns, 351
microorganisms (microbes), 351. See also bacteria; pathogens
"middle molecule" wastes, 265, 267
mineral bone disorder (MBD), 33–34
modality, definition of, 351
mole, definition of, 91
molecular weight cutoff, 351
molecular weight, definition of, 351
molecules, definition of, 351
money concerns, 7, 61
monitoring, definition of, 182. See also patient monitoring
monitors and alarms, 114–117, 127–128, 246–247
    access surveillance, 182–184
    air detectors, 128–129, 247, 333
    alarm safety check, 227–229
    blood leak detectors, 116–117, 122, 177, 336
    blood volume monitoring, 129
    conductivity, 115, 339
    dialysate alarms, 228
    extracorporeal alarms, 126–129, 228
    flow rate, 116
    infiltration, 176
    pH, 117
    power outage, 114
    predialysis treatment procedures, 227
    pressure alarms, 126–127, 176, 177, 244, 246
    pyrogen filters, 117

Index

resistivity meters, 292–293
temperature, 116, 360
venous bloodline alarms, 128
water outage, 115
mood of patients, 63
morbidity, definition of, 351
mortality, definition of, 351. *See also* deaths
MRSA (Methicillin-Resistant Staphylococcus Aureus), 216
muscle cramps, 259
muscle pain (myalgia), 351
My Life, My Dialysis Choice, 73, 237
myalgia. *See* muscle pain
myocardial infarction ("heart attack"), 351. *See also* arrhythmia
myocardial stunning, 252. *See also* organ stunning

N

NANT (National Association of Nephrology Technicians/Technologists), 14
nasogastric tubes, 351
natural disasters, 307. *See also* emergency planning and response
nausea, 260
needle fear, helping patients with, 169–171
needle placement, 161–168. *See also* buttonhole technique; cannulation
aneurysms and, 179
"area puncture," 162
blood clotting at site, 182
for fistulas, 159, 164–165
flipping, 176
for grafts, 174–175
hubbing, 166
infiltration by, 176
insertion by patients, 170
removing needles, 171
re-touching a needle site, 160
rope ladder technique, 162–165
single needle option, 168
taping, 167–168, 244
watching needles during treatment, 178
needle protectors, 165
needle site rotation. *See* rope ladder (needle site rotation)
needle stick injuries, 165, 213
needles, 162, 218
back-eye needles, 162
length and gauge, 162, 200, 218
pain from, 166, 169–171, 198
sharp vs. blunt tips, 162
sterile items, 212
negative pressure, 352
neointimal hyperplasia, 172, 181, 352
nephrologists, 50, 352
nephrology, definition of, 352
nephrons, 22, 23, 25, 352
neuropathy (nerve damage), 35, 178, 354
new patients, special concerns for, 236–237
nitrates, testing for, 298

NKF (National Kidney Foundation), 9–10, 25, 73
DOQI, 9
KDIGO, 10
KDOQI, 9–10, 189, 193–194, 266
NNCC (Nephrology Nursing Certification Commission), 14, 15
NNCO (National Nephrology Certification Organization, Inc.), 15, 16
nocturnal home HD, 48, 168, 177, 275, 352
nocturnal in-center HD, 46–47, 352
non-tunneled catheters, 154
normal saline, 352
nosocomial, definition of, 352
nurses, 50, 315
nutritionists, 50–51, 322. *See also* food and drink

O

obesity, 53
OneSite single needle, 168
one-site-itis, 180
online technician discussions, 14
opportunistic illnesses, 352
organ stunning, 32, 236, 252
avoiding, 93–94
definition of, 353
organic chemical contamination. *See* contamination
organizations
emergency planning and response, 321
patient organizations, 73–74
orthostatic hypotension, 353
OSHA environmental exposure limits, 143
osmolality, 353
osmosis, 85–86, 90–94, 97. *See also* reverse osmosis (RO)
definition of, 353
osmotic gradient, 353
osmotic pressure, 353
osteosclerosis, 297
outflow stenosis, 180
overweight, 53
oxygen in blood (hypoxemia), 258–259

P

pain
from needles, 166, 169–171, 198
Pain Assessment Scale, 63
palpate, definition of, 353
palpitations, 353
paper charting, 224
papilla/papillae, 22
parathyroid hormone, 39, 353
patent, definition of, 353
pathogens, 137, 209. *See also* bacteria; bloodborne diseases; infection
definition of, 353
patient education, 66–68, 170. *See also* communication
on access ruptures, 177, 243

answers, 66–67
attitude, 66
belief, 68
on catheter care, 190
for emergencies, 314–315
on feeling the thrill, 174
hope, 67
language level, 67
monitoring and protecting fistulas or grafts, 187
readiness, 67
repetition, 68
self-cannulation, 198–205
patient evaluation, 299–302
blood pressure, 230–232
body temperature, 232–233
edema, 230
physical and emotional health, 233–234
predialysis, 227–241
pulse, 230
respiration rate, 232
vascular access, 233
vital signs, 227
water quality and, 299
weight, 228–230
patient monitoring, 242–247
anticoagulation, 245–246
definition of, 182
general patient condition, 243–244
giving medicines, 243–244
machine monitoring, 246–247
patient comfort and safety, 244–245
taking vital signs, 242
vascular access, 243
water quality and, 299
patient organizations, 73–74
patient outcomes, 353
patient resources, 72–74
patients. *See also* self-cannulation
access planning roles, 155–156
active in own care, 170, 204–205, 243
body image, 156
in care team, 49
comfort and safety, 244–245
in emergency planning, 316–317, 318–320, 322–324
evaluating, 227–241
helping patients cope, 59–63
lifting and moving, 220–223
monitoring during dialysis, 243–247
needle fear, 169–171
new patients, 51, 54, 236
patient time in-center vs. time on own, 65
phosphorus management, 58
potassium management, 57
professional boundaries, 13–14
PTSD, 318–319
screaming patients, 71
self-management, 65–66
vital papers, 314
payment for dialysis and transplant, 6–8
PD (peritoneal dialysis), 5–6, 42–45, 96–98. *See also* adequacy
adsorption in, 98

369

Index

catheters, 43, 44
continuous ambulatory PD, 44
convection in, 98
definition of, 354
dialysis technician's role in, 6
diffusion in, 97
osmosis in, 97
PDCA ("Plan, Do, Check, Act") cycle, 12
peracetic acid, 142, 143, 296
percutaneous, definition of, 353
pericardial effusion, 353
pericarditis, 33, 353
peripheral, definition of, 353
peripheral neuropathy, 35, 354
peripheral vascular resistance, 354
peritoneal dialysis. See PD
peritoneum, definition of, 354
peritonitis, 354
permeable, definition of, 354
person with kidney failure, 20–79. See also kidney functions
goal of caring for, 21–22
personal hygiene, 214
personal protective equipment, 159, 213
pH, 83, 84. See also acid-base balance; buffers
definition of, 354
monitors and alarms, 117
phosphate binders, 29, 58, 59, 354
phosphorus, 29, 39, 111, 354
patient management of, 58
physical activity, 69
PKD (polycystic kidney disease), 27, 74, 355
plasma refill rate, 92–93, 354
plastic, toxins in, 106
plasticizers, 354
platelets (thrombocytes), 88, 181, 355
pneumothorax, 187, 355
pores, definition of, 355
portable lift devices, 223
positional, definition of, 355
positive pressure, 355
post-, definition of, 355
post trauma resources, 321
post-dialysis pressure. See venous pressure
post-dialysis procedures, 240, 263–264
post-pump (arterial) pressure. See predialyzer pressure
potassium, 39, 111, 355
dialysate levels of, 28–29
nutrition and, 57
testing for, 297
potency test strips or ampules, 144
pre-, definition of, 355
precipitate (scale), 84, 89, 358
predialysis procedures, 224–227
pre-dialyzer pressure, definition of, 355
preprocessing, definition of, 355. See also dialyzer reprocessing
pre-pump arterial pressure, definition of, 355
prescriptions for dialysis, 224, 226
pressure, definition of, 355
pressure gradient. See transmembrane pressure
pressure monitors, 126–127, 185, 355
presternal PD catheters, 356
priming, 227, 356
privacy, maintaining, 13–14, 64, 71–72
procedures. See dialysis; post-dialysis procedures; predialysis procedures
product water, 280, 356. See also water treatment systems
professionalism, 12–14
proof of identity, 314
proportioning system, 113, 115, 356
protective eyewear, 213
protein
nutrition, 52
in the urine, 25
proteinuria, definition of, 356. See also microalbuminuria
proximal (near) convoluted tubule, 23
proximal, definition of, 356
pruritus (itching), 35–36, 260–261
definition of, 356
pseudoaneurysms, 179–180, 356
PTSD (post-traumatic stress disorder), 318–319
pulmonary (lung) TB, 217
pulmonary edema, 51, 356
pulse, 129, 230. See also thrill, bruit and pulse
apical pulse, 334
brachial pulse, 336
pulse oximeters, 232
pump occlusion, 124–125, 356
pumps
dialysate mixing, 113
extracorporeal circuit, 124–126
ultrafiltration, 119–120
purpura, definition of, 356
pyramids, 22
pyrogen, definition of, 356
pyrogenic reactions, 137, 233, 277, 356
pyrogen filters, 117

Q
QIP (Quality Incentive Program), 8, 10
quality, 9–12
assurance and control, 145–147
CQI (continuous quality improvement), 11–12, 192–193, 339
ESRD Networks, 9
ESRD Quality Improvement Initiative, 10
guidelines for dialysis care, 9–10
QAPI (Quality Assessment and Performance Improvement), 12, 193
QI in emergency planning, 319–320
Quality Assurance Audit Schedule, 146
quality standards for dialysis, 10–11

R
radial pulse, 356
radiocephalic fistulas, 155, 356. See also fistulas
RD/RDN (renal dietitians/nutritionists), 50–51, 322
reagents, definition of, 357
recirculation, 178, 183–184, 227, 240, 357
record keeping, 224, 314
recovery plans, after emergencies, 316–319
red blood cells, 88
anemia and, 30–31
Redsense, 177
rehabilitation, 65–66
reject water, definition of, 357
rejection, definition of, 357
relationships with patients, boundaries in, 13–14
renal dietitians/nutritionists (RD/RDN), 50–51, 322
renal osteodystrophy, 357
Renal Physicians Association (RPA), 12
Renal Support Network (RSN), 74
RenalWEB, 14
renin-angiotensin system, 24, 357
reprocessing, definition of, 357. See also dialyzer reprocessing
resistance, definition of, 357
resistivity, definition of, 357
resources, 72–74, 321
respiration rate, 232
retrograde placement, 163, 175, 357
reuse, definition of, 357. See also dialyzer reprocessing
reverse osmosis (RO), 280–281, 282–283
definition of, 357
monitoring, 288, 291–292
portable systems, 281–282
RO water quality, 293
water softeners, 283–284, 290
rinsebacks, 140, 263, 357
roller pumps, 124–125, 357. See also blood pumps
rope ladder (needle site rotation), 162–165, 175
definition of, 352

S
Safe Drinking Water Act (1974), 273–274
safety, 209. See also infection; monitors and alarms
dialysis precautions, 211, 229
hazardous material handling training, 143
saline solutions, 241
IV solutions, using, 220
normal saline, 352
saline infusion lines, 123, 357
scab removal, 167, 204
screaming, 71
secondary hyperparathyroidism, 33–34, 358
secondary hypertension, 27
sediment filters, 287, 290
seizures, 261, 358
selenium, 299, 300
self-cannulation, 187
buttonhole technique, 198–205

Index

choosing not to, 202
gloves, 203
infiltration and, 176
needle insertion, 170
needle length, 200
pre-cannulation education, 199–200
reading glasses for, 200
single needle option, 168
tandem-hand cannulation, 201–202
touch cannulation, 167, 202
use of word "stick, 199
semipermeable membranes, 23, 84, 107, 358
sepsis (blood infection), 25, 137, 185, 358
serum, 358
sexuality, 62–63
shivering. *See* chills
shopping lists, 324
short daily home HD, 358
shunts, 358
sieving coefficient (SC), 94, 108–109, 358
"skin freezing" spray, 169, 171
skin itching. *See* pruritus
sleep problems, 36
slide boards, using, 222–223
sling lifts, 223
soap and water hand hygiene, 212
social media, 14
social workers, 50, 71, 315
sodium, 28, 111, 358
    diet and, 56
    testing for, 39, 297
sodium bicarbonate. *See* bicarbonate concentrate
sodium hypochlorite (bleach), 250, 296
sodium modeling, 55, 94, 120, 239, 359
solubility, 83
solutes, 83, 84
    definition of, 359
    in dialysate, 90, 91
    molecular weight cutoff, 107
solutions, 83, 85, 88–89. *See also* medications and solutions, giving
    definition of, 359
solvents, 83, 84
    definition of, 359
spores, 359
spread plate technique, 296
staffing, during emergencies, 316, 317
stand and pivot technique, 222
standard home HD, 47, 51, 359
    definition of, 359
standard in-center HD, 46, 51
    definition of, 359
    first 90 days, 51
    nutrition for patients on, 51, 55
    nutrition for people on, 52–59
    organ stunning during, 32
    safe vascular access, 51
    tailoring the first treatments, 51
    weekly time in-center, 65
standing orders, 359
state surveyors, 10
steal syndrome, 158, 160, 178

definition of, 359
stenosis, 36, 180–181
    arm elevation test, 158
    catheters and, 154, 188
    central venous, 180, 192
    definition of, 359
    fistulas and, 156, 160, 180–181
    grafts and, 153, 181
    signs of, 181
stents, 181, 359
sterilants, 360
sterile items, 212
    definition of, 360
sterile technique. *See* aseptic technique
sterilization, 360
stretcher-to-bed (lateral) transfers, 223
stretcher-to-chair transfers, 223
stunning damage. *See* organ stunning
subclavian catheters, 153, 180, 188, 360
subclavian veins, 188
subcutaneous, definition of, 360
submicron filters, 284, 292
sulfates, testing for, 298
supplies. *See* equipment and supplies
surface area, definition of, 360
surface water, 273
surgery, 156–157, 194–195
surveillance, definition of, 182
survival rates. *See also* deaths
    BMI and, 53
    dialyzer reuse, 136
    HD (hemodialysis), 46–48, 93, 265
    transplants, 41
swelling. *See* edema
synthetic membranes, 105
syringes, 218
systemic, definition of, 360
systolic, definition of, 360
systolic blood pressure, 230

T

tandem-hand cannulation, 201–202. *See also* self-cannulation
tap water. *See* water
taping technique, 167–168, 244
target (dry) weight, 54–55, 92
    assessing, 228, 235
    definition of, 360
    factors affecting, 228–230
    nutrition and, 54–55
    post-dialysis procedures, 263
technical complications, 261–262
technicians. *See* dialysis technicians
telephone "call trees," 310–311
temperature. *See also* body temperature
    metric system conversions, 99
    monitors and alarms, 116, 360
temperature blending valve, 287
temporary catheters, 360
test tubes, 240
The Joint Commission (TJC), 308
thermometer types, 233
thermometers, 116
thin film composite (TFC), 280
thirst, 94
thrill, bruit, and pulse

definition of bruit, 336
definition of thrill, 360
fistulas and, 157, 158, 160
grafts and, 174
thrombectomy, 360
thrombolysis, 360
thrombosis (blood clots), 181–182
    anticoagulation, 245–246
    definition of, 360
thrombus, 360
TJC (The Joint Commission), 10
topical lidocaine creams or gels, 169–170
total cell volume. *See* fiber bundle volume
total parenteral nutrition, 53, 360
touch cannulation. *See* self-cannulation
toxins in plastic, 106
trace metals, 299, 300
training, 143. *See also* patient education
transducer protectors, 361
transfusions, to treat anemia, 31
Transmembrane pressure, 92, 110
transmembrane pressure, 118, 361
    UFR and, 237
transonic HD monitors, 183–184
transplants, 37, 40–41
    blood transfusions and, 31
    definition of, 350
    payment for, 6–8
transportation, during emergencies, 316–317
travel, helping patients cope, 61–62
treatment options, 4, 37–49. *See also* dialysis; transplants
    medical management without dialysis, 4, 48–49
    stopping treatment, 48–49
treatment plans, 224, 226
treatment procedures. *See* dialysis; post-dialysis procedures; predialysis procedures
Trendelenburg position, 361
triage, during emergencies, 315
Triferic, iron, 31
Troponin T, 32
tuberculosis (TB), 217
tubular system/tubules, 23
Twardowski, Dr. Zbylut, 202
tympanic thermometers, 233
type A dialyzer reactions, 106
type B dialyzer reactions, 106

U

ultrafilter, definition of, 361
ultrafiltration (UF), 87, 234–235. *See also* membrane filters
    blood pressure and, 32
    chair positions, 238
    charting, 238
    control systems, 117–121
    definition of, 361
    in HD, 90–94
    management programs, 238
    new patients, 236–237
    organ stunning and, 32

Index

profiling, 121, 237
pumps, 119–120
replacing fluid, 237, 239
reverse, 141
transmembrane pressure and, 237
water removal calculation, 234–239
ultrafiltration (UF) coefficients, 110
ultrafiltration rate (UFR), 92–93
    definition of, 361
    drops in blood pressure and, 93
    UFR calculator, 93
ultrasound, 183–184
urea, 29–30. See also BUN (blood urea nitrogen)
urea kinetic modeling (UKM), 265, 266, 267
    definition of, 361
uremia, 25, 29–30, 361
USRDS (United States Renal Data System), 11
UV (ultraviolet light), 284, 292, 361

V

vapo-coolant sprays, 169, 171
VASA (Vascular Access Society of the Americas), 194
Vasc-Alert, 185
vascular access, 150–195, 151. See also cannulation; catheters; fistulas; grafts; infection
    connecting, 239
    CQI and, 192–193
    definition of, 361
    HD, 45, 51
    improving outcomes, 192–194
    monitoring, 182–184, 187, 233, 243–244
    planning, 154–155
    rupture, patient reactions to, 243
    sites, 151
    troubleshooting problems, 244
    types of, 151
vascular surgeons, selecting, 194–195
vasoconstrictors, 24
vasoconstrictors, definition of, 361
vasovagal responses, 169

veins. See also fistulas; grafts
    for catheters, 188–189
    definition of, 361
    for fistulas, 151–152, 156
venipuncture, 362
venograms, 181
venous bloodline alarms, 128
venous line clamps, 126
venous pressure, 362
venous pressure high/low alarm, 362
vessel mapping, 156–157
viruses, 362. See also bloodborne diseases; pathogens
vital signs, 234, 242, 263
vitamins, 24, 59
volumetric, definition of, 362
volumetric UF control systems, 118–120
vomiting, 260
VRE (Vancomycin-Resistant Enterococcus), 216

W

walkers, patients with, 221–222
washing hands. See hand hygiene
waste disposal, 130, 136
water. See also water treatment systems
    AAMI standards for, 140–141, 275–277
    after emergencies, 318
    contaminants in, 273, 295–299
    DI water quality, 293
    disposal, 130
    patient monitoring and, 299
    quality analysis, 293–299
    RO water quality, 293
    tap water, 273–274, 277, 288, 300–302
    ultrapure dialysate, 277
    water supply, 273–277
water outage monitors, 115
water removal. See ultrafiltration
water softeners, 283–284, 290
    definition of, 362
water treatment systems, 272–302
    calculating EBCT, 283
    components, 277
    design of, 277–279
    direct feed system, 279, 285–286
    disinfectants compatible with, 290
    distribution system, 278, 284–286, 290, 294–295
    home dialysis, 275
    indirect feed system, 279, 284, 286
    local water supply, 277
    monitoring, 287–295
    objectives, 272
    organization resources, 321
    parts of, 280–286
    pretreatment components, 278, 281–284
    purification components, 278, 284, 294–295
water weight
    assessing, 228
    fluid intake and, 53–54
    reducing gain of, 55
website resources, 72–73
    emergency planning and response, 321
    government resources, 74
weight measurement, 55, 263. See also dietitians; target (dry) weight; water weight
wet cannulation, 164
white blood cells, 88

X

X-ray (fistulogram or venogram), 181

Z

zinc, 298–299